Introduction to
Emergency Medicine

Introduction to Emergency Medicine

Elizabeth L. Mitchell, M.D.

Assistant Professor

Boston University School of Medicine

Department of Emergency Medicine

Boston Medical Center

Boston, Massachusetts

Ron Medzon, M.D.

Assistant Professor

Boston University School of Medicine

Department of Emergency Medicine

Boston Medical Center

Boston, Massachusetts

LIPPINCOTT WILLIAMS & WILKINS
A **Wolters Kluwer** Company

Philadelphia • Baltimore • New York • London
Buenos Aires • Hong Kong • Sydney • Tokyo

Acquisitions Editor: Charlie Mitchell and Donna Balado
Managing Editor: Elena Coler
Marketing Manager: Scott Lavine
Designer: Doug Smock
Compositor: Nesbitt Graphics, Inc.
Printer: Quebecor / Versailles

Copyright © 2005 Lippincott Williams & Wilkins

351 West Camden Street
Baltimore, MD 21201

530 Walnut Street
Philadelphia, PA 19106

Printed in the United States of America

ISBN# 0-7817-3200-X

Library of Congress Cataloging-in-Publication Data
Introduction to emergency medicine / [edited by] Elizabeth Mitchell, Ron Medzon.
   p. ; cm.
  Includes bibliographical references and index.
  ISBN 0-7817-3200-X
  1. Emergency medicine. I. Mitchell, Elizabeth, 1957– II. Medzon, Ron.
   [DNLM: 1. Emergency Medical Services—methods—Case Reports. 2.
Emergency Medicine—methods—Case Reports. 3. Emergencies—Case
Reports. WB 105 I615 2005]
RC86.7.I586   2005
616.02'5—dc22

The publishers have made every effort to trace the copyright holders for borrowed material. If they have inadvertently overlooked any, they will be pleased to make the necessary arrangements at the first opportunity.

To purchase additional copies of this book, call our customer service department at **(800) 638-3030** or fax orders to **(301) 824-7390**. International customers should call **(301) 714-2324**.

Visit Lippincott Williams & Wilkins on the Internet: http://www.LWW.com. Lippincott Williams & Wilkins customer service representatives are available from 8:30 am to 6:00 pm, EST.

04 05 06 07 08
1 2 3 4 5 6 7 8 9 10

Contributors

L. Kristian Arnold, M.D., F.A.C.E.P.
Assistant Professor (Retired)
Department of Emergency Medicine
Boston University School of Medicine
Boston Medical Center
Boston, Massachusetts

William E. Baker, M.D.
Assistant Professor
Department of Emergency Medicine
Boston University School of Medicine
Boston Medical Center
Boston, Massachusetts

Brook D. Beall, M.D.
Attending Physician
Emergency Department
St. Lukes Hospital
New Bedford, Massachusetts

Edward Bernstein, M.D.
Professor and Vice Chair for Academic Affairs
Department of Emergency Medicine
Boston University School of Medicine
Boston, Massachusetts
Professor of Social and Behavioral Sciences
Boston University School of Medicine
Boston, Massachusetts

Darcey Q. Bittner, M.D.
Clinical Instructor
Section of Emergency Medicine
Brown University School of Medicine
Providence, Rhode Island

Keith S. Boniface, M.D.
Assistant Professor
Associate Residency Director
Department of Emergency Medicine
George Washington University Medical Center
Washington, DC

Edward W. Boyer, M.D., Ph.D.
Chief, Division of Medical Toxicology
University of Massachusetts Medical School
Worcester, Massachusetts
Assistant in Pediatrics
Children's Hospital
Boston, Massachusetts
Harvard Medical School,
Boston, Massachusetts

Mark Bracken, M.D.
Clinical Instructor
Department of Emergency Medicine
Boston University School of Medicine
Boston Medical Center
Boston, Massachusetts

Kathryn Brinsfield, M.D., M.P.H., F.A.C.E.P.
Assistant Professor
Department of Emergency Medicine
Boston University School of Medicine
Boston Medical Center
Boston, Massachusetts
Associate Medical Director
Boston EMS
Boston, Massachusetts

Frank Michael Carrano, M.D.
Attending Physician
Emergency Department
Newton-Wellesley Hospital
Newton, Massachusetts

Merle A. Carter, M.D.
Associate/Assistant Residency Director
Department of Emergency Medicine
Albert Einstein Medical Center
Philadelphia, Pennsylvania

Karen Ann Casper, M.D.
Attending Physician
Emergency Department
Martha's Vineyard Hospital
Oak Bluffs, Massachusetts

Robert S. Chang, M.D.
Staff Physician
Emergency Department
South Shore Hospital
Weymouth, Massachusetts

Lamont G. Clay, M.D.
Attending Physician
Emergency Department
Christ Medical Center
Chicago, Illinois

Robert P. Collins, M.D.
Attending Physician
Emergency Department
Emerson Hospital
Concord, Massachusetts

Edward P. Curcio, III, M.D.
Attending Physician
Emergency Department
Mt. Auburn Hospital
Cambridge, Massachusetts
Division of Emergency Medicine
Harvard Medical School
Boston, Massachusetts

Robert Dart, M.D.
Chief of Emergency Services
Quincy Medical Center
Quincy, Massachusetts
Associate Professor of Emergency Medicine and
    Vice-Chair
Department of Emergency Medicine
Boston University School of Medicine
Boston Medical Center
Boston, Massachusetts

Ami K. Davé, M.D.
Assistant Director
Emergency Medicine Residency
Assistant Professor
Department of Emergency Medicine
New York University/Bellevue Hospital Center
New York, New York

Andreas Dewitz, M.D.
Director
Department of Emergency Medicine
Division of Emergency Ultrasonography
Boston Medical Center
Boston, Massachusetts
Assistant Professor
Boston University School of Medicine
Boston, Massachusetts

Lynn C. Dezelon, M.D.
Assistant Professor
Department of Emergency Medicine
Case Western Reserve University School of Medicine
Cleveland, Ohio
Director
Medical Student Education
Emergency Department
MetroHealth Medical Center
Cleveland, Ohio

Tara D. Director, M.D.
Assistant Professor
Department of Emergency Medicine
Emory University School of Medicine
Crawford-Long and Grady Hospitals
Atlanta, Georgia

K. Sophia Dyer, M.D., F.A.C.E.P.
Assistant Professor
Department of Emergency Medicine
Boston University School of Medicine
Boston, Massachusetts
Medical Toxicologist/Attending Physician
Boston Medical Center
Boston, Massachusetts
Assistant Medical Director
Boston EMS
Boston, Massachusetts

Laura J. Eliseo, M.D., M.P.H.
Emergency Medicine Resident
Boston Medical Center
Boston, Massachusetts

Peter W. Emblad, M.D., F.A.C.E.P.
Attending Physician
Emergency Department
Kaiser Permanente
San Francisco, California

Jeffrey A. Evans, M.D.
Attending Physician
Emergency Department
Mount Auburn Hospital
Cambridge, Massachusetts
Clinical Instructor
Department of Medicine
Division of Emergency Medicine
Harvard Medical School
Boston, Massachusetts

James A. Feldman, M.D.
Vice Chair, Research
Department of Emergency Medicine
Boston Medical Center
Boston, Massachusetts
Associate Professor, Emergency Medicine
Boston University School of Medicine
Boston, Massachusetts

Michael R. Filbin, M.D.
Clinical Instructor
Department of Emergency Medicine
Harvard Medical School
Massachusetts General Hospital
Boston, Massachusetts

James S. Ford, Jr., M.D.
Assistant Professor
Department of Emergency Medicine
University of Hawaii Medical School
Oahu, Hawaii

Rohit Gupta, M.D.
Instructor
Department of Emergency Medicine
University of Chicago
Chicago, Illinois

Mary Hancock, M.D., F.A.C.E.P.
Attending Physician
Emergency Department
MetroHealth Medical Center
Cleveland, Ohio
Assistant Professor
Department of Emergency Medicine
Case Western Reserve University School of Medicine
Cleveland, Ohio

Patricia Mather Harrison, R.N., M.S., A.C.N.P.,
    C.C.R.N., C.E.N.
Nurse Practitioner
Department of Surgery
Division of Trauma
Boston Medical Center
Boston, Massachusetts

Diane B. Heller, M.D., J.D.
Attending Physician
Emergency Department
Morristown Memorial Hospital
Morristown, New Jersey

Brian J. Hession, M.D.
Attending Physician
Emergency Department
Holyoke Medical Center
Holyoke, Massachusetts

Benjamin Honigman, M.D.
Professor and Chair
Division of Emergency Medicine
Director
Colorado Center for Altitude Medicine and Physiology
University of Colorado School of Medicine
Denver, Colorado

Robert L. Hood, M.D., Ph.D., F.A.C.E.P.
Associate Medical Director
Emergency Department
Munroe Regional Medical Center
Ocala, Florida

Alexander P. Isakov, M.D., M.P.H.
Co-Director
Section of Prehospital and Disaster Medicine
Department of Emergency Medicine
Emory University School of Medicine
Atlanta, Georgia

Thea James, M.D.
Assistant Professor
Department of Emergency Medicine
Boston University School of Medicine
Boston Medical Center
Boston, Massachusetts

Nicholas J. Jouriles, M.D.
Emergency Department
Akron General Medical Center
Akron, Ohio
Professor
Emergency Medicine
Northeast Ohio University College of Medicine
Akron, Ohio

Fred N. Jones, M.D.
Clinical Instructor
Department of Emergency Medicine
Boston University School of Medicine
Boston Medical Center
Boston, Massachusetts
Emergency Department
Quincy Medical Center
Quincy, Massachusetts

Christopher Kabrhel, M.D.
Clinical Instructor
Department of Emergency Medicine
Harvard Medical School
Massachusetts General Hospital
Boston, Massachusetts

Joseph H. Kahn, M.D., F.A.C.E.P.
Associate Clinical Professor of Emergency Medicine
Boston University School of Medicine
Boston, Massachusetts
Director
Medical Student Education
Department of Emergency Medicine
Boston Medical Center
Boston, Massachusetts

Sangeeta Kaushik, M.D.
Major
United States Army
U.S. Army Research Institute of Environmental Medicine
Natick, Massachusetts

Michelle Fischer Keane, M.D.
Clinical Instructor
Department of Emergency Medicine
Boston University School of Medicine
Boston Medical Center
Boston, Massachusetts
EMS Fellow
Boston EMS
Boston, Massachusetts

Amy Kontrick, M.D.
Assistant Professor of Medicine
Department of Emergency Medicine
Northwestern University
Feinberg School of Medicine
Chicago, Illinois

Melisa W. Lai, M.D.
Instructor
Harvard Medical School
Boston, Massachusetts
Fellow
Harvard Medical Area Fellowship in Medical Toxicology
Boston, Massachusetts
Emergency Physician
Mount Auburn Hospital
Cambridge, Massachusetts

Eric Legome, M.D.
Assistant Professor of Emergency Medicine
New York University School of Medicine
New York, New York
Director
New York University/Bellevue Emergency Medicine Residency
New York, New York

Judith A. Linden, M.D.
Associate Residency Director
Emergency Department
Boston Medical Center
Boston, Massachusetts
Assistant Professor of Emergency Medicine
Boston University School of Medicine
Boston Medical Center
Boston, Massachusetts

Robert Lowenstein, M.D.
Clinical Instructor
Department of Emergency Medicine
Boston University School of Medicine
Boston Medical Center
Boston, Massachusetts

Nannette M. Lugo-Amador, M.D., M.P.H.
Assistant Professor
Department of Emergency Medicine
University of Puerto Rico
University of Puerto Rico Hospital
Carolina, Puerto Rico

Brendan G. Magauran, Jr., M.D., M.B.A.
Assistant Clinical Professor
Department of Emergency Medicine
Boston University Medical School
Boston Medical Center
Boston, Massachusetts

Medical Director
East Newton Pavilion Emergency Department
Boston, Massachusetts

Katherine Manzon, M.D.
Assistant Professor
Department of Emergency Medicine
Case Western University School of Medicine
Cleveland, Ohio

Attending Emergency Physician
MetroHealth Medical Center
Cleveland, Ohio

Kerry K. McCabe, M.D.
Assistant Professor of Emergency Medicine
Boston University School of Medicine
Boston Medical Center
Boston, Massachusetts

Ron Medzon, M.D.
Assistant Professor
Department of Emergency Medicine
Boston University School of Medicine
Boston Medical Center
Boston, Massachusetts

Elizabeth L. Mitchell, M.D.
Assistant Professor
Department of Emergency Medicine
Boston University School of Medicine
Boston Medical Center
Boston, Massachusetts

Robert E. Murray, M.D.
Attending Emergency Physician
South Shore Hospital
Weymouth, Massachusetts

Attending Physician
Emergency Department
Massachusetts General Hospital
Boston, Massachusetts

Mark B. Mycyk, M.D.
Assistant Professor
Division of Emergency Medicine
Northwestern Memorial Hospital
Chicago, Illinois

Attending Physician
Section of Toxicology
Cook County Hospital
Chicago, Illinois

Sandra Najarian, M.D.
Assistant Professor
Department of Emergency Medicine
Case Western University School of Medicine
MetroHealth Medical Center
Cleveland, OH

Assistant Residency Director
Department of Emergency Medicine
MetroHealth Medical Center
Cleveland, OH

Vicki E. Noble, M.D.
Clinical Instructor
Department of Emergency Medicine
Massachusetts General Hospital
Boston, Massachusetts

David A. Peak, M.D.
Clinical Instructor
Department of Emergency Medicine
Harvard Medical School
Massachusetts General Hospital
Boston, Massachusetts

Thomas Perera, M.D.
Residency Director
Department of Emergency Medicine
Albany Medical Center
Albany, New York

Niels K. Rathlev, M.D.
Associate Professor and Vice-Chair
Department of Emergency Medicine
Boston University School of Medicine
Boston Medical Center
Boston, Massachusetts

Peter Rosen, M.D.
Senior Lecturer
Harvard University
Cambridge, Massachusetts

Visiting Professor
University of Arizona
Tucson, Arizona

Attending Emergency Physician
Beth Israel/Deaconess Medical Center
Boston, Massachusetts

Teaching Faculty
Massachusetts General Hospital
Boston, Massachusetts

Attending Emergency Physician
St. John's Hospital
Jackson, Wyoming

Todd C. Rothenhaus, M.D.
Assistant Professor of Emergency Medicine
Director of Medical Informatics
Boston University School of Medicine
Boston Medical Center
Boston, Massachusetts

Simon Roy, M.D.
Attending Physician
Emergency Department
South Shore Hospital
Weymouth, Massachusetts

David Schindler, M.D.
Clinical Instructor
Department of Emergency Medicine
Quincy Medical Center
Quincy, Massachusetts
Boston Medical Center
Boston, Massachusetts

Jeffrey I. Schneider, M.D.
Clinical Instructor
Department of Emergency Medicine
Boston University School of Medicine
Boston Medical Center
Boston, Massachusetts

J. Matthew Scholl, M.D., M.P.H.
Clinical Instructor
Department of Emergency Medicine
Maine Medical Center
Portland, Maine

Rishi Sikka, M.D.
Clinical Instructor
Department of Emergency Medicine
Boston University School of Medicine
Boston Medical Center
Boston, Massachusetts

Corey M. Slovis, M.D., F.A.C.P., F.A.C.E.P.
Professor of Emergency Medicine and Medicine
Vanderbilt University School of Medicine
Nashville, Tennessee
Chairman
Department of Emergency Medicine
Vanderbilt University School of Medicine
Nashville, Tennessee
Medical Director
Metro Nashville Fire Department
Nashville, Tennessee

Michael Snyder, M.D.
Clinical Instructor
Department of Emergency Medicine
Quincy Medical Center
Quincy, Massachusetts
Boston Medical Center
Boston, Massachusetts

Rebecca M. Steinberg, M.D.
Resident in Family Practice
University of Minnesota
Waseca-Mankato Rural Family Practice Program
Waseca, Minnesota

John M. Swanson, M.D., F.A.C.E.P.
Clinical Assistant Professor
Department of Internal Medicine
University of Nevada School of Medicine
Reno, Nevada

Todd W. Thomsen, M.D.
Attending Physician
Emergency Department
Mount Auburn Hospital
Cambridge, Massachusetts
Instructor in Medicine
Harvard Medical School
Boston, Massachusetts

Rebecca Tipton, M.D.
Attending Physician
Emergency Department
MetroWest Medical Center
Framingham, Massachusetts

Tri C. Tong, M.D.
Attending Physician
Emergency Department
University of California San Diego Medical Center
San Diego, California

J. David Walsh, M.D.
Emergency Physician
Midwest Regional Medical Center
Midwest City, Oklahoma

Joel M. Wassermann, M.D.
Emergency Department
Virginia Mason Medical Center
Seattle, Washington
Emergency Department
Group Health Cooperative
Seattle, Washington
Emergency Department
Swedish Medical Center
Seattle, Washington

Steven Wexler, M.D., F.A.A.E.M.
Assistant Director
Emergency Department
Waterbury Hospital
Waterbury, Connecticut

Kevin G. Wheeler, M.D.
Attending Physician
Emergency Department
North Shore Medical Hospital
Union Hospital Campus
Lynn, Massachusetts

Deborah R. Wong, M.D.
Attending Physician
Emergency Department
Mount Auburn Hospital
Cambridge, Massachusetts
Clinical Instructor
Department of Medicine
Division of Emergency Medicine
Harvard Medical School
Boston, Massachusetts

Janet Simmons Young, M.D.
Assistant Professor of Emergency Medicine
University of North Carolina at Chapel Hill
Chapel Hill, North Carolina

Acknowledgments

To Karyn, Daniel, and Noah—thank you for your love and support. Thanks to my parents, Ted and Ori, for always being there. Thank you to Java and Jasper for sharing their experiences with rabies vaccinations. Special thanks to Sydney Miller and Larry Lemish for their unsurpassed technical advice and for being available 24/7.

RM

To Peter Rosen and John Marx—for their intelligence and wit and for the great kindness and compassion they show to patients, students, residents, and colleagues. To my parents, for their unending support and for living life in a way I can only hope to emulate. To my husband Ned, for his never-ending patience, encouragement, and love, and to my darling Rees, who has made my heart grow larger than I ever thought possible. Dedicated to Jesse the best ball throwing, smiling Labrador, who went to medical school, finished residency, and left his paw print on the planet.

ELM

Foreword

When I was a junior in medical school, I had this terrible feeling that I had missed some critical lecture during one of the many periods when someone came in, turned off the lights, and started lecturing in some language that was supposed to be English. It may well have been just the turning off of the lights, but I was usually in delta wave before any memorable communication had been made. Nevertheless, as I began my clinical rotations, I always had the feeling that everyone around me had stayed awake for that lecture. They knew how to start; they seemed to be able to talk like they knew a lot about whatever service we were on, and I felt like I hadn't learned anything since orientation on opening day.

Every rotation seemed to be dependent on the one I hadn't yet experienced, and when I did arrive at the last of the rotations, I could no longer use the excuse that I was going to learn everything I needed to know on the next service.

The feeling was most acute when I was in the emergency department (ED). There of course was no such thing as a field of emergency medicine, but I was constantly being told to go see a patient, start the work-up, and talk to the resident when I had "things going."

Today there is a field. There is a literature. There are textbooks. There are, unfortunately, no easy ways into the subject. Many students either arrive on their first rotation in the ED or, in some schools, come from an in-patient service to pick up a patient. I see many senior students who have a look on their face that I well relate to and remember. How do I start?

The answer is here, with this book. It is entirely appropriate to find a concise overview of the important aspects of the field and dive in. The encyclopedic discussions of the major texts in the field are of course useful for those who will make emergency medicine their specialty. The "5-minute consult" is fine for an individual problem, but for a way to an overview to prevent that feeling of total incapacitating ignorance, this book is the place to start. Even if one isn't aware of it until the first day of rotation in the ED, it is comprehensible and able to be assimilated into usable knowledge in a finite and compressed time frame.

I think this book will become standard reading for all medical students, and I hope it will appear in everyone's library.

Now, even if you slept through the introduction to clinical emergency medicine, you can catch up and feel like making a competent start into the biology of emergency medicine.

Peter Rosen MD
Attending Emergency Physician
Beth Israel/Deaconess Hospital
Boston, Massachusetts
Associate Professor Emergency Medicine
Harvard University
Senior Lecturer
Harvard University
Cambridge, Massachusetts

Preface

We are pleased to introduce this new book to the increasing numbers of students interested in the field of emergency medicine. We have taken great care to create a text that students at any level can understand and learn from. First- and second-year medical students will find this book ideal for learning core concepts of emergency medicine practice and the relationship of clinical practice and pathophysiology. Third- and fourth-year students should find the clinical scenarios and procedure sections particularly useful during clinical rotations. In addition, physician assistants and nurse practitioners who practice in emergency departments and ambulatory care settings may find this book a helpful learning tool.

This book was born out of the desire to create a work that introduces the discipline of emergency medicine in a meaningful and substantial way. It takes you through critical emergency care topics by teaching you how to approach and manage a patient and how to perform procedures, while introducing aspects unique to the specialty of emergency medicine, such as prehospital care, disaster medicine, trauma, toxicology, environmental injuries—to name just a few.

The book begins with a brief history of the specialty and then covers the basic principles of resuscitation and shock. The concepts of resuscitation recur frequently in all critically ill patients, whereas shock is the final common pathway for most patients whose organ systems are unable to cope with severe illness. This information is best read before the clinical case studies, because many of the patients discussed will show signs of shock and require resuscitation, and the reader can refer back to these chapters as needed.

The clinical case studies are the most unique aspect of the book. One of the challenges of being a medical student, especially in the preclinical years, is finding ways to relate the basic science material that you are being taught to its clinical application. The case studies are focused on ten common complaints for seeking emergency care. Each patient possesses all of the typical symptoms and signs of that particular disease process. While reading the rest of the chapter, you should have a clear mental picture of the prototypical patient and hopefully be able to associate the relevant history, physical findings, diagnostic evaluation, treatment, and pathophysiology to that patient. When you see an actual patient in the emergency department, you will be able to draw on that experience in a meaningful way. Topics unique to emergency medicine follow the case scenarios.

Because of space constraints, some topics found in larger emergency medicine texts could not be included. Our decisions regarding the topics that were included were based on how significant those topics are to a student being introduced to emergency medicine. Particular attention was given to interpretation of common laboratory analyses and procedural issues in an emergency context.

A book of this kind cannot be realized without the help and dedication of numerous individuals, too many to mention by name. Our heartfelt thanks go to each of them. Their expertise and hard work is greatly appreciated. We wish to acknowledge the many contributors to the text with special thanks to the editors of the clinical case studies, whose work provided cohesiveness and clarity to their sections. Thanks are also extended to the reviewers of the book, whose comments were immensely helpful, and to the staff at Lippincott, Williams & Wilkins, whose superb editorial work brought the writing in this book to a higher level. We thank in particular Elena Coler for pulling all its disparate threads together and for weaving it into a tightly knit book.

Thank you to Lois Lombardo at Nesbitt Graphics, Inc. for immeasurably improving the book. A special thanks to Vicky Heim for creating the artwork for the figures. Last but not least, we thank the students whose infectious enthusiasm made our work most enjoyable and inspired us to write this book.

Ron Medzon
Elizabeth L. Mitchell

Contents

PART I

Basic Principles of Emergency Medicine

Introduction

CHAPTER 1

History of Emergency Medicine

Benjamin Honigman, MD

History

Caring for the critically ill and injured has occurred for centuries, during wars on battlefields, in hospitals, and in people's homes. However, the development of emergency medicine as a specialty that cares for these patients is a phenomenon of the last 40 years. Emergency medicine developed largely because of patient demand. It is a specialty "of the people, by the people, and for the people." Unlike most other disciplines that grew out of the academic origins and interests of the physicians, emergency medicine grew from a unique set of circumstances based on the needs and desires of patients. Emergency medicine is a time-dependent specialty of the severely ill and injured.

In addition, it serves as a safety net for anyone without access to other providers, whether resulting from lack of insurance or inability to access one's own physician. It is a specialty that enables the practicing emergency physician to have a finger on the pulse of the nation's health care needs.

The First Hospital Emergency Departments (EDs)

Before the organization of an emergency medicine specialty, the hospital ED was considered an afterthought. Often referred to lovingly as "the pit," it was commonplace to have long waits and misdiagnoses. It has been described as the "rawest interface" of the hospital with the community. Nurses would often staff the emergency room (ER) without physicians and would call for physician or housestaff assistance, based on the nurse's initial assessment.

The makeup of the physician staff varied widely from hospital to hospital. At community hospitals, physicians who were just starting or ending their practice often worked in the ED. Other community hospitals had locum tenens physicians or providers who would occasionally staff the department. At university hospitals, it was considered to be the intern's domain. Many academic medical centers had 24-hour shifts for interns and junior housestaff and senior residents would avoid the ED for more glamorous sites of clinical practice.

Although the transportation of ill and injured patients to health care providers has occurred for centuries during war and peacetime, prehospital care before the 1960s was usually done with minimal standards. Ambulances often functioned as hearses, and it was not uncommon to see a Cadillac owned by a funeral home director, who employed high school students as drivers. This was a true "load-and-go" operation.

Cultural Changes 1960s to 1970s

During the 1960s, changes in the culture of the American medical community increased the demand for emergency services. Solo practitioners began to merge into group practices. Physicians looked for ways to reduce their after-hours and on-call duties. The ratio of specialists to general practitioners increased. In addition, patients moved more frequently in search of employment and did not establish roots in their communities. This resulted in more patients who did not have a primary care physician and, therefore, required medical care from emergency centers. Patients developed a "fast-food" mentality, in which they demanded immediate care in all clinical practice settings (whether in a physician's office or at the hospital). These changes combined to vastly increase the numbers of patients being treated in EDs. By the mid-1970s, more than 80 million patients were seen in U.S. EDs on an annual basis.

In addition to patient and physician changes, other events fueled the increase in ED visits. Insurance companies began to reimburse at a higher rate for hospital and emergency visits than they did for office-based practices. Malpractice claims rose, and there were increased awards paid for cases seen in the ED. These changes began to create a demand for high-quality and competent care in the emergency setting.

There were several important clinical, academic, and social changes during the 1960s and 1970s that further advanced the development of the field of emergency medicine. Acute care medicine became increasingly sophisticated. Cardiopulmonary resuscitation (CPR) research was in its infancy, but in the early 1970s there was enough scientific background to develop advanced cardiac life support (ACLS) programs on a national level. The Vietnam war changed the concepts of triage, stabilization, and transport to specialized field hospitals from the front lines. This led to the beginnings of trauma regionalization, which blossomed in the 1980s. Mobile cardiac care units (CCUs) were established in New York City and Miami in the 1960s. At the same time, the landmark report from the National Research Council in 1966 entitled "Accidental Death and Disability: the Neglected Disease of Modern Society" helped spur legislation establishing prehospital care and emergency medical services. The National Highway Acts of 1966 and 1973 established financial resources for emergency medical service (EMS) systems to be developed on a regional basis. Finally, during the 1960s, an increasing number of hospitals realized that they required more highly trained and skilled providers in the ED. Many changed their bylaws and regulations to demand that their facilities be staffed by physicians.

The First Emergency Medicine Organizations

All of these conspiring factors led to the establishment of the first recognized ED clinical practices, the beginnings of emergency medicine as we know it today. In Pontiac, Michigan, the "Pontiac Plan" provided staffing in the ED with surgeons and internists who each shared call to supplement their private practice. In Alexandria, Virginia, the "Alexandria Plan" was the first ED to be staffed by full-time emergency physicians. Several hospitals followed these staffing patterns, and by 1968, 32 physicians from 19 states met in Alexandria, Virginia to form a national organization of emergency providers. This meeting became the nidus for the American College of Emergency Physicians and for the organized practice of emergency medicine.

As patient and hospital demands for qualified health care providers in the ED grew, the membership of the American College of Emergency Physicians (ACEP) also grew. In 1970, a new organization developed, which was called the University Association for Emergency Medical Services

(UAEMS). Most of the members of this organization were academic physicians, predominantly surgeons, who were assigned responsibility for running their EDs in the early part of their academic careers. Although the beginnings of this organization focused on trauma and surgical emergencies, the interest levels broadened to include physicians who were practicing emergency medicine and residents training in emergency medicine. An increased number of emergency medicine residents joined this organization and formed the Emergency Medicine Residents Association (EMRA). This organization provided resident representation to UAEMS and to ACEP and obtained important information that could be disseminated to emergency medicine residents nationally. The first elected official of EMRA to UAEMS was Joseph Wackerle, M.D., who later became the editor of the *Annals of Emergency Medicine*, one of the premier journals of the specialty.

The First Residency

The academic infrastructure of emergency medicine also began in the 1970s. The first formal residency program for emergency medicine began at the University of Cincinnati in 1972. Before this there were "training fellowships." In the next 3 years, 10 new programs developed in such cities as Philadelphia, Louisville, Los Angeles, and Chicago. The first two independent academic departments of emergency medicine at U.S. medical schools were established in 1971 at the University of Southern California and the University of Louisville.

Specialty Designation

As the specialty gained popularity, it required a formal recognition within the American Medical Association (AMA). This was accomplished through a coalition of UAEMS, ACEP, and the Society of Critical Care Medicine, which formed a federation for Emergency and Critical Care Medicine in 1973. During that time, the AMA sponsored a conference to identify the parameters of undergraduate,

graduate, and continuing education for emergency medicine. This eventually led to a formal section on Emergency Medicine, which was ultimately approved in 1976. It took another 3 years for the American Board of Emergency Medicine (ABEM) to be formally recognized as a conjoint specialty board by the American Board of Medical Specialties (ABMS). Emergency Medicine became the 23rd academic specialty in the House of Medicine. The first certification examination was in February 1980, when more than 600 emergency physicians sat for the examination.

American Board of Emergency Medicine (ABEM)

Residency training also began looking for ways to increase its credibility. In 1976, a liaison committee was established with representatives from ACEP, UAEMS, and EMRA. This was the first time that any residency review committee had resident representation, which is now a standard for all residency review committees. The American College of Graduate Medical Education assumed full responsibility for the accreditation process of residencies in emergency medicine in 1981. Until that time, the 10 programs that were training residents were voluntarily endorsed by the LREC. It took 10 years from the original approval as a conjoint board for the ABMS to finally approve the ABEM as a full primary board on September 22, 1989.

Important Legislation

During the 1980s, several significant events occurred that began to change the practice of emergency medicine and the specialty as a whole.

The Libby Zion Case

In 1987, a young woman named Libby Zion took an overdose of several medications and was taken to a hospital in New York City. She was initially treated only by housestaff in both the ED and on the wards and eventually died. Her family sued the hospital and the providers and not only won their malpractice claim but also changed the practice of emergency medicine. The state of New York established a requirement that all housestaff must have faculty supervision in their clinical settings, including EDs. This soon became the national standard in all communities.

Emergency Medical Treatment and Active Labor Act (EMTALA)

The EMTALA of 1985 is commonly known as the federal anti-dumping law. The initial purpose of this law was to deter and to punish hospitals that were "dumping" indigent patients from their ED to nearby public institutions. EMTALA requires that the patient be stabilized before any such transfers. Although originally intended as a piece of social welfare legislation to aid patients with little or no health insurance, all individuals who have a genuine and serious emergency medical condition or who are in active labor are protected under the law. The penalties for both the institution and the health care provider are far reaching, including financial penalties, incarceration, and loss of Medicare licensure.

EMTALA is the single most significant piece of medical legislation in American history, establishing broad legal obligations relating to medical care misconduct and failure to provide appropriate treatment. There is no national law of this type applicable to any other specialty or hospital service.

Trauma System Legislation

In 1970, "Injury in America," a publication from the National Institutes of Health, identified trauma as the leading cause of death in patients between the ages of 1 and 45. With the aid of state laws, and federal and state dollars, the establishment of state trauma systems blossomed in the 1980s and 1990s to provide for regionalization of trauma care.

Principles of the Specialty

Clinical Principles

The clinical principles and curricula of emergency medicine continued to evolve in the

1970s and 1980s. The foundations of the clinical practice became vital not only in daily practice but also in the teaching of emergency medicine in residency programs. The overarching principle of emergency medicine views the whole person in the context of potential threats to life and limb in a temporally demanding setting. Dr. Peter Rosen, one of the fathers of academic emergency medicine, once described this as the need to rescue a mountain climber who is hanging on to the edge of a cliff. The rescuer's primary mission is to bring the mountain climber back to a safe place, not necessarily to ask why the climber fell or who pushed him or her. Although a diagnosis can be made in the ED in many instances, it is not always necessary to treat and stabilize the patient. The basic tenets of emergency medicine are to identify and treat immediate threats to the life of the patient, using the skills of a comprehensive team of providers.

An emergency physician must also be able to prioritize multiple patient encounters caused by a multiple-casualty incident or simply by heavy patient volume. The characteristics of the practice also include the principle that the patient defines the emergency. This has evolved to the level of legislation in several states, defining emergencies according to a "prudent layperson definition." This establishes for the patient, the providers, and insurance payor a standard definition that states that an emergency is anything that would be viewed as such by a layperson under similar conditions. Another basic feature of our practice is that we are available 24 hours per day, 365 days per year. Physicians function in a time-dependent process of initial evaluation, recognition, stabilization, and disposition with an unrestricted patient population. This is true for patients who have injuries and illnesses and for those who have behavioral problems. In fact, chief complaints run the entire spectrum of human diseases and calamities.

Health Care Access

In the 1990s, several other aspects of emergency systems and emergency care began to influence the specialty. Access to care became a significant problem. Urgent care centers developed to handle the large populations of urgent problems, as opposed to true emergencies. Several studies show that only 10% to 15% of patients who arrive in the ED have true life or limb-threatening emergencies, whereas 50% to 60% have emergent problems. Those remaining have urgent problems. However, the use of EDs has continued to grow to more than 100 million patients nationally in 1999. Access to care is particularly problematic for the indigent population, which has also grown dramatically in the 1990s. This has led to increased waiting times, unavailability of beds in both the ED and the hospital, and an increasing number of patients who are left without being seen (LWBS). Research in the 1980s showed that LWBS patients did not usually have an emergent medical problem; however, more recent research suggests that a high percentage of these patients actually do have serious medical problems.

Access to health care providers has also been affected by health maintenance organizations (HMOs). Their impact on the practice has been significant, not only in the payment structure of emergency physicians and facilities but also in their attempts to divert patients away from EDs and into private physician's offices. Despite the predictions that HMOs would decrease ED use, the opposite has occurred, creating overloaded emergency systems and a high volume of patients requiring care. This has led to problems particularly in major urban centers, causing ambulance diversions.

Several authors have pointed out that ED care may not be as expensive as was once believed. Because there is a fixed overhead expense associated with maintaining an open ED for 24 hours per day, many economists and health care experts now suggest that use of these EDs to their maximum is more economical than trying to divert patients to minimize patient volumes. The other impact that HMOs have had on our practice has been to try to make emergency medical systems more efficient by decreasing inappropriate use of ambulance ser-

vices. Emergency medical dispatch, a subspecialty of emergency medical systems, are now offering other, less expensive transportation options to patients, when specialized ambulances are not needed.

Academics

As the clinical practice of emergency medicine evolved, so too did the national organizations and academic practices. UAEMS continued to evolve and changed its name to the University Association for Emergency Medicine (UAEM), which began to emphasize research at its annual meetings. The Society of Teachers of Emergency Medicine (STEM) was formed to provide representation to the American Association of Medical Colleges. It became the focus for educational activities within emergency medicine. STEM and UAEM merged in 1989 and formed the Society for Academic Emergency Medicine (SAEM) because it was apparent to both groups that education and research were vitally linked. As an organization for academic emergency physicians, the annual SAEM meeting continues to provide the best forum for researchers and academicians in emergency medicine, while promoting academic emergency medicine through education and research.

At the medical school level, the number of academic departments of emergency medicine in the U.S. medical schools expanded with the help of the Association of Academic Chairs of Emergency Medicine, which was founded in 1989. The number of academic departments more than doubled from 1990 to 1994 and reached 57 in 1999. This has significantly enhanced the education and training of emergency physicians and advanced knowledge through emergency medicine research activities. In 1996, a document was developed by the Josiah Macy Junior Foundation, which published a report of a conference entitled "Research Directions in Emergency Medicine." Recommendations from this report included ways to enhance support for basic clinical and basic health services research, to promote collaborative interdisciplinary research, to develop new systems to manage clinical information, to develop new methods to assist the outcomes of emergency care, and to secure increased funding for emergency medicine research.

The maturation of emergency medicine as a specialty has generated the formation of subspecialties, including pediatric emergency medicine, sports medicine, medical toxicology, EMS, and hyperbaric medicine. Fellowships have evolved that provide subspecialty training to emergency physicians in these areas.

The Practice of Emergency Medicine Today

Over the last 40 years we have witnessed the growth of a specialty, which began from people's demands for a higher quality of care in EDs to an academic discipline within the House of Medicine. In the last 10 years, emergency medicine has attracted the best and the brightest of medical students and has become an increasingly popular specialty. Through its clinical practice, it offers a challenging and diverse clinical environment. It affords the ability to care for a breadth of medicine that cannot be found in any other field of practice. Although HMOs, insurance companies, and federal regulations have changed the face of emergency practice, is

still affords the opportunity to care for all patients who enter our doors. As emergency medicine physicians, we can continue to provide care to our patients, educate our students and future physicians, and ask questions to expand our knowledge base to learn more about disease and injury processes. It is truly an exceptional field of practice.

Suggested Readings

Committee on Trauma Research Commission on Life Sciences National Research Council and the Institute of Medicine. *Injury in America. A continuing Public Health Problem.* Washington, D.C.: National Academy Press, 1985.

Gallagher EJ, Schropp MA, Henneman PL. Changing status of Academic Emergency Medicine (1991–1996). Task Force on the Development of Emergency Medicine. *Acad Emerg Med* 1997;4:746–751.

Josiah Macy Jr. Foundation. The role of emergency medicine in the future of American medical care. *Ann Emerg Med* 1995;25:230–233, 1995.

Rosen P. History of emergency medicine. New York, NY: Josiah Macy Jr. Foundation conference on "The Role of Emergency Medicine in the Future of American Medical Care," April 17–20, 1997.

Rosen P. The biology of emergency medicine. *JACEP* 1979;8:280–283.

Principles of Resuscitation

Joseph H. Kahn, MD, FACEP

Chapter Outline

Resuscitation refers to the aggressive management of critically ill patients and patients in cardiac or respiratory arrest, regardless of the cause. Causes may include cardiac dysrhythmia, myocardial infarction, heart failure, dehydration, vascular emergencies, electrolyte imbalances, overwhelming infection, renal failure, shock, liver failure, drowning, electrocution, choking, head trauma, spinal trauma, hemorrhage, chest trauma, and abdominal trauma. The treatment administered in the first hour to critically ill patients may significantly impact their outcome. Management of patients already in cardiac or respiratory arrest is the highest priority in both prehospital and in-hospital emergency care, because any chance of survival is predicated on reversing the arrest state within minutes.

It is optimal to begin the resuscitation of a patient at the scene where the patient is found. Survival to hospital discharge rates for patients found in cardiac arrest vary from 2% to 33%, and one of the factors that affects outcome is bystander cardiopulmonary resuscitation (CPR). Communities in which a large percentage of the citizens are trained in CPR have been shown to have better survival rates after out-of-hospital cardiac arrest.

In order for resuscitation to begin at the scene where the patient is found, the scene must be safe for the victim and the rescuer. In general, moving trauma patients without adequate immobilization risks exacerbation of spinal injuries. However, when the environment is unsafe the patient should be moved to safety, using care to flex or extend the spine as little as possible. This chapter attempts to describe the principles of resuscitation, including the primary survey (ABCDE) and secondary survey. In adult victims outside the hospital, the American Heart Association (AHA) advises calling emergency medical services (EMS) once unresponsiveness is determined. In children up to age 8, the AHA advises 1 minute of resuscitation before activating EMS. If there is more than one person present, EMS can be activated immediately regardless of the age of the victim, because one bystander can start resuscitating while the other calls EMS. When EMS is activated, there may be a one-

or two-tiered response, depending on the community. Emergency medical technicians (EMTs) can provide life-saving care in many situations and are capable of providing Basic Life Support (BLS), including the use of the automatic external defibrillator, airway management, cardiopulmonary resuscitation, stroke recognition, control of bleeding, extrication, and transport of patients. Paramedics can start intravenous (IV) lines; provide advanced airway management; interpret cardiac rhythms; deliver synchronized cardioversion; perform cricothyrotomies and chest decompressions; and treat with many medications, either by standing order or with medical direction via two-way radio.

In any resuscitation, an organized approach is essential for any possibility of a successful outcome for the patient. This organized approach was initially provided by the AHA and then modified by the American College of Surgeons. It can be summarized as the primary survey or the ABCDE of resuscitation: Airway, Breathing, Circulation, Disability, Exposure/Environmental control (Table 2.1). As the primary survey proceeds, treatment must be instituted for any serious abnormalities found.

Primary Survey

Airway

The approach to the critically ill patient and the patient in cardiac and respiratory arrest is different from the typical doctor-patient interaction. In resuscitating critically ill or injured patients, the history, physical examination, tests, and treatment all occur rapidly

---

Table 2.1.

The ABCDEs of the primary survey

Airway
Breathing
Circulation
Disability (neurological)
Exposure/environmental control

---

and simultaneously. The first area to assess is the patient's airway.

The airway may be obstructed for a variety of reasons. The patient may be unconscious, with loss of airway reflexes and settling of the tongue in the posterior pharynx. The patient may have blood or vomitus pooled in the mouth and pharynx, obstructing ventilation. Witnesses may reveal that the patient choked on a piece of meat or other foreign body before collapsing. Traumatic etiologies may include blunt or penetrating trauma to the face or neck, destroying bony and/or cartilaginous integrity of the airway; burns to the airway with subsequent edema; or corrosive ingestions. Infectious causes include epiglottitis, retropharyngeal abscesses, and submandibular space infections (Ludwig's angina).

The most common cause of airway obstruction in an unconscious patient is the tongue sliding back and blocking the pharynx. In this situation if there is no obvious history or sign of trauma, the head tilt-chin lift maneuver should be used to reposition the tongue away from the posterior pharynx. This is done by lifting the chin up with one hand while holding downward pressure on the forehead. When trauma is suspected, the airway should be opened using the jaw-thrust maneuver, which can be accomplished without moving the neck. This maneuver is accomplished by pulling the jaw forward with one hand grasping the angles of the mandible while maintaining cervical spine immobilization with the other hand.

Once the airway has been opened using the head tilt-chin lift or the jaw-thrust maneuver, the airway can be kept patent by inserting an oropharyngeal airway. The oropharyngeal airway is a curved structure, which keeps the tongue out of the posterior pharynx and allows for better oxygenation, ventilation, and suctioning. The patient must have a depressed gag reflex to tolerate an oropharyngeal airway. If an oropharyngeal airway cannot be inserted either because the mouth will not open or the patient has a gag reflex, and there is no suspicion of midface fractures, a nasopharyngeal airway can be inserted instead.

Opening the airway can be much more difficult when the obstruction is from causes other than the tongue sliding back into the posterior pharynx. If there is blood or vomitus obstructing the airway, suctioning may clear it. Because these fluids tend to reaccumulate, the suctioning may need to be repeated frequently. If there is inflammation and edema from trauma, chemical or thermal burns, infection, or other causes, endotracheal intubation may be required to control the airway.

Breathing

Once the airway has been opened, the rescuer should ascertain whether the patient is breathing. This is best accomplished with the "look, listen, and feel" method outlined by the AHA. The rescuer places her or his ear near the mouth and nose of the victim, with eyes looking toward the patient's chest. The rescuer can look at the chest for rising and falling, while simultaneously listening for and feeling air movement from the nose and mouth. This evaluation should take no longer than 10 seconds, and once it is determined that the patient is not breathing, rescue breathing should be initiated. Rescue breathing refers to several types of ventilation, including mouth-to-mouth, mouth-to-nose, mouth-to-mouth-and-nose (infants), mouth-to-stoma, and mouth-to-mask. Mouth-to-mouth ventilation poses a risk of transmission of infectious diseases to the rescuer. This has stimulated studies looking at chest compressions and mouth-to-mouth ventilation versus chest compressions alone. There is some early evidence that mouth-to-mouth ventilation may not improve survival, but the results are not convincing, and mouth-to-mouth ventilation is still recommended by the AHA when a mask is not available.

The specific recommendations for mouth-to-mouth ventilation include pinching the victim's nose shut, positioning the head so that the airway is open, and sealing the rescuer's mouth around the patient's. The rescuer delivers two slow breaths in rapid succession, followed by one slow breath every 4 or 5 seconds in an adult (12/minute), or every 3 to 5 seconds in children (20/minute). Clearly mouth-to-mask or mouth-to-face shield ventilation has the advantage of protecting the rescuer from infectious diseases. Pocket masks are readily available and can be carried in the rescuer's pocket or car. For prehospital and hospital personnel, the bag-valve-mask (BVM) device is widely used. The BVM device consists of a facemask, a one-way valve, and a self-inflating bag, which should be attached to oxygen if available. The facemask is held firmly over the patient's mouth and nose with one hand while the bag is squeezed with the other hand. If there are enough rescuers available, the facemask can be held in place with both hands by one rescuer, while another compresses the bag. All medical personnel should become facile in the use of the BVM device. This device has many useful features: high-flow oxygen can be delivered to the patient, it can be used in conjunction with chest compressions if the patient is in cardiac arrest, and its rapid application can be used to preoxygenate patients while preparing for endotracheal intubation.

Patients who do not begin breathing spontaneously within a few minutes of BVM ventilation will require endotracheal intubation. Endotracheal intubation is also recommended for patients who are breathing spontaneously but who are unconscious with an absent gag reflex or inability to handle secretions both of which could lead to aspiration of gastric and oral contents. Intubation may be required in patients with severe respiratory distress resulting from asthma, chronic obstructive pulmonary disease (COPD), congestive heart failure (CHF), pneumonia, and other causes. It may be performed as a protective measure in those patients whose upper airways (pharynx, larynx, and trachea) are at risk for compromise, such as burn victims, victims of facial and neck trauma, victims of corrosive ingestion, patients with upper airway infections, and patients with upper airway angioedema.

The principle of endotracheal intubation is the insertion of a semirigid plastic tube through the patient's mouth or nose into the trachea allowing delivery of oxygen directly to the patient's lungs, without the simultaneous delivery of oxygen to the stomach. It helps prevent aspiration of vomitus, blood, and other fluids into the trachea, via inflation of the cuff, which is located near the distal tip of the endotracheal tube. In children younger than 8 years, the tube fits snugly enough through the cricoid cartilage so that it aids in aspiration prevention without a cuff. In patients other than those in cardiac arrest, premedication is usually required. This may vary from sedation and analgesia to rapid sequence induction (RSI) with neuromuscular blockade.

If indicated, nasotracheal intubation may be performed instead of orotracheal intubation. This technique can be useful in asthma exacerbations, COPD exacerbations, and CHF. The technique, which is blind, requires a patient with intact respiratory effort. There are more complications with nasotracheal than with orotracheal intubations; the most common complication is nosebleeds and the second most common is pharyngeal perforation. Contraindications to nasotracheal intubation include cerebrospinal fluid (CSF) rhinorrhea, suspected midface fractures, epiglottitis, retropharyngeal abscess, neck trauma, bleeding diathesis, suspected foreign body, bilateral large nasal polyps, or no respiratory effort.

Cricothyrotomy may be required in the patient who cannot be intubated and requires definitive airway control. The inability to intubate may be due to technical difficulties, trauma, edema, or infection. Cricothyrotomy can be performed with a needle or surgically. Two other techniques used in difficult intubations include fiberoptic intubation and the laryngeal mask airway (LMA), which can be inserted without visualizing the larynx and can allow for adequate oxygenation and ventilation. It has been used successfully in neonates, as well as in children and adults.

If the patient is breathing, adequacy of oxygenation and ventilation must be assessed. The clinician should percuss and auscultate the chest, listening for abnormal sounds, such as wheezing (bronchiolar constriction), rhonchi (mucus in bronchi), rales (fluid in alveoli), or stridor (upper airway constriction). Respiratory status can further be assessed by patient's skin color and oxygen saturation. Oxygen should be used readily in the resuscitation of critically ill or injured patients in respiratory distress.

While assessing the patient's breathing, the examiner may find evidence of pathology that requires emergent intervention. Examples include wheezing and prolonged expiration suggestive of asthma or COPD; inspiratory rales suggestive of pulmonary edema or pneumonia; pneumothorax or hemothorax suggested by the absence of breath sounds; and tension pneumothorax that also includes tracheal deviation, jugular venous distension, and hemodynamic instability. All of these entities are discussed in detail elsewhere in the book. In this chapter, the principle they illustrate is that treatment must occur simultaneous to evaluation.

Circulation

Basic Life Support (BLS)

Determining the presence or absence of a pulse is the next step. If the patient is not breathing, the health care worker should check for pulses immediately after rescue breathing has begun. This can be accomplished by palpating for the carotid pulse in adults and in children older than 1 year and by feeling for the brachial pulse in infants (umbilical pulsation in neonates). If there is no pulse felt within 10 seconds, external chest compressions should be initiated. According to the 2000 AHA guidelines, lay people (people who are not health care workers) should begin chest compressions without a pulse check, if the patient is not breathing and not moving. In adults, chest compressions involve depression of the sternum $1\frac{1}{2}$ to 2 inches, using two hands, with the heels of the hands on the lower half of the sternum. The recommended compression rate in adults is 100 per minute. After every 15 compressions, two rescue breaths should be given, in both one and two person CPR. In children aged 1 to 8 years, the sternum is depressed $1–1\frac{1}{2}$ inches by the heel of one hand on the lower half of the child's sternum. The recommended compression rate is 100 compressions per minute, and one ventilation every five compressions. In infants, the lower half of the sternum should be depressed ½–1 inch by the rescuer's two thumbs (with hands wrapped around the chest) or two fingers. The compression rate in infants is at least 100 compressions per minute (120 compressions per minute in neonates), with a 5:1 compression to ventilation ratio (3:1 in neonates). The rescuer should check for return of pulse and breathing after 1 minute of CPR and every few minutes thereafter.

Early defibrillation has been shown to increase survival in cardiac arrest victims. In one study, 66% of adults with out-of-hospital cardiac arrest who survived to hospital admission had ventricular fibrillation (VF) as their presenting rhythm. The AHA recommends defibrillation within 5 minutes of the EMS call. Early defibrillation can be more realistically achieved with automatic external defibrillators (AEDs). If applied properly, the AED will determine whether the patient is in VF and, if so, will advise the rescuer to deliver an electric shock and defibrillate the patient. Because of their ease of use and effectiveness, AEDs are now used by many airlines, public buildings and offices, and hospital inpatient wards and outpatient clinics. The AHA now recommends that use of AED be taught as part of BLS courses, so that professionals trained in BLS, such as police, firefighters, basic EMTs, and other health care workers, and lay people, can properly use an AED.

Advanced Cardiac Life Support (ACLS)

Once it is established that the victim is in cardiac arrest, EMS has been activated, and CPR has begun, AED has been applied (if available), and shocks delivered (if advised), Advanced Cardiovascular Life Support (ACLS) treatments should be initiated. A complete review of this topic is beyond the scope of this book but can be readily accessed by the AHA's publications of ACLS protocols. ACLS treatments may be started

by the paramedics when they arrive or in the hospital emergency department (ED) when the patient arrives. These include rhythm interpretation and treatment, airway management with BVM device or endotracheal intubation, and initiation of IV access and medication administration. If peripheral IV access cannot be achieved because of technical reasons, central access should be attempted via the internal jugular, subclavian, or femoral veins. In children younger than age 6, intraosseous cannulation can be used if peripheral IV access cannot be obtained. While IV access is being attempted, several resuscitation medications can be administered down the endotracheal tube. These can be easily remembered by the mnemonic NAVEL: naloxone, atropine, diazepam, epinephrine, and lidocaine.

If the cardiac arrest victim is found to be in VF or ventricular tachycardia (VT) without a pulse, the patient should be immediately defibrillated with 200 joules (J) of electricity. If the patient remains in VF or pulseless VT, the patient should be shocked again at 200 to 300 J. If the patient remains in VF or pulseless VT, 360 J should be delivered. If these three shocks have failed to change the rhythm, the airway is secured and an IV line started. Epinephrine, 1 mg, can be given intravenously and repeated every 3 to 5 minutes. New AHA guidelines allow the one-time administration of vasopressin, 40U IV, as an alternative to the first dose of epinephrine. Other medications used to treat VF and pulseless VT include amiodarone, lidocaine, magnesium, and procainamide. The patient should be shocked at 360 J after each medication administered.

Other than VF and pulseless VT, in which defibrillation precedes other treatments, all patients in cardiac arrest should have immediate airway management, CPR, and IV access. If the monitor reveals pulseless electrical activity (PEA), the patient should be treated as any other pulseless arrest with intubation, IV access, CPR, epinephrine, and possibly atropine, while an etiology for the PEA is sought. The clinician should consider the following diagnoses and treat them if appropriate: hypovolemia, hypoxia, acidosis, hyperkalemia, hypokalemia, hypothermia, poisoning, cardiac tamponade, tension pneumothorax, myocardial infarction, and pulmonary embolism (Table 2.2).

If the cardiac monitor reveals no electrical activity in at least two leads, the cardiac arrest victim is in asystole. The use of a transcutaneous pacemaker to provide electrical stimulation to the heart should be considered. Medications for asystole include epinephrine and atropine.

Circulatory resuscitation of the patient with a palpable pulse mandates appropriate diagnosis of cardiac arrhythmias or other causes. Once a pulse is established, a blood pressure should be obtained and the patient evaluated for adequate perfusion. Cardiac arrhythmias associated with chest pain, shortness of breath, depressed level of consciousness, low blood pressure (hypotension), poor peripheral perfusion, or CHF require emergent intervention. For the patient with bradycardia, or slow heart rate, options include atropine, transcutaneous pacing, dopamine, and epinephrine. Pacemakers are also indicated for Type II second-degree atrioventricular (AV) block and third-degree AV block.

The unstable tachycardic patient may not have an arrhythmia but rather a sinus tachycardia. In this instance, it is imperative to determine the cause and institute treatment. Tachycardia and hypotension may be due to many causes, including blood loss, septic shock, dehydration, overdose, cardiogenic shock, and pulmonary embolism. A thorough evaluation and emergent treatment must be instituted.

Assessing the patient's circulatory status involves more than just checking for pulse and blood pressure. In addition, capillary refill should be assessed. If gentle pressure is applied to the fingertip to cause blanching, the color should return in less than 2 seconds. Delayed capillary refill time indicates decreased peripheral perfusion, which may be due to dehydration, blood loss, or shock. In addition, skin color, temperature, and moistness should be noted. Cool, moist skin may be secondary to the poor peripheral perfusion seen in many types of shock, whereas hot skin may indicate infection, certain poisonings, heat stroke, or neurogenic shock. Profusely diaphoretic skin is consistent with CHF, myocardial infarction, and profound hypoglycemia. Bleeding may be noted resulting from penetrating trauma.

During resuscitation of circulation in the critically ill or injured patient, remember that during the primary survey treatment occurs simultaneously with diagnosis. If the patient is dehydrated, IV fluids should be infused. When the patient is bleeding externally, direct pressure should be applied, and fluid (and possibly blood) replacement therapy begun. If internal bleeding is suspected, IV fluids (normal saline or Ringer's lactate) and possibly blood infusion should begin immediately, and emergent surgical consultation should be obtained. Type O-negative blood or type-specific blood can be infused while the laboratory is preparing typed and cross-matched blood.

There are many other diagnoses requiring treatment. Examples include antibiotics and fluid resuscitation in a patient suspected of having serious infection; consideration of antidotes and charcoal in the overdose patient; and in a patient with an acute myocardial infarction, nitrates, aspirin, blood thinners, beta blocking medications, thrombolytics, and potentially cardiac catheterization. Appropriate, rapid diagnosis and treatment is critical to the morbidity and mortality of these patients.

Table 2.2.

The differential diagnosis of pulseless electrical activity (remember Ts and Hs)

Hypoxia
Hypovolemia
Hydrogen ions, acidosis
Hyperkalemia and hypokalemia
Hypothermia
Thrombosis, coronary
Thrombosis, pulmonary
Tamponade, cardiac
Tension pneumothorax
Tablet overdose

Disability

Once the ABCs of the primary survey are complete, the patient is evaluated for neurological disability. In trauma resuscitations, early neurosurgical treatment of intracranial injuries is essential, and ATLS (Advanced Trauma Life Support) has long recognized the importance of neurological evaluation. Since thrombolytic therapy for stroke was introduced, early neurological assessment has recently taken on greater importance in medical resuscitations as well. The neurological assessment in the primary survey is threefold: pupillary response, level of alertness, and Glasgow Coma Score.

Pupillary Response

Pupillary assessment begins by checking whether the pupils are equal in size in both eyes and whether their shape is round. Response is assessed by shining a bright light into one pupil and then the other, watching for reaction. In the setting of head trauma, a large, nonreactive pupil on one side may indicate intracranial hemorrhage with rapid, compartmentalized increase in intracranial pressure (ICP) leading to brain herniation. This is rapidly fatal unless treated immediately with hyperventilation, osmotic diuresis, and definitively, neurosurgical decompression. Unequal pupils may have many other causes: intracranial aneurysm, eye injury, stroke, tumor, cranial nerve abnormality, medications, and nontraumatic causes of herniation. Approximately 4% of the population has a 1-mm difference in pupillary size at baseline. In that case, the pupils should both be briskly reactive.

Level of Alertness

The AVPU scale can be used to rapidly assess level of alertness. A for alert, refers to a patient who is awake and appropriately conversant with the staff while being evaluated. V stands for verbal and means that the patient appears to be lying quietly on the stretcher and speaks or moves only when spoken to (responds to verbal stimuli). P stands for painful and means that a painful stimulus must be applied to the patient to get her or him to move or speak (responds to painful stimuli). U stands for unresponsive and means that a patient is unconscious and does not speak or move even when a painful stimulus is applied.

Glasgow Coma Scale

The Glasgow Coma Scale (GCS) can be determined rapidly and gives a significant amount of information. The GCS assesses the patient's eye-opening ability, motor response, and verbal response. The GCS can range from 3 (unable to open eyes, move, or speak) to 15 (eyes open without stimulation, follows commands, alert and oriented) (Table 2.3). In addition it should be noted whether the patient is able to move one side better than the other, because this may represent stroke, intracranial mass, or intracranial hemorrhage.

Stroke

If the patient is thought to have a stroke, based on difficulty speaking and difficulty

Table 2.3.	
The Glasgow Coma Scale	
Eye Opening (E)	
Spontaneous	4
To speech	3
To pain	2
None	1
Best Motor Response (M)	
Obeys commands	6
Localizes pain	5
Normal flexion (withdraws from pain)	4
Abnormal flexion (decorticate)	3
Abnormal extension (decerebrate)	2
None (flaccid)	1
Verbal Response (V)	
Oriented	5
Confused conversation	4
Inappropriate words	3
Incomprehensible sounds	2
None	1
Glasgow Coma Score = (E + M + V)	

moving one side of the face or body, time of onset is critical. If the patient has stroke symptoms and signs for less than 6 hours, rapid head computed tomography (CT) scan and emergent neurological consultation are indicated, to determine whether the patient is a candidate for thrombolysis. Thrombolysis for stroke may be IV (up to 3 hours) or intra-arterial (up to 6 hours).

Seizure

Other neurological abnormalities requiring immediate treatment, such as seizures, may be noted during the primary survey. In the ill or traumatized patient, a seizure may be difficult to diagnose. A seizure may present with subtle signs such as rapidly fluttering eye movements or jaw clenching. If the seizure lasts longer than a few minutes, treatment should be initiated because prolonged seizures can cause long-term morbidity.

Glucose and Naloxone

During the brief neurological assessment, any abnormality of mental status should be noted. This may range from agitated delirium to coma. All these patients should have their blood glucose level checked. If the blood glucose level is low, this can be corrected with IV dextrose infusion. Low blood glucose level (hypoglycemia) should always be considered in diabetic patients on insulin or oral diabetic medications. Hypoglycemia frequently complicates pediatric resuscitations, especially in children with sepsis (infection), and blood glucose level should always be checked. High blood glucose level may also alter the patient's mental status.

In addition to checking the glucose on any patient with altered mental status, consideration should be given to narcotic overdose and treatment with naloxone (Narcan). Naloxone is a competitive antagonist of opioid receptors. Because it has relatively few side effects at therapeutic doses, it is used frequently in both the prehospital environment and the ED as both a diagnostic and therapeutic intervention.

Exposure/Environmental Control

The patient's clothes should be removed so that the patient can be adequately examined and treated. During the course of any resuscitation, the patient should be evaluated for trauma that may not have been reported. Routinely rolling the cardiac arrest victim onto the side to examine the back will occasionally reveal a gunshot or knife wound. Undressing the patient may also reveal rashes that may suggest a cause for the patient's critical condition, such as infection or anaphylaxis (severe allergic reaction). In certain cases of hazardous exposures, special care must be taken in the decontamination of the patient and in clothes removal.

Care must be taken to prevent causing hypothermia in critically ill or injured patients. After removing the clothing and examining the patient, the patient should be covered with warm, dry sheets and blankets. The resuscitation room should be warm.

Diagnostic Tests

Diagnostic tests may be obtained or ordered during the primary survey as indicated by the patient's clinical condition. The clinical laboratory might include complete blood count, electrolytes, amylase, liver function tests, pregnancy test, blood type and crossmatch, arterial blood gases, toxic screen, and urinalysis. Radiological studies may include chest x-ray films, lateral cervical spine and pelvis x-rays films (in the setting of multiple trauma), head CT (for suspected intracranial hemorrhage or stroke), bedside limited cardiac echocardiogram, and bedside abdominal ultrasound (FAST, Focused Abdominal Sonography in Trauma, examination). It is important to remember that diagnostic testing should not be ordered as a "shotgun" approach but only when clinically indicated. A nasogastric tube may be inserted during the primary survey if clinically indicated, such as in determining whether the patient has a massive upper gastrointestinal bleed or in preventing aspiration. A urinary catheter may be inserted during the primary survey if monitoring of urine output is essential, as in CHF or shock.

Secondary Survey

After the primary survey (ABCDEs) is completed and resuscitative measures are well under way, the clinician should move on to the secondary survey. The American College of Surgeons has defined the secondary survey as a head-to-toe evaluation. It is a thorough but rapid history and physical examination, with frequent rechecking of vital signs.

History

The history should include whether the patient has any medical problems, current medications, and allergies. The patient or family member should also be asked how and when the present critical illness or injury began. If the patient is a woman of childbearing age, it should be ascertained whether she is pregnant. If the patient may require an operation, the time of the last meal is important.

Head

The head should be carefully examined, with attention to the conjunctivae (pink, pale, presence of subconjunctival hemorrhages), sclera (clear or yellow), pupils (round regular, equal, reactive to light), and extraocular movements. Careful inspection of the face and head for bruises, lacerations, and fractures is essential. The ears should be examined for blood, hemotympanum, pus, or CSF. The clinician should check the nose for bleeding, CSF, deformity, and septal hematoma. The mouth and oropharynx should be observed for patency, bleeding, foreign bodies (including tooth fragments), mandible fractures, or edema. In trauma, the signs of basilar skull fracture should be sought: hemotympanum, bilateral periorbital ecchymosis (raccoon's eyes), swelling over the mastoid (Battle's sign), blood or CSF coming from the ears or nose, and abnormalities of extraocular movements. Presence of the signs of basilar skull fracture requires CT scan of the head and neurosurgical consultation.

Neck

Examination of the neck is the next step. Presence of jugular venous distention may indicate CHF or pericardial tamponade. Both carotid arteries should be palpated and auscultated. Absence of one carotid pulse may indicate aortic or carotid dissection, either spontaneous or resulting from trauma. A carotid bruit may indicate the presence of a plaque in the carotid artery; pieces of plaque can break off and cause a stroke. Stridor, a high-pitched sound on inspiration, indicates upper airway compromise and may be due to infection, inflammation, edema, or foreign body. If there is no suspicion of trauma, the clinician can determine whether the neck is supple or stiff. The neck may be stiff in the setting of meningitis or subarachnoid hemorrhage. In the setting of trauma, the neck should not be moved until it has been assessed for fracture. Penetrating injuries to the neck require emergent surgical consultation and may require imaging studies or operative exploration to determine depth of injury and underlying structures involved.

Chest

Careful examination of the chest is an essential portion of the secondary survey in any resuscitation. During the initial survey, a quick assessment of the chest was done to determine the presence of breathing and abnormal breath sounds. In the secondary survey, more careful inspection, palpation, percussion, and auscultation are indicated. Inspection may reveal a thoracotomy scar, tracheal deviation (tension pneumothorax), retractions (respiratory distress), asymmetric chest movement (splinting), paradoxical chest movement (flail chest), or evidence of blunt or penetrating trauma. Palpation of the chest may reveal fractures of the ribs, sternum, clavicles, or scapulae. Percussion may reveal hyperresonance (pneumothorax) or dullness (pleural fluid). Auscultation may reveal adventitious sounds, such as wheezing in COPD exacerbation or asthma or rales in CHF or pneumonia. Auscultation may also reveal absent breath sounds, as in pneumothorax or hemopneumothorax. A chest x-ray film may help clarify what the disease process is. A chest tube is indicated for pneumothorax or hemopneumothorax. If a tension pneumothorax is present with hemodynamic instability, needle decompression is performed while preparing to insert the chest tube. If the chest x-ray film shows a widened mediastinum in the absence of trauma, aortic dissection should be suspected and either chest CT scan with IV contrast or transesophageal echocardiogram obtained. A wide mediastinum in the presence of trauma is suspicious for aortic rupture, and CT scanning or aortogram of the chest is indicated. Air along the mediastinum, or pneumomediastinum, seen on chest x-ray film may indicate esophageal perforation or rupture, a dire emergency causing gastric contents to spill into the chest cavity, with rapid progression to shock and death. Treatment involves supporting the patient with fluids and antibiotics and rapid surgical repair.

Heart

The cardiac examination should focus on the rhythm, extra heart sounds, and the quality of the heart sounds. A murmur in the setting of prior valve replacement may indicate a failing valve and requires emergent echocardiography and cardiology and possibly cardiothoracic surgery consultation. If an aortic dissection is suspected, the presence of an aortic insufficiency murmur may indicate proximal dissection with loss of competence of the aortic valve and impending pericardial tamponade. If the heart sounds are muffled, this may indicate a pericardial effusion, and an echocardiogram should be performed.

Abdomen

The abdomen is one of the most crucial and most difficult regions to evaluate. A patient may complain of abdominal pain, low back pain, or groin pain or show signs of abdominal distention, abdominal tenderness, or abdominal trauma. A careful physical examination with selective laboratory and imaging aids will help narrow the diagnosis. The patient with hematemesis and melena may have an upper gastrointestinal (GI) bleed from the esophagus, stomach, or duodenum, requiring fluid and blood infusion and esophagogastroduodenoscopy (EGD) to locate and cauterize the bleeding. The patient with hematochezia may have a lower GI bleed from the large intestine, requiring fluids, blood, colonoscopy, or a bleeding scan. The patient with a diffusely tender, rigid abdomen may have a perforated viscus, from a duodenal ulcer or diverticulum, requiring emergency surgery. Free air from the perforation may be seen on an upright chest x-ray film. The patient with abdominal or back pain and hypotension may have a leaking abdominal aortic aneurysm, which may be diagnosed clinically, by bedside ultrasound or by abdominal CT scan and requires emergent surgical repair. The appendix, gallbladder, or diverticula may become inflamed, requiring antibiotics and surgery. Inflammation of the pancreas may progress to massive fluid losses and require careful IV fluid and electrolyte management. Abdominal pain and vomiting in an older patient or a patient with prior surgery may be due to a bowel obstruction. Abdominal x-ray films may aid in this diagnosis. The young woman with low abdominal pain may have a ruptured ectopic pregnancy and may require infusion of fluids and blood, rapid ultrasound for diagnosis, and emergent gynecological consultation for surgical treatment. The older patient or patient in atrial fibrillation who presents with abdominal pain out of proportion to examination and metabolic acidosis may have mesenteric ischemia, requiring anticoagulation, fluid repletion, and surgery. Gun shot wounds to the abdomen always require operative exploration. Stab wounds often require surgery but can be managed nonoperatively with the aid of laboratory studies, ultrasound, diagnostic peritoneal lavage, abdominal CT scanning, and serial clinical examinations. Blunt trauma to the abdomen is a particular challenge to manage. Depending on the patient's clinical condition, the patient may require immediate surgery, diagnostic peritoneal lavage, ultrasound, CT scan, or observation. The secondary survey includes a rectal, genital, perineal, and pelvic examination if clinically indicated.

Musculoskeletal Examination

Examination of the musculoskeletal system should include inspecting and palpating all four extremities for fractures, dislocations, lacerations, pulses, motor function, and sensation. X-ray films for suspected fractures and dislocations are warranted. Dislocations should be immediately reduced, and fractures splinted, pending orthopedic evaluation. Open fractures require IV antibiotic administration and operative repair by an orthopedic surgeon. Careful evaluation of the thoracic and lumbar spine involves palpating and inspecting for deformity and tenderness. X-ray evaluation may be required for suspected fractures, with magnetic resonance imaging (MRI) indicated for suspected spinal cord injury or compression by an abscess or hematoma. In the trauma patient, careful palpation of the pelvis for fracture is essential, with x-ray imaging if there is any question of a fracture on clinical examination. A fractured pelvis can cause life-threatening internal bleeding and can be difficult to diagnose clinically; therefore, the American College of Surgeons recommends a pelvis x-ray film for all multiple trauma patients.

Neurological Examination

During the secondary survey, a more complete neurological examination should be performed, building on the initial neurological evaluation in the primary survey. The level of consciousness should be assessed, including orientation. Pupils and cranial nerves should be reevaluated. Motor and sensory examination and reflexes should be noted. If the patient has a sensory level below which there is no feeling or movement, a presumptive diagnosis of spinal cord injury can be made, with administration of high-dose steroids and emergent neurosurgical/orthopedic consultation. Unilateral pupil-

lary, cranial nerve, and motor-sensory findings suggest intracranial pathology, requiring head CT scanning and neurological or neurosurgical consultation.

Summary

The successful resuscitation of a critically ill or injured patient or a patient in cardiac or respiratory arrest demands careful attention to the principles outlined by the AHA (BLS, Basic Life Support, ACLS, Advanced Cardiac Life Support, and PALS, Pediatric Advanced Life Support), and the American College of Surgeons (ATLS). The primary survey (ABCDE) is a rapid assessment of critical signs that reveals life-threatening problems and initiates treatment. Once the primary survey is complete and treatment is under way, the secondary survey should be performed. The secondary survey involves a history and a head-to-toe examination of all systems, with institution of diagnostic studies, consultation, and treatment as abnormalities are discovered. Although there is never a guarantee of a successful outcome from a resuscitation, preservation of life and body functions can be maximized by following these principles.

Suggested Readings

American Academy of Pediatrics, American Heart Association. *Pediatric Advanced Life Support*. Dallas: AMA, 1997.

American College of Emergency Physicians. Discontinuing resuscitation in the out-of-hospital setting [policy statements]. *Ann Emerg Med* 1998;312:152.

American College of Surgeons. *Advanced Trauma Life Support Program for doctors: instructor course manual*, 6th ed. Chicago: ACS, 1997.

American Heart Association. *Advanced Cardiac Life Support*. Dallas: AMA, 1997.

American Heart Association, International Liaison Committee on Resuscitation. Guidelines 2000 for cardiopulmonary resuscitation and emergency cardiovascular care. *Circulation* 2000;102(Suppl).

Camp BN, et al. Effect of Advanced Cardiac Life Support training on resuscitation efforts and survival in a rural hospital. *Ann Emerg Med* 1997;29: 529–533.

Chochinov AH, et al. Recovery of a 62-year-old man from prolonged cold water submersion (case report). *Ann Emerg Med* 1998;31:127–131.

Cummins RO, et al. In-hospital resuscitation: executive summary. *Ann Emerg Med* 1997;29: 647–649.

Cummins RO, et al. Advisory Statements of the International Liaison Committee on Resuscitation [Ilcor Advisory Statement]. *Circulation* 1997;95:2172–2173.

Dorfsman ML et al. Two-thumb vs two-finger chest compression in an infant model of prolonged cardiopulmonary resuscitation. *Acad Emerg Med* 2000;7:1077–1082.

Doron MW, et al. Delivery room resuscitation decisions for extremely premature infants. *Pediatrics* 1998;102:574–582.

Gandini D, et al. Neonatal resuscitation with the laryngeal mask airway in normal and low birth weight infants. *Anesth Analg* 1999;89:642–645.

Haddad B, et al. Outcome after successful resuscitation of babies born with Apgar scores of 0 at both 1 and 5 minutes. *Am J Obstet Gynecol* 2000;182:1210–1214.

Handley AJ, et al. Single-rescuer adult Basic Life Support: an advisory statement from the Basic Life Support Working Group of the International Liaison Committee on Resuscitation [Ilcor Advisory Statement]. *Circulation* 1997;95:2174–2179.

Helmer SD, et al. Family presence during trauma resuscitation: a survey of AAST and ENA members [annual meeting articles]. *J Trauma* 2000; 48:1015–1024.

Hilty WM, et al. Real-time ultrasound-guided femoral vein catheterization during cardiopulmonary resuscitation. *Ann Emerg Med* 1997;29: 331–336.

Hirshon JM. Cardiopulmonary resuscitation in adults. *Tintinalli's emergency medicine: a comprehensive study guide*, 5th ed. New York: McGraw-Hill, 2000:44–49.

Kattwinkel J, et al. Resuscitation of the newly born infant: an advisory statement from the Pediatric Working Group of the International Liaison Committee on Resuscitation [Ilcor Advisory Statement]. *Circulation* 1999;99: 1927–1938.

Kloeck W, et al. Special resuscitation situations: an advisory statement from the International Liaison Committee on Resuscitation [Ilcor Advisory Statement]. *Circulation* 1997;95:2196–2210.

Lindner KH, et al. Randomised comparison of epinephrine and vasopressin in patients with out-of-hospital ventricular fibrillation [early report]. *Lancet* 1997;349:535–537.

Losek JD. Hypoglycemia and ABCs (sugar) of pediatric resuscitation. *Ann Emerg Med* 2000;35: 43–46.

Mace SE. The laryngeal mask airway: guidelines for appropriate usage. *Resident Staff Physician* 2001;47:30–40.

Milzman DP, ed. Critical resuscitations. *Emerg Med Clin North Am* 1996;14:1–253.

Parish DC, et al. Resuscitation in the hospital: differential relationships between age and survival across rhythms [clinical investigations]. *Crit Care Med* 1999;27:2137–2141.

Porter JM, et al. In search of the optimal end points of resuscitation in trauma patients: a review [review article]. *J Trauma* 1998;44: 908–914.

Ruth WJ, et al. Intravenous etomidate for procedural sedation in emergency department patients. *Acad Emerg Med* 2001;8:13–18.

Schierhout G, et al. Fluid resuscitation with colloid or crystalloid solutions in critically ill patients: a systematic review of randomised trials. *BMJ* 1998;316:961–964.

Spaite DW, et al. Prehospital Advanced Life Support for major trauma: critical need for clinical trials. *Ann Emerg Med* 1998;32:480–489.

Stratton S, et al. Effects of adding links to the "chain of survival" for prehospital cardiac arrest: a contrast in outcomes in 1975 and 1995 at a single institution. *Ann Emerg Med* 1998; 31:471–477.

Thompson RJ, et al. Prediction of death and neurologic outcome in the emergency department in out-of-hospital cardiac arrest survivors. *Am J Cardiol* 1998;81:17–21.

Walls RM. Airway management. *Rosen's emergency medicine: concepts and clinical practice*, 4th ed. St. Louis: Mosby-Year Book, 1998:2–24.

York J, et al. Fluid resuscitation of patients with multiple injuries and severe closed head injury: experience with an aggressive fluid resuscitation strategy. *J Trauma* 2000;48:376–380.

Shock

Robert S. Chang, MD

Chapter Outline

Shock is defined as the clinical condition whereby the circulatory system is unable to adequately maintain tissue perfusion or remove toxic metabolites. A complex cascade of cellular events ensues resulting in alteration of all aspects of cellular function. Shock can be described as a transition between illness and death; rapid identification and aggressive treatment is necessary to optimize patient outcome.

Shock is classified into three categories: hemorrhagic and hypovolemic (failure of adequate circulatory volume), cardiogenic (failure of the heart's pump function), and distributive/vasogenic (failure of adequate distribution of blood flow). Although the etiology of shock may be different, the final common pathway is similar. Initially, heart rate and systemic vascular resistance increase in an effort to increase cardiac output. This intrinsic compensatory mechanism serves to maintain perfusion and thus protect the most vital organ functions—the brain and heart. The release of endogenous vasoactive hormones such as norepinephrine, epinephrine, and dopamine results in arteriolar vasoconstriction allowing shunting of blood flow from the skin, skeletal muscle, kidney, and intestine. There is constriction of venous capacitance vessels in an attempt to increase venous return. Water and sodium retention is achieved when antidiuretic hormone is released and the renin-angiotensin-aldosterone axis is activated. As shock progresses, intrinsic compensatory mechanisms are no longer able to maintain adequate tissue perfusion and anaerobic metabolism ensues with resultant lactic acid build-up and release of proteolytic enzymes leading to cell death. Systemic acidosis contributes to cardiac dysfunction by acting as a myocardial depressant. Death occurs when the imbalance of cellular perfusion and metabolism causes irreversible damage to the brain and heart.

It is important to note that shock is often but not always associated with hypotension, defined as a systolic blood pressure (SBP) of less than 90 mm Hg. As blood pressure is a measure of the product of cardiac output and systemic vascular resistance, a decrease in cardiac output may not reflect a decrease in blood pressure if the systemic vascular resistance is increased. Similarly, tissue hypoperfusion may be present in the face of a normal blood pressure. Thus, hypotension is not a sensitive sign of shock until late in the disease process.

Certain physiological changes may occur in the early stages of shock providing sensitive clinical indicators. These include tachycardia (heart rate greater than 90 beats per minute), and tachypnea (respiratory rate greater than 20 breaths per minute). If shock is due to infection other indicators include temperature greater than 38°C or less than 36°C and white blood cells greater than 12×10^3 or greater than 10% bands.

In the emergency department (ED), a careful history and physical examination will often elicit the etiology of shock. A patient with pale, cold, clammy skin and tachycardia following trauma suggest hemorrhagic shock. The same patient with the complaint of severe chest pain may well be experiencing cardiogenic shock. Fever or hypothermia and altered mentation suggest septic shock. Shock that followed a dose of penicillin is likely due to acute anaphylaxis.

Hypovolemic and Hemorrhagic Shock

Acute blood loss may occur from a variety of surgical and medical conditions. They include major trauma, vascular catastrophes, and reproductive and gastrointestinal tract diseases (Table 3.1). The body can compensate for up to 15% of volume loss before clinical signs develop. With further volume loss, there is a decrease in blood pressure triggering the body's intrinsic compensatory mechanism. Baroreceptors in the carotid artery sinus and aortic arch cause a reflexive decrease in vagal tone and release of norepinephrine. In response, heart rate, vascular resistance, and cardiac output increase. With a blood volume loss of greater than 30%, the pulse pressure narrows, stroke volume decreases, and tachycardia alone cannot compensate for the decreased cardiac output and blood pressure. Myocardial perfusion and oxygenation decrease leading to acidosis, which further depresses myocardial function. Vascular smooth muscle ultimately exhibits pathological vasodilation termed vascular decompensation. Mortality at this stage is 100% (Table 3.2).

The classic clinical signs of hemorrhagic shock are tachycardia, tachypnea, narrow pulse pressure, poor capillary refill, cold and clammy skin, decreased urine output, low central venous pressure (CVP), hypotension, and altered mental state. Not every patient will manifest every sign. Patients taking β-blockers or calcium channel blockers may not have tachycardia in the setting of acute blood loss. In addition, elderly patients may

Table 3.1.

Etiologies of hypovolemic and hemorrhagic shock

Trauma
Solid organ injury
Major vascular injury
Cardiac rupture
Pelvic fracture
Hollow viscus injury
Scalp lacerations

Vascular Conditions
Ruptured and leaking aneurysm
Aortic dissections

Reproductive System Conditions
Ruptured ectopic pregnancy
Hemorrhagic ovarian cyst
Placenta previa
Retained products of conception

Gastrointestinal System Conditions
Diverticulitis
Arteriovenous malformation
Hemorrhoid
Malignancy
Peptic ulcer disease
Esophageal varices
Esophageal tear (Mallory-Weiss tear, Boerhaave's syndrome)

Table 3.2.

Classification of hemorrhagic shock

Class	% Blood Loss	Clinical Signs
I	<20	Asymptomatic
II	20–30	Cool, clammy skin Decreased capillary refill Tachycardia
III	30–40	Tachycardia Tachypnea Hypotension Decreased urine output Altered mental status
IV	>40	Marked tachycardia Unobtainable diastolic blood pressure No urine output Unconsciousness

develop more severe signs and symptoms with less blood loss when compared with younger patients who can appear clinically well despite significant volume loss. It is possible to predict the percent of hypovolemia based on clinical signs. For example, a young patient with a 20% blood loss may exhibit cool, clammy skin; tachycardia; and decreased capillary refill, yet maintain a normal blood pressure.

The treatment and management of the critically ill patient in the ED begins with the careful assessment and management of the ABCs: Airway patency, adequate work of Breathing, and stabilization of the Circulation. The patient is placed on oxygen, two large-bore intravenous (IV) lines (14 to 18 gauge) are established, and the patient is placed on continuous cardiac and pulse oximeter monitoring. If a peripheral line is unobtainable due to vasoconstriction or poor IV access, other choices include an external jugular line, or a Cordis, a single-lumen, large-gauge central line, usually placed in the femoral vein. A triple-lumen central line is less desirable because the length and smaller gauge make it less efficient to infuse large volumes of fluid quickly. The approach to the patient with hemorrhagic shock hinges on controlling hemorrhage and providing adequate volume repletion with crystalloid (0.9% normal saline or Ringer's lactate) and blood. Traditionally, fluid resuscitation consisted of giving 3 L of crystalloid (or three 20 mL/kg crystalloid boluses in children) over 10 to 20 minutes. Because roughly 30% of crystalloid remains in the intravascular space, restoration of blood volume with crystalloid requires approximately three times that of lost blood. There is evidence to support that early resuscitation with blood (packed red blood cells) may be most beneficial in the setting of acute hemorrhage. This may be especially important in the elderly or those with significant cardiopulmonary disease, because their ability to tolerate a decreased oxygen-carrying state is significantly impaired. Surgically correctable causes of bleeding should be treated emergently with surgical consultation and operative intervention. In addition, upper and lower gastrointestinal bleeding may require gastroenterology consultation for emergent fiberoptic scoping.

Ancillary tests are useful in confirming diagnosis and aiding in management. In the setting of acute blood loss, the judicious use of radiological studies is warranted to localize the source of bleeding and direct whether the condition will require an operative intervention. These tests include plain radiographs, computed tomography (CT) scan, ultrasound, nuclear scan, and angiogram. In some cases, patients may be too unstable for CT scanning. Ultrasound and even diagnostic peritoneal lavage (DPL) may be the only viable choices for locating blood loss.

Successful resuscitation cannot be accomplished without adequate hemodynamic monitoring. Most patients in shock can be effectively stabilized and monitored with peripheral IV access, pulse oximetry, frequent SBP measurement by cuff sphygmomanometer, and a Foley catheter to gauge urine output. Limitations with cuff sphygmomanometry include overestimation of the SBP, inaccuracies related to arrhythmias (rapid atrial fibrillation), peripheral vascular disease, and appropriate cuff size. In certain patients, in particular those with chronic organ dysfunction (e.g., congestive heart failure [CHF] or renal failure), adequate resuscitation may require continuous monitoring of the CVP to guide fluid replacement. Normal CVP is approximately 10 to 12 mm Hg and measured through a central line placed in the subclavian or internal jugular vein. A pulmonary artery (Swan-Ganz) catheter may provide more extensive hemodynamic measurements, but its role is more appropriate in the intensive care unit than the ED.

Cardiogenic Shock

Shock occurs when the heart fails to be an effective pump. The result is a reduction in myocardial contractility and stroke volume with subsequent global tissue hypoperfusion. Cardiogenic shock predominantly occurs following an acute myocardial infarction (AMI);

however, valvular abnormalities, drugs, and extracardiac obstruction must always be considered in the differential diagnosis (Table 3.3). As with the sequence of events described in hypovolemic shock, autonomic responses are activated in an effort to increase cardiac output. The larger the area of left ventricular (LV) myocardial damage, the greater the risk of developing shock. Other risk factors for the development of cardiogenic shock include prior AMI, multivessel coronary artery disease, advanced age, previous CHF, female gender, and diabetes. The systolic blood pressure is often less than 90 mm Hg with concomitant tachycardia. However, reflexive bradycardia and hypotension may occur with inferior and posterior wall infarcts. Additional clinical findings include tachypnea; cool, clammy skin; decreased urine output; prolonged capillary refill time; anxiety; and confusion. Pulmonary edema occurs with severe LV dysfunction manifested by tachypnea, rales, and wheezing. The patient with right ventricular (RV) infarct may present with hypotension and jugular venous distension with no evidence of pulmonary edema. Extracardiac, obstructive causes of shock include massive pulmonary embolus and acute pericardial tamponade. On physical examination, the patient may have jugular venous distension in the face of hypotension, distant heart sounds, tachycardia, and tachypnea. Mitral regurgitation secondary to ruptured chordae tendonae will produce a characteristic holosystolic murmur that radiates to the axilla.

History and physical examination findings may point to a diagnosis and with the help of ancillary tests direct treatment and management. The 12-lead electrocardiogram is useful in evaluation of an AMI (ST-segment elevation) or arrhythmia (third-degree heart block, ventricular fibrillation). A normal or nonspecific electrocardiogram in the setting of shock may suggest extracardiac causes.

Plain radiographs of the chest confirm fluid overload (pulmonary edema) and evaluate heart size (cardiomegaly suggests previous CHF, cardiomyopathy, or chronic pericardial effusion) and the mediastinum (widened mediastinum suggest aortic dissection). An echocardiogram is an invaluable tool in the setting of cardiogenic shock. In particular, it aids the diagnosis of acute pericardial tamponade, aortic dissection and aneurysm, ventricular and septal wall motion abnormalities, and valvular dysfunction. In addition, elevated RV and pulmonary artery pressures suggest pulmonary embolism.

The treatment and management of the patient in cardiogenic shock depends on the etiology of the underlying disorder. In a patient with severe LV infarct and pulmonary edema, IV fluids must be administered judiciously while a patient with RV infarct may require a large volume of fluids to maintain preload. Profound hypoxia or increasing work of breathing despite supplemental oxygen may require endotracheal intubation and mechanical ventilation. Pharmacological adjuncts useful in treating refractory shock include dobutamine, dopamine, norepinephrine, phenylephrine (Neo-Synephrine), and epinephrine (Table 3.4). These agents are used when there is an inadequate response to fluid resuscitation or a contraindication to volume infusion. Additional treatment modalities include use of an intraaortic balloon pump, which improves coronary artery perfusion during diastole and decreases afterload. These measures provide only temporary stabilization and definitive treatment

Table 3.3.
Etiologies of cardiogenic shock

Decreased Myocardial Contractility
Myocardial infarction
Cardiomyopathy
Myocardial contusion

Extracardiac Obstruction
Pulmonary embolism
Pericardial tamponade
Tension pneumothorax

Valvular Abnormalities
Aortic, mitral, and tricuspid stenosis
Mitral insufficiency
Ruptured chordae tendineae

Table 3.4.

Pharmacological agents useful in shock

Drug	Dosage	Physiological Effects
Dobutamine	5–10 µg/kg/min 15–20 µg/kg/min	Inotropic Vasodilatation
Dopamine	1–3 µg/kg/min 5–10 µg/kg/min 10–20 µg/kg/min	Renal vasodilatation Inotropic Vasoconstriction
Norepinephrine	2–8 µg/min	Vasoconstriction
Phenylephrine	20–200 µg/min	Vasoconstriction
Epinephrine	1–8 µg/min	Vasoconstriction

often requires immediate revascularization of the coronary artery either through angioplasty or coronary artery bypass graft surgery. Although early recognition leading to early reperfusion therapies has proven effective in improving patient outcome, once cardiogenic shock develops, the mortality is extremely high, between 70% to 80%.

Distributive/Vasogenic Shock

Septic Shock

Sepsis is defined as a clinical syndrome caused by any variety of microorganisms; gram-negative and gram-positive bacteria are the most common. These organisms release exogenous toxins into the systemic circulation, and the host responds by releasing endogenous mediators. They include cytokines, arachidonic acid metabolites, myocardial depressant substances, and nitric oxide. These mediators are responsible for depressing myocardial function, decreasing peripheral vascular resistance, and damaging the vascular endothelium leading to a process termed the systemic inflammatory response syndrome. Despite autonomic reflexes, a dysregulation of blood flow occurs leading to inadequate tissue perfusion, multiorgan failure, shock, and death.

The clinical features of septic shock often include tachycardia, tachypnea, hyperthermia or hypothermia, mental status changes, and hypotension. There is usually an associated focus of infection such as meningitis, pneumonia, pyelonephritis, and soft tissue infections. It is important to note that the very young, the elderly, and the immunosuppressed may not manifest fever or an elevated white blood cell count, and the infection is often occult. In early septic shock, vasodilation predominates and the skin appears warm and flushed. Cardiac output and stroke volume is increased with associated tachycardia. Because of myocardial depression, a significant volume of fluid (4 to 6 L) may be required to reverse the hypotension. Other organ systems affected include the lungs. The patient may develop the acute respiratory distress syndrome (ARDS) characterized by pulmonary edema secondary to increased permeability of the alveolar capillary endothelium. Acute renal failure is a result of hypoperfusion of the kidneys and a direct toxic insult from various endogenous mediators. Clinically, the patient presents with azotemia, oliguria/anuria, and increased urine sedimentation. Blood dyscrasias such as leukocytosis with left shift, thrombocytopenia, and disseminated intravascular coagulation are common findings in septic shock. Consumption of clotting factors and platelets with diffuse microvascular thrombi deposition contributes to multiorgan failure.

The organisms responsible for sepsis are mainly the gram-positive and gram-negative bacteria. Some of the more common include *Streptococcus pneumoniae* or *Neisseria meningitidis* in bacterial meningitis; bacterial pneumonia with *S. pneumoniae*, *Staphylococcus aureus*, gram-negative rods, and *Legionella*; pyelonephritis with gram-negative enteric species (*Escherichia coli*); and soft tissue infections with *S. aureus* or *Streptococcus pyogenes*.

Ancillary studies in the ED may help identify sepsis and localize an infectious source. Laboratory tests include a complete blood count (CBC) with differential; coagulation panel; liver function profile; chemistry including blood urea nitrogen (BUN) and creatinine; arterial blood gas; urinalysis; and cultures of sputum, blood, and urine. In addition, a lumbar puncture may be needed to obtain cerebrospinal fluid (CSF) for analysis and culture. Radiographic studies may include chest and abdominal x-rays and CT scan of the head if there is reason to suspect increased intracranial pressure.

Treatment begins with the universal ABCs of critical care management. Achieving adequate ventricular filling to allow tissue perfusion is the treatment goal in septic shock. Fluid replacement with crystalloid is rapidly infused via two large-bore IV lines. As much as 4 to 6 L of fluid may be needed to reverse the hypotension. Maintaining adequate urine output, improving mentation, and stabilizing vital signs will guide resuscitation efforts. Blood products should be considered to maintain a hematocrit between 30% to 35%. Inotropic agents are added if hypotension persists despite adequate volume replacement or in cases of fluid overload (e.g., pulmonary edema). Vasopressors include dobutamine, dopamine, and norepinephrine (see Table 3.4).

Antibiotic therapy should be initiated early in an attempt to combat infection. In the ED, a broad coverage antibiotic should be chosen if the source is not known. Usually this will be a third-generation cephalosporin or antipseudomonal penicillin with β-lactamase inhibition along with an aminoglycoside. A single agent such as imipenem or meropenem is also acceptable. If an anaerobic source is suspected, metronidazole or clindamycin should be added.

Anaphylactic Shock

This clinical entity is defined as a severe life-threatening systemic hypersensitivity reaction characterized by either hypotension or airway compromise produced by an immune response. An allergen triggers the release of IgE mediators from mast cells leading to the exaggerated immune response. Table 3.5 lists selective agents known to cause anaphylaxis. The most important mediator is histamine, which acts on various organ systems. It relaxes vascular smooth muscle, constricts bronchial smooth muscle, and depresses cardiac function. Although anaphylaxis is at one end of the hypersensitivity spectrum, it is important to note that even a

Table 3.5.

Common agents causing anaphylactic shock

Antibiotics
Penicillins
Cephalosporins
Tetracyclines
Sulfonamides
Chloramphenicol
Bacitracin

Foreign Proteins
Hymenoptera venom (bees, wasp, hornet)
Fire ant
Snake venom
Equine-derived antivenoms
Pollen
Egg-based vaccines

Foods
Milk
Egg white
Shellfish
Nuts
Chocolate
Mango
Citrus fruits

Other Causes
Radiopaque contrast dye
Exercise-induced
Local anesthetics
Latex (rubber gloves)

Table 3.6.

Pharmacological adjuncts in anaphylactic shock

Drug	Dosage
Epinephrine	IV: 0.1 mg (1:10,000) over 5–10 min ×1 dose Infusion: 1–8 μg/min SC: 0.3–0.5 mL (1:1000)
Diphenhydramine (Benadryl)	25–50 mg IV, IM
Ranitidine (Zantac)	50 mg IV
Methylprednisolone (Solu-Medrol)	125 mg IV
Albuterol	2.5 mg via nebulizer (0.5 mL 0.5% solution)
Glucagon	1 mg IV every 5 min until hypotension resolves Infusion: 5–15 μg/min

IM, intramuscular; IV, intravenous; SC, subcutaneous.

seemingly mild allergic reaction may rapidly evolve into anaphylaxis.

In cases in which there is a clear history of exposure to environmental (bee sting), food (shellfish or nuts), or iatrogenic (antibiotic) sources, the diagnosis is simple. Symptoms usually begin 30 to 60 minutes from time of exposure. The faster the onset of symptoms, the greater the likelihood of a severe reaction. Patients with an acute allergic reaction usually present to the ED with pruritus, flushing of the skin, and urticarial rash. As the disease progresses, there may be an associated sensation of shortness of breath, fullness in the throat, or tightness in the chest. These symptoms in association with wheezing, hoarseness, stridor, and air hunger portend acute laryngeal edema and airway compromise.

Treatment of anaphylaxis hinges on rapid recognition and stabilization of the airway and circulation. IV access, oxygen administration, and cardiac and pulse oximetry monitoring are obtained immediately. If there is evidence of airway compromise (i.e., angioedema), immediate tracheal intubation is indicated. Epinephrine is the first-line pharmacological agent used in anaphylaxis. It may be given by the subcutaneous, IV, or endotracheal route. In severe anaphylaxis with respiratory failure and circulatory collapse, IV epinephrine is indicated followed by crystalloid volume replacement. Table 3.6 lists other drugs in the treatment of allergic reaction and anaphylaxis and in the prevention of recurrences. These include antihistamines, corticosteroids, albuterol, and glucagon. All patients with anaphylaxis should receive histamine blockers and corticosteroids; nebulized albuterol may be added if there is evidence of bronchospasm manifested by wheezing. Glucagon may be helpful when patients taking β-blockers present with refractory hypotension.

Neurogenic Shock

The hallmarks of neurogenic shock are hypotension and bradycardia occurring after an acute spinal cord injury. This results from the disruption of the sympathetic outflow with unopposed vagal tone. This is not synonymous with spinal shock, which is a loss of spinal reflexes that occurs at a level below where the spinal cord is injured.

Blunt trauma from motor vehicle collision, falls, or sporting activity is the most common cause of acute spinal cord injury. Penetrating trauma accounts for less than 15% of cases. The cervical spine is the most frequently injured, followed by the thoracolumbar, thoracic, and lumbar segments.

The sympathetic nervous system is responsible for the "fight-or-flight" response. Through the release of natural sympathomimetics, vascular constriction and increases in heart rate, cardiac output, and stroke volume occur. The sympathetic outflow tracts originate in the hypothalamus and medulla and descend into the lateral gray matter of the spinal cord. These efferent fibers exit the cord to synapse with ganglia located in the paraspinal sympathetic trunk, which span the entire length of the vertebral column. From here, the nerve fibers travel throughout the body to innervate respective organs. The heart and thoracic blood vessels are innervated by fibers from T1 to T8; spinal cord injuries anywhere proximal to T1 will have a high likelihood of complete sympathetic disruption and associated bradycardia, whereas injuries distal to T1 to L3 have less profound hypotension and bradycardia resulting from partial sympathetic loss. Therefore, the higher the level of spinal cord injury, the greater the likelihood of developing neurogenic shock.

Hypotension occurs soon after acute spinal injury. Loss of sympathetic tone results in vascular dilatation manifested by warm and dry skin. In addition, hypothermia may occur from failure to redistribute heat from the periphery to the body's core. Treatment begins with adherence to the tenets of initial trauma management: ABCDEs (where D represents disability or neurological deficit and E stands for exposure or removal of clothing). In a multi-injured trauma patient, shock secondary to acute spinal cord injury is diagnosed by excluding all other possible causes first, specifically hemorrhagic or hypovolemic shock. As previously discussed, clues to the diagnosis of neurogenic shock include hypotension in the face of bradycardia and warm, dry skin. Hypotension often responds to placing the patient in the Trendelenburg position (feet at an angle higher than the head) and modest crystalloid volume replacement. The goal is to maintain SBP greater than 90 mm Hg to maintain adequate perfusion pressure of the spinal cord. Hypotension unresponsive to adequate fluid replacement will require pharmacological support, with ephedrine, phenylephrine, and dopamine useful for their vasoconstrictive effects. Blood pressure and CVP measurements and measurement of urine output are helpful in monitoring the response to resuscitation. In cases in which neurogenic shock is associated with severe bradycardia or heart block, atropine is given as the first-line agent. The patient with persistent bradycardia or with evidence of complete heart block will require a pacemaker. In the ED, a transcutaneous pacer may be used until a permanent pacemaker can be placed. Neurogenic shock is often transient and sympathetic responses may return after 3 to 4 days.

Disposition

All patients presenting in shock to the ED require admission to an intensive care unit (ICU). Patients in cardiogenic shock would be best cared for in a coronary care unit (CCU). All trauma patients with shock are admitted to the surgical intensive care unit (SICU). Anaphylactic patients may also benefit from a SICU, if there is concern about the potential for a swelling airway in the nonintubated patient. Patients in neurogenic shock benefit from specialized rehabilitation services. All other patients in shock are admitted to a medical ICU. Some community hospitals do not possess the capabilities to adequately care for the patient in shock, and the patient should be transferred to a nearby capable facility once stabilized.

Suggested Readings

Court O, Kumar A, Parrillo JE, Kumar A. Clinical review: myocardial depression in sepsis and septic shock. *Crit Care* 2002;6:500–508. (Epub 2002 Sep 12)

Dellinger RP. Cardiovascular management of septic shock. *Crit Care Med* 2003;31: 946–955.

Domsky MF, Wilson RF. Hemodynamic resuscitation. *Crit Care Clin* 1993;9:715–726.

Falk JL, O'Brien JF, Kerr R. Fluid resuscitation in traumatic hemorrhagic shock. *Crit Care Clin* 1992;8:323–340.

Rosen P, et al. *Emergency medicine: concepts and clinical practice,* 4th ed. New York: Mosby-Year Book, 1998.

Tintinalli JE, et al. *Emergency medicine, a comprehensive study guide,* 5th ed. New York: McGraw-Hill, 2000.

Vincent JL, de Carvalho FB, De Backer D. Management of septic shock. *Ann Med* 2002;34:606–613.

Wilson M, Davis DP, Coimbra R. Diagnosis and monitoring of hemorrhagic shock during the initial resuscitation of multiple trauma patients. *J Emerg Med* 2003;24:413–422.

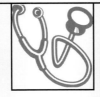

PART II

Case Studies in
Emergency Medicine

Chest Pain

Thanks to the human heart by which we live,
Thanks to its tenderness, its joys, and fears
Wordsworth 1807

INTRODUCTION
James A. Feldman, MD
Section Editor

Chest pain is a common emergency department complaint, with diagnoses ranging from immediate life threats to minor illness. Because many life-threatening diseases including acute coronary syndromes (unstable angina and acute myocardial infarction), pulmonary embolism, and aortic dissection routinely enter the differential diagnosis, a carefully obtained, structured history of the patient's pain remains a key diagnostic tool for the chest pain evaluation.

The complaint of chest pain should be carefully explored and documented using open-ended questions. This point cannot be overly emphasized to the student. Failure to obtain a careful history of pain is a common source of error. It may be helpful to use a structured pain history such as the suggested "PQRST" approach, whereby:

P = precipitant/provokers/previous

Q = quality/quantity (pain scale)

R = radiation/relievers

S = associated symptoms/severity

T = time/time intensity curve/previous tests (e.g., cardiac catheterization, ETT [exercise treadmill test], gastrointestinal [GI] endoscopy) and treatments

This approach will prevent the tunnel vision or anchoring bias that can easily lead clinicians astray.

Additional key sources of information include all written descriptions of the presenting complaint, including referral notes, emergency medical service (EMS) reports, and nursing notes. In addition, the family may offer information that a patient is unwilling or reluctant to provide. Take into consideration that patients may minimize or deny important symptoms.

Finally, if a language or communication barrier exists, assume a significant source of chest pain until it can be excluded.

Chest pain results from a stimulation of pain receptors arising from structures within or outside the thorax. Pain impulses travel along dorsal roots to the spinal cord and along the ascending spinal tracts via the thalamus to the frontal and somatosensory cortex in the brain where the pain signal is interpreted. The pain that is experienced from deep visceral structures such as the heart is poorly localized. The pain sensation may be generated from contiguously stimulated structures such as the parietal pleura or diaphragm. Contiguous dermatomal routes can also be stimulated within the thoracic spinal cord because sensory inputs overlap or provide input to the same neuron. This is why heart pain is often referred to the shoulders or arms. Pain can arise from structures outside the thorax and referred to the chest, and patients may have multiple components of their pain, further confusing the clinician. For example, patients with myocardial infarction may also report some component that appears to suggest a chest wall problem and is worsened by moving or palpation. This may lead the patient to try self-medication to treat the self-perceived musculoskeletal or gastrointestinal source. The complexity of chest pain challenges both the patient and physician.

In the clinical scenarios presented in this section, the focus is always on identifying and treating or excluding serious underlying conditions. The student should read and consider each of these clinical scenarios with this perspective in mind.

CHAPTER 4

Myocardial Infarction

James S. Ford, Jr., MD

Clinical Scenario

A 50-year-old man presents to the emergency department (ED) complaining of crushing substernal chest pain that began while he was shoveling snow 3 hours before arrival. He initially thought he felt gas-type pain and indigestion and took several Rolaids without relief. The pain increased in intensity and became more pressure-like, radiating to his left arm and jaw. He began to experience shortness of breath, nausea, and diaphoresis; became worried; and drove himself to the ED.

His cardiac risk factors include poorly controlled type II diabetes mellitus, hypercholesterolemia, hypertension, a 60-pack-year smoking history, and a family history of premature ischemic heart disease (the patient's father died from a myocardial infarction [MI] at age 45).

He has no history of angina, MI, or cardiovascular testing. In the past, he was told that he had a hiatal hernia with reflux. He takes glyburide, diltiazem, and pravastatin and has no medication allergies.

The patient is immediately triaged into a resuscitation area, and a physician is called for an immediate evaluation.

Physical examination reveals a pale, diaphoretic, obese man in moderate distress, clenching his left chest. Vital signs include a blood pressure of 160/95 mm Hg, heart rate of 94 beats/minute, temperature 98.6°F, respiratory rate 20 times/minute, and oxygen saturation of 94% on room air. The heart examination is noted to be rapid and regular. His lungs are clear, the abdomen is soft, and no extremity edema or tenderness is noted. The blood pressure is symmetric in both arms, and all pulses are checked and noted to be intact.

Simultaneous to the physician's evaluation, a 12-lead electrocardiogram (ECG) is performed. The ECG reveals sinus rhythm at 90 beats/minute with 5-mm ST elevations in leads V_1 to V_3 and upright T waves, indicating an acute anterior wall MI (see Figure 4.2).

The triage nurse has already placed the patient on monitors (cardiac, intermittent blood pressure cuff, and continuous pulse oximetry), started two large-bore intravenous (IV) access sites, and given the patient two baby aspirin to chew and swallow and 0.4-mg nitroglycerin sublingually (NTG SL). An anteroposterior (AP) upright portable chest x-ray film reveals no mediastinal widening and no evidence of heart failure.

The ED physician immediately notifies the cardiac catheterization team that a patient with an anterior wall ST-elevation acute MI (AMI) with 3 hours of pain and without contraindications to thrombolysis is in the ED. The patient is treated according to the ST-elevation pathway (Table 4.2) with morphine, IV nitroglycerin, metoprolol, and unfractionated heparin while awaiting transport to the cardiac catheterization laboratory.

At catheterization, a completely occluded left anterior descending (LAD) coronary artery is successfully ballooned and stented. The time from ED arrival to balloon reperfusion is 50 minutes.

Clinical Evaluation

Introduction

AMI is the development of myocardial necrosis that results from an imbalance in the oxygen supply and demand of the myocardium. It is the leading cause of morbidity and mortality in the United States, annually accounting for 1.3 million nonfatal MIs (incidence 600 per 100,000 people) and for 500,000 to 700,000 deaths.

You must rapidly identify patients with evident ST-elevation MI (STEMI). The National Heart Attack Alert working group has suggested administration of a thrombolytic within 30 minutes or balloon angioplasty reperfusion within 90 minutes of ED arrival to patients with STEMI. It is equally important to identify suspected non-Q wave AMI or active unstable angina pectoris with prolonged rest pain and dynamic (changing) ST or T-wave abnormalities. This chapter discusses the approach to these important disease processes.

History

AMI is considered part of the spectrum of acute coronary syndrome (ACS) (includes unstable angina and MI). This spectrum, based on ECG findings and test results, includes STEMI, non-Q wave AMI (ST depression, T-wave inversion, or no ECG changes), and unstable angina.

Although chest pain is the most common presenting complaint, one must consider the diagnosis of ACS in all patients with acute cardiovascular symptoms. AMI may also present atypically with unexplained weakness or confusion in an elderly patient or as a silent precipitant of diabetic ketoacidosis (DKA) in a diabetic patient. Cardiac chest pain is more likely to be atypical in women as well. AMI can complicate other disease processes. Examples include shock from any cause, poisoning from such agents as carbon monoxide, severe anemia, chest trauma, aortic dissection, a congenital abnormality, or an arteritis such as Kawasaki's disease. The history should be detailed, because it holds the key to the diagnosis of the chest pain's etiology.

Precipitants should be looked for. Is the pain precipitated by exertion, especially using the upper extremities or by anger (emotion), sex, large meals, or cocaine use? Does the patient experience prolonged or severe pain at rest, especially with prior history of angina? Does rest relieve the pain or is it like their prior AMI?

Patients with a prior history of MI, percutaneous transluminal coronary angioplasty (PTCA), coronary artery bypass graft (CABG), or nitroglycerin use have confirmed coronary artery disease and should be presumed to have a new ischemic event unless another cause of chest pain is evident. Patients with prior stable angina who develop a change in symptoms (change in severity, duration, or onset of pain), especially new rest pain within 48 hours of presentation (i.e., unstable angina) are at high risk.

The quality of the pain should be determined. Is it severe, 10/10 on a scale of one to ten, pressure-like, dull, aching, burning, or like gas or indigestion? The quality can be quite variable. It can be sharp; painless; or a chest pain equivalent including jaw pain, shoulder pain, and shortness of breath.

Ask whether the pain radiates outside of the left chest area. Ask whether the pain moves to the arms, back, or jaws. Ask if it is relieved by NTG SL. If so, a cardiac source is more likely; however, esophageal spasm is also relieved by NTG, so be cautious with response to NTG.

Ask if there is associated shortness of breath, sweating, syncope, heart skipping palpitations, or nausea. Prominent gastrointestinal (GI) features such as nausea and vomiting may be associated with a large infarction or diaphragmatic irritation with an inferior wall infarct.

Ask about the timing of the pain. The pain of a MI is usually prolonged, greater than 20 minutes, and progressive. Sudden and severe pain may suggest dissection.

Classic risk factors for coronary artery disease can be explored. These include the following:

Age: Male older than 33 years, female older than 40

Family history: First-degree relative who sustained their first AMI before the age of 45 for a man, or 55 for a woman

Hypercholesterolemia (high low-density lipoprotein (LDL)/low high-density lipoprotein) HDL cholesterol level)

Hypertension

Diabetes

Smoking

Left ventricular (LV) hypertrophy

The clinical scenario illustrates a patient with AMI who does not have previously confirmed coronary artery disease but who has multiple risk factors for coronary artery disease and many historical features that point to an acute cardiac event.

Physical Examination

As demonstrated with our patient, the physical examination integrates evaluation and stabilization in a patient with chest pain who appears acutely ill. The primary survey is performed, vital signs are obtained, and the heart and lungs (and usually abdomen) are examined. The examination may identify complications of AMI, such as congestive heart failure or a new systolic murmur from papillary muscle dysfunction, or suggest alternative diagnoses by finding a pericardial rub, aortic insufficiency murmur, absent breath sounds in a hemithorax (pneumothorax), or signs of an acute abdominal process.

The physical examination can be unremarkable. Patients may appear pale and diaphoretic because of sympathetic stimulation from catecholamines and parasympathetic response from stimulation of the vagus nerve as in an inferior MI (IMI) or patients presenting in shock.

Pulses can be within a normal rate range. They can be slow because of calcium or β-blockade or because of IMIs with bradycardia resulting from parasympathetic stimulation or conduction block. The pulses may be fast because of pain, catecholamine release, or dysrhythmia, or they may be irregular because of underlying disorders such as atrial fibrillation or ventricular ectopy.

Blood pressure can be high because of hypertension as a pre-existing condition or because of pain, anxiety, or heart failure. Blood pressure is low in ventricular dysfunction secondary to ischemia, involvement of the right ventricle with poor filling, or abnormally fast or slow heart rates. Beware of "normotension" (normal blood pressure) in a patient with prior hypertension. This may indicate that the patient you are treating is in fact hypotensive relative to their average daily pressures.

Jugular venous distention (JVD) is seen as elevated neck veins. This is measured by having the patient lie at 30 degrees in the stretcher and measuring the column of blood from the right atrium (angle of Louis, or second costochondral line) to the highest visible pulsation of the internal jugular vein. If the jugular venous pressure (JVP) is elevated, consider pre-existing failure of the right or both ventricles (biventricular), an infarct involving the right ventricle, or pericardial tamponade.

Cardiopulmonary findings include a new mitral regurgitation murmur if the area of infarction includes the papillary muscle, or rales or wheezes on pulmonary examination, indicating LV failure.

Bilateral edema of the extremities suggests prior heart disease (failure). Levine's sign is found if a patient clenches a fist over the chest when describing pain and is considered highly suggestive of anginal chest pain.

Clinical features (quality of pain such as pleuritic), physical findings such as chest wall tenderness, and response to therapies directed toward noncardiac diagnoses cannot be used to exclude the diagnosis of AMI. A classic example of clinician misdirection is a patient's relief from the "GI cocktail," a mixture of viscous lidocaine and liquid antacids. A patient with acid reflux and esophageal spasm will get relief from this cocktail; however, this does not rule out the existence of heart disease.

In the setting of cardiogenic shock (see Chapter 3) a patient will present with some or all of the following: altered mentation, hypotension, cool clammy skin, diaphoresis, poor peripheral pulses, and mottled extremities.

Diagnostic Evaluation

Obtain an ECG as soon as possible (within 5 minutes) after a patient enters the ED. The ECG should be repeated at frequent intervals, approximately every 15 minutes, or after any change in symptoms or by continuous 12-lead monitoring for patients whose initial ECG is considered normal or nondiagnostic. A prior tracing, if available, may be useful in identifying changes from baseline. The location of an STEMI can be classified by the location of the ST elevations on the ECG (Figs. 4.1, 4.2, and 4.3):

Inferior: II, III, aVF.

Lateral: I, aVL, (possibly V_4 to V_6, some use only I,L for true lateral). This tracing shows evidence of inferior and lateral infarction.

Anteroseptal: V_1 to V_3.

Anterolateral: V_1 to V_6.

Right ventricular (RV): suggested by ST elevation III greater than II in limb leads, ST elevation RV_4, RV_5 (right-sided chest leads).

Posterior: R/S ratio greater than 1 in V_2 and V_3 and upright T waves in V_1, ST depressions V_1 to V_3.

Combinations of locations (inferolateral, inferior-posterior) and multidistribution can occur.

Identification of ST elevation in bundle branch block or with prior abnormal conduction such as with a pacemaker is beyond the scope of this chapter. In the presence of a bundle branch block, the diagnosis of AMI becomes more complicated.

Chest x-ray may reveal an alternative diagnosis such as aortic dissection, pneumothorax, or perforated abdominal viscus or suggest a complication of AMI such as pulmonary edema. In addition, heart size may be useful in assessing long-standing hypertension, cardiomyopathy, and other pathology.

In our patient with clear-cut symptoms and diagnostic ECG, cardiac markers are not required for diagnosis or treatment. Markers may be obtained to measure infarct size but are not clinically necessary in the ED. Many markers of cardiac injury have been studied.

Troponin I (Tr I)

Tr I is a regulatory protein spaced along the actin filaments of cardiac muscle cells that is not normally found in the serum unless there

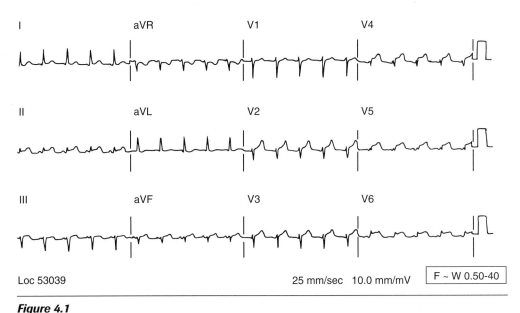

Loc 53039   25 mm/sec   10.0 mm/mV   F ~ W 0.50-40

Figure 4.1
This electrocardiogram shows evidence of inferior and lateral infarction. Note the "tombstones" in leads V_4, V_5, and V_6, and the elevation in 2, 3, and aVF.

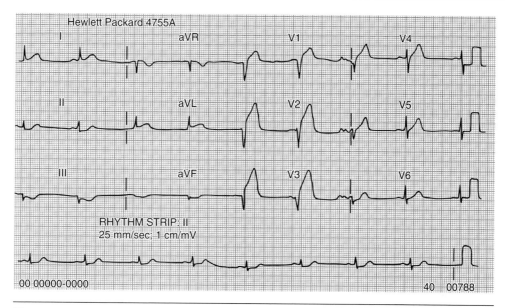

Figure 4.2
This electrocardiogram shows elevations and peaking in the anterior leads consistent with acute anterior infarction. In addition, there are reciprocal changes (inversion) in the inferior leads.

is cardiac muscle injury. The sensitivity is superior to that of creatinine phosphokinase, myocardial fraction (CPK-MB). It is detectable in the serum 3 to 6 hours post-AMI, and the level remains elevated for up to 2 weeks. Troponin T has similar specificity for myocardial necrosis but is slightly less sensitive than Tr I within the first 6 hours.

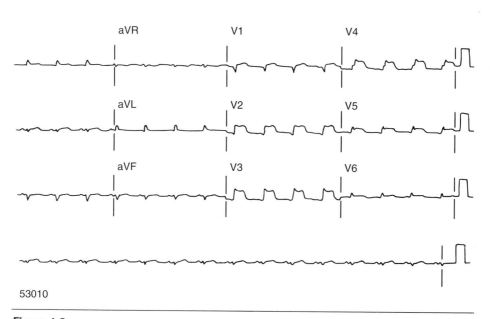

Figure 4.3
This electrocardiogram shows an acute anteroseptal infarction with "tombstone" elevation in V_1 to V_5.

Creatinine Phosphokinase Fraction (CPK-MB)

Although somewhat less specific than Tr I, CPK-MB levels rise within 4 hours of injury, peak at 18 to 24 hours, and subside over 3 to 4 days. The MB fraction is calculated as a percentage of the total CPK. An MB fraction of greater than 5% is considered positive for myocardial injury. CPK-MB is elevated in AMI and in other conditions.

Myoglobin

Myoglobin is an extremely sensitive, early marker of acute myocardial necrosis. The problem is that it is not specific for myocardial cell necrosis.

Laboratory Tests

Laboratory tests that may be useful in a patient with AMI include a complete blood count (CBC) to identify anemia; electrolytes including magnesium especially in patients with diabetes, hypertension, or diuretic use; coagulation studies; and a blood bank specimen especially if thrombolysis or angioplasty is a consideration or if the patient has anemia or active bleeding. Selected studies (carbon monoxide level, toxicology) are drawn as clinically appropriate.

Echocardiography

Echocardiography should be considered in all patients with AMI complicated by acute LV failure, new murmur, shock, or possible tamponade.

Other Diagnostic Tests

Other diagnostic tests can be considered should a patient appear to have an AMI but have normal or nondiagnostic initial and repeat ECGs. These include myocardial perfusion imaging, combination of markers and dynamic testing, or diagnostic catheterization.

Differential Diagnosis

The differential diagnosis of acute chest pain is illustrated in Table 4.1.

Table 4.1.

Differential diagnosis of acute chest pain

Vascular Causes
Aortic dissection
Pulmonary embolus

Cardiopulmonary Causes
Pneumothorax
Pneumonia
Mitral valve prolapse
Pericarditis

Gastrointestinal Causes
Esophageal rupture
Esophagitis
Esophageal spasm
Peptic ulcer disease
Biliary colic

Musculoskeletal Pain
Costochondritis
Pectoralis strain

Panic Disorder, Anxiety, Stress

Treatment

Patients with suspected AMI must be placed immediately in a resuscitation area. A monitor defibrillator must be immediately available should the patient develop a rhythm disturbance such as ventricular tachycardia or ventricular fibrillation during the early phase of an AMI. Our patient arrived in the ED with severe chest pain and "looked sick." He was rapidly evaluated and treated for prolonged ischemic chest pain with STEMI.

The primary goal of all of the treatment regimens is to minimize injury and relieve pain (Table 4.2). The initial treatment includes the following:

- Oxygen: Indicated in the first few hours of AMI and in patients with low oxygen saturation.
- Aspirin: Should be administered as soon as possible to inhibit thromboxane A_2 production. Aspirin can be administered via nasogastric tube or rectally in patients unable to take it orally (post arrest, intubated). Ticlopidine or clopidogrel are approved antiplatelet agents that may be

Table 4.2.

Treatment of acute myocardial infarction

Oxygen

Intravenous access (preferably two lines)

Vital signs with continuous monitors (cardiac, O_2
saturation, BP)

Blood specimens

12-lead ECG, repeat every 15 minutes
or continuously

Avoidance of invasive lines and/or arterial
puncture if patient is possible thrombolytic
candidate

Drugs

Aspirin 325 mg

Nitroglycerin sublingual repeated at 5-minute
intervals, IV for first 24–48 hours if no
contraindications (do not use with IMI and
evident or suspected RV infarct)

Morphine 2–5 mg IV repeated until pain
controlled (or meperidine IV)

Anticoagulation (unfractionated heparin or
low-molecular-weight heparin)

β-blockade: metoprolol 5 mg IV repeated every
5 minutes for three doses

Consideration of glycoprotein IIb/IIIa inhibitor

Thrombolysis versus cardiac catheterization

Other (vasopressors/IABP for cardiogenic
shock), dysrhythmia management

BP, blood pressure; ECG, electrocardiogram; IABP,
intraaortic balloon pump; IMI, inferior myocardial
infarction; IV, intravenous; RV, right ventricular.

considered for a patient with a true aspirin allergy.

- Nitroglycerin (mechanism described in Chapter 8): Nitrates may occasionally reverse ischemia when due to spasm, as in variant (spasm) angina or subtotal occlusion. Because coronary thrombosis most commonly (>90%) causes ST elevation, prolonged efforts with repeated nitroglycerin administration (i.e., every 5 minutes repeated three times) should not delay rapid preparations for reperfusion therapy. Hypotension is the most important complication from nitroglycerin use and it should be used carefully in patients older than 60 years (consider 1/200 gr. or administer with patient supine). It is *contraindicated* in those patients with suspected RV infarct (either IMI with ST elevation III greater than II or ST elevation in lead V_4 with right-sided ECG leads) and severe aortic stenosis.

- Morphine (or meperidine): For severe pain unless immediately responsive to initial nitrate therapy and may be useful with AMI complicated by pulmonary congestion or agitation.

- Anticoagulation: With either unfractionated heparin (see Table 4.2) or low-molecular-weight heparin (LMWH). The advantages of LMWH are twice daily intramuscular (IM) dosing (as opposed to constant IV infusion) and usually less time to achieve therapeutic levels.

- β-Adrenoreceptor blockers (β-blockers): β-blockers act as both negative inotropes and chronotropes on the heart, thus reducing myocardial oxygen demand. If there are no contraindications (hypotension, bradycardia, severe asthma or pulmonary congestion), give in the acute setting and continue postinfarction.

- Glycoprotein IIb/IIIa antagonists: The glycoprotein (GP) IIb/IIIa receptor is an integrin receptor found on the platelet membrane. When platelets are activated by stimuli (including thrombin, collagen, adenosine diphosphate, and epinephrine), the GP IIb/IIIa receptor changes conformation to be receptive to one end of a fibrinogen dimer. Occupation by another IIb/IIIa receptor to the other end of the fibrinogen leads to platelet aggregation. The antagonists prevent this process. These are indicated when chest pain persists despite appropriate administration of all the medications listed previously.

- Thrombolytics: The indications for thrombolysis for AMI are ST elevation (greater than 0.1 mV in two or more contiguous leads) or a new bundle branch block in a patient presenting within 12 hours of symptom onset.

- Primary and rescue PTCA (or cardiac catheterization): Acute catheterization can identify the source of the problem, reperfuse the occluded artery with lower risk of hemorrhagic stroke, and identify patients whose anatomy favors emergent surgical revascularization. Because patency rates are higher than achieved with thrombolytics, many centers where rapid access to cardiac catheterization is available may consider this the preferred strategy for reperfusion. Rescue PTCA describes the use of PTCA when thrombolysis has failed because of either inadequate relief of patient discomfort or persistent ST elevations on ECG.

The management of patients with AMI, including the patient described in the clinical scenario, is very dynamic. Strategies that combine low-dose thrombolytics with PTCA or combine different thrombolytics with anticoagulants or antiplatelet agents require

the student to review updated management guidelines on a periodic basis. (See Table 4.3 for contraindications to thrombolytics.)

Disposition

All patients with STEMI should be admitted to an intensive care unit (ICU). Many centers manage patients with uncomplicated non-Q MI and unstable angina patterns that have been stabilized in the ED in a lower intensity setting such as a step-down or telemetry service. A patient as described in the clinical scenario would have postinfarct care and predischarge testing according to well-defined guidelines.

Pathophysiology

ACS usually occurs as the result of a dynamic change in an atherosclerotic plaque. With STEMI, as in the clinical scenario, plaque rupture and coronary thrombosis are found. With non-Q AMI and unstable angina, an acute change in a plaque with subtotal occlusion is usually found, although abnormal coronary artery constriction may contribute.

AMI most commonly occurs when there is an abrupt interruption of the coronary blood flow by a thrombotic occlusion of an already narrowed, atherosclerotic artery. High-grade atherosclerotic narrowing of the coronary vessels does not directly cause AMIs because their prolonged time course of narrowing allows time for collateral circulation to develop.

When an atherosclerotic plaque fissures, ruptures, or ulcerates, the local arterial environment is such that the vessel wall enters a thrombogenic state, leading to a mural thrombus at the site of the rupture that can then form a site of occlusion. A monolayer of platelets covers the surface of the ruptured plaque (platelet adhesion), and more platelets are recruited to the site (platelet aggregation). Fibrinogen crosslinks the platelets and thrombin is generated, further activating the coagulation cascade. It is at this early stage that the antiplatelet agents (aspirin and GP IIb/IIIa inhibitors) are thought to be most effective. An intermittently occlusive

Table 4.3.

Absolute and relative contraindications for thrombolysis

Absolute Contraindications
Active internal bleeding (except menses)
Previous hemorrhagic stroke at any time
Other cerebrovascular events within 1 year
Suspected aortic dissection
Known intracranial neoplasm
Acute pericarditis

Relative Contraindications
Age >75 years
History of chronic, severe hypertension
Uncontrolled hypertension on presentation
 (blood pressure >180/110 mm Hg after
 treatment)
On anticoagulants
Recent internal bleeding (2 to 4 weeks)
Known bleeding problems (hemophilia, platelet
 disorders)
Recent major surgery (within 3 weeks)
Recent trauma (2 to 4 weeks) including head
 trauma or traumatic or prolonged (>10
 minutes) cardiopulmonary resuscitation (CPR)
Puncture of noncompressible vascular site
Prior exposure to streptokinase (5 days to
 2 years), if that agent is to be administered
Pregnancy
Active peptic ulcer
Cardiogenic shock

thrombus may lead to myonecrosis of a distinct region supplied by the occluded artery, leading to a non-Q-wave MI. If there is prolonged thrombus occlusion, a transmural or STEMI results.

The symptoms and signs of AMI are related to the complex interplay between the sites of infarction; associated sympathetic or parasympathetic stimulation; and patient-specific factors such as age, medications, and preexisting cardiac disease.

Suggested Readings

ACC/AHA guidelines for the management of patients with acute myocardial infarction: executive summary and recommendations. 1999 update. Acute coronary syndromes, *Circulation* 2000;102:1–172.

American College of Emergency Physicians. Clinical policy for the initial approach to adults presenting with a chief complaint of chest pain, no history of trauma. *Ann Emerg Med* 1995;25:274–299.

Collins R, et al. Aspirin, heparin and fibrinolytic therapy in suspected acute myocardial infarction. *N Engl J Med* 1997;336:847–860. (Available at http://circ.ahajournals.org/cgi/content/full/100/9/1016).

Lee T, Goldman, L. Evaluation of the patient with acute chest pain. *N Engl J Med* 2000; 342:1187–1195.

Norris RM. The natural history of acute myocardial infarction. *Heart* 2000;83:726–730.

CHAPTER 5

Pulmonary Embolus

David Schindler, MD

Clinical Scenario

A 63-year-old woman presents to the emergency department (ED) with sudden onset of shortness of breath and pleuritic chest pain. She flew into Boston from Fargo, North Dakota 3 days ago. She is here to be evaluated for an experimental treatment for her newly diagnosed pancreatic cancer. The pain occurred while trying to stretch her nagging right calf, which has been bothering her for 2 days. She arrives by ambulance after calling 911.

Past medical history reveals hypertension. Her medications include a thiazide diuretic and hormone replacement therapy. She has no known drug allergies. She has a family history of breast and colon cancer. She is a heavy smoker.

Physical examination reveals an anxious woman in moderate respiratory distress. Vital signs include a blood pressure of 130/70 mm Hg, heart rate 110 beats/min, a temperature of 100.1°F, respiratory rate of 28 breaths/minute, and oxygen saturation of 100% on 2 L of oxygen (O_2). On cardiovascular examination, there is no jugular venous distension (JVD). The patient is tachycardic with no additional heart sounds, rubs, or murmurs. The lung examination is normal, with equal breath sounds bilaterally, and no dullness to percussion. Lower extremity examination is notable for marked swelling and tenderness of the left calf.

The patient is given 2 L of O_2 per minute via nasal cannula, an intravenous catheter (IV) is inserted, and blood for laboratory tests is drawn. She is placed on a cardiac monitor, which shows a sinus tachycardia.

An electrocardiogram (ECG) shows no evidence of cardiac ischemia or strain. She is sent for a posteroanterior (PA) and lateral chest x-ray examination, which are normal. The physician has a high clinical suspicion that the patient has a pulmonary embolism (PE), so he starts her on intravenous (IV) heparin. He also orders a nuclear scintigraphic ventilation perfusion (V/Q) scan. The patient returns from the study an hour later with the test showing a high probability of PE. The patient appears stable and is transferred to the intensive care unit (ICU). Despite the therapy given, she has a complicated course in the ICU and suffers a cardiorespiratory arrest the next morning. Resuscitation efforts are unsuccessful. An autopsy is performed, which showed total occlusion of the left pulmonary artery, as well as multiple foci of smaller clots in every other pulmonary vessel. It also showed a large area of thrombus extending from the right posterior tibial vein up into the femoral vein.

Clinical Evaluation

Introduction

PE is one of the most difficult diagnoses to make in emergency medicine. Most patients present with nonspecific complaints that are found in many disease states. Patients with PE may appear to be having an acute coronary syndrome or pneumonia. They may have underlying chronic diseases such as emphysema (chronic obstructive pulmonary disease [COPD]), asthma, or heart failure; presentation of these diseases can mimic PE, thus distracting the clinician from considering PE in the differential diagnosis.

History

The history should focus on the onset and timing of the symptoms. The symptoms of PE are classically described as abrupt onset of pleuritic chest pain and shortness of breath, as in our patient. The clinician should ask about recent prolonged immobility such as long trips, or bed-bound postoperatively, because of illness or long bone casts. Past medical history plays an important role in risk stratifying the patient (Table 5.1). Previous PE or deep venous thrombosis (DVT) are strong risk factors. Malignancy, hypercoagulable states (e.g., lupus, inflammatory bowel disease), smoking, estrogens, and oral contraceptive use are all contributors to PE risk. According to one study, PE is the leading cause of death in pregnancy. Family history may reveal hereditary coagulopathy. Dyspnea is present in more than half (60%) of patients with PE. Chest pain, typically pleuritic, is another common symptom in PE.

Physical Examination

The most common physical finding is a respiratory rate greater than 16 breaths/minute (90% of patients). Other vital sign abnormalities include a heart rate greater than 100 beats/minute (40% of patients) and a low-grade fever greater than 37.8°C. The temperature may be helpful in differentiating

Table 5.1.

Risk factors for deep venous thrombosis (DVT) and pulmonary embolism

1. Prolonged immobilization
2. Surgery lasting more than 30 minutes within the last 3 months
3. History of DVT or pulmonary embolus
4. Malignancy
5. Pregnancy or recent pregnancy
6. History of pelvis or lower extremity trauma
7. Oral contraceptive use combined with cigarette smoking
8. Congestive heart failure
9. Chronic obstructive pulmonary disease
10. Obesity

PE from pneumonia. PE rarely causes a high fever, whereas it is a common finding in patients with pneumonia.

The lung examination is usually normal, as in our clinical scenario. Patients can develop wheezing or rales, which may lead to the inappropriate diagnosis of COPD or an infection. Patients may have palpable chest tenderness, which should not be mistaken for a muscle strain. It is important to remember that the clot lodges in the pulmonary vasculature, not the parenchyma, and that, initially, there may be no physical findings at all.

Significant PE may lead to acute elevation in pulmonary artery pressures and right ventricular dysfunction. On physical examination, one may hear a loud P_2 (pulmonary component of the second heart sound) or a systolic murmur, or one may see JVD (see Chapter 4). Massive PE may also present with syncope and shock (see Chapter 3) secondary to poor blood flow to the brain because of right ventricular outflow obstruction.

DVT and PE are intimately related. The majority of emboli that are found in the lungs originate in the veins of the legs and pelvis. Unfortunately, in most patients with proven PE, DVT is never found on ultrasound. This is most likely because the clot developed in a deep pelvic vein or has already embolized to the lungs. A patient with a DVT may present with calf swelling, tenderness, or venous engorgement of one extremity. Homans's sign, calf pain with dorsiflexion of the foot, may be elicited and is highly suggestive for DVT. Unfortunately, like PE, the classic signs of DVT occur too infrequently to be considered reliable in diagnosing thrombosis.

Diagnostic Evaluation

Initial testing strategies on patients suspected of PE are influenced by clinical stability. A patient who presents with symptoms and signs suggestive of massive or submassive PE is brought to a resuscitation room and given cardiorespiratory support until stabilized and is then evaluated for etiologies of the shock state (i.e., acute coronary syndrome, aortic dissection, and PE). The availability and accessibility of certain modalities in each particular institution also influence testing strategies in many EDs.

A chest x-ray film and ECG are useful as initial screening tests. These are helpful in identifying non-PE diagnoses such as myocardial infarction (ECG) and pneumonia, pneumothorax, or dissection (x-ray findings). Although abnormalities on ECG or chest x-ray film may suggest a diagnosis of PE, none are sensitive nor specific enough to make a definitive diagnosis of PE without further testing.

In PE, the chest x-ray film may show atelectasis or focal infiltrates, but 30% of the time is completely normal. There are three classic but uncommon findings on x-ray film that can be associated with PE: Hampton's hump, Westermark's sign, and Palla's sign. Hampton's hump is a wedge-shaped density emanating from the pleura and is usually contiguous with the diaphragm. It is caused by an infarction of lung tissue and is seen in 4% of patients with PE. Westermark's sign consists of pulmonary vessel oligemia caused by distal clot resulting from thrombus (12% of patients with PE). Palla's sign is seen as an enlarged right descending pulmonary artery (25% of patients with PE).

Patients suspected of PE should have an ECG. The $S_1Q_3T_3$ pattern (deep S wave in lead I, and a large Q wave and inverted T wave in lead III) is a classic finding suggestive of PE. It is seen in less than 10% of patients with PE. The most common ECG patterns are sinus tachycardia and T-wave inversion in the anterior leads. Another suggestive ECG finding is a rightward axis.

Arterial blood gas (ABG) analysis is insensitive for diagnosing PE. The partial pressure of oxygen in the blood (PaO_2) cannot be used to rule out a PE if the value is normal. Alveolar-arterial gradients (A-a gradients) are calculated based on the difference between the calculated PaO_2 and measured PaO_2. They are a measure of gas exchange, but unfortunately patients with small PEs may have normal A-a gradients because gas exchange is not impaired. Thus, a normal ABG and/or A-a gradient does not rule out PE.

V/Q scan has historically been the most frequently used diagnostic study for stable patients with suspected PE. A radioactive dye is infused intravenously containing labeled aggregates of albumin. A nuclear scanner is then placed over the chest of the patient. The resulting image delineates the pulmonary arterial tree. If the albumin is unable to reach an area because of clot, it shows up on the scan as an area of perfusion defect. A radioactive gas is then inhaled, and the lungs are scanned to assess if a ventilation defect matches any defect in perfusion.

The landmark Prospective Investigation of Pulmonary Embolism Diagnosis (PIOPED) trial showed that the V/Q scan is useful in only two situations. In a patient with a high clinical probability of PE and a high probability V/Q scan, there is a 96% likelihood of PE. Conversely, in patients with low clinical suspicion and normal or low probability VQ scan, there is only a 2% to 4% likelihood of clinically significant PE. Unfortunately, many scans are read as intermediate probability or indeterminate, especially in those patients with comorbidities, such as emphysema. This forces you to either treat empirically or send the patient for a pulmonary angiogram.

Spiral computed tomography pulmonary arteriogram (CTPA) scan is replacing V/Q as the initial screening test for PE. It allows physicians to actually visualize a PE and it also detects other important, unsuspected diseases such as mediastinal tumors, aortic dissection, and lung cancers. CTPA misses PEs in smaller segments of the lungs. Whether these emboli are significant is a controversial topic. Until further study of the newer generation of CT scanners is more conclusive, it may be prudent to do duplex ultrasonography of both legs with a negative CTPA, even in the patient you deem to have low probability of a PE.

The pulmonary angiogram is still considered the "gold standard" in testing for PE. The main drawback of the test is its 3- to 4-hour duration in a less than ideal monitoring environment, and it has a 0.5% mortality rate. It is considered the standard of care for patients with nondiagnostic V/Q scans, especially if anticoagulation will present a significant risk because of the patient's comorbidities.

A recent addition to the testing arsenal is the D-dimer serum test. All blood clots undergo some degree of fibrin breakdown after forming. D-Dimer is a fibrin degradation product that is released into the circulation when fibrin cross-links are cleaved by plasmin during fibrinolysis. Circulating D-dimer then remains in the blood for 7 days after a PE. The electrophoresis immunosorbent assay (enzyme-linked immunosorbent assay [ELISA]) method of this test has been found to have high sensitivity and strong negative predictive value for patients with a low clinical probability of PE. In some centers, it is being used as an initial screening test to rule out PE in low-risk patients. There is no strong evidence to support this practice.

Echocardiography is often considered in the diagnosis of PE, especially in the evaluation of unstable patients. Frequently these patients are too unstable to leave the resuscitation room to undergo V/Q scan or pulmonary angiogram. Echocardiography can be done at the bedside to look for signs of PE, such as right ventricular overload.

Differential Diagnosis

The differential diagnosis of acute chest pain is illustrated in Table 5.2.

Treatment

The treatment of PE is currently a controversial topic (Table 5.3). PE is often treated empirically based on clinical suspicion. An untreated embolism has a high morbidity and mortality, and diagnostic studies are often not available routinely after hours in many community hospitals. Provided the patient is considered a low risk for anticoagulation, heparin is started until an appropriate imaging study confirms the diagnosis. If PE is ruled out, the treatment is immediately stopped.

Most experts agree that therapy should be based on the patient's degree of hemodynamic instability. If there is even minimal

---

Table 5.2.

Differential diagnosis of pulmonary embolism

Pneumonia/bronchitis
Pneumothorax
Lung cancer
Tuberculosis
ARDS*
Asthma or COPD† exacerbation
Angina or myocardial Infarction
Aortic dissection
Aortic insufficiency
Atrial fibrillation
Myocarditis
Pericarditis/pericardial tamponade
Congestive heart failure
Anemia
Pancreatitis
Salicylate intoxication
Septic shock
Costochondritis/chest wall pain
Anxiety

*ARDS, acute respiratory distress syndrome; †COPD, chronic obstructive pulmonary disease

---

Table 5.3.

Treatment for pulmonary embolism

Hemodynamically Stable
Supplemental O_2
IV heparin or subcutaneous low-molecular-weight heparin (anticoagulation may be started in high and/or intermediate clinical probability of PE before testing—anticoagulation stopped if tests are negative)
Vena cava filter—if anticoagulation is contraindicated

Hemodynamically Unstable
Supplemental O_2
If persistently hypoxic or in shock, intubation required
IV fluids
IV heparin or subcutaneous low-molecular-weight heparin
Massive PE* and shock—consideration of thrombolysis

IV, intravenous; *PE, pulmonary embolism.

suspicion that PE has occurred, it is appropriate to start anticoagulation with unfractionated or low-molecular-weight heparin (LMWH). LMWH is easier to titrate and requires less invasive monitoring than unfractionated heparin. Anticoagulation reduces death resulting from PE from 30% to less than 10%. Heparin prevents continued formation of an existing clot and acts as prophylaxis to avoid the formation of new clots. It does not dissolve existing emboli.

Supportive care should be given to all patients. For example, patients with pleuritic chest pain should receive analgesics. Oxygen should be provided to the patient with low oxygen saturation. Supplemental oxygen is thought to benefit patients with normal oxygen saturation by acting as a pulmonary vasodilator, although this has never been scientifically substantiated.

In hemodynamically unstable patients, the initial therapy includes monitoring airway, respiratory status and cardiovascular support, if needed (ABCs). The patient may require intubation and mechanical ventilation, and, if hypotensive, may require a vasopressor medication such as dopamine.

Currently, if the patient shows signs of shock, consider thrombolysis. A thrombolytic agent is given to any patient decompensating from a PE who does not meet any exclusion criteria for the drug (see Chapter 4, Table 4.3). Thrombolysis itself carries a considerable risk of internal hemorrhage; thus, it is essential that you are certain a PE has occurred before starting this medication. The use of thrombolytics is also being considered in a select class of stable patients at high risk of mortality. Studies have shown rapidly improved right ventricular function and pulmonary perfusion among patients with PE in patients who are clinically stable but have evidence of right ventricular dysfunction. A precise definition of the patient requiring thrombolysis remains controversial.

Following PE, there is a 25% risk of recurrence. There are two methods for preventing recurrence: prevent the formation of thrombus in the legs (DVT) or prevent the thrombus from traveling to the lungs. In patients with a history of recurrent thrombus, or those with contraindications to anticoagulation, a vena cava filter is placed. The femoral vein is catheterized and an "umbrella" net is placed in the inferior vena cava to prevent recurrence of emboli. To prevent DVT, many patients are given gradient compression stockings to wear. These effectively increase blood flow in the lower extremities fivefold and have been proven in multiple studies to reduce the recurrence of PE. Studies have also shown that following thromboembolic events, anticoagulation reduces the incidence of recurrence. Most patients are being discharged from the hospital with LMWH and then placed on oral warfarin, which they take for at least 6 months, to prevent recurrence.

Disposition

Currently all patients with a PE are admitted to the hospital. Stable patients are admitted to the general medical floor. Any patient who is unstable or has signs of shock is at risk of sudden cardiovascular collapse and requires admission to an intensive care setting.

Pathophysiology

The majority of PEs are in reality the endpoint of another pathological entity, DVT. The well-known triad of Virchow, which is hypercoagulability, stasis, and endothelial injury, is responsible for all episodes of DVT. In a patient with malignancy, it is thought that neoplastic cells produce procoagulants, leading to the formation of thrombin and the hypercoagulable state. Patients requiring a long hospital stay are at increased risk for DVT, because of their immobility and the stasis and pooling of blood in their lower extremities. The risk of thromboembolism is exponentially higher for patients undergoing orthopedic procedures, because of the concomitant endothelial injury. Thrombus usually begins in the legs, most commonly the calf veins, and often extends upward into the popliteal and thigh veins before dislodging and traveling to the lungs.

DVTs commonly form around a venous valve. Platelets aggregate initially and are eventually surrounded by fibrin, forming a thrombus. At that point, the thrombus is unstable and continues to grow through fibrin and platelet adherence. It may break off and embolize in this stage. Otherwise, fibrinolysis and resolution may occur, or the thrombus may organize and turn into a plaque adhering to the endothelium. Studies show that on a microscopic scale this occurs continuously in the venous circulation. It is when one of Virchow's rules is broken that trouble occurs.

Suggested Readings

American College of Emergency Physicians. Clinical policy for the initial approach to adults presenting with a chief complaint of chest pain, with no history of trauma. *Ann Emerg Med* 1995;25:274–299.

Fedullo P, Tapson F. The evaluation of suspected pulmonary embolism. *N Engl J Med* 2003; 349:1247–1256.

Ferrari E, Imbert A, Chevalier T, et al. The ECG in pulmonary embolism: predictive value of negative T waves in precordial leads—80 case reports. *Chest* 1997;111:537–543.

Ginsberg JS. Management of venous thromboembolism. *N Engl J Med* 1996;335:1816–1828.

Goldhaber SZ. Medical progress: pulmonary embolism. *N Engl J Med* 1998;339:93–104.

Holbert JM, Costello P, Federle MP. Role of spiral computed tomography in the diagnosis of pulmonary embolism in the emergency department. *Ann Emerg Med* 1999;33:520–528.

Hull R, Hirsh J, Sackett DL, et al. Clinical validity of a negative venogram in patients with clinically suspected venous thrombosis. *Circulation* 1981;64:622–625.

Jones JS, Neff TL, Carlson SA. Use of the alveolar-arterial oxygen gradient in the assessment of acute pulmonary embolism. *Am J Emerg Med* 1998;16:333–337.

Kline JA, Johns KA, Colucciello S. New diagnostic tests for pulmonary embolism. *Ann Emerg Med* 2000;35:168–180.

Miniati M, Prediletto R, Formichi B. Accuracy of clinical assessment in the diagnosis of pulmonary embolism. *Am J Respir Crit Care Med* 1999;159:864–871.

PIOPED Investigators. Value of the ventilation/perfusion scan in acute pulmonary embolism: results of the prospective investigation of pulmonary embolism diagnosis (PIOPED). *JAMA* 1990;263:2753–2759.

Pneumothorax

Rishi Sikka, MD

Clinical Scenario

A 20-year-old man is brought by ambulance to the emergency department for chest pain and shortness of breath. While stretching in the gym, he developed a sudden, sharp, moderately severe left-sided chest pain and difficulty breathing. The pain was initially sharp and worsened by deep breathing. The pain gradually improved and is now described as a dull, left-sided ache. Past medical and surgical history is unremarkable. He does not take any medications and he has no known drug allergies. He denies any illicit substance abuse but admits to smoking one pack of cigarettes a day for the past 2 years. There is no family history of any pulmonary diseases or connective tissue disorders. Physical examination reveals a tall, thin man in mild respiratory distress. Vital signs include a blood pressure of 120/65 mm Hg, heart rate of 112 beats/minute, temperature 98.6°F, respiratory rate 22 times/minute, and oxygen saturation of 92% on room air, 100% on non-rebreathing face mask. On cardiovascular examination, there is no jugular venous distention (JVD); the heart is tachycardic with no additional heart sounds, rubs, or murmurs. On lung examination, there are decreased breath sounds and hyperresonance over the left side of the chest. The patient is placed on a cardiac monitor with an intermittent blood pressure cuff and continuous pulse oximetry, along with 100% oxygen via a non-rebreathing facemask. An intravenous (IV) access site with normal saline is placed. The rhythm on the cardiac monitor is sinus tachycardia. An anteroposterior (AP) upright portable chest x-ray film reveals a sharp visceral pleural line associated with a distal hyperlucency and absent lung markings. There is collapse of approximately 40% of the left lung with volume loss and some mediastinal shift toward the left. These findings are consistent with a pneumothorax without tension.

The patient has a small-caliber chest tube placed under conscious sedation. Repeat chest x-ray film shows complete resolution of the pneumothorax. He is admitted to the hospital, has the chest tube pulled the next morning, and leaves the hospital later that day. In some hospitals he would have had a one-way (Heimlich) valve placed by interventional radiology and been discharged with follow-up for valve removal.

Clinical Evaluation

Introduction

Pneumothorax is the presence of air in the pleural space. It can be classified as traumatic, iatrogenic, or spontaneous. Traumatic pneumothorax occurs from blunt or penetrating trauma to the chest wall. Diagnostic and therapeutic interventions, such as thoracentesis, central venous line placement, and positive pressure ventilation, are responsible for cases of iatrogenic pneumothorax. Spontaneous pneumothorax lacks an apparent precipitating event. It can be further subdivided into primary and secondary causes. Primary spontaneous pneumothorax occurs in individuals without pre-existing lung disease. Secondary spontaneous pneumothorax occurs in individuals with underlying pulmonary disease. In some pneumothoraces, a one-way pleural valve forms that allows air to enter but not to leave the pleural space. This potentially rapidly fatal phenomenon is known as a tension pneumothorax. Regardless of the type of pneumothorax, the primary management goal is re-expansion of the collapsed lung.

History

Many cardiac and pulmonary disorders, including pneumothorax, can present with chest pain and shortness of breath. A thorough history should focus on the onset and quality of the pain and any precipitating, exacerbating, or relieving factors. Information should also be obtained regarding past medical history, medications, and allergies. This should include a history of significant cardiovascular and pulmonary disease, including coronary artery disease, asthma, emphysema, connective tissue disease, malignancy, or immunodeficiency. Use of tobacco and cocaine are risk factors for many cardiopulmonary diseases and should not be forgotten in the history.

As in our clinical scenario, primary spontaneous pneumothorax tends to occur at rest and is associated with chest pain and shortness of breath. The chest pain initially can be described as sharp and localized to the side of the chest with the pneumothorax. The intensity of the pain usually varies with inspiration, a quality known as pleuritic chest pain. Both the degree of chest pain and dyspnea are positively correlated with the size of the pneumothorax. These clinical manifestations may spontaneously improve over 24 hours even if the pneumothorax does not resolve.

Secondary spontaneous pneumothorax has a more dramatic presentation because the patient's underlying pulmonary function is already compromised. This diagnosis must always be considered in the evaluation of patients with chronic lung disease, such as chronic obstructive pulmonary disease (COPD) or asthma, with increased shortness of breath. Patients complain of new onset or worsened dyspnea and localized, pleuritic chest pain. Unlike primary spontaneous pneumothorax, these symptoms do not spontaneously improve.

Tension pneumothorax presents as an immediate, life-threatening event. Typically, the degree of dyspnea and clinical instability prevents the patient from articulating any history. Tension pneumothorax must be in the differential of any patient with respiratory distress and hemodynamic instability in the setting of mechanical ventilation or injury to the thorax.

Physical Examination

A patient with a suspected pneumothorax should undergo a thorough examination of the thorax, including auscultation, palpation, and percussion. Particular emphasis should be placed on apical auscultation to detect subtle, asymmetrical breath sounds. The physical findings are closely related to the size of the pneumothorax. A patient with a small, primary spontaneous pneumothorax may have an unremarkable examination, whereas a patient with a tension pneumothorax may have a dramatic clinical presentation and specific examination abnormalities.

The young man in the clinical scenario has a number of classic examination findings associated with pneumothorax. Although many patients may present with normal vital signs, our patient's pneumothorax is of sufficient size to cause tachycardia and tachypnea. He has the most common physical examination abnormalities: decreased breath sounds over the affected lobe and hyperresonance of the chest wall. The normal percussion note from the lung is described as resonance, whereas the percussion note over the gastric air bubble is known as tympany. In a lung with a pneumothorax, percussion of the overlying chest wall yields a sound between resonance and tympany known as hyper-resonance.

Two additional physical examination findings of pneumothorax are decreased tactile fremitus and bell tympany. These abnormalities are infrequently demonstrated in the emergency department because the clinical picture and availability of chest radiography enable a rapid diagnosis. Fremitus describes the sensation of vibratory palpation. To test for vocal fremitus, the examiner places the palms of the hands symmetrically against the chest wall while asking the patient to repeat the words "ninety-nine." The examiner compares the quality of vibration in both hands while palpating down the chest wall. A pneumothorax obstructs transmission of the sound and yields decreased vocal fremitus. The coin test takes advantage of this phenomenon. While the physician auscultates the lungs, an assistant places a coin flat against the anterior chest wall and strikes it with the edge of a second coin. If the two coins are struck over a pneumothorax, there is a clear, ringing sound called bell tympany.

Additional physical findings may be present with traumatic pneumothorax. The air from a traumatic pneumothorax can enter the subcutaneous tissue and the mediastinum and cause subcutaneous emphysema and pneumomediastinum. Palpation over an area of subcutaneous emphysema yields a crackling sound accompanied by the feeling of small, fluctuant nodules. Pneumomediastinum may manifest on auscultation as a crunching sound caused by the heart's movement of mediastinal air, known as Hammon's crunch.

Although a tension pneumothorax shares many of the physical findings associated with primary and secondary pneumothorax, there are several unique examination abnormalities associated with this disorder. Unlike a spontaneous pneumothorax, a tension pneumothorax creates increased positive pressure within the pleural space. This pressure can compress mediastinal structures; impede venous return to the heart; cause hemodynamic compromise; and lead to hypotension, tachypnea, and tachycardia. On examination, there can be respiratory distress, cyanosis, neck vein distention, and absent or decreased breath sounds over the affected lung. Tracheal deviation away from the affected hemithorax is a late and infre-

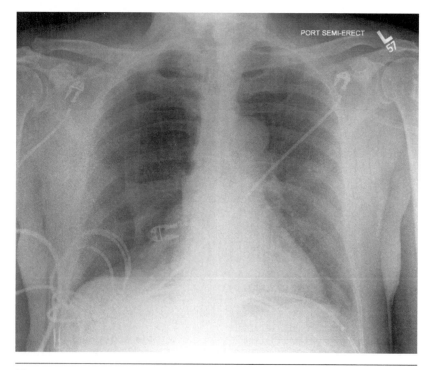

Figure 6.1
Radiograph of a pneumothorax. The radiograph demonstrates a radiolucent, visceral pleural line with absent distal lung markings delineating the edge of the collapsing lung tissue.

quent finding. Patients with tension pneumothorax appear clinically unstable and require rapid evaluation and treatment without confirmatory studies. Rapid decompression of the pleural space with the release of air under pressure and the subsequent improvement in clinical status serves as a valuable therapeutic and diagnostic maneuver.

Diagnostic Evaluation

Although the history and physical examination can provide compelling evidence of a pneumothorax, chest radiography remains the mainstay for diagnosis. It is a sensitive screening test for pneumothorax that also can identify other disorders causing chest pain and dyspnea. A portable upright AP chest radiograph is often sufficient to confirm the diagnosis of a clinically significant pneumothorax. The radiograph reveals a radiolucent, visceral pleural line with absent distal lung markings (Fig. 6.1). There can be volume loss and shift toward the side of a simple pneumothorax. Although skin folds and borders of ribs and scapula may also present as thin, linear lines, these normal anatomic shadows have lateral lung markings and often extend beyond the thoracic cavity.

These radiographic signs are difficult to appreciate in the recumbent patient, such as a patient with trauma who cannot be seated upright. In the supine position, the air of a pneumothorax rises to the anterior costophrenic angle, the highest point in the hemithorax. On an AP view of the chest, this produces a wide and deep costophrenic angle, known as the deep sulcus sign. The air within the pleural space may also cause increased lucency over the ipsilateral upper quadrant of the abdomen and sharp definition of the anterior diaphragmatic surface (Fig. 6.2). If chest radiography is normal but clinical suspicion of pneumothorax is high, decubitus and expiratory views of the chest may be helpful. During expiration, the lung volume decreases while the size of the pneumothorax remains constant. As a result, the radiolucent, visceral pleural line shifts farther out from the chest wall and is more

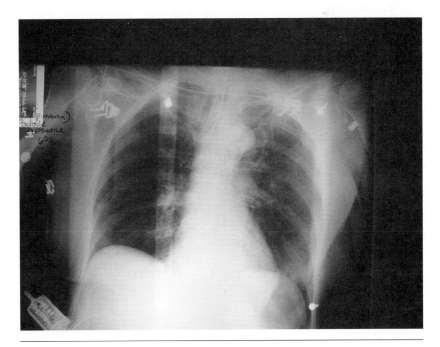

Figure 6.2
A deep sulcus sign shows a wide and deep costophrenic angle. The air within the pleural space may also cause increased lucency over the ipsilateral upper quadrant of the abdomen and sharp definition of the anterior diaphragmatic surface.

visible. If the presence of a pneumothorax is still in doubt, computed tomography (CT) of the chest can provide definitive visualization. CT of the chest is also valuable to distinguish a giant bulla from a pneumothorax in a patient with bullous lung disease.

A tension pneumothorax displays even more dramatic radiographic abnormalities. Chest radiography reveals a shift of the mediastinum away from the pneumothorax, widening of the ipsilateral rib spaces, and depression of the ipsilateral diaphragm. Although a tension pneumothorax is sometimes identified by radiography, this disorder should be principally diagnosed by history and examination and treated before obtaining films in an unstable patient. Treatment of a tension pneumothorax should not be delayed for a radiological study.

If the history and the physical examination are strongly suggestive of a pneumothorax, then chest radiography is the only required diagnostic study. Laboratory specimens, including preoperative studies, are appropriate for patients who may require hospital admission and specialty consultation. This includes patients with bilateral pneumothoraces, tension pneumothorax, and recurrent pneumothorax.

Differential Diagnosis

The differential diagnosis for acute chest pain is illustrated in Table 6.1.

Table 6.1.

Differential diagnosis for pneumothorax

Ischemic chest pain
Pericarditis
Myocarditis
Esophageal rupture (Boerhaave's syndrome)
COPD/asthma exacerbation
Aortic dissection
Pericardial tamponade
Pneumonia
Hemothorax/hydrothorax
Pulmonary embolism
Costochondritis/chest wall pain
Other causes of chest pain and/or dyspnea

COPD, chronic obstructive pulmonary disease.

Treatment

The goal of treatment for pneumothorax is the removal of air from the pleural space. This can be accomplished with supplemental oxygen, catheter aspiration, or chest tube thoracostomy. Pleura reabsorb air at a rate of approximately 2% per day. Supplemental oxygen increases reabsorption fourfold and accelerates resolution of a pneumothorax. Catheter aspiration augments this process by directly removing the air. An IV catheter is introduced in the midclavicular line of the second intercostal space, and air is aspirated with a syringe until there is resistance. Chest tube thoracostomy can speed the resolution of a pneumothorax. In this procedure, a small-bore chest tube is introduced through the chest wall and into the pleural space and is attached to low suction.

The specific treatment of a pneumothorax varies because of controversy over management strategies. In general, the treatment approach depends on the type of pneumothorax and the clinical setting, including the patient's age, underlying medical conditions, and the need for surgery or medical transfer (Table 6.2). Patients with a small primary spontaneous pneumothorax (defined as involving less than 15% of the hemithorax) should be placed on supplemental oxygen and observed for 6 hours. If a repeat chest radiograph shows no expansion of the pneumothorax and the patient is considered reliable, has a support network, and has close access to medical care, the patient may be discharged. However, patients with pneumothorax expansion and patients with a large, primary spontaneous pneumothorax should undergo needle catheter aspiration. If a repeat chest radiograph 6 hours after the procedure shows improvement, the patient can be discharged with close medical follow-up. If the lung does not re-expand after aspiration, the needle catheter can be attached to a water seal device and function as a chest tube. In contrast, secondary spontaneous pneumothorax, bilateral pneumothorax, and pneumothorax in patients on mechanical ventilation must be managed initially with chest tube thoracostomy. All patients with a chest tube require hospitalization.

Table 6.2.

Treatment guidelines for pneumothorax

All Types of Pneumothorax
Supplemental oxygen
Chest radiograph

Primary Spontaneous Pneumothorax
Observation if small pneumothorax (<15%) or
    else consideration of needle catheter
    thoracostomy
If the lung fails to re-expand, consideration of
    adding suction or performing chest tube
    thoracostomy

Secondary Spontaneous Pneumothorax
Chest tube thoracostomy

Tension Pneumothorax
Needle catheter thoracostomy followed by chest
    tube thoracostomy

Pneumothorax in a Patient on a Ventilator
Chest tube thoracostomy. If tension
    pneumothorax, needle thoracostomy
    followed by chest tube thoracostomy

Tension pneumothorax should be treated immediately with a needle catheter thoracostomy in the midclavicular line of the second or third intercostal space. This interspace is identified by palpating along the sternum to the angle of Louis, then following the adjacent interspace over the affected side laterally to the midclavicular line. The needle catheter then should be inserted over the rib and into the pleural space. The needle does not damage lung and underlying structures because the pleural space is filled with air under pressure. This potentially life-saving procedure decompresses the pressure within the pleural space and improves respirations and hemodynamics. Needle thoracostomy should be followed by more definitive chest tube thoracostomy. The management of chest tubes is beyond the scope of this chapter.

Disposition

Pneumothorax recurrence is the most significant long-term complication. The risk of recurrent primary and secondary spontaneous pneumothorax is approximately 30% and 40%, respectively. Most recurrent primary spontaneous thoraces (pleural) occurs within the first year.

These risks can be minimized with referral for definitive surgical management. This can include pleurodesis (the use of sclerosing agents to seal the pleural space), video-assisted thoracoscopy or thoracotomy to resect bullae, or a combination of surgical resection and pleurodesis. Treatment recommendations are variable and are determined by the consultant.

Pathophysiology

The pleural space is the potential space between the visceral pleura, which covers the surface of the lung, and the parietal pleura, which covers the chest wall, diaphragm, and mediastinum. This space is normally filled with a few milliliters of fluid. If either pleural surface ruptures, air enters the pleural space down a subatmospheric pressure gradient, causes partial or total lung collapse, and results in a pneumothorax.

Primary spontaneous pneumothorax accounts for most cases of spontaneous pneumothorax. Like the young man in our clinical scenario, the classic patient is a tall, thin young man. Smoking increases the risk of primary spontaneous pneumothorax by about 20 times in men and by about 9 times in women in a dose-dependent manner. Primary spontaneous pneumothorax is thought to result from a combination of subpleural blebs and distal airway inflammation.

Secondary spontaneous pneumothorax occurs in individuals with underlying pulmonary disease. It tends to occur in an older cohort than primary spontaneous pneumothorax. The most frequent underlying etiologies are COPD and *Pneumocystis carinii* pneumonia (PCP) infection in patients with acquired immunodeficiency syndrome (AIDS). Additional pulmonary pathology responsible for secondary spontaneous pneumothorax includes airway disease (asthma, cystic fibrosis), interstitial lung disease (idiopathic pulmonary fibrosis, sarcoid), infection (tuberculosis, fungal pneumonia), connective tissue disease (Marfan's syndrome, rheumatoid arthritis, scleroderma), and malignancy. Secondary spontaneous pneumothorax can also occur in neonates secondary to meconium aspiration. Although less common, the air causing a pneumothorax can enter the pleural space from a nonpulmonary source, such as an esophageal rupture (Boerhaave's syndrome).

Tension pneumothorax can occur in any type of pneumothorax but is most commonly associated with traumatic pneumothorax and with pneumothorax in patients on mechanical ventilation with positive end-expiratory pressure (PEEP). As the volume of air in a tension pneumothorax increases, pressure builds up, which compresses mediastinal structures, impedes venous return to the heart, and ultimately leads to circulatory and respiratory collapse. A tension pneumothorax is a life-threatening emergency that requires immediate intervention.

Suggested Readings

Sahn SA, Heffner JE. Spontaneous pneumothorax. *N Engl J Med* 2000;342:868–874.

Schramel FMNH, Postmus PE, Vanderschueren RGJRA. Current aspects of spontaneous pneumothorax. *Eur Respir J* 1997;10:1372–1379.

Spillane RM, Shepard JO, Deluca SA. Radiologic aspects of pneumothorax. *Am Fam Physician* 1995;51:459–464.

Vukich DJ. Pneumothorax, hemothorax and other abnormalities of the pleural space. *Emerg Med Clin North Am* 1983;1:431–448.

CHAPTER 7

Atypical Chest Pain

Rohit Gupta, MD

Clinical Scenario

A 43-year-old man presents to the emergency department (ED) complaining of constant, burning, substernal chest pain lasting for several hours. The pain began while the patient was reclining in bed shortly after eating a spicy meal. The pain does not radiate. He denies nausea, vomiting, or diaphoresis. He reports experiencing similar episodes of pain in the past, but none was as severe or long lasting as the present episode. There is no relation to exertion. He took several antacid tablets at home and felt some relief. However, when the pain did not resolve completely, he came to the ED for further evaluation. The patient has a prior diagnosis of gastroesophageal reflux disease (GERD) controlled by antacids.

His cardiac risk factors include hypertension and a 20-pack-year history of smoking. He denies diabetes mellitus, hyperlipidemia, or family history of early myocardial infarction (MI). The patient takes hydrochlorothiazide for hypertension. He has no drug allergies.

He is sitting comfortably on a stretcher in no apparent distress. His vital signs are normal. On examination, the neck reveals no carotid bruits; the cardiac examination is normal with no murmurs, rubs, or gallops; and the lungs are clear. The patient's pain is not reproducible on palpation of the chest wall. The abdomen is soft but mildly tender in the epigastrium. On rectal examination stool is guaiac negative.

The patient's electrocardiogram (ECG), obtained immediately on arrival, reveals normal sinus rhythm with a rate of 68 beats/minute, normal axis, normal intervals, and no changes of the ST intervals. Similarly, the patient's complete blood count (CBC) and electrolytes are normal. Finally, his chest x-ray film reveals a normal heart size and mediastinum and clear lung fields.

He is placed on a cardiac monitor. He is treated with oxygen via nasal cannula and normal saline intravenous (IV). Although his chest pain syndrome is very suggestive of a possible gastrointestinal (GI) source such as reflux disease or peptic ulcer disease, he is treated for possible acute coronary syndrome (ACS) with aspirin, a trial of nitroglycerine, and serial examinations. The patient is also given Maalox and famotidine. As a patient assessed with low risk for coronary disease, he is admitted to either the chest pain unit or telemetry service as available. His primary care physician is uncertain of the need to admit a patient with a probable GI source of pain. However, she agrees after discussion with the ED physician that, although the patient appears at low risk, the accelerated diagnostic pathway prevents an inappropriate discharge of a patient with missed ACS.

Clinical Evaluation

Introduction

Chest pain is the second most common presenting complaint to EDs in the United States. Chest pain, more than most complaints, has many serious causes that can lead to severe morbidity or mortality if not treated aggressively. All patients with chest pain require a targeted history, focused physical examination, and rapid ECG to risk stratify the pain and identify life-threatening causes, especially cardiac ischemia. The focus of this chapter is the approach to the clinically stable patient whose chest pain has features that are atypical of cardiac ischemia.

History

A detailed history is the cornerstone of any chest pain evaluation, providing information that is vital to quick and accurate risk stratification. Chest pain is categorized as ischemic, atypical, or noncardiac based on three attributes of the history. Ischemic pain is brought on or worsened by exertion, is substernal in location, and is relieved by rest or nitroglycerin. When only one or two of the attributes are present, the pain is described as being atypical. If none of the attributes are present, the pain is noncardiac.

The American Heart Association's unstable angina guidelines suggest using the four-way classification system from Coronary Artery Study System (CASS), in which a patient's chest pain is classified as definite angina, probable angina, probably not angina, and definitely not angina. Historical features suggesting a nonischemic etiology include pleuritic pain that is sharp, knife-like, or related to respiratory movements or cough; pain that is primarily located in the mid or lower abdomen; constant pain lasting for days; fleeting pain lasting for a few seconds or less; or pain radiating to the lower extremities or above the mandible.

In addition to specific characteristics of the pain, a patient's prior history of cardiac evaluation can also aid in risk stratification. An adequate, recent stress test, coronary catheterization, or other objective evaluation that is negative for coronary artery disease greatly reduces the chance that the pain is of ischemic cardiac etiology.

Physical Examination

The physical examination is less informative than the history when evaluating chest pain. Nonetheless, vital signs, general appearance, and chest and cardiovascular examinations provide useful information. Vital signs and general appearance allow assessment of the severity of disease. Patients with abnormal vital signs, especially tachycardia, hypoxia, or hypotension, or a distressed appearance, including anxiety, diaphoresis, visible shortness of breath, should be stratified as being high risk. Serious causes of morbidity and mortality such as aortic dissection, pulmonary embolus, tension pneumothorax, pericardial tamponade, congestive heart failure, and acute MI (AMI), should be individually sought and excluded in the evaluation.

In a patient with stable vital signs and a reassuring general appearance, the physical examination of the chest wall, lungs, and heart often provides diagnostic clues. Chest pain that can be reproduced by palpation or movement of the chest wall and that can be localized with one finger, suggests a nonischemic etiology. However, it is important to remember that ischemic chest pain has been associated with findings of chest wall pain in 10% to 15% of patients. Examination of the lungs can provide evidence of pneumothorax, pneumonia, or congestive heart failure (as discussed elsewhere). The cardiac examination may reveal a pericardial rub to suggest the diagnosis of pericarditis; a midsystolic click, to suggest mitral valve prolapse (MVP); or a systolic ejection murmur, to suggest aortic stenosis. Each of these findings is discussed in detail later in the chapter and elsewhere.

Diagnostic Evaluation

The primary diagnostic test that must be ordered in the initial evaluation of chest pain is an ECG. The initial ECG should be completed within 10 minutes of a patient's arrival into the ED. ECG changes suggestive of ACS are discussed in detail elsewhere. Only the absence of ischemic changes allows the physician to consider common causes of atypical chest pain as discussed later in this chapter. Other diagnostic tests to consider depend on the character of the pain and associated symptoms and may include chest x-ray film, arterial blood gas, hematocrit, pulse oximetry, serum potassium, and echocardiography.

Differential Diagnosis

When ischemic cardiac and other life-threatening causes of chest pain can be excluded, the evaluation can focus on identifying the

Table 7.1.

The differential diagnosis of noncardiac chest pain

Gastrointestinal Causes
Esophageal spasm
Gastroesophageal reflux disease
Peptic ulcer disease
Gastritis
Mallory-Weiss tears

Pulmonary Causes
Pneumonia
Pleurisy
Tracheobronchitis

Non-ischemic Cardiac Causes
Pericarditis
Mitral valve prolapse
Other valvular disorders (IHSS*)

Musculoskeletal Causes
Costochondritis
Rib fracture
Muscle strain
Sickle cell disease
Herpes zoster

Psychiatric Causes
Anxiety disorder
Depression
Panic disorder

*IHSS, idiopathic hypertrophic subaortic stenosis.

actual cause of pain. Table 7.1 lists by system the extremely large differential diagnosis for noncardiac chest pain. Clearly, chest pain can originate from any structure within the chest as well as from many systemic and psychological disorders. The remainder of this chapter further discusses several of the common etiologies in Table 7.1.

Treatment

Table 7.2 summarizes the primary treatments for each disorder discussed. It is important to note that risk stratifying chest pain does not exclude a diagnosis of significant coronary artery disease.

Gastroesophageal Reflux Disease

Heartburn is the classical manifestation of GERD. It is usually described as a sharp,

retrosternal, burning pain, which may radiate to the epigastrium, neck, throat, or back. Frequently, heartburn occurs after meals and is worsened by lying back or bending over. Patients may report effortless regurgitation of acid especially after meals and at night. Water brash, the appearance of salty or sour taste from salivary glands in response to intraesophageal acid, also suggests GERD. Other less frequent symptoms include dysphagia and odynophagia. Extra-esophageal complaints associated with reflux include asthma and laryngitis. The physical examination is not helpful in diagnosing GERD.

When the clinical presentation is highly suggestive of GERD, a trial of therapy may be initiated based on history alone. The mainstay of treatment for patients with GERD is targeted at reducing the quantity and acidity of refluxed contents. Lifestyle modifications can be helpful. Patients should be instructed to elevate the head of the bed, remain upright for several hours after meals, avoid large meals, lose weight, and avoid eating before sleeping. Patients should be counseled to avoid certain foods, beverages, and medications including, caffeine products, alcoholic beverages, spicy foods, non-steroidal anti-inflammatory medications, and cigarettes. Pharmacotherapy of GERD includes acid-neutralizing agents and acid-reducing agents. Antacids and acid-neutralizing agents provide fast relief of mild, infrequent reflux symptoms. Acid-reducing agents consisting of histamine-2 (H$_2$) antagonists and proton pump inhibitors, are the mainstays of treatment. H$_2$ receptor antagonists are well tolerated, safe, and effective. Proton pump inhibitors are even more potent.

Patients with GERD may be safely discharged home. They should be advised to follow-up with their medical doctors. Further exploration via endoscopy or 24-hour pH monitoring does not occur in the ED and, if indicated, can be arranged by the patient's primary physician.

Esophageal Spasm

A second important GI cause of atypical chest pain is diffuse esophageal spasm. Classically, esophageal spasm causes chest pain that

62   CHEST PAIN

Table 7.2.

Treatment and disposition summary for noncardiac chest pain

Diagnosis	Treatment	Disposition
GERD	Lifestyle modification Antacids, H_2 blockers, proton pump inhibitors	D/C with instructions to F/U with PCP or GI specialist
Esophageal spasm	Calcium-channel blocker Nitroglycerin	Frequent admission to telemetry unit
Acute pericarditis	Pain control with NSAIDs	D/C with F/U
Mitral valve prolapse	No emergent therapy indicated	D/C with F/U
Costochondritis	Pain control with NSAIDs	D/C with F/U
Psychiatric	Reassurance and encouragement	D/C with F/U with psychiatry

D/C, discharge; F/U, follow-up; GERD, gastroesophageal reflux disease; GI, gastrointestinal; H_2, histamine-2; NSAIDs, nonsteroidal anti-inflammatory drugs; PCP, primary care physician.

is very similar to ischemic cardiac pain. Often described as a pressure, the pain of esophageal spasm is substernal and frequently radiates to the back, neck, jaw, and arms. It can range in intensity from a mild discomfort to an agonizing pain similar to that of an MI or a dissecting aortic aneurysm. The pain may be transient, lasting only seconds, or long lasting. MI pain is anything greater than 20 minutes, spasm pain can last hours, and pain in absence of ECG changes is suggestive of noncardiac pain. It usually occurs at rest, may be triggered by emotional upset, and frequently improves with nitroglycerin. Patients with esophageal spasm may also report intermittent dysphagia, heartburn, or regurgitation. As in GERD, the physical examination is not useful in diagnosis.

The test of choice to diagnose esophageal spasm is manometry, especially when the patient is having an attack. In esophageal manometry, pressure and pH are measured at multiple locations along the esophagus. Abnormal motor activity or drops in intraesophageal pH accompanying chest pain strongly suggest the diagnosis of esophageal spasm. Manometry is not performed in the ED.

Treatment of esophageal spasm is difficult. Pharmacological therapy uses nitroglycerin, anticholinergics, or calcium-channel antagonists with varying rates of success. The patient with known esophageal spasm, potentially from previous history, may be safely discharged from the ED. However, because differentiation between cardiac ischemia and esophageal spasm may be impossible on clinical grounds, many patients need to be admitted for further testing.

Acute Pericarditis

Pericarditis is an important cause of atypical chest pain. Pericarditis refers to inflammation of the pericardium, a two-layer serous membrane that surrounds the heart. Inflammation of the pericardial membranes can cause a pericardial effusion, the accumulation of fluid within the pericardial space. Whenever the diagnosis of pericarditis is being considered, pericardial tamponade must be excluded. In tamponade, the virtual space between the parietal and visceral membranes becomes filled with fluid under enough pressure to prevent proper cardiac function. Impaired cardiac filling leads to decreased cardiac output, hypotension, and cardiogenic shock.

The chest pain of pericarditis is severe, substernal or left precordial, and sharp or stabbing in quality. It can be sudden or gradual onset. It frequently radiates to the back along the trapezius ridge, to the neck, or to the top of the shoulders. The pain is pleuritic, worsening with deep inspiration, coughing, and movement. Classically, lying back worsens the pain, while sitting forward eases it. Associated symptoms often include low-grade fevers, dysphagia, or dyspnea. On occasion, it may be possible to obtain a history of a viral upper respiratory tract infection in the weeks before presentation.

The pathognomonic finding of pericarditis is a pericardial friction rub. The rub is characteristically described as a triphasic scratching sound and is heard best with the diaphragm of the stethoscope over the left sternal border with the patient sitting forward. The three phases correspond to atrial systole, ventricular systole, and rapid filling in ventricular diastole. The rub of pericarditis is notoriously transient.

Signs suggestive of a significant pericardial effusion include a resting tachycardia, jugular venous distension, and distant heart sounds. If there is a pericardial effusion, a pulsus paradoxus should be measured to assess for tamponade. The pulsus paradoxus is the normal physiological variation in peak systolic blood pressure of less than 10 mm Hg with respiration. In patients with a pericardial effusion, the pulsus increases. If it increases above 20 mm Hg, the patient is at risk for impending tamponade. A pulsus can be measured using a manual blood pressure cuff. The cuff must be deflated slowly so that the interval when the first Korotkoff sound disappears with inspiration can be measured.

The ECG is useful in diagnosing acute pericarditis. The characteristic ECG changes of pericarditis progress systematically over weeks. They are as follows: (1) diffuse PR segment depression or diffuse, concave upward ST segment elevation in leads I, II, III, aVF, and V_2 to V_6 with reciprocal changes in aVR and V_1; (2) the ST and PR segments

return to baseline; (3) global T-wave inversion; and (4) complete normalization.

AMI and the normal variant of early repolarization are two causes of abnormal ECGs that must be distinguished from acute pericarditis. Most importantly, in contrast to AMI, the changes in acute pericarditis occur globally and are not localized to traditional ischemic territories. In addition, in acute pericarditis, ST segments are concave not convex, ST segments are rarely elevated above 5 mm, the QRS complexes do not change, Q waves do not develop, and the changes evolve slowly over a much longer time frame.

Occurring in 2% of healthy young adults, the normal variant of early repolarization is a common cause of abnormal ECGs with ST-segment elevation. A reliable indicator to differentiate early repolarization from acute pericarditis is the ST segment to T-wave amplitude ratio in leads I, V_5, and V_6. Measured as the height of the ST-segment elevation over baseline divided by the peak amplitude of the T wave, a ratio exceeding 0.24 is highly suggestive of acute pericarditis.

Although history, physical examination, and the ECG in most instances allow the diagnosis of pericarditis, the echocardiogram is the procedure of choice for evaluation and follow-up. Small pericardial effusions, seen as echo-free spaces on the echocardiogram, strongly suggest the diagnosis. Echocardiograms can accurately quantify the amount of fluid, determine whether the fluid is hemodynamically significant (causing tamponade), and serially follow the amount of fluid over time. In cases of viral pericarditis, an echocardiogram is not obtained. Echocardiography should be performed if purulent pericarditis, large pericardial effusion, or tamponade is suspected.

Unlike the ECG and echocardiogram, laboratory data frequently confound the diagnosis of pericarditis. Acute pericarditis frequently causes a modest rise in serum transaminases and creatine kinase levels. The rise is believed to stem from diffuse involvement of the epicardium. The rise in cardiac enzymes makes distinguishing pericarditis from ACS even more difficult. Additional laboratory tests consisting of human immunodeficiency virus (HIV) serology, antinuclear antibody titer, tuberculin skin test, and blood cultures may be indicated if the history is appropriate.

Most patients with acute pericarditis do not require specific therapy. Patients with idiopathic or viral pericarditis improve with time, although symptoms may last as long as 3 weeks. Therapy is supportive consisting primarily of pain control with nonsteroidal anti-inflammatory drugs. Patients with uncomplicated acute pericarditis of presumed viral etiology do not need to be admitted to the hospital and can be safely discharged. Acute pericarditis from malignancy or autoimmune disease must be treated more aggressively. These patients should be admitted for an inpatient workup. Patients with large pericardial effusions, tamponade at presentation, persistent symptoms, or possible myocarditis also require admission.

Mitral Valve Prolapse

MVP is movement of one or both of the mitral valve leaflets into the left atrium past the mitral valve annular plane during systole. It varies in significance from being simply a normal variant to being an important cause of atypical chest pain. MVP is usually asymptomatic but in rare cases can be associated with mitral regurgitation, atrial fibrillation, syncope, sudden cardiac death, and chest pain. When chest pain does occur, it may occur in association with palpitations and syncope. On physical examination, the classical findings are a midsystolic click and a late systolic murmur. The click occurs when the chordae tendineae are stretched taut by the mitral valve leaflets in midsystole. As the leaflets prolapse, they permit mitral regurgitation and cause the late systolic murmur. Echocardiography is the diagnostic test of choice. It not only proves whether prolapse is present but it can also measure the amount of regurgitation and its physiological effects.

Most patients with MVP have a benign clinical course and do not require therapy. MVP has not been shown to increase the risk of MI and is not associated with increased morbidity or mortality. Patients believed to have MVP may be safely discharged from the hospital. They should be advised to follow up with their primary physician or a cardiologist for further testing and recommendations regarding antibiotic prophylaxis.

Neuromusculoskeletal Causes of Chest Pain

Neuromusculoskeletal (NMS) causes encompass many different types of chest pain originating from the nerves, muscles, bones, and bony articulations that compose the chest wall. Costochondritis is one of the most common chest wall pain syndromes.

Costochondritis is inflammation of the costochondral and chondrosternal joints. Positive diagnosis is difficult because history, physical examination, and radiographical findings are all nonspecific. It occurs in patients of all age groups and equally in both sexes. Its primary symptom, pain, is located in the anterior chest wall, most frequently affecting the third through fifth costochondral joints. The pain is usually described as being sharp or stabbing and is extremely well localized. Its onset may be gradual or sudden and may be related to recent trauma or increased or unaccustomed physical activity. Movement, coughing, and deep inspiration usually exacerbate the pain. On physical examination palpation of the chest wall frequently reproduces the pain. Diagnostic laboratory and radiographic tests are not useful.

Patients with costochondritis may be safely discharged from the ED and, as always, be provided with appropriate discharge instructions and warning symptoms of when to return to the ED. Costochondritis resolves spontaneously but may require several weeks to resolve completely. The mainstay of therapy is pain relief using non-steroidal anti-inflammatory medications. Additional therapeutic measures include application of heat and rest. Patients must be reassured that the pain is not due to a serious, life-threatening etiology.

Psychiatric Causes of Chest Pain

Psychiatric disorders are frequently diagnosed in patients with chest pain. Multiple studies suggest that the prevalence of panic disorders, anxiety, or depression in patients with noncardiac chest pain may be as high as 60% to 70%. Patients who have had negative coronary angiography and normal endoscopy and esophageal pH monitoring have a higher incidence of these psychiatric disorders. Although a direct causal relationship is difficult to establish, psychiatric disorders, particularly depression, anxiety, and panic disorder, are clearly important causes of chest pain.

Patients with psychiatric causes of chest pain are more frequently young and female. On history, they tend to relate a higher number of autonomic symptoms including tachycardia, dyspnea, dizziness, and paresthesias. They usually have fewer cardiac risk factors and often possess a prior psychiatric history. A full psychiatric evaluation with reference to the *Diagnostic and Statistical Manual of Mental Disorders*, 4th edition (DSM-IV) criteria is required to make the diagnosis.

The emergency physician may safely discharge patients with suspected psychiatric chest pain. The prognosis for patients with psychiatric causes of chest pain is excellent. Long-term follow-up reveals that psychiatric chest pain does not significantly impact longevity. Nonetheless, significant morbidity can result. Patients with psychiatric causes of chest pain continue to experience pain, continue to seek medical attention, and frequently contemplate suicide. On discharge, it is incumbent on the emergency medicine physician to provide referral and encouragement for psychiatric follow-up.

Disposition

Table 7.2 summarizes the dispositions for each disorder discussed. Patients with atypical chest pain often require admission to either a chest pain unit or telemetry service or evaluation via exercise testing or perfusion imaging to exclude an ischemic cardiac cause of chest pain. This is because no feature of the history, physical examination, or ECG can reliably exclude ACS. Reliance on clinical features and response to a therapeutic trial such as an antacid can lead to misclassification and inappropriate discharge. Patients

with atypical chest pain frequently have ACS or other life-threatening causes of chest pain.

Clear discharge instructions must be provided to all patients with atypical chest pain syndromes. In patients with atypical chest pain in which a serious disorder is not considered likely, discharge instructions are important for patient management and risk management. These instructions should indicate explicit follow-up plans and explicit criteria to return to the ED, such as centralizing or worsening pain, fever, or dyspnea. Patients may evolve the skin lesions of Herpes zoster or later have a lung cancer or complication from GERD identified in follow-up. Thus, it is essential that evaluation and treatment continue beyond the ED evaluation for all causes of atypical chest pain.

Pathophysiology

The pathophysiology of atypical chest pain cannot be neatly summarized, because it is a diagnosis with multiple etiologies. A more complete discussion of pathophysiology of some of these entities may be found in other parts of this book. Here, we briefly discuss some of the pain pathways and pathophysiology of entities mentioned in this chapter.

Gastrointestinal Conditions

GERD is one of the most common causes of atypical chest pain. It may account for up to 60% of cases. GERD refers to the clinical and histopathological sequelae of the movement of gastroduodenal contents into the esophagus. It can vary from simple heartburn resolving with antacids to debilitating symptoms that do not respond to potent antireflux agents and produce severe morbidity.

Cardiac Conditions

In general, the pathophysiology of chest pain is complex and not well understood. The heart has no sensation to cold, heat, touch, or incision. The pain of ischemia results from stimulation of pain fibers in the myocardium by the accumulation of metabolic products.

The axons of these nerve fibers enter the spinal cord at T1 to T4 or T5 on the left. Pain can be referred to areas supplied by the T1 to T4 spinal roots. Pain can be felt in the chest, shoulders, jaw, neck, left arm, back, epigastrium, or, in cases of silent infarction, not at all.

Pericardial Conditions

Acute inflammation of the pericardial sac has many different etiologies: infectious (viruses, including HIV, bacteria, tuberculosis, and fungi); malignancy (leukemia, lymphoma, and lung and breast cancer); autoimmune (rheumatoid arthritis, Lyme disease); and following MI, uremia, and drug reactions, to name a few. Despite full evaluation, the etiology of pericarditis is never established in fully two thirds of patients. These idiopathic cases usually have a viral etiology, most commonly echovirus or Coxsackie virus. Inflammation of the pericardial sac causes a transudative fluid, ranging from nondetectable to the large amounts sometimes seen in chronic pericarditis.

Mitral Valve Prolapse

Although pain is not a common symptom of MVP, it does occur. The exact cause of chest pain has been difficult to establish. It may be associated with the presence of true ischemia in the papillary muscles despite normal epicardial coronary arteries, perhaps because excessive tension on the papillary muscles increases oxygen consumption.

Neuromuscular Conditions

Neuromuscular pain syndromes account for 10% to 30% of patients with non-cardiac chest pain. Chest discomfort may arise from multiple specific NMS disorders including compression of nerve roots through cervical disc disease, shoulder arthritis, overuse myalgia, trauma to bony structures, herpes zoster, and costochondritis.

Thoracic spinal nerve roots divide into anterior and posterior divisions immediately after passing through the vertebral foramina. The dorsal (posterior) division supplies the muscles, bones, joints, and skin of the back. The ventral (anterior) division of thoracics 1 to 11 enters the spaces between the ribs, known as the intercostal space. A typical intercostal nerve enters the space between the parietal pleura and the internal intercostal membrane and has branches to both skin and muscle. This explains why inflammation, irritation, or injury to ribs, intercostal muscle, parietal pleura, or skin may all be felt as pain with inspiration (pleuritic pain), pain with movement, or palpation. Pain can also be referred to the thoracic and abdominal walls. The phrenic nerve supplies mediastinal and central aspects of the parietal pleura. When irritation occurs here, pain can be referred to the neck or shoulder.

Suggested Readings

Bass C, Wade C. Chest pain with normal coronary arteries: a comparative study of psychiatric and social morbidity. *Psychol Med* 1984;14:51–61.

Braunwald E, Jones R, Mark D, et al. Diagnosing and managing unstable angina. Agency for Health Care Policy and Research. *Circulation* 1994;90:613–622.

Disla E, Rhim HR, Reddy A, et al. Costochondritis: a prospective analysis in an emergency department setting. *Arch Intern Med* 1994;154:2466–2469.

Fam AG. Approach to musculoskeletal chest wall pain. *Primary Care* 1988;15:767–782.

Fennerty MB, Castell D, Fredrick AM. The diagnosis and management of gastroesophageal reflux disease in a managed care environment: suggested disease management. *Arch Intern Med* 1996;156:477–484.

Kahrilas PJ. Gastroesophageal reflux disease. *JAMA* 1996;276:983–988.

Katon W, Hall ML, Russo J, et al. Chest pain: relationship of psychiatric illness to coronary angiographic results. *Am J Med* 1988;84:1–8.

Mittal B. Mechanisms of disease: the esophagogastric junction. *N Engl J Med* 1997;336:924–932.

Chest Pain
Questions and Answers

Questions

1. An 88-year-old woman presents to the emergency department in acute respiratory distress, hypotensive with a blood pressure of 70/30 mm Hg, O_2 saturation of 85%, and a heart rate of 120 beats/minute. She has a history of lung cancer, is bedridden because of a recent fall, and has an obviously swollen left calf. The first thing you do is intubate the patient. Your next action should be:

A. Pulmonary angiogram

B. V/Q scan

C. Thrombolysis

D. Aspirin

E. Heparin

2. A 27-year-old woman presents with acute onset pleuritic chest pain and shortness of breath. She has had an unusual swelling in her left calf for 1 week. On physical examination, she is noted to be tachypneic, to be tachycardic with a heart rate of 100 beats/minute, and to have a normal oxygen saturation of 97% on room air. Which of the following statements is correct?

A. In a patient with high clinical probability of pulmonary embolism, a negative D-dimer test is useful to rule out a pulmonary embolism.

B. Spiral computed tomography (CT) scan is more sensitive than V/Q scan in the diagnosis of small, subsegmental emboli.

C. Aside from sinus tachycardia, the electrocardiogram is normal in most patients with a pulmonary embolism.

D. Most chest x-ray films demonstrate either "Hampton's hump" or "Westermark's sign" in patients with a pulmonary embolism.

E. Most patients with pulmonary embolism will have a negative Doppler ultrasound study of their lower extremities.

Directions: There are two sets of response options for the following scenario. You will be required to select one best answer from each question set.

3. A 25-year-old male unrestrained driver is brought to the emergency room after sustaining a front-end collision against a tree. On arrival, vital signs are blood pressure 80/40 mm Hg, heart rate 30 beats/minute, respiratory rate 40 breaths/minutes, and oxygen saturation of 92% on 100% nonrebreathing facemask. On physical examination, there is tracheal deviation to the right, distended neck veins, and absent lung sounds over the left hemithorax. The remainder of the examination is unremarkable.

3.1. The most likely diagnosis in this patient is:

A. Traumatic rupture of the aortic arch

B. Pericardial tamponade

C. Tension pneumothorax

D. Hemothorax

3.2. The most appropriate next step in the management of this patient is:

A. Pericardiocentesis

B. Needle thoracostomy

C. Intravenous fluids and blood

D. Chest tube thoracostomy

4. A 45-year-old man presents to the emergency department complaining of chest pain. Which of

the following statements would be appropriate for his workup and treatment?

A. One millimeter of ST-segment elevation in two contiguous leads is insufficient evidence of an acute myocardial infarction (MI) to begin thrombolysis.

B. Aspirin, β-blockers, nitroglycerin, antibiotics, and heparin are all used in an acute MI

C. A negative troponin I test 4 hours after onset of chest pain is sufficient to eliminate MI as a possibility.

D. Immediate catheterization is equally effective as thrombolysis.

5. A 60-year-old man with no prior medical history arrives at the emergency department complaining of severe substernal chest pain. The pain has been present for almost 24 hours, worsens with movement and deep inspiration, and is sharp in quality. He cannot recall having the pain before and was not exerting himself when the pain began. He denies nausea, vomiting, and shortness of breath. The patient has no past medical history or known cardiac risk factors; however, he has not seen a physician in more than 40 years. On examination, the pain is reproducible with palpation and localizable with one finger. Finally, the patient has only nonspecific T-wave changes on his electrocardiogram (ECG). What is the correct further management of the patient?

A. Admit the patient to overnight telemetry or a chest pain unit for cardiac evaluation.

B. Discharge home with a diagnosis of costochondritis, reassurance, and a prescription for ibuprofen.

C. Discharge with a diagnosis of atypical chest pain and referral to a primary care physician with a recommendation for outpatient cardiac testing.

D. A thorough diagnostic workup including laboratory work, a chest x-ray examination, repeat ECGs, and a trial of ketorolac (Toradol) in the emergency department. If the workup is normal and the Toradol is effective in relieving pain, then discharge to home.

Directions: There are three sets of response options for the following scenario. You will be required to select one best answer from each question set.

6. A 50-year-old man with a history of hypertension is brought to the emergency department after the sudden onset of severe squeezing left-sided chest pain associated with diaphoresis and nausea. His physical examination is remarkable for a blood pressure of 90/50 mm Hg and heart rate of 50 beats/minute. He is pale and uncomfortable. His lungs are clear, and cardiac and abdominal examinations are normal. An electrocardiogram (ECG) reveals an acute ST-elevation myocardial infarction (MI) in the inferior leads.

6.1. What is the first medication that should be given to this patient?

A. Sublingual nitroglycerin (NTG)

B. Intravenous nitroglycerin

C. Aspirin

D. Atropine

E. Heparin

6.2. Which of the following ECG findings are consistent with this patient's infarction?

A. Elevation of V_1, V_2, V_3

B. Elevation of I, aVL, V_5, V_6

C. Depression of II, III, and aVF

D. Elevation of II, III, and aVF

E. Depression of V_1, V_2, and V_3

6.3. Which coronary artery is usually responsible for the inferior MI?

A. Left circumflex

B. Right coronary

C. Left anterior descending

Answers and Explanations

1. C. In a patient with a high likelihood of pulmonary embolism (PE) with abnormal vital signs, securing the airway, followed by thrombolysis, is the only acceptable choice. A hemodynamically unstable patient should NOT be sent for diagnostic testing. Heparin does not dissolve an existing thrombus and is most useful in preventing further clot formation. Aspirin is not indicated for either acute PE or prevention of recurrent PE or deep venous thrombosis (DVT).

2. C. The most common findings on electrocardiogram (ECG) in this disease are sinus tachycardia and occasionally, ST-T wave changes. Hampton's hump (a wedge-shaped pleural density) and Westermark's sign (a thickening of the pulmonary vasculature) are rare, late findings in pulmonary embolism (PE). The use of a D-dimer test, accompanied by a low clinical probability of PE, is highly sensitive in ruling out the disease. There are a number of D-dimer tests on the market, mostly latex agglutination tests, which are less sensitive. The enzyme-linked immunosorbent assay (ELISA) method of running this test, which is more expensive and time consuming, is not readily available in all centers. The drawback of spiral computed tomography (CT) is that it misses small, subsegmental emboli. The morbidity related to these emboli is still controversial. Rarely one may see evidence of acutely elevated pulmonary artery pressures (i.e., new onset atrial fibrillation or ST depressions in the anterior leads resulting from compression of the right coronary artery by the right ventricle). Most PEs originate from deep venous thromboses (DVTs); thus the lower extremity ultrasound examination is often positive. Most chest x-ray films in patients with PE are completely normal.

3.1. C. Tension pneumothorax occurs when so much air is trapped outside the lung parenchyma, but inside the lung cavity, that the mediastinal contents are physically shifted to the opposite side of the chest cavity. The pressure on the left atrium reduces filling pressures, resulting in backup of flow, hence the jugular venous distension and hypotension. The lung collapse is responsible for the hypoxia. Pericardial tamponade would produce hypotension but does not affect the lung sounds. Hemothorax would produce decreased lung sounds and hypotension; however, this volume is not sufficient to cause tracheal deviation. Traumatic rupture of the aortic arch typically does not produce tracheal deviation on physical examination.

3.2. B. The patient has a pneumothorax and will require chest tube thoracostomy; however, because

he is unstable, it is much faster to do a needle decompression of the chest to alleviate the tension on the mediastinum. This provides you with adequate time to do the chest tube thoracostomy with a patient who is more stable. Needle decompression is a temporizing measure. Depending on its success, the patient may indeed "stabilize," but this is not a given. Although cardiac tamponade will cause decreased filling of the left atrium and resultant hypotension, tachycardia, and jugular venous distension, it would not cause a decrease in breath sounds or hypoxia, which is due to the pneumothorax; therefore, pericardiocentesis is not the correct answer. Although fluids and/or blood are used to resuscitate trauma patients who are in shock, clearly the primary concern for this patient is tension pneumothorax, and this is the first issue to be approached. He may well have blood in his chest cavity and require resuscitation, but the decompression is of primary importance.

4. C. Although troponin I is a sensitive assay for destroyed myocardial cells, a single measure does not rule out the possibility of an acute myocardial infarction (MI). Furthermore, a patient may be experiencing unstable angina, in which case the troponin I would be normal in a patient who has significant and dangerous cardiac disease. ST-segment elevation greater than 1 mm in two contiguous leads is sufficient evidence to treat for an acute MI. Cardiac catheterization has been shown to produce better results in reinfarction and mortality if performed within 90 minutes of presentation. It eliminates the risk of significant intracranial hemorrhage that is brought about by using thrombolytics. Although studies are attempting to link coronary thrombosis to infectious agents, there are still no indications for antibiotics in acute coronary syndromes. Aspirin, β-blockers, nitroglycerin, and heparin are all used in an acute MI.

5. A. Focus on getting the patient pain free in the emergency department. Then, admit the patient to a low-risk chest pain unit where he can be monitored, ruled out for acute coronary syndromes, and receive cardiac testing to assess for coronary artery disease. Although the chest pain history given by the patient is somewhat atypical for acute coronary syndrome, he has an abnormal electrocardiogram (ECG) with chest pain. Cardiac chest pain may be reproducible, and the patient may have unstable angina, which would produce normal cardiac laboratory values, but it is still an entity requiring urgent testing.

6.1. C. This patient is having an acute myocardial infarction (MI) with bradycardia and hypotension. Aspirin is the first medication that should be given, for three reasons. First, it has no hemodynamic consequences and, therefore, can be given even in the hypotensive patient. It does not require an intravenous (IV) catheter, which means it can be given quickly without waiting for an IV line to be established. Finally, it has been shown to improve outcome in patients with acute MI, particularly when given early. Nitroglycerin (NTG) would be dangerous with a blood pressure of only 90/50 mm Hg. Atropine is not indicated with a heart rate of 50 beats/minute. The patient should receive a bolus of normal saline to see if there is

improvement in the blood pressure. Heparin is indicated; however, it is not a first-line medication in the treatment of acute MI.

6.2. D. An acute inferior myocardial infarction (MI) has the pattern of elevation of the ST segments of limb leads II, III, and aVF. Depression is a sign of ischemia not infarction. ST elevation in leads V_1, V_2, and V_3 is consistent with an anterior MI, and ST elevation in leads I, aVL, V_5, and V_6 is consistent with a lateral infarction.

6.3. B. The right coronary artery supplies the atrioventricular (AV) node and inferior wall of the left ventricle in most patients. In a small percentage of patients, the left circumflex artery will supply these areas. The left anterior descending artery is responsible for the anterior and anterolateral walls of the left ventricle and most of the intraventricular septum.

Shortness of Breath

How art thou out of breath, when thou hast breath to say to me that thou art out of breath?

William Shakespeare

INTRODUCTION
Ron Medzon, MD and Elizabeth L. Mitchell, MD

Section Editors

We spend most of our lives entirely unaware that we are breathing. Dyspnea is a subjective, unpleasant sensation that we are having difficulty breathing. Breathing is normally an unconscious activity, and, when respiration is impaired, the patient suddenly becomes aware of breathing, experiencing it as anything from mild discomfort to feelings of suffocation. Shortness of breath can be both chronic and acute and can run the spectrum from life threatening to slight breathlessness.

Breathing is a complex, multifactorial activity. Impairment can occur in ventilation (the work of breathing), perfusion to and from the lungs, metabolic function, or the central nervous system (CNS). Derangement in any component may lead to the sensation of dyspnea.

The medulla oblongata in the brain is the central respiratory control center. It interprets information from the afferent sensors and determines the respiratory rate. There is a pneumotaxic center in the pons that switches inspiration to expiration. There are cortical elements that can override the medulla sending their commands via the corticobulbar and corticospinal tracts and change the respiratory pattern.

There are many sensors for respiration. There are chemoreceptors that lie in the CNS situated near the medulla that respond primarily to changes in the partial pressure of carbon dioxide in the blood (pCO_2). Peripheral chemoreceptors in the carotid bodies, chest wall, airways, and lungs are stimulated by a drop in arterial partial pressure of oxygen (PaO_2). There are also various stretch receptors that can stabilize the chest wall in response to lung volume changes and chemoreceptors that can detect noxious stimuli. Most of the information is carried to the brain via the vagus nerve, through the carotid body and carotid sinus, through the glossopharyngeal nerve, and on to the medulla.

The efferent pathways control the muscles of respiration. The phrenic nerve (C3 to C5) is the only motor neuronal connection to the diaphragm, and it also conducts sensory information from the diaphragm back to the brain. The intercostal muscles receive their motor stimuli via the thoracic nerves (T1 to T12). The scalene muscles elevate the sternum and ribs 1 and 2 via fourth through eighth cervical nerve roots (C4 to C8). The sternocleidomastoid muscle receives its innervation via the spinal accessory nerve (cranial nerve [CN] XI).

Respiration is a complex multilevel process involving central medulla monitoring of pCO_2, which can be overridden by the cortex when necessary. The peripheral levels of oxygen as monitored in the carotid bodies are integrated with this, while the intercostal muscles keep watch on chest wall tension. This sensory information is processed in the brain, and the effectors keep the muscles of respiration in a smooth, cyclical pattern in the healthy individual. Any disturbance in pCO_2 or PaO_2 detected by the chemosensors, or any disease process that affects the pulmonary muscles, will send a ripple through the fine-tuned neurological circuit indicating an imbalance has occurred.

Emergency department management of the patient with dyspnea must always begin with evaluation of airway, breathing, and circulation (the ABCs). Protecting the airway and assisting ventilation may be the first step in managing a patient with respiratory distress, with diagnosis coming later.

This section explores a few common disease processes that cause dyspnea, their pathophysiology, and the clinical approach to their diagnosis and treatment.

CHAPTER 8

Congestive Heart Failure

Ron Medzon, MD

Clinical Scenario

A 72-year-old woman presents to the emergency department (ED) complaining of acute shortness of breath. She states that she was in her usual state of health until 15 minutes before calling for the ambulance, when, while walking vigorously, she had sudden onset of left substernal chest pressure, radiating to her left jaw and left arm. She became light-headed, broke out into a cold sweat, and began to have difficulty catching her breath. She describes the chest pain as feeling like her usual angina. She has a history of mild heart failure. She does not have difficulty lying flat in bed at night, nocturia, or paroxysmal nocturnal dyspnea (PND). Past medical history is significant for prior myocardial infarction (MI), angina, mild congestive heart failure (CHF), adult-onset diabetes, and hypertension. She currently takes an aspirin a day, furosemide, diltiazem, glyburide, and occasional acetaminophen for pain.

Physical examination reveals a 72-year-old woman in moderate to severe respiratory distress. She is using accessory muscles to breathe while sitting upright in the stretcher. Vital signs are blood pressure (BP) of 180/105 mm Hg; heart rate (HR) of 104 beats/minute; temperature of 98.7°F; respiratory rate of 36 times/minute; and oxygen saturation of 89% on room air, 94% on a non-rebreathing oxygen mask. Pertinent positive findings are crackles heard on lung examination two-thirds from the bases bilaterally and an S_3 gallop on heart auscultation. There is no jugular venous distension (JVD) or peripheral cyanosis. There is mild peripheral edema.

She is continued on a non-rebreathing oxygen facemask. An intravenous (IV) line is placed in her left arm. Continuous pulse oximetry and continuous cardiac monitoring are instituted. An electrocardiogram (ECG) and stat portable chest x-ray examination are ordered. While she is in the ED, 80 mg of furosemide are administered IV, 325 mg of aspirin (ASA) po (orally) is given, and 0.4 mg sublingual nitroglycerin (NTG) tablets are administered every 5 minutes for three doses.

The patient states that the chest pressure has resolved and her breathing has eased somewhat. Chest x-ray examination reveals Kerley B lines and infiltrates consistent with acute pulmonary edema. ECG revealed ST-segment depressions in the precordial leads, which have returned to baseline on repeat ECG after the pain has resolved. The patient is admitted to a telemetry unit where an MI is ruled out. During her hospital stay, she successfully undergoes cardiac catheterization to reopen an occluded coronary artery and is discharged 2 days later on an adjusted regimen of cardiac medications.

Clinical Evaluation

Introduction

Heart failure occurs when the heart as a pump cannot keep up with the blood supply demands of the body. The clinical scenario describes a patient who experienced acute pulmonary edema and heart failure from an acute episode of cardiac ischemia. The Framingham Heart Study shows that the 5-year mortality for heart failure is 50%, highlighting the seriousness of the illness. The prognosis depends on the person's exercise tolerance, ejection fraction, heart size on chest x-ray examination, plasma norepinephrine levels, and presence of ventricular arrhythmias.

History

This clinical scenario demonstrates many of the classic features of a person who is experiencing ischemic chest pain leading to acute heart failure. For a patient whose cardiac function exists in a tenuous equilibrium, an ischemic event can compromise the forward flow of blood, resulting in fluid quickly backing up into the lungs. The patient then experiences acute shortness of breath.

Questioning should be directed toward all possible precipitants of heart failure such as ischemia and angina, systemic hypertension, systemic infection, dietary indiscretion (high sodium), and dysrhythmia. You should ask if the patient has had cardiac surgery or catheterization recently. Exploration of the patient's medications may also provide additional information. For example, furosemide is a diuretic, diltiazem is an antihypertensive, and glyburide is an oral hypoglycemic agent. You can infer that she has hypertension and diabetes and may have a history of heart failure or fluid overload.

Orthopnea is dyspnea experienced when lying down. When supine, there is increased venous return to the heart, which increases diastolic pressure and can lead to pulmonary congestion. PND is breathlessness that causes the patient to be awakened from sleep. When supine, venous pressure in the legs decreases. Interstitial fluid is reabsorbed into the circulation, which increases plasma volume. Nocturia (waking at night to void) is caused by the same physiological mechanism as PND. You should also ask the patient if he or she has noticed increased leg swelling or recent weight gain, which are evidence of fluid retention. This is particularly helpful in the patient who has had CHF in the past and is on diuretic therapy.

Physical Examination

Initial evaluation begins with the vital signs and the general appearance of the patient.

Tachycardia, tachypnea, low oxygen saturation on pulse oximetry, and extreme hypertension are all abnormal signs that alert you to a potentially very ill patient. Patients may appear sweaty, ashen, or fatigued merely from the exertion of trying to breathe. These patients need immediate attention.

The physical examination should focus primarily on the heart and lungs. The cardiac examination may reveal a third heart sound, an S_3, also called a gallop. This is heard shortly after the second heart sound and is caused by the blood striking the left ventricle, which is noncompliant and is suddenly restricting blood flow. Acute rupture of the papillary muscles in MI reveals the murmur of mitral regurgitation. A loud diastolic murmur may indicate aortic regurgitation, which can present with pulmonary edema. Displaced point of maximal impulse by palpating the chest wall indicates cardiomegaly.

Inspiratory crackles on lung examination are sometimes referred to as rales and reflect alveolar flooding. Interstitial edema causes narrowing of the airways, and it is not uncommon for bronchoconstriction to occur with wheezing evident on physical examination. JVD is measured by having the patient lying at 30 degrees in the stretcher and measuring the column of blood from the right atrium (angle of Louis, or second costochondral line) to the highest visible pulsation of the internal jugular vein. Hepatojugular reflux can be assessed while the patient is still in this recumbent position. The examiner applies pressure in the patient's right upper quadrant, taking care that the patient is relaxed and not performing a Valsalva maneuver that elevates the right-sided pressures and causes JVD. Elevated right-sided pressures are transmitted via the inferior vena cava through the superior vena cava and into the jugular veins.

In addition, it is important to look for other signs of fluid retention, such as peripheral pitting edema.

Diagnostic Evaluation

Continuous pulse oximetry is used to monitor the patient's oxygenation using the light

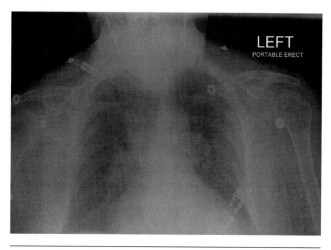

Figure 8.1
X-ray film of a patient with congestive heart failure. Interstitial pulmonary edema appears on the x-ray film as an increase in the number and size of upper lobe blood vessels. The vessel margins are blurred and indistinct because the interstitium is retaining fluid.

absorption spectra of oxyhemoglobin to calculate saturation of hemoglobin with oxygen. An ECG is obtained for evidence of ischemia, infarction, or arrhythmia.

A chest x-ray film should be obtained (Fig. 8.1). Interstitial pulmonary edema appears on a x-ray examination as an increase in the number and size of upper lobe blood vessels. The vessel margins are not sharp. Instead, they are blurred and indistinct because the interstitium retains fluid. Small pleural effusions may be evident. The cardiac silhouette is enlarged, if the disease is chronic. There may be Kerley A and Kerley B lines, which are irregular, coarse, thin, linear densities usually present in the upper lobes but also visible in other parts of the lungs. They are produced by abnormal amounts of edema fluid that have collected in the lymphatic system because of the elevated pulmonary venous pressure. Alveolar pulmonary edema occurs when the pulmonary venous pressure is greater than 30 mm Hg. Radiographically, there is almost complete obliteration of the vascular markings. There is a coarse alveolar pattern that may coalesce, and there may be pleural effusions not only at the costophrenic angles but also in the interlobar fissures. There may be a

"butterfly" pattern to the infiltrate, extending out from the hilum on either side.

Useful laboratory data include a complete blood cell count (CBC), electrolytes, and blood urea nitrogen (BUN)/creatinine levels. Electrolyte values are particularly useful in the patient taking diuretics, because patients may become hypokalemic and hyponatremic. When cardiac ischemia is suspected, a sample for creatinine phosphokinase (CPK), myocardial-specific CPK (CPK-MB) and troponin should be obtained. An arterial blood gas examination may be helpful in evaluating the patient who does not appear to be responding, remains persistently hypoxic, or is fatiguing. The clinical scenario dictates the need for additional testing.

B-natriuretic peptide (BNP) is secreted by the left ventricle in response to an elevated left ventricular pressure resulting from volume overload. Studies have shown that an elevated BNP level may be helpful to differentiate those patients in whom you cannot tell clinically whether they are clearly having a pulmonary respiratory issue such as chronic obstructive pulmonary disease (COPD) versus a CHF exacerbation. Thus, the treatment of a patient with unexplained shortness of

Table 8.1.

Differential diagnosis for congestive heart failure

Cardiogenic Causes	Noncardiogenic Causes
Acute myocardial infarction (MI)	Sepsis
Ischemia	Shock
Valvular disease	Toxins and drugs
Cardiomyopathy	Neurogenic
Hypertensive emergency	High altitude
	Aspiration syndrome
	Fat embolism syndrome

Table 8.2.

Treatment of congestive heart failure (CHF)

All Patients with CHF
IV access
Oxygen: non-rebreather facemask
Cardiac monitor
Continuous pulse oximetry
ECG
Portable chest x-ray examination
Test for arterial blood gas?
Intubation necessary?
Furosemide IV
Sublingual nitroglycerin $+/-$ nitroglycerin IV
Sodium nitroprusside (if unresponsive to nitrates or severe hypertension)
Morphine sulfate IV

Patients with Arrhythmia
Checking of digitalis level
Correction of abnormal electrolyte (K^+, Mg^{2+}) levels
Amiodarone for atrial fibrillation and ventricular arrhythmia

Patients with Cardiogenic Shock
All of the above
Intubation
Dopamine
Dobutamine (in acute MI)
Intraaortic balloon counterpulsation if other modes fail (for patients with reversible cause CHF or as bridge to transplant)
Thrombolysis or urgent cardiac catheterization if MI suspected

ECG, electrocardiogram; IV, intravenous; MI, myocardial infarction.

breath and no history of CHF may be dramatically altered if the BNP level was elevated. The BNP level can increase considerably in those patients with pulmonary embolism; thus, it is not a definitive assay for CHF.

Differential Diagnosis

The differential diagnosis for CHF is illustrated in Table 8.1.

Treatment

A patient who is short of breath and hypoxic is treated initially with the following interventions irrespective of underlying diagnosis (Table 8.2). A facemask with 100% oxygen is placed, preferably with a non-rebreather bag to maximize the concentration of oxygen delivered. At least one large-bore IV catheter is placed so medications can be given quickly. Blood specimens are often drawn out of the IV catheter to be sent for laboratory tests. The larger bore IVs decrease the chances of shearing on the blood sample, which causes hemolysis and affects the results of some electrolyte levels. The patient is placed on continuous cardiac monitoring and continuous pulse oximetry. Urine output is essential to follow fluid status. If necessary, place a Foley catheter. Order a stat portable chest x-ray examination and ECG. A blood gas may be useful to determine how hypoxic and acidotic the patient has become.

If the patient is still short of breath despite the facemask, an attempt at continuous positive airway pressure (CPAP) by means of a tight-fitting mask is a stopgap measure that may avoid the need to intubate the patient. Assessing the need for intubation is a clinical call, which is aided by the data you have collected from your clinical assessment and laboratory tests. These include the following:

- A pO_2 less than 60 mm despite 100% oxygen by facemask

- Persistently elevated respiratory rate and patient fatigue

- Evidence of end-organ hypoperfusion (shock) including change in mental status, poor urine output, cool and clammy skin
- BP less than 90 mm Hg
- A rising pCO_2
- Worsening acidosis

Drugs to treat heart failure should optimally decrease both preload and afterload, be easy to titrate, and have a low toxicity profile. The following medications are used to treat acute CHF.

Morphine Sulfate

Morphine is a narcotic medication that is a sympatholytic. It causes peripheral vasodilatation, decreasing central venous return, which decreases preload. It also decreases HR, BP, and contractility, which decrease myocardial oxygen consumption. It also relieves the anxiety associated with having difficulty breathing.

Nitrates

Nitrates act intracellularly to stimulate guanosine 3′,5′-cyclic monophosphate (cGMP). This induces the sarcoplasmic reticulum to sequester calcium. In turn, there is relaxation of vascular smooth muscle. In lower doses, it acts primarily as a venodilator, decreasing preload, which is good for treating acute pulmonary edema. In higher doses intravenously, NTG causes arteriolar dilation, which decreases both afterload and BP. Therefore, forward pumping action is enhanced while decreasing oxygen demand simultaneously. An added benefit is that NTG also acts directly on the coronary arteries to dilate them. If administered sublingually, a tablet lasts 30 minutes; the spray, which is commonly used on ambulances, lasts 2 hours. Although transcutaneous NTG is thought to provide a sustained release of drug, it is not recommended by the American Heart Association for the treatment of acute heart failure. In acute pulmonary edema, the patient clamps down peripherally, so there is likely suboptimal absorption of medications through the skin, and this should be kept in mind. IV NTG can easily be titrated to BP and desired effect, and IV is an excellent route of administration. The drips are usually started at 10 to 20 µg/kg/minute. The patient with angina typically require 50 to 90 µg/kg/minute, and a patient with a hypertensive urgency may require as much as 200 to 300 µg/kg/minute. Nitrates should be avoided in right ventricular MI.

Loop Diuretics

Furosemide and bumetanide inhibit resorption of sodium at the ascending loop of Henle. This increases the renal sodium and water excretion and lowers the plasma volume, thereby decreasing preload and pulmonary congestion. Their onset of action is 5 to 10 minutes; however, clinically an effect is seen earlier than this. This is believed to be caused by a humoral change induced by the diuretic. The dose in acute pulmonary edema is 1 mg/kg in hypertensive patients. In patients with abrupt onset of heart failure, the cause may not be related to volume overload, and in these cases diuretics will not help. Potassium and magnesium are excreted in higher concentrations, and those levels must be checked if patients are placed on diuretics. Diuretics are to be avoided in right ventricular MI.

Nitroprusside

Nitroprusside is a potent direct smooth muscle relaxant. It is administered by continuous infusion and requires continuous BP monitoring. It reduces both preload and afterload. It is the drug of choice in acute pulmonary edema in the setting of a hypertensive crisis. Its side effects include hypotension, and patients with renal failure may experience cyanide toxicity.

Digitalis

Digitalis is a cardiac glycoside, which acts by blocking sodium-potassium adenosine triphosphatase (ATPase) in the myocardial membrane. This increases intracellular calcium and increases the slow inward Ca^{2+} current during the myocardial action potential. The effect of these actions is to increase myocardial contractility (positive inotrope) and to slow the HR (negative chronotrope), both advantageous in CHF. Any patient known to be taking digitalis should have a level checked. Recent studies of heart failure patients in sinus rhythm do not benefit from digitalis and may have an increased mortality rate. Digitalis should be reserved for patients refractory to other CHF-related medications.

Class III Antiarrhythmic Drugs

The class III antiarrhythmic drugs, bretylium, amiodarone, and sotalol, all act to prolong the cardiac action potential duration. Amiodarone has been extensively studied in ventricular arrhythmias, and data also indicate it is a safe antiarrhythmic for patients with atrial fibrillation who are in CHF.

Treatment for Cardiogenic Shock

Cardiogenic shock is defined by pulmonary congestion, hypotension, and decreased peripheral perfusion. Initial therapy includes 500 mL of IV normal saline run over 1 hour. If the patient is low on volume, this measure will help temporarily. If the patient is volume overloaded, then the other interventions you will use will take care of the small excess of fluid that you have introduced.

Intraarterial balloon pumps are used as temporizing measures in patients in shock. If a definitive treatment can reverse the cause of heart failure, it should be provided urgently. These include cardiac catheterization and/or thrombolysis for acute MI and urgent valve replacement in patients with mitral regurgitation after papillary muscle rupture in acute MI, for example.

Dopamine

Dopamine is a naturally occurring catecholamine, which is a precursor to norepinephrine. It exhibits dose-dependent effects. At 2 to 5 µg/kg/minute, its effect is primarily on the receptors in the kidney. It causes renal vasodilatation and increases urine output. At 5 to 15 µg/kg/minute, its effect is on β-adrenergic receptors, which increase cardiac contractility and increase the HR. Pulmonary artery opening pressure may decrease secondary to better ejection fraction and peripheral vasodilation. At greater than 15 µg/kg/minute, its effect is to vasoconstrict all vascular beds, similar to norepinephrine. Therefore, increasing doses of dopamine can increase the HR and cause peripheral vasoconstriction, which may precipitate ischemia or arrhythmia. Adding NTG when high doses of dopamine are used may help.

Dobutamine

Dobutamine is a synthetic catecholamine that stimulates the β-1 catecholamine receptor responsible for increasing HR and contractility. At doses of 5 to 25 µg/kg/minute, it acts as an inotrope and as a vasodilator. Dobutamine is effective in patients with MI, acute pulmonary edema, and left ventricular dysfunction.

Disposition

Few patients presenting with heart failure are stable enough to discharge after treatment in the ED. Patients with chronic heart failure who have had a recent dietary indiscretion (too much salty food) or have stopped their regular medication, for example, may respond to diuresis in the ED sufficiently to discharge them on their usual medications with an increased dose or with an additional medication, provided that their workup in the ED is negative. Any first time presentation of heart failure should be admitted for an evaluation of the cause of the failure.

Stable patients are patients whose oxygen saturation remains higher than 95% on 2 to 4 L/minute of oxygen delivered by nasal cannula. They can be admitted to a general medical floor. If there is no suspicion of underlying arrhythmia or ischemia, then they do not require telemetry. They need strict observation of fluid input and urinary output and daily weights to follow the success or failure of treatment. If ischemia or arrhythmia is suspected in an otherwise stable patient, then the patient should be placed on telemetry.

Patients who require intensive care are those whose oxygenation is inadequate despite oxygen and a trial of the treatment medications described previously or those who are on IV drips requiring frequent monitoring (e.g., NTG). Respiratory rates greater than 30 breaths/minute, oxygen saturations less than 90% despite oxygen, persistent hypoxia and acidosis on the blood gas analysis despite treatment, and evidence of ischemia on ECG are all signs that the patient is too ill to be admitted to the general medical floor. The decision to intubate can be made clinically by obvious respiratory fatigue in the patient, a pO_2 less than 60 mm, a rising pCO_2, worsening acidosis, or declining mental status.

Pathophysiology

Cardiogenic Pulmonary Edema

Cardiogenic pulmonary edema arises from acute MI, ischemia, cardiomyopathies, valvular disease, and hypertensive emergencies. The accumulation of fluid first in the pulmonary interstitium and then in the alveoli is described by the Starling equation:

Total Flow of Fluid
    = Hydrostatic Pressure Gradient
    − Osmotic Pressure Gradient

A balance between colloid osmotic pressure and hydrostatic pressure is what determines fluid and protein traffic across the pulmonary capillary membrane. The pulmonary circulation is a low-pressure system with a high-protein interstitium. In cardiogenic pulmonary edema, an increase in pulmonary capillary hydrostatic pressure forces the low-protein plasma ultrafiltrate across the pulmonary capillary membrane into the pulmonary interstitium. The immediate response of the body is to drain this excess fluid away from the lung via the lymphatic system. As one can imagine, this drainage can easily be overwhelmed, and the excess fluid accumulates inside the alveoli.

Preload

Preload refers to the force that stretches the myofibril before contraction. The amount of force in turn obviously depends on the health of the myocardium and the volume of blood that stretches the myocardium.

Contractility

Contractility (or inotropy) relates to the ability of the contractile proteins in the myocytes to generate force. The Frank-Starling relationship describes the intricate relationship between preload and contractility, that

is, the force of ventricular contraction is directly related to the end-diastolic length of cardiac muscle. The more the sarcomere is stretched, the better contact the actin-myosin filaments have, and the stronger the contraction. This logically holds true to a maximum stretch beyond which there is detriment to the ventricle's capacity to generate pumping force.

Afterload

Afterload is the amount of pressure that the heart as a pump must generate to create forward flow of blood. Put another way, it is the amount of tension placed on the wall of the myocardium during contraction. The amount of peripheral vascular resistance (PVR) against which the ventricle is trying to eject the blood and the size of the ventricular chamber determines the afterload. The PVR is a function of the cross-sectional area of the circulation and other factors such as blood viscosity.

The BP is a function of cardiac output (CO) and systemic vascular resistance (SVR):

$$BP = CO \times SVR$$

The body must maintain a BP sufficient to perfuse the vital organs. The failing heart is a low CO state. The body compensates by increasing SVR with peripheral vasoconstriction. The ventricle cannot overcome this high SVR and it begins to dilate. Initially, the Frank-Starling relationship holds and the heart compensates for its failure with the increased stroke volume (SV).

CO is a function of both SV and HR:

$$CO = HR \times SV$$

As you can see, the failing heart tries to maintain CO by increasing SV. When this fails, the HR increases. Because myocardial perfusion occurs in diastole, it becomes impaired by severe tachycardia, usually greater than 150 beats/minute. At the end of diastole, the atria contract producing a small ejection of blood into the ventricle, also known as the atrial "kick." At very fast HRs, the atrial kick is lost, and this has a significant impact on the failing heart.

The heart's primary compensation for pump failure is to hypertrophy. The number of myofibrils per cell increases. Initially, there is better contractility at a higher energy cost. The persistent volume overload leads to such hypertrophy that eventually the blood supply to the muscle tissue diminishes and there ensues myocyte death and fibrosis. Thus, what begins as compensation ends in destruction.

Humeral Response

When the heart goes into failure, the kidneys are underperfused. This decrease in glomerular filtration rate (GFR) decreases renal excretion of sodium. There is a reflex increase in renin release, leading to increased angiotensin I, which is converted into angiotensin II by angiotensin-converting enzyme. Angiotensin II is a potent vasoconstrictor that stimulates aldosterone release, causing an increase in sodium (and therefore water) retention.

In the central nervous system (CNS), heart failure stimulates the sympathetic nervous system and inhibits the parasympathetic nervous system. The pituitary releases arginine vasopressin (antidiuretic hormone), which increases contractility and renal water retention that lowers serum sodium concentrations.

The heart releases atrial natriuretic peptide in response to atrial stretch. This inhibits the activation of the renin-angiotensin axis, induces vasodilatation, and improves the sodium homeostasis by enabling salt wasting.

The true significance of identifying the pathophysiological process behind each patient with heart failure lies not in better "roundsmanship" but in tailoring the most effective treatment for the patient.

Coronary Artery Disease

Atherosclerotic coronary artery disease is the leading cause of heart failure in developing countries. The atherosclerotic plaque ruptures, and a thrombus forms, occluding the artery. The muscle distal to the occluded artery infarcts, leading to a focal abnormality of ventricle wall motion (dyskinesis). There is a resultant lowering of the ejection fraction, the ability of the ventricle to eject blood. Over time, the ventricle dilates, and there is reactive hypertrophy.

Cardiomyopathies

These disease states exclude coronary artery disease, valvular disease, and pericardial disease.

Dilated cardiomyopathy is the most common cardiomyopathy. Its etiology is most often unknown, but common causes include chronic alcohol abuse, viral damage, cocaine use, other toxins, and occasionally as a postpartum complication. Usually all four chambers are enlarged, and there is systolic pump dysfunction. Mural thrombi are frequent complications.

Hypertrophic cardiomyopathy is caused by hypertension, valvular disease, or aortic stenosis. It is familial in half of the cases. Anatomically there is left ventricular hypertrophy without enlargement of the ventricle's chamber. There is primarily diastolic dysfunction. In 25% of cases, the systolic motion of the anterior leaflet of the mitral valve moves in such a way that it obstructs normal outflow of blood. This creates a harsh systolic murmur heard at the left sternal border. It can present as exertional syncope but is frequently clinically silent.

Restrictive cardiomyopathy is cardiac muscle that is invaded by foreign materials such as iron (hemachromatosis), protein (amyloidosis), or granulomatous tissue (sarcoidosis). The cardiac chambers are stiff and experience abnormalities in diastole. Clinically, patients may experience ascites, congestive hepatomegaly, and peripheral edema.

Myocarditis

Myocarditis is an acute inflammatory reaction in the myocardium. Often it goes clinically unnoticed, but presents with dyspnea and fatigue, and usually resolves spontaneously. Rarely, patients experience life-threatening arrhythmias. The most common cause is viral. It may present with sinus tachycardia and symptoms similar to pericarditis, which include shortness of breath and discomfort while breathing (pleuritic chest pain). The chest x-ray film reveals an enlarged cardiac silhouette, and there may be ST-T changes on ECG. Some forms of myocarditis respond to steroid therapy.

Valvular Heart Disease

Acute valvular failure usually results in regurgitant blood flow. If the damage is severe, over time the retrograde portion of flow will cause pulmonary congestion and pulmonary edema. In acute MI, the papillary muscles are prone to rupture. If they do, the mitral valve is no longer anchored and mitral regurgitation ensues. Patients with bacterial endocarditis or aortic dissection may experience aortic insufficiency.

In patients with chronic valvular diseases, an accurate physical examination can help dictate appropriate treatment. Chronic mitral insufficiency is improved by vasodilator therapy. On the other hand, patients with aortic stenosis should not be given vasodilators because this can lead to syncope and inadequate coronary artery perfusion and MI.

The normal pericardial sac contains 20 mL of fluid and can accommodate up to 100 mL of pericardial fluid without hemodynamic compromise. Excess fluid accumulates in numerous clinical conditions including uremia, trauma, malignancy, infection, and rheumatological diseases. Patients experience shortness of breath, which typically worsens when supine. Physical examination reveals elevated jugular venous pressure, tachycardia, pulsus paradoxus, and hypoperfusion. In patients who are significantly compromised (that is, hypotensive), it may be necessary to perform pericardiocentesis, which is therapeutic and may be diagnostic in some cases. The least invasive, most accurate modality to diagnose the effusion is cardiac ultrasound.

Under the rubric of heart failure exist many subclasses of the disease. The following is a guide to the terminology and classification of different forms of heart failure.

High-Output Failure

High-output failure is a hyperdynamic state with supernormal CO. If the end-diastolic pressures are high, patients may experience pulmonary congestion and peripheral edema. Diastolic dysfunction eventually leads to systolic dysfunction, and CO is compromised. Clinical situations that can cause this include beriberi, hyperthyroidism, anemia, arteriovenous (AV) fistula, pregnancy, cirrhosis, and Paget's disease.

Low-Output Failure

We have discussed previously the conditions that lead to heart failure as a result of low-output states. Clinical entities include ischemic heart disease, valvular heart disease, and cardiomyopathy.

Acute Heart Failure

Acute heart failure is the sudden onset of symptoms, usually leading to an ED visit, which are most often secondary to ischemic or valvular malfunction.

Chronic Heart Failure

Patients with chronic heart failure experience symptoms of fluid retention, but perfusion is compensated. Patients experience gradual decline in cardiac function, including a slow decline in exercise tolerance resulting from shortness of breath and progressively worsening peripheral edema. Examples include post-MI patients and those with dilated cardiomyopathy.

Right-Sided Heart Failure

The differentiation between right- and left-sided heart failure is somewhat contrived, because obviously the circulation is a closed circuit in which right and left sides are intimately related. Clinical signs of right-sided heart failure include passive congestion of the lungs and hepatomegaly. Patients are short of breath, but physical examination reveals clear lung fields.

Left-Sided Heart Failure

Patients with left-sided heart failure present with shortness of breath on exertion and have passive congestion of the lungs. Physical examination reveals crackles and possibly an S_3 gallop. Chest x-ray examination demonstrates pulmonary venous congestion, Kerley B lines, and cephalization, which is evidence of pulmonary venous congestion.

Forward Heart Failure

Forward heart failure refers to inadequate systemic perfusion resulting from low CO. Symptoms of weakness, oliguria, fatigue, and prerenal azotemia may be present. Patients with advanced cases demonstrate hypotension and shock.

Backward Heart Failure

The term "backward heart failure" refers to the symptoms caused by backward pressure that builds up behind a failing chamber. Patients may have pulmonary edema, extremity edema, and hepatomegaly.

Systolic Dysfunction

Systolic dysfunction refers to a situation of impaired contractility leading to a decrease in stroke output and forward flow of blood. It is caused by myocyte death, as seen in MI and myocarditis.

Diastolic Dysfunction

Diastolic dysfunction is a scenario in which the ventricles are unable to relax and fill normally. Often systolic function is maintained, as is the case with hypertrophic and restrictive cardiomyopathy. Chronic valvular disease, hypertension, and aortic stenosis can cause diastolic dysfunction. Impaired relaxation of the myocardium leads to higher filling pressures and later congestive symptoms. Because patients usually have intact myocardium, treatment is aimed at decreasing myocardial oxygen demand with the use of β-blockers or calcium channel blockers.

Suggested Readings

Coodley E. Newer drug therapy for CHF. *Arch Intern Med* 1999;159:1177–1183.

Francis GS, et al. Comparative hemodynamic effects of dopamine and dobutamine in patients with acute cardiogenic circulatory collapse. *Am Heart J* 1982;103:995–1000.

Morrison LK, et al. Utility of a rapid B-natriuretic peptide assay in differentiating congestive heart failure from lung disease in patients presenting with dyspnea. *J Am Coll Cardiol* 2002;39:202–209.

Singh SN, Fletcher RD. Symptomatic systolic ventricular failure. *Curr Cardiol Rep* 1999;1:20–28.

Singh SN, et al. Amiodarone in patients with congestive heart failure and asymptomatic ventricular arrhythmia. Survival trial of antiarrhythmic therapy in congestive heart failure. *N Engl J Med* 1995;333:77–82.

Wiliams JF, et al. Guidelines for the evaluation and management of heart failure. Report of the American College of Cardiology/American Heart Association Task Force on Practice Guidelines (Committee on Evaluation and Management of Heart Failure). *Circulation* 1995;92:2764–2784.

9

Asthma

Rebecca Tipton, MD

Clinical Scenario

A 25-year-old woman with a history of asthma presents to the emergency department (ED) in respiratory distress. She is sitting upright and can speak in only two-word sentences. Her friend states she was exposed to a cat today. She has used her albuterol nebulizer machine at home without relief. She has been hospitalized for her asthma several times, most recently 6 months ago, and required intubation once about 5 years ago. Her usual triggers are change in weather, infection, and cats. She has not been on corticosteroids recently.

Her past medical history is otherwise unremarkable. Her medications include nebulized albuterol and an inhaled corticosteroid. She denies any drug allergies or illicit drug use. She does smoke half a pack of cigarettes a day.

On examination, she is in severe respiratory distress, diaphoretic, and anxious and is using accessory muscles to breathe. Her vital signs include a temperature of 99.1°F, blood pressure of 150/80 mm Hg, heart rate of 125 beats/minute, respiratory rate of 34 breaths/minute, and arterial oxygen saturation (SaO_2) of 90% on room air. On lung examination, she has decreased air movement with minimal wheezing and an inspiratory to expiratory ratio (I:E ratio) of 1:3. No rales or rhonchi are appreciated. On cardiac examination, she is tachycardic with no murmurs, rubs, or gallops. The abdomen is soft and nontender. Extremities show no edema.

A peak expiratory flow shows only 150 L/minute with good effort. She is immediately begun on an albuterol nebulizer treatment and oxygen.

The patient is having a severe asthma exacerbation. She has a history of severe asthma requiring intubation and presents in respiratory distress with tachycardia, tachypnea, decreased air movement, and an increased expiratory phase. She will require rapid treatment with oxygen, nebulized albuterol and ipratropium bromide, and steroids, and may require mechanical ventilation with an intensive care admission.

Clinical Evaluation

Introduction

Asthma is a very common disease, affecting 4% to 8% of adults in the United States. Despite increased understanding of the disease and the availability of new treatment options, asthma mortality rates have increased 40% from 1982 to 1991. Asthma will continue to be a common disease treated in the ED. In addition to providing treatment, the emergency physician must be able to identify a patient in impending respiratory failure, assess response to treatment, and ultimately decide if a patient can be safely discharged to home or requires admission to the hospital.

History

Symptoms of asthma include cough, wheezing, dyspnea, and chest tightness, as seen in this clinical scenario. The history of a patient who is wheezing and dyspneic can be difficult to obtain. A complete history is often deferred until treatment has been initiated. By obtaining certain components of the history, the severity of the asthma exacerbation can be more completely understood. The duration of symptoms helps determine if this process is acute, subacute, or chronic. A subacute or chronic course may incite a prolonged inflammatory response. The subjective severity of dyspnea is often helpful. A patient may be able to characterize the attack as mild, moderate, or severe in comparison with past exacerbations.

Identifying inciting causes or triggers in past exacerbations and recent exposure to those triggers can help explain the cause for the attack and identify specific environments to avoid. Common triggers for patients with asthma include respiratory infection, change in weather, allergens such as pollen or animal dander, cigarette smoke, chemical fumes, aspirin or nonsteroidal anti-inflammatory drug (NSAID) use, and exercise. A history of prior hospitalizations, ED visits, and need for intubation help characterize the severity of the patient's illness. Current or recent steroid use may indicate a severe unresponsive asthma exacerbation. Frequency of medication use can also clarify the severity of disease and help guide treatment in the ED. For example, a patient who has used his or her albuterol inhaler every 5 minutes for the past hour and is still wheezing is more worrisome than one who has used an inhaler twice in the past day. Other medical problems are important to determine, including cardiac history, diabetes, and pregnancy, because these patients may require further diagnostic tests, altered treatments, closer follow-up, or change in disposition.

Medication allergies, cigarette smoking, and illicit drug use are important components of the history. Finally, it is helpful to record the patient's best peak flow reading so that it can be compared to readings obtained during the current exacerbation.

Physical Examination

The severity of an exacerbation is often apparent by the general appearance of a patient. A patient who is having a mild exacerbation may look comfortable and be able to talk in full sentences. However, a patient having a severe attack may be anxious, diaphoretic, sitting forward, talking in one- or two-word sentences, or using accessory muscles to breathe. As a patient worsens, his or her mental status may decline and he or she may become tired, confused, or lethargic. A pediatric patient may present with grunting, nasal flaring, and supraclavicular and intercostal muscle retractions.

Vital signs are often abnormal in an exacerbation. An increased temperature may indicate an infection. Blood pressure, heart rate, and respiratory rate are often elevated. A heart rate of 120 beats/minute or higher, a respiratory rate of greater than 30 breaths/minute, or a SaO_2 on room air of less than 91% are all signs of a severe exacerbation.

Examination of the ears, nose, and throat may reveal an infectious cause for the exacerbation. On lung examination, breath sounds and wheezing should be equal in lung fields. Wheezing in one area indicates a separate process from asthma, such as foreign body aspiration, pneumonia, or neoplasm. The loudness of the wheezing can range from a mild end-expiratory wheeze to a more severe loud wheeze throughout inhalation and exhalation. A patient who is in near respiratory arrest may have no wheeze on auscultation resulting from the lack of air movement. The I:E ratio is normally about 1:1, although patients with asthma have a longer expiratory time. In a severe exacerbation, the I:E ratio can be 1:3 or higher. Auscultation of rales or rhonchi may indicate another cause for symptoms, such as congestive heart failure (CHF) or pneumonia. Finally, a complete cardiac examination should document any abnormal sounds, and an extremity examination should note any cyanosis or edema.

Documenting the presence or absence of pulsus paradoxus may be valuable in determining the severity of disease. Normally, there is a decrease in systolic blood pressure on inspiration of less than 10 mm Hg. In a moderate to severe asthma exacerbation, there is a greater decrease in blood pressure with inspiration, with values of 12 to 30 mm Hg. To perform this test, have the patient breathe quietly. Slowly lower the pressure of the blood pressure cuff and note the level when the first sounds are heard, which will be on expiration. Lower the cuff pressure again slowly until the sounds can be heard throughout the respiratory cycle. The difference of the two is the pulsus paradoxus. A pulsus paradoxus of 12 to 30 mm Hg can be seen in asthma and in other entities including pericardial tamponade and emphysema.

Diagnostic Evaluation

In general, very few diagnostic tests are needed when a patient with known asthma presents with an asthma exacerbation to the ED. One test that is useful in all cases of asthma is a peak expiratory flow rate (PEFR), or peak flow. The PEFR is measured by having a patient take a deep breath then forcefully exhaling into a portable peak flow meter. The resultant number is the measure of the maximal airflow rate achieved. This test gives an objective assessment of airflow and the degree of bronchospasm but is limited by patient effort. Some patients know their best peak flow; alternatively, basic reference charts of predicted peak flow values based on age, sex, and height may be used. In general, a normal PEFR is 450 to 600 L/minute in men and 350 to 500 L/minute in women. You can compare the patient's peak flow in the ED to his or her personal best or best-predicted PEFR. The value expressed as a percent can be used to assess the severity of the exacerbation and to monitor improvement with treatment. A peak flow less than 100 L/minute or less than 50% maximal indicates a severe exacerbation.

Obtaining an arterial blood gas (ABG) sample should be considered when a patient has severe respiratory distress, has a decrease in alertness, or is not responding to therapy. In moderate to severe exacerbations, the patient's respiratory rate increases. Respiratory alkalosis with a partial pressure of carbon dioxide (pCO_2) less than 35 mm occurs as the patient expires carbon dioxide. When the patient fatigues, the respiratory rate slows, and as the patient retains carbon dioxide, the pCO_2 normalizes and then rises. This may cause a carbon dioxide narcosis and a respiratory acidosis will develop. In addition to the respiratory acidosis, a metabolic acidosis may

occur because of lactic acid build up in respiratory muscles (hypoxia interferes with the breakdown of lactic acid to carbon dioxide and water). Thus, an ABG result showing acidosis, normal or elevated pCO_2, and/or low pO_2 is cause for concern, and intubation should be considered.

A chest x-ray examination is generally not recommended in known asthma exacerbations. A typical chest x-ray film in a patient with asthma may show hyperinflation. However, an x-ray film can be helpful when a patient has new-onset wheezing, evidence of infection on history or physical, or lack of response to therapy or when the diagnosis is not clear.

Blood test results are usually not helpful in the diagnosis or treatment of asthma. A complete blood count (CBC) may be useful as an indication of infection, although an increased white blood cell count can relate to recent corticosteroid use or increased stress. A low hematocrit indicates anemia, which can cause shortness of breath. Electrolyte levels generally are normal. Frequent β_2-agonist administration may cause hypokalemia, although this rarely produces any clinical effects. A glucose level may be elevated in patients with diabetes who are taking corticosteroids. A patient on theophylline may benefit from a theophylline level to monitor toxicity and guide therapy.

An electrocardiogram (ECG) can be considered in patients in severe respiratory distress, in older persons, or in patients with heart disease. A typical ECG in a patient with asthma shows sinus tachycardia.

Differential Diagnosis

The differential diagnosis for asthma is illustrated in Table 9.1.

Treatment

The goal of treatment in asthma is to promote bronchodilation and reverse inflammation to allow greater oxygenation and ventilation (Table 9.2). Medications such as oxygen, β_2-agonists, corticosteroids, and anticholinergics are used to reverse airflow obstruction and hypoxia.

Table 9.1.

Differential diagnosis of asthma (includes other causes of wheezing, dyspnea, cough, or chest tightness)

Chronic obstructive pulmonary disease
Foreign body aspiration
Pneumonia
Congestive heart failure/pulmonary edema
Pneumothorax
Anaphylaxis/allergic reaction
Upper airway obstruction
Pericarditis
Pericardial tamponade
Pulmonary embolism
Bronchitis
Valvular disease
Neoplasm
Acute respiratory distress syndrome
Ischemic chest pain

Table 9.2.

Treatment guidelines for asthma exacerbations

Mild to Moderate Exacerbation
Supplemental oxygen as needed to keep SaO_2 ≥ 95%
Nebulized albuterol (2.5–5.0 mg every 20 minutes)
Corticosteroids (60 mg po prednisone)
Antibiotics if infection suspected

Severe Exacerbation
Continuous pulse oximetry
Placement of IV catheter
CBC if infection suspected
Chest x-ray film, if infection suspected
Consideration of ABG sample
Continuous nebulized albuterol
Nebulized ipratropium bromide (0.5 mg)
Prednisolone 125-mg IV
Epinephrine 1:1000 (0.3–0.5 mg subcutaneous)
Theophylline, if the patient is taking the drug as an outpatient
Magnesium (2 g IV)
Heliox
Intubation for respiratory fatigue, falling O_2 saturation, and rising pCO_2 on ABG sample

ABG, arterial blood gas; CBC, complete blood count; IV, intravenous.

Oxygen is required to prevent hypoxia and should be administered to patients to maintain a SaO_2 of 95% or above.

Short-Acting β₂-Agonists

A short-acting β₂-agonist, most commonly albuterol, is the first-line agent used to relax bronchial smooth muscle. β₂-receptors relax airway smooth muscle and inhibit the release of bronchoconstricting substances from mast cells. The most common route used to deliver a β₂-agonist is by inhalation, because the medication can act directly on the β₂-receptors in the lung. Subcutaneous administration of terbutaline can be considered in a patient with severe asthma who is not breathing well and thus cannot receive adequate medication through inhalation.

In the ED, the most common β₂-agonist used for asthma exacerbations is short-acting inhaled albuterol. Long-acting β₂-agonists such as salmeterol are not used for acute attacks. Two inhalation devices can be considered for delivery of albuterol: the nebulizer and metered-dose inhaler (MDI). Nebulized albuterol is most often used in the ED because it is easier to deliver and requires little patient effort. However, with correct technique and medication dose, a MDI with spacer is as effective as a nebulizer. Reviewing the technique with the patient may also improve medication delivery at home. In the nebulized form, albuterol is given 2.5 mg to 5.0 mg every 20 minutes for three doses, then as needed based on symptoms and side effects. In severe cases, continuous albuterol nebulization is effective. The MDI with spacer is dosed with albuterol as 4 to 8 puffs every 20 minutes for three doses, then as needed. The common side effects of β₂-agonists are tremors, tachycardia, and anxiety.

Nonspecific β-Adrenergic Agents

Nonspecific β-adrenergic agents are not used for first-line treatment. However, a 1:1000 concentration of epinephrine given 0.3 to 0.5 mg subcutaneously can be used in severe cases, often as a last resort before intubation Epinephrine must be used with caution because the β_1 effects can cause cardiac stimulation including tachycardia, arrhythmias, or angina.

Corticosteroids

Corticosteroids decrease airway inflammation and mucus production. Most patients who present to the ED should receive steroids, with the exception of the patient with a mild exacerbation that reverses after one albuterol nebulized treatment. Oral prednisone (40 to 60 mg) is used in the ED for most cases of asthma, unless the patient has decreased intestinal absorption, difficulty swallowing, or vomiting. Intravenous (IV) methylprednisolone (80 to 125 mg) is the alternative medication The effect of corticosteroids may not be evident in the ED because the peak effect is seen 6 to 12 hours after the dose; however, it is important to administer corticosteroids early. Side effects of short-course therapy include hyperglycemia, peptic ulcer disease, hypertension, weight gain, psychosis, and increased risk of infection. Side effects are less common when steroids are given for short courses.

Anticholinergic Medication

Anticholinergic medication, such as ipratropium bromide, inhibits the action of acetylcholine at parasympathetic sites in the bronchial smooth muscle causing bronchodilation. Although ipratropium is not as effective as albuterol, it can be added to albuterol in nebulized form and may cause additional bronchodilation. The dose of ipratropium bromide is 0.5 mg, administered by a nebulizer with a dose of albuterol. Because the effect of ipratropium lasts up to 6 hours, usually one dose is adequate in the ED. Side effects are minimal and include narrow-angle glaucoma and urinary retention.

Theophylline

Theophylline is not recommended as first-line therapy in acute exacerbations. Theophylline is a bronchodilator and also increases the contractility of the diaphragm.

In patients who are on theophylline, a theophylline level can be measured to monitor toxicity and guide therapy. Patients with moderate to severe exacerbations who have a low theophylline level can be given a bolus of IV aminophylline or oral theophylline. However, the drug interactions and side effects are numerous, and the therapeutic index is narrow with severe toxicity including seizures and cardiac arrhythmias. In addition, patients who are on oral theophylline may not comply with their current outpatient dose, so care must be taken before increasing their dose at discharge. Serum levels may be increased from medications such as macrolide antibiotics, ciprofloxacin, cimetidine, isoniazid, allopurinol, propranolol, and oral contraceptives. In contrast, serum levels may be decreased by increasing the clearance of theophylline, as seen with smoking, carbamazepine, phenobarbital, phenytoin, rifampin, and furosemide. Side effects include tachycardia, tremor, anxiety, nausea, and vomiting.

Intravenous Magnesium

IV magnesium inhibits smooth muscle contraction and increases bronchodilation. Although magnesium may not be helpful in all cases, it can be used in severe exacerbations unresponsive to other medications. The dose of magnesium is 2.0 g IV over 20 minutes. Common side effects are flushing, hypotension, drowsiness, and vomiting.

Heliox

Heliox, a helium-oxygen mixture, is less dense than oxygen and improves laminar flow in the airways. In addition, it increases the amount of medication delivered to the airways. Despite these advantages, preliminary studies show that heliox may only have use in patients with severe asthma who have not responded well to inhaled β_2-agonists, while waiting for the corticosteroid effect.

Antibiotics

Antibiotics are required only if a concurrent infection is diagnosed in addition to the asthma exacerbation.

Mechanical Ventilation

Patients with severe asthma exacerbations unresponsive to medications may require mechanical ventilation. The decision to intubate is often difficult. Absolute indications for intubation include cardiac or respiratory arrest and change in mental status, but it must be considered in patients with progressive hypercarbia, severe metabolic acidosis, worsening mental status, or profound patient exhaustion despite maximal medical therapy.

Although most of the usual principles of rapid sequence induction (RSI) and ventilator management apply in asthma, a few specifics should be taken into consideration. For RSI, ketamine, an induction agent, should be considered because of its bronchodilation properties. Succinylcholine remains the most common agent for neuromuscular paralysis. Because of the risk of barotrauma and hypotension in mechanical ventilation, airway pressures must be kept at a minimum, using continued sedation and paralysis, controlled hypoventilation (respiratory rate of 6 to 10 breaths/minute), and an I:E ratio of 1:3 to 1:6.

Complications

Complications of asthma include pneumothorax and infection. Pneumothorax can occur in any patient with asthma but is most commonly seen in intubated patients with asthma. A pneumothorax should be considered in a patient with chest pain, asymmetric breath sounds, tracheal deviation, subcutaneous emphysema, and/or hypotension. The diagnosis can be confirmed with a chest radiograph if the patient is stable, or decompression with a large-gauge needle placed in the second intercostal space in the midclavicular line if the patient is unstable. Infection such as pneumonia must be suspected in a patient with asthma who has fever, chest pain, productive cough, and/or abnormal lung findings. A chest x-ray film helps confirm the diagnosis.

Disposition

Patients who require intubation and those who continue to have peak flows of less than 50% of predicted after adequate treatment should be hospitalized. On the other hand, if symptoms are minimal or absent and the peak flow is greater than 70% of predicted, patients can be discharged. The difficulty comes with the patient who has improved with medication but is still wheezing, dyspneic, and/or has a peak flow between 50% to 69% of predicted. A re-evaluation after extended observation and treatment in the ED may be helpful. Ultimately, the decision to admit or discharge will rely on the patient's subjective feeling of improvement, severity and duration of symptoms, severity of disease in the past, medication use at home, and ease of follow-up.

A patient who is discharged to home must have proper medications and follow-up. β_2-agonists should be continued with a MDI and/or spacer at increased frequency. If a patient is given corticosteroids in the ED, continued prednisone should be prescribed. Because adrenal-pituitary suppression is usually not seen until after 2 weeks of therapy, it is reasonable and less complicated if a short "burst" of prednisone is given, usually 40 mg orally once a day for 4 to 6 days. In patients who have recently received steroids or are on chronic continuous steroid therapy, a longer course with taper is needed. Adding an inhaled corticosteroid to a patient's long-term regimen should be considered. A follow-up appointment with the primary care doctor in 3 to 5 days is necessary, and the patient should be advised to stop smoking and avoid asthma triggers.

Pathophysiology

Asthma is a disease of airway obstruction. Biopsies of lung tissue from a patient with asthma show that no damage occurs at the level of the alveoli; all of the changes occur at the level of the airway. There are three components to the obstructive process. They are smooth muscle contraction, which causes bronchoconstriction; swelling (edema) of the airways; and mucus secretion, which plugs the airways.

The inflammatory response is still being defined at the cellular and molecular level.

What is known is that high numbers of eosinophils and lymphocytes bearing the TH2 subtype are found in the airway walls in patients with asthma. The lymphocytes in particular are responsible for the release of several interleukin subtypes and chemotactic molecules. These cytokines ostensibly signal the plasma cells to differentiate with the ability to produce IgE against the antigens that were introduced to the T lymphocytes. These IgE molecules find the mast cells in the circulation and attach to them. When the mast cell is sensitized, it releases histamine, bradykinin, chemotactic factors, and arachidonic acid metabolites such as prostaglandins and leukotrienes. The result is attraction of eosinophils, promotion of additional mast cell production, and differentiation of the TH2 lymphocytes. Several drugs that attack asthma at the level of leukotrienes and eosinophil activity have been recently introduced. Montelukast (Singulair) may be of benefit in mild asthma prevention and stabilization of some types of more severe asthma.

Specific agents responsible for initiating this inflammatory reaction vary among patients with asthma. Infection, change in weather, seasonal allergies, animal dander, and house dust are common precipitants. Medications such as aspirin and NSAIDs can cause an exacerbation. Exercise may provoke an asthma attack, which may be due to thermal changes in the airways. Emotional stress can worsen or even precipitate an exacerbation. In many cases, no specific trigger can be identified.

Suggested Readings

Bates B. *A guide to physical examination and history taking*, 5th ed. Philadelphia: JB Lippincott, 1991:303.

Edmond SD, Camargo CA, Nowak RM. 1997 National Asthma Education and Prevention Program Guidelines: a practical summary for emergency physicians. *Ann Emerg Med* 1998;31:579–589.

Harwood-Nuss A, Wolfson AB, Linder CH, et al. eds. *The clinical practice of emergency medicine*, 2nd ed. Philadelphia: Lippincott-Raven, 1996:653–657.

Henderson SO, Acharya P, Kilaghbian T, et al. Use of heliox-driven nebulizer therapy in the treatment of acute asthma. *Ann Emerg Med* 1999;33:141–146.

Kardon EM. Acute asthma. *Emerg Med Clin North Am* 1996;14:93–114.

Kass JE, Terregino CA. The effect of heliox in acute severe asthma: a randomized controlled trial. *Chest* 1999;116:296–300.

McFadden ER-FR, Warren EL. Observations on asthma mortality. *Ann Intern Med* 1997;127:142–147.

CHAPTER 10

Chronic Obstructive Pulmonary Disease

Elizabeth L. Mitchell, MD

Clinical Scenario

A 62-year-old man is brought to the emergency department (ED) by ambulance. He complains of 3 days of increased sputum production. Today, he became extremely short of breath. He has used his home nebulizer without relief. He notes recent cold symptoms without fever or chills.

Past medical history includes chronic obstructive pulmonary disease (COPD) and hypertension. He has never been intubated but has had multiple hospital admissions for wheezing. The last one was 1 month ago.

He has a 60-pack-year history of smoking but states he quit 1 month ago. His medications include ipratropium bromide (Atrovent), albuterol, clarithromycin, aspirin, and hydrochlorothiazide. He has no known drug allergies.

Physical examination reveals a thin male sitting bolt upright in bed, with lips pursed, and speaking only a few words at a time using his accessory muscles of respiration. Vital signs are blood pressure of 160/110 mm Hg, heart rate of 100 beats/minute, respiratory rate of 40 breaths/minute, temperature of 98.6°F, and room air oxygen saturation of 84%.

The head, ears, eyes, nose, and throat (HEENT) examination is normal, and his neck is without jugular venous distension (JVD). Very distant breath sounds with a few diffuse wheezes and little air movement are heard over his lungs. There is decreased excursion of the diaphragms on percussion. There are no rales or rhonchi appreciated. Cardiovascular sounds are distant, with a regular rate and rhythm. The abdomen is soft, nontender, and nondistended. His extremities show clubbing but no cyanosis or edema.

The patient is immediately placed on 2 L of oxygen by nasal cannula. A nebulized treatment of albuterol and ipratropium (Atrovent) is begun on forced air. He is given 60 mg of prednisone orally. He shows little improvement after the first treatment. An arterial blood gas (ABG) sample is drawn, an intravenous (IV) line is placed, and a chest x-ray film ordered. He is admitted to the hospital with a diagnosis of COPD exacerbation. He is discharged after 2 days in hospital fully recovered.

Clinical Evaluation

Introduction

COPD affects up to one fourth of the adult population of the United States. It is a title for several entities whose pathophysiology differs, but the end result is airway obstruction. It is responsible for countless days of lost work, and many individuals are admitted to the hospital each year with COPD exacerbations. COPD is the fifth leading cause of death in the United States. Smoking is still the leading cause of COPD; thus, as inroads are made into tobacco smoking prevention, we will hopefully see a decline in morbidity and mortality from COPD. As discussed later, this disease has a vast spectrum from minimal symptoms to respiratory failure. In the ED, prompt and aggressive treatment may be necessary to prevent intubation and mechanical ventilation.

History

The spectrum of disease can range from asymptomatic to respiratory failure, depending on the extent of pulmonary destruction and complicating factors such as infection. Clinical presentation depends somewhat on the variable components of the disease. Patients may present to the ED during any phase of the disease. A patient with no history of COPD but a long history of smoking may present with complaints of dyspnea on exertion (DOE), wheezing, recurrent infection, or shortness of breath even at rest. As the disease progresses, patients may go from noting shortness of breath only during exercise to a state of chronic dyspnea. Patients will have poor exercise tolerance and increasing episodes of decompensated states with less responsiveness to treatment.

The patient in this clinical scenario has a number of features common to patients with COPD. Perhaps the most important is a history of cigarette use. It is very important to elicit a history of smoking, secondhand exposure, or occupational exposure in a patient you suspect of having COPD or other acquired lung diseases. Often a patient denies smoking if he or she has recently quit. Thus, any patient who responds, "No, I don't smoke," must be asked the follow-up question, "Have you ever smoked?" The patient in the clinical scenario also notes increased sputum production and cold symptoms. This is perhaps the etiology of his exacerbation. Respiratory infection is often the culprit in worsening of a patient's respiratory health. One can judge the severity of the patient's illness in part by a history of many hospital and ED admissions. This patient has not reached the point of intubation but has a relatively advanced state of disease. Patients may present with insidious worsening of baseline symptoms over hours to days. The inciting factor may be identified by a good history, such as seasonal allergens, smoking, secondhand smoke, animal exposure, or upper respiratory infection (URI). Careful attention to a patient's medications may reveal poor compliance or sedatives and narcotics, which can inhibit respiratory drive.

Patients with COPD are subject to other complications of the disease as well. Because the patient with COPD has a decreased ability to clear normal pulmonary pathogens, he or she is at risk not only for bronchitis but also for life-threatening episodes of pneumonia.

Pneumothorax is another complication of emphysematous COPD. The destruction of the alveolar wall leads to changes that result in loss of normal lung tissue. Enlarged fibrotic air spaces, known as blebs, are at risk for rupturing, creating a pneumothorax. This air leak out of the lung leads to pulmonary collapse and loss of aeration of lung tissue. This can be catastrophic for the patient with COPD and requires urgent reinflation with a chest tube. Any patient with sudden severe shortness of breath and chest pain should be suspected of having a pneumothorax.

Chronic lung disease and pulmonary hypertension cause cor pulmonale, or right-sided heart failure. A patient may complain of fluid retention. These patients also have an increase in their hematocrit in response to chronic hypoxia and an increased circulating volume. They require careful fluid management and optimization of pulmonary function.

Physical Examination

Physical findings are variable and may depend on the stage of disease. In early stages, the examination may be normal except for prolonged expiration. Rhonchi or wheezing may be present or the chest examination may be unusually quiet. As the disease progresses and the lungs become overinflated, the diaphragms lower with decreased excursion on inspiration. With percussion, there may be decreased area of cardiac dullness and hyperresonance of the chest. There may also be decreased transmission of the sounds of consolidation and tactile fremitus. The patient tends to sit in a stooped posture, leaning on the elbows when sitting. With chronic hypoxia, there may be clubbing of the nails. The distal phalanx is enlarged and rounded, with pronounced rounded fingernails. The lips may be pursed, and there may be obvious labored breathing. The patient may use accessory muscles of respiration (intercostal, sternomastoids, and abdominal). Finally, patients may have findings of cardiac decompensation from pulmonary hypertension. These include right-sided heart failure (lower extremity edema, increased jugular venous pressure, and tricuspid regurgitation) or biventricular failure with left-sided heart failure and pulmonary edema.

Note the vital signs in the clinical scenario. The patient is mildly hypertensive and tachycardic, which may signal distress. His respiratory rate is markedly elevated, and his oxygen saturation is very low. In addition, his physical examination shows him sitting in a position common to patients in respiratory distress, known as tripoding. He sits bolt upright, leaning slightly forward on his arms. This allows maximum aeration of the lungs and opening of the upper airway. He can only manage a few words at a time, and he is using the accessory muscles of respiration. In addition, little air movement is appreciated on auscultation. The decreased diaphragmatic movement is evidence of enlarged emphysematous lungs that are hyperexpanded. Heart sounds become distant when listening through a larger volume of air. This patient is noted to have clubbing of his fingertips.

Diagnostic Evaluation

The diagnostic workup of patients with COPD exacerbation may be delayed to initiate therapy in a patient who is in profound distress. Attention must be paid to the airway, breathing, and circulation (ABCs). Airway should be checked for patency; lungs examined to assess the possibility of pneumonia, collapse, or pneumothorax; and IV access should be obtained for circulatory support and medication delivery. A chest x-ray film should be obtained early to rule out treatable causes of the exacerbation, such as a pneumothorax or pulmonary edema. An ABG sample is useful in the evaluation, treatment, and disposition of the patient. An ABG result tells you how hard the patient is working to maintain adequate oxygenation. It tells you if the patient is retaining CO_2, and it gives valuable information about the patient's acid-base status. In addition, you can obtain other helpful information such as the hemoglobin and electrolytes. Intubation should not be delayed for an ABG sample in a patient who shows clinical signs of respiratory failure.

Careful attention to the patient's history may help direct the workup. Any patient who has sudden acute decompensation should be evaluated for potentially catastrophic events such as pulmonary embolus, pneumothorax, or lung collapse. Patients with subacute deterioration should be carefully questioned as well to rule out treatable causes. A patient with recent trauma should be assessed for hemothorax, rib fractures, and anemia. A patient with chest pain, pulmonary edema, or irregular heart rate should have an electrocardiogram (ECG) to evaluate for coronary ischemia or arrhythmia. Any patient with suspected metabolic disturbance or comorbid disease should have the appropriate serum chemistry tests performed. A hematocrit should be obtained if anemia is suspected. In addition, polycythemia (increased numbers of red cells in reaction to chronic hypoxia) may be helpful in judging the severity of disease. A white blood cell (WBC) count may help in the face of infection, with the caveat that both stress and steroids (part of the treatment) can elevate the WBC.

The extent of airway obstruction can be measured using spirometry. In obstructive pulmonary disease, the speed of forced expiration is decreased because of reduced lung recoil and compressibility, high airway resistance, and collapse of small airways. One such measure used to determine extent of illness is the ratio of the forced expiratory volume at one second (FEV_1) to the forced vital capacity (FVC), FEV_1/FVC. The finding of a low ratio is usually indicative of disease.

In the ED, a peak flow is a more practical tool to evaluate the patient's disease and progress while being treated.

Differential Diagnosis

The differential diagnosis for COPD is illustrated in Table 10.1.

Table 10.1.

Differential diagnosis of COPD

Asthma
Bronchiectasis
Tuberculosis
Sarcoidosis
α-1 Antitrypsin disease
Congestive heart failure
Pneumonia

COPD, chronic obstructive pulmonary disease.

Treatment

Treatment of acute COPD exacerbation can be difficult and complex (Table 10.2). Acute exacerbations may present in life-threatening respiratory failure. Skilled airway management, rapid clinical assessment, and understanding of the pulmonary pathophysiology are essential for the successful treatment of the many and varied presentations of this disease.

For the emergency physician, oxygenation and ventilation are the most important initial considerations. Patients with severely advanced disease may present with ineffective, low-volume respirations and cyanosis. They may appear exhausted, confused, and lethargic. These patients require emergent intubation and mechanical ventilation. If

Table 10.2.

Treatment guidelines for COPD

Respiratory Failure
Consideration of intubation

Moderate Exacerbation
Oxygen by nasal cannula or rebreather mask
  to keep saturation above 90%—monitor
  mental status.
Albuterol 2.5 mg + ipratropium bromide 0.5 mg
  in 5 mL of normal saline nebulized; follow by
  repeated doses of albuterol as needed
Prednisone 60 mg po or prednisolone 125 mg IV
Monitoring of CO_2 and acidosis by arterial blood
  gases
Consideration of CPAP

COPD, chronic obstructive pulmonary disease; CPAP, continuous positive airway pressure; IV, intravenous.

they are not sufficiently sedated, they should be intubated with rapid-sequence induction. For the patient who is not clearly end stage, the indications for intubation can be more difficult. Serial ABG results along with clinical status may be helpful in determining a patient's need for mechanical ventilation. Often a trial of aggressive therapy may obviate the need for intubation. In addition to the therapies discussed later, these patients may benefit from nasal continuous positive airway pressure (CPAP). CPAP helps decrease the work of breathing by counteracting the intrinsic increased peak expiratory pressures found in COPD.

Oxygen therapy is required in most patients. The oxygen saturation should be maintained above 90%. Often this can be accomplished with a nasal cannula and low oxygen flow. High-flow oxygen is rarely needed and can be dangerous in the patient who is hypoventilating and retaining CO_2. This patient may require hypoxia to stimulate the respiratory drive, and too much oxygen will cause the patient to retain more CO_2. These patients can be extremely frustrating to manage during an exacerbation, requiring you to walk a fine line between too much and too little oxygen. These patients, and really all patients with COPD, must be monitored carefully for clinical deterioration and improvement. Signs of fatigue, lethargy, increased or decreased respiratory rate, paradoxical abdominal breathing, and decreasing oxygenation despite treatment may point to a required intubation and mechanical ventilation.

Bronchodilators are the first line of drug therapy in COPD exacerbations. β_2-agonists are the mainstay of therapy. These drugs work by β_2-receptor activity causing bronchial smooth muscle relaxation. They are given in nebulizer (inhaled) form and can be given in rapid succession. They can be given to mechanically ventilated patients as well. Side effects are caused by the cardiostimulatory effects of β-agonists and include tremor, tachycardia, and ventricular ectopy. Albuterol is the most commonly used β-agonist. The dose is 2.5 to 5.0 mg in 5 mL of saline. Anticholinergic bronchodilators can be used concurrently with β_2-agonists. They work by blocking muscarinic receptor sites and preventing smooth muscle contraction. In addition, they decrease release of secretions in submucosal glands. The medication ipratropium bromide (Atrovent) can be used simultaneously with albuterol and is thought to have synergistic effects. The dose is 0.5 mg in nebulizer form. Unlike albuterol, it has not clearly been shown to be helpful when given in a continuous fashion. The usual protocol is a combination (albuterol/Atrovent) nebulizer for the first treatment and albuterol alone subsequently. Subcutaneous epinephrine and terbutaline are bronchodilators used rarely as adjunct therapy in COPD exacerbations. They have significant cardiac side effects and are contraindicated in any patient at risk for cardiac disease.

Corticosteroids are thought to work by antiinflammatory action. They have benefits for the acute exacerbation, decreased relapse rate, and long-term maintenance. Although it takes approximately 4 hours for the full benefit of steroid therapy, they are standard therapy in any moderate to severe COPD exacerbation. Steroids can be given in IV form as prednisolone (Solu-Medrol) 125 mg, oral prednisone 60-mg loading dose, or as an inhaler for maintenance therapy. Patients who require admission are usually given the IV dose of prednisolone, although the onset of action for both the PO (oral) and IV routes are the same. Patients who receive steroids in the ED and are discharged must be discharged on oral prednisone. In general, patients are given 5 to 7 days of 40 mg of prednisone or are given a tapering dose. The decision whether to taper is still controversial, but it is clear that there are no harmful adrenal effects if a short course of prednisone is offered without a taper. No particular tapering regimen has been demonstrated as superior to another.

Methylxanthines (aminophylline and theophylline) are rarely used in the acute setting. These medications are mired in controversy. Although beneficial in maintenance therapy, the acute benefits have not been decisively shown. These medications require careful administration and dosing and have serious side effects when levels are too high. Their beneficial effects include bronchodilation, improved diaphragm contractility, improved respiratory drive, and improved mucociliary function. Patients on maintenance therapy should have a level checked before beginning IV aminophylline.

Antibiotics should be started on any patient with evidence of bronchitis or pneumonia.

Disposition

Any patient who does not readily improve with treatment in the ED should be considered for hospital admission. The more difficult question can be where to admit the patient. Any patient in respiratory failure or on the verge of respiratory failure should be admitted to the medical intensive care unit (MICU). Depending on the services of a particular hospital, moderate exacerbations may require a step-down unit rather than a general medical floor, for frequent nebulizer therapy, pulmonary toilet, and close observation. Those patients who have had good response to ED treatment and are close to their baseline may be discharged to home on indicated medications (bronchodilators, steroids, and antibiotics). All patients should have follow up planned. If they are smoking, they should be advised to quit.

Pathophysiology

COPD is a disease seen most commonly in smokers between the ages of 55 and 65 years. Although smoking is the greatest risk factor for development of COPD, there is likely to be a genetic predisposition as well. Other risk factors include environmental pollutants and passive smoking. There are three basic components to the disease: reactive, chronic obstructive bronchitis, and emphysematous. Most patients have disease that includes all three components to greater or lesser degrees. It is helpful to understand the pathophysiology of each component to appreciate the spectrum of disease.

The reactive component of asthma is reversible bronchoconstriction. Patients tend to have "twitchy" lungs, that is, they respond to a number of stimulants by constricting and can be treated with bronchodilator therapy with reversal of the symptoms. The reactive component in COPD is not identical to asthma. COPD has different, more poorly defined, mediators than those found in asthma. In addition, unlike asthma, there does not appear to be a component of atopy determined by a lack of IgE and eosinophil elevation.

The inflammatory component, also known as chronic obstructive bronchitis, is characterized by inflamed, edematous bronchioles. It is defined by a productive cough for more than 3 months' duration for two successive years. There is increased mucus production and decreased ability of the cilia to clear either mucus or pathogens. Bronchioles become narrowed by inflammation and may be obstructed by mucus secretion.

The emphysematous airway can be described as a disease of the small airways: narrowing of the bronchioles and destruction of the alveoli. The alveolar wall is dilated and ultimately destroyed. This leads to enlargement of air spaces and destruction of lung parenchyma. In addition, there is loss of the elasticity of the wall and collapse of air spaces with forced expiration. Eventually the capillary bed is affected as well.

These components coexist in most patients but may occur as primarily bronchitic or primarily emphysematous. The patient who is primarily emphysematous has profound dyspnea and air hunger and suffers from pulmonary wasting. The bronchitic patient has a somewhat different clinical picture. This patient has both profound hypoxia (low oxygenation) and hypercapnia (excess carbon dioxide). He or she is unable to increase the minute volume appropriately, and chronic hypoxia leads to pulmonary hypertension. This patient usually suffers from profound CO_2 retention and acidosis during exacerbations. Patients may fall into the category of "pink puffer" or "blue bloater." These terms refer to extremes of two spectrums of the disease. The pink puffer tends to hyperventilate to maintain normal arterial oxygenation, and the blue bloater tends to be chronically hypoxic and cyanotic. These distinctions have clinical implications, because some patients need to be somewhat hypoxic to stimulate their respiratory drive. Too much oxygen can cause them to retain CO_2 and cause further decompensation.

Suggested Readings

American Thoracic Society. Standards for the diagnosis and care of patients with chronic obstructive pulmonary disease. *Am J Respir Crit Care Med* 1995;152:S77–S121.

Barnes PJ. Chronic obstructive pulmonary disease. Review article. *N Engl J Med* 2000;343:269–279.

Mandavia DP, Dailey RH. Chronic obstructive pulmonary disease. In: *Rosen emergency medicine*, 4th ed., Eds. P. Rosen and R. Barkin. St. Louis: Mosby, 1998:1494–1511.

Martin L. *Pulmonary physiology in clinical practice.* St. Louis: Mosby, 1987.

Palm KH, Decker WW. Acute exacerbations of chronic obstructive pulmonary disease. *Emerg Med Clin North Am* 2003 May;21(2) 331–352.

CHAPTER 11

Pneumonia

Darcy Q. Bittner, MD

Clinical Scenario

A 62-year-old woman presents with fever, cough with thick greenish sputum, and fatigue for 2 days. She has pain with deep inspiration and mild shortness of breath. She also describes a loss of appetite. She has no relief of her cough with over-the-counter medicines. There is no blood in the sputum. She denies night sweats.

Her past medical history includes adult-onset diabetes, hypertension, and hypothyroidism. Her medications are atenolol, glyburide, and levothyroxine (Synthroid), and she has no known drug allergies. She lives alone, is a 25-pack-year smoker, and does not drink alcohol.

On physical examination, her vital signs are blood pressure of 154/86 mm Hg, heart rate of 90 beats/minute, respiratory rate of 36 breaths/minute, temperature of 101.1°F, and room air oxygen saturation of 93%. She is in mild respiratory distress. She is flushed and slightly sweaty. Her head, ears, eyes, nose, and throat (HEENT) examination is normal. There is no jugular venous distension (JVD). The lungs are dull to percussion over the right base, with E to A sound changes in the right base. There are decreased breath sounds in the right base with crackles and no wheezes. Heart and abdominal examination is unremarkable. Her extremities show no edema, cyanosis, or clubbing.

The patient is placed on 2 L/minute of oxygen by nasal cannula and continuous pulse oximetry. Intravenous (IV) access is obtained, and laboratory samples are sent for complete blood count (CBC) with differential, blood cultures, and metabolic panel.

A chest x-ray film is obtained. One gram of acetaminophen (Tylenol) is given. The chest x-ray film shows a right lower lobe infiltrate with loss of definition of the right hemidiaphragm. The patient's lung examination and chest x-ray film confirm that she has lobar pneumonia. Antibiotic therapy is initiated, and she is admitted to the hospital. She has an uneventful recovery and is discharged 3 days later to home on oral antibiotics.

Clinical Evaluation

Introduction

Approximately 3 million people of all ages contract pneumonia each year in the United States. Approximately 20% require admission for their symptoms. Pneumonia remains a significant cause of death particularly in the elderly and immunocompromised patients. Although the diagnosis of pneumonia is often obtained through history and physical examination, identification of the culprit organism is difficult and may not occur despite appropriate efforts. Treatment is directed against the most common bacteria, but the patient's history remains vital to the direction of antimicrobial treatment.

History

Symptoms of pneumonia range from a mild febrile illness to septic shock. Common symptoms of pneumonia include fever, productive cough, and dyspnea. Patients may describe the onset of their dyspnea as progressive (insidious) and associated with cough. Sometimes pneumonia begins precipitously with rigors (shaking chills) and a cough. The cough may be productive of colored sputum (red, brown, green, yellow, or white), or there may be no sputum at all, as is seen in *Mycoplasma* pneumonia. The patient may not have a cough. The location of the infection may produce pain in a particular area. Pneumonias irritating the diaphragm may present with shoulder pain or abdominal pain, lower lobe infiltrates may present with back pain, or the patient may complain of chest pain in a variety of locations. Pain is usually pleuritic, increasing with inspiration. Other symptoms include those of systemic illness: myalgias, arthralgias, chills, and other generalized complaints.

Typically, cough is reported 80% of the time. Sixty-five percent of patients with pneumonia describe sputum production. As people age, there is a significant reduction in the percentage of patients who report pleuritic chest pain. In general, advanced age is associated with reporting of lower lobe symptoms and increasingly vague symptoms and physical findings.

In addition to gathering symptom history, it is important to elicit information regarding risks and immune status. This will help to guide antibiotic choices. Immune-system compromise can include human immunodeficiency virus (HIV) infection or acquired immune deficiency syndrome (AIDS), oncological causes, steroids, alcoholism, or other illnesses. Other risk factors for pneumonia include recent hospitalization, nursing home residence, and comorbid conditions such as chronic obstructive pulmonary disease (COPD) or diabetes.

Physical Examination

Patients may appear well or markedly ill. Vital signs may show tachycardia, fever, and tachypnea. Patients may be volume depleted or septic and manifest a low blood pressure. Pulse oximetry may be low or normal. On general inspection, notice the skin, particularly the lips and fingers, which may be cyanotic. Patients may also splint toward the side of the pneumonia in an attempt to limit the air entry and subsequent discomfort.

The lung examination has multiple facets. During auscultation, listen for bronchial breath sounds, which are higher pitched and louder during expiration. A pleural rub can sometimes be heard in pneumonia. This is produced by inflammation of the pleura and is a creaking sound. Egophony may be present, elicited when a patient says "E" and it sounds like "A" over an area of consolidation. Overall, the consolidation causes increased transmission of sound through the fluid. Crackles or rales, which sound like small popping noises, remain the most reliable predictor of pneumonia. Another component of the lung examination is palpation and the diagnosis of tactile fremitus. Tactile fremitus involves placing the ulnar side of the palm against the back horizontally and asking the patient to say "ninety-nine." The hand detects changes in vibration. It is increased in pneumonia but decreased in pneumothorax, pleural effusion, and COPD. A third diagnostic maneuver is percussion. When percussing over a consolidated area of lung, it is often dull or thudding when compared to clear areas of lung. Dullness to percussion is a common finding in pleural effusion.

Diagnostic Evaluation

The chest x-ray film must have positive findings to diagnose pneumonia; however, it is only marginally helpful in determining the causative organism. If the patient is stable, obtain a posterior-anterior (PA) and lateral film, because it increases the diagnostic findings over the portable x-ray film (Table 11.1).

A CBC can assist in the diagnosis when elevated levels of white blood cells with a left shift appear. This does not help in determining etiology and does not change management, but it may give you clues as to the patient's immune status and severity of disease.

Sputum Gram stain and culture is difficult to obtain in the emergency department (ED) and cannot be relied on.

Blood cultures should be drawn in the ED before initiation of antibiotics. Although culture results rarely result in a change in the management of the patient, it is still considered standard of care to draw cultures on all admitted patients. If a patient is clinically well enough to be treated as an outpatient, cultures are rarely necessary.

Arterial blood gas results in the sicker patient can help guide management by showing

Table 11.1.

Relationship between x-ray findings of pneumonia and the causative organisms

Radiograph Appearance	Etiological Agents
Lobar	Pneumococcus, Klebsiella
Bronchopneumonia: fluffy or patchy infiltrates	Chlamydia pneumoniae, Mycoplasma pneumoniae, Legionella, viruses
Interstitial	M. pneumoniae, Pneumocystis carinii, viruses
Disseminated nodules: miliary	Mycobacterium tuberculosis, fungi
Posterior upper/superior lower consolidations	Aspiration
Peripheral infiltrates	Staphylococcus aureus due to hematogenous spread
Apical infiltrates	M. tuberculosis
Mediastinal lymphadenopathy	M. tuberculosis, fungi
Cavitation	Anaerobes, gram-negative organisms, fungi, S. aureus, M. tuberculosis

hypoxemia, hypercarbia, or ventilation-perfusion mismatch.

There are other laboratory tests that may be of value, including a lactate dehydrogenase (LDH) level, which is elevated in Pneumocystis carinii pneumonia (PCP) and may be useful in the evaluation of metabolic and renal functions. Elevated levels of blood urea nitrogen (BUN) and creatinine may be a marker of severity of dehydration and a useful evaluation of kidney function. Serum sodium level may be decreased in Legionella pneumonia and again may be helpful in assessing dehydration.

Differential Diagnosis

The differential diagnosis for pneumonia is illustrated in Table 11.2.

Treatment

Treatment is driven by the severity of the illness (see Table 11.3 for general treatment guidelines). For patients who appear well with no significant comorbidities, treatment is aimed at appropriate antibiotic therapy as an outpatient (Table 11.4). Ill or hypoxic patients require inpatient treatment (Table 11.5). Once you have decided to admit the patient, prompt administration

Table 11.2.

Differential diagnosis of pneumonia

COPD
CHF
Bronchiolitis obliterans
Endocarditis
Pulmonary embolism
Silicosis
Chemical or toxin exposures
Tumors
Aspiration of foreign bodies
Immunological diseases: sarcoid, Wegener's granulomatosis and Goodpasture's disease

CHF, congestive heart failure; COPD, chronic obstructive pulmonary disease.

Table 11.3.

Treatment plan for pneumonia

Oxygen: nasal cannula or face mask
IV access
Blood cultures, CBC, electrolytes specimens
IV fluids if necessary
Cardiac monitor
Continuous pulse oximetry
Portable CXR or PA/lateral film if stable enough
ABG sample
Suctioning necessary if aspiration known
Intubation if necessary
Bronchodilators if bronchospasm evident
Empiric antibiotic therapy

ABG, arterial blood gas; CBC, complete blood count;
CXR, chest x-ray; IV, intravenous; PA, posterior-anterior.

Table 11.4.

Outpatient antibiotics options

Healthy Young Person with Nonproductive Cough
Suggestive of Atypical Organisms
Erythromycin, levofloxacin, azithromycin,
clarithromycin

COPD Patients with Mild Illness
Levofloxacin, azithromycin, clarithromycin

Possible Bacterial Etiology
Levofloxacin, ß-lactam, trimethoprim/
sulfamethoxazole, amoxicillin/clavulanate

COPD, chronic obstructive pulmonary disease.

of IV antibiotics is necessary. Administration of antibiotics in the ED greatly decreases the time to first receipt of antibiotics and decreases hospitalization duration.

Disposition

The first decision that must be made involves determining how ill the patient is on presentation and how likely he or she is to get worse. The patient's vital signs will direct you to admit or discharge. A scoring system used to identify low-risk patients was developed by Fine et al. and is known as the Pneumonia

Table 11.5.

Inpatient antibiotic options

CAP
Levofloxacin (Levaquin) or second- or third-
generation cephalosporin plus erythromycin

Aspiration
Second- or third-generation cephalosporin plus
clindamycin or metronidazole or a combination
ß-lactamase (i.e., ampicillin/sulbactam)

Nursing Home/Hospitalization
ß-lactam or first-generation cephalosporin plus
aminoglycoside and antipseudomonal such as
ticarcillin/clavulanate or piperacillin/tazobactam

CAP, community-acquired pneumonia.

Outpatient Research Team (PORT) Criteria. They developed a two-tiered scoring system that stratifies patients into five severity classes. Patients are classified as risk class I (low risk) if they are age 50 or younger, with no history of five comorbid conditions (neoplastic disease, liver disease, heart failure, cerebrovascular disease, or renal disease), normal mental status, and normal or only mildly abnormal vital signs. Patients who have not been assigned to class I are assigned to risk classes II to V based on the number of points according to age; place of residence (e.g., apartment or house vs. nursing home); and presence of five comorbid conditions, five physical examination findings, and seven laboratory or radiographic findings. Class I and II are considered stable for outpatient treatment, class III is treated as either outpatient or inpatient, and classes IV and V require inpatient treatment. In general, for most clinicians, the parameters for admission include those that predispose a patient toward a higher likelihood of mortality: pulse higher than 125 beats/minute, systolic blood pressure less than 90 mm Hg, respiratory rate greater than 30 breaths/minute, pulse oximetry less than 90%, altered mental status, temperature less than 35°C or more than 40°C, or PO_2 less than 60 mm Hg. The patient's baseline health status may require admission as well (e.g., the elderly; young children; pregnant patients; patients with previous pneumonias, immunosuppression, or obstructed airways). Multilobar involvement and pleural effusions on chest x-ray examination usually require admission.

Pathophysiology

Pathophysiology is based on the host, organisms, and spread of infection. Essentially, the respiratory system protects itself from infection via structures such as nasal cilia, mucus, gag reflex with cough, surfactant, and the immune system. Cellular defenses include the IgA and IgG pathways and alveolar macrophages that also protect the airways. Anything that impairs the host can lead to pneumonia. Some patients have difficulty protecting the airway secondary to altered mental status, drugs, alcohol, coma, or indwelling devices such as endotracheal tubes. In addition, a loss of ciliary mobility can lead to complications as in cystic fibrosis, viral infections, smoking, or COPD. Inoculation of a pathogen is required to seed an infection. Each person has, on average, 1 billion bacteria in each milliliter of saliva. Everyone aspirates as they sleep, but if one has a large enough bolus of bacteria and a loss of normal immune defenses, pneumonia can develop. A significant aspiration can also occur with a healthier host who is intoxicated. Aspirated vomitus damages the airways with acidic stomach contents and increases the likelihood of infection. Pathogens can also be inhaled from the environment.

Pathogens

Table 11.6 summarizes patient conditions and traits that increase the likelihood that particular infectious organisms will cause pneumonia.

Community-Acquired Pneumonia

One fourth of the cases of CAP requiring hospitalization is caused by *S. pneumoniae* and *H. influenzae*. Combined *Legionella*, *Mycoplasma*, and *C. pneumoniae* constitute approximately one sixth of hospitalized patients with CAP. Viral etiologies make up another sixth of pneumonias. The following is a brief description of organisms in order of most frequent to least in the general population.

Streptococcus pneumoniae

S. pneumoniae is the most common cause of community-acquired pneumonia (CAP). It can sometimes be distinguished by rust-colored sputum. The use of vaccination has been instituted for at-risk groups including the elderly and patients with sickle cell disease.

Haemophilus influenzae

H. influenzae often affects smokers and patients with COPD. It is an encapsulated organism and is frequently isolated. *H. influenzae* may become less common as a cause for pneumonia with the routine vaccination of children.

Mycoplasma pneumoniae

M. pneumoniae is common in those younger than 40 years. Patients may present with clear or purulent sputum, a multiforme-type rash, pharyngeal erythema, and a chest x-ray film more abnormal than expected based on physical examination. Treatment is usually outpatient.

Viral Causes

Viral causes of pneumonia or pneumonia symptoms include respiratory syncytial virus (in infants and small children), parainfluenza, influenza, and adenovirus.

Legionella

Legionella is famous for its initial outbreak at a Legionnaire's convention in Philadelphia and is often associated with epidemics. It is an intracellular organism, and it spreads through water droplets (classically found in air conditioning systems). Patients classically have a nonproductive cough and may have mental status changes or a relative bradycardia.

Table 11.6.

Patient conditions and traits that increase the likelihood of pneumonia with particular infectious organisms

Associated Conditions	Organism
Alcoholism	Oral anaerobes, gram-negative rods
COPD	*Streptococcus pneumoniae, Haemophilus influenzae, Moraxella catarrhalis*
AIDS or other immune compromise	*Pneumocystis carinii, Mycobacterium tuberculosis*, cryptococcus varicella, fungi
Influenza	*Staphylococcus aureus*
Homelessness	*M. tuberculosis*
Geographic exposure	Endemic mycoses (coccidioidomycosis, histoplasmosis, blastomycosis)
Hospital/nursing home	Gram-negative rods, *Pseudomonas aeruginosa, S. aureus*
IV drug use	*S. aureus*
Exposure to rodent droppings	Hantavirus
Cystic fibrosis	*P. aeruginosa, S. aureus*
Travel or residence in endemic areas	*M. tuberculosis*

AIDS, acquired immunodeficiency syndrome; COPD, chronic obstructive pulmonary disease; IV, intravenous.

Chlamydia pneumoniae

C. pneumoniae is highly prevalent especially in younger populations. It is associated with typical upper respiratory symptoms (bronchitis, wheezing, and pharyngitis). Overall, it is difficult to distinguish from other pneumonias.

Aspiration Pneumonia

The severity of aspiration pneumonia depends on the amount of gastric contents aspirated. It can progress rapidly from tachycardia and tachypnea to respiratory failure. Most cases begin with crackles on examination and evolve to wheezing and frothy or bloody sputum. The right middle lobe is often affected because of the structure of the airway and because of gravity. Oral anaerobes are seen in aspiration pneumonias.

Mycobacterium tuberculosis

M. tuberculosis can sometimes be distinguished by the description of weight loss, known tuberculosis contacts, recent immigration, hemoptysis, and night sweats.

Pneumocystis carinii

P. carinii can be the first presenting illness of a patient with AIDS. It can sometimes be distinguished radiographically by a characteristic "ground-glass" appearance on chest x-ray examination. However, it is important to note that the most common pneumonia in an AIDS patient is CAP.

Staphylococcus aureus

S. aureus can be particularly concerning because it often strikes immunocompromised patients, patients with hospital exposure, and IV drug users through hematogenous spread. It can be associated with tricuspid valve disease, empyemas, and necrotizing cavitary pneumatoceles requiring surgical intervention. It is also seen following a prior viral pneumonia.

Klebsiella pneumoniae

K. pneumoniae strikes a patient population that is commonly seen in the ED: alcoholic patients, diabetic patients, and patients with chronic illnesses. Currant-jelly sputum is the classic description because of the necrotizing nature of the infection.

Suggested Readings

Fine MJ, et al. A prediction rule to identify low-risk patients with community-acquired pneumonia. *N Engl J Med* 1997;336:243–250.

Harwood-Nuss A, Wolfson AB, Linden CH, Shepherd, SM, Luten RC. Pneumonia. In: *The clinical practice of emergency medicine.* Philadelphia: Lippincott-Raven Publishers, 1996:643–649.

Holmes WF, et al. Providing better care for patients who may have pneumonia. *Thorax* 1999;54:925–928.

Margolis P, et al. Does this infant have pneumonia? *JAMA* 1998;279:308–313.

Marino P. *The ICU book.* Baltimore: Williams & Wilkins, 1990:516–529.

Marrie TJ, et al. A controlled trial of critical pathway for treatment of community-acquired pneumonia. *JAMA* 2000;283:749–755.

Metlay JP, et al. influence of age on symptoms at presentation in patients with community-acquired pneumonia. *Arch Intern Med* 1997; 157:1453–1459.

Niederman MS. Community-acquired pneumonia: a North American perspective. *Chest* 1998; 113:179S–182S.

Schwartz DN, et al. Preventing mismanagement of community-acquired pneumonia at an urban public hospital: implications for institution-specific practice guidelines. *Chest* 1998;113: 194S–198S.

Shortness of Breath
Questions and Answers

Questions

1. A 65-year-old woman is brought to the emergency department in respiratory distress and with chest pain. She has a history of chronic obstructive pulmonary disease (COPD). She is a 60-pack-year smoker and has a history of hypertension and diabetes. On physical examination, she has a rapid respiratory rate, a heart rate of 120 beats/minute, and an oxygen saturation of 80%. She is using accessory muscles of respiration and has decreased air movement and diminished lung sounds throughout. She is placed on oxygen 100% rebreather and begun on a Combivent nebulizer. The patient suddenly deteriorates with a decreasing saturation, hypotension, and altered mentation. What should you do next?

A. Obtain an electrocardiogram (ECG) to rule out myocardial ischemia.

B. Obtain a chest x-ray examination to rule out pneumothorax.

C. Intubate of the patient.

D. Perform needle thoracostomies to alleviate any tension pneumothorax.

E. All of the above.

2. You are examining the patient in question 1. When listening to the lungs, you note decreased breath sounds on the right. In addition, you note tracheal deviation to the left and increased venous distension. Her vital signs have not improved. What should you do?

A. Obtain a stat chest x-ray film.

B. Obtain a stat echocardiogram.

C. Give steroids.

D. Put a chest tube in the right side.

3. A 72-year-old woman presents with shortness of breath worsening over the past 2 weeks. She was on vacation and was unable to refill her prescriptions for Lasix furosemide and isosorbide dinitrate. On physical examination, she has prominent jugular venous distension, crackles at both lung bases, and oxygen saturation of 90% on room air. Which of the following statements about treatments for congestive heart failure (CHF) is most correct?

A. Morphine sulfate increases preload, heart rate, contractility, and anxiety associated with heart failure.

B. Nitroprusside is a smooth muscle relaxant and is excellent for treating CHF related to hypertension, especially if needed for prolonged administration in the intensive care unit (ICU).

C. Furosemide is a loop diuretic that reduces preload and helps the patient to rid the body of excess fluid.

D. Dobutamine is used in cardiogenic shock because it is a negative inotrope, increases heart rate, and also reduces afterload.

4. A 62-year-old man with a history of hypertension present in congestive heart failure. An echocardiogram reveals a thickened left ventricle, which appears stiff during contraction. Which statement about this patient is true?

A. The Frank-Starling relationship states that the force of ventricular contraction is directly related to the end-systolic length of cardiac muscle.

B. Cardiac output is the product of heart rate and systemic vascular resistance.

C. Afterload is the amount of tension placed on the wall of the myocardium during contraction.

D. Blood pressure is directly related to the product of heart rate and systemic vascular resistance.

5. A 55-year-old man with a history of asthma presents to the emergency department with a nonproductive cough and shortness of breath. He denies fever, chills, vomiting, and chest pain. He has increased his use of his albuterol inhaler at home and takes no other medication. He has no history of intubation and has been hospitalized once in the past. On examination, the patient is afebrile, and his vital signs are as follows: blood pressure 130/85 mm Hg, heart rate 105 beats/minute, respiratory rate 20 breaths/minute, and O_2 saturation 94% on room air. Peak flow is 250 L/minute. He has expiratory wheezing with inspiratory to expiratory ratio (I:E ratio) of 1:2. With treatment of nebulized albuterol and prednisolone 125 mg intravenous (IV), he improves. His heart rate is 95 beats/minute, his O_2 saturation is 95%, and he has only faint end-expiratory wheezing. His peak flow is 350 L/minute. On which of the following medications should he be discharged?

A. Oxygen

B. Theophylline

C. Prednisolone

D. Antibiotics

E. Prednisone

Directions: There are two sets of response options for the following scenario. You will be required to select one best answer from each question set.

6. A 45-year-old man with a history of hypertension, diabetes, and coronary artery disease arrives in the emergency department with shortness of breath. He states that for the last several days it has been getting worse and worse, particularly at night when he finds he cannot lie flat. He says he has been coughing up a lot of reddish white sputum. His medications include atenolol, aspirin, glyburide, and hydrochlorothiazide. He is not a smoker. He denies chest pain. His vital signs include blood pressure 160/110 mm Hg, heart rate 112 beats/minute, respiratory rate 28 breaths/minute, temperature 99.9°F, and O_2 saturation of 89%.

6.1. What is the most likely disease process in this patient from the following differential diagnosis?

A. Congestive heart failure (CHF)

B. Pneumonia

C. Ischemic heart disease

D. Acute asthma attack

E. Pulmonary embolus

6.2. On physical examination, you find jugular venous distension, rales bilaterally halfway up both lung fields, an S_3 gallop on cardiac examination, and slight pitting edema. Based on these findings, which of the following procedures would be appropriate?

A. Chest x-ray film

B. Electrocardiogram (ECG)

C. Admission to the hospital

D. Oxygen by nasal canula

E. All of the above

Directions: Match the following patients with their most likely causative organism.

7.1. A 25-year-old otherwise healthy man who has had a cough and shortness of breath for 1 week. His chest x-ray film has bilateral patchy infiltrates.

7.2. A 35-year-old intravenous drug user presents with fatigue and a temperature of 102.4°F. His chest x-ray film shows a peripheral patchy infiltrate.

7.3. A 45-year-old homeless woman, who emigrated from South America 15 years ago, has a 2-cm nodule in the right apex on her chest x-ray film.

7.4. A 65-year-old female smoker, who has been coughing up yellow sputum. Her chest x-ray film shows a left lower lobe infiltrate.

A. *Streptococcus pneumoniae*

B. *Mycobacterium tuberculosis*

C. *Mycoplasma pneumoniae*

D. *Staphylococcus aureus*

Answers and Explanations

1. C. The airway should be the first priority in any patient who is rapidly decompensating. Although this patient may be having a myocardial infarction (MI) and may have a pneumothorax, the airway should be managed first. Once the airway is secured, an electrocardiogram (ECG) and chest x-ray film are warranted. There is no evidence by history or physical examination for a pneumothorax; thus, needle decompression is not warranted.

2. D. This patient has all the signs of tension pneumothorax. Waiting for a chest x-ray film may be too long a delay, allowing for external pressure to increase on the heart to prevent meaningful filling and precipitate cardiac arrest. Although you might consider placing an Angiocath in the right anterior 2nd intercostal space in an attempt to alleviate the tension, you will ultimately have to place a chest tube. In addition needle thoracostomy may be placed outside the chest accidentally and cause unnecessary delays before chest tube insertion. Steroids have no role for this patient. Her problem is not of an obstructive nature as seen in chronic obstructive pulmonary disease (COPD) or asthma. An echocardiogram is appropriate if the presentation suggested cardiac tamponade. The patient would have had distant heart sounds, elevated jugular venous pressures, hypotension, and tachycardia. She would have had clear lung sounds and no tracheal deviation.

3. C. Furosemide is a loop diuretic that reduces preload and helps the patient to rid the body of excess fluid. It is used frequently for outpatient management of congestive heart failure (CHF). Nitroprusside is an excellent medication for patients in CHF who are acutely hypertensive. When used at higher rates than 2 μg/kg/minute or for greater than 24 to 48 hours, the body may not be able to keep up with the metabolism of cyanide, a byproduct of nitroprusside degradation. Morphine sulfate actually decreases preload, heart rate, contractility, and anxiety associated with heart failure. Dobutamine is a positive inotrope giving the myocardium better contraction. It does increase the heart rate and reduce afterload.

4. C. Afterload is the amount of pressure that the heart as a pump must generate to create forward flow of blood, which is another way of saying that it is related to the tension placed on the wall of the myocardium. The Frank-Starling relationship states that the force of ventricular contraction is directly related to the end-diastolic length (i.e., degree of maximal stretch) not systolic length of cardiac muscle. Cardiac output is the product of heart rate and stroke volume. Blood pressure is directly related to heart rate and stroke volume because the pressure is the product of cardiac output and systemic vascular resistance.

5. E. This patient is having an asthma exacerbation, and prednisone is indicated for treatment to decrease inflammation. Oxygen is not indicated because his O_2 saturation is 95%. Theophylline is generally not a first-line medication for asthma in the emergency department (ED). Although prednisolone can be given intravenously in the ED, it is not given as outpatient therapy. Finally, antibiotics are not indicated because he has no history of fever or productive cough and no rales or evidence of consolidation on physical examination.

6.1. A. This patient's medical history puts him at risk for congestive heart failure (CHF) and ischemic heart disease. He does not describe the classic anginal symptoms of ischemic chest pain; although he could be experiencing ischemia, it would be leading to the CHF, which he is clearly experiencing. He has symptoms that could be found in either CHF or pneumonia, including difficulty lying flat, productive cough, and dyspnea. The reddish sputum is the pink frothy sputum commonly found in CHF; furthermore, he has no fever and is not primarily complaining of an infectious cough, which must put pneumonia lower on the list compared with CHF. Pulmonary embolus is a more difficult disease to diagnose but should at least be considered in anyone with dyspnea. It typically has an acute onset, presents with hypoxia and tachycardia, but does not produce orthopnea or paroxysmal nocturnal dyspnea that this patient has. Asthma would be very unlikely in this patient with no history of smoking or reactive airways disease. He does not describe symptoms common to an acute asthma attack: tightness, wheezing, or nonproductive cough.

6.2. E. This patient has classic findings of congestive heart failure. He should have an x-ray film to confirm the diagnosis and evaluate heart size. An electrocardiogram (ECG) should be done to rule out acute myocardial infarction (MI), arrhythmia, or ischemia. Oxygen should be placed, and the patient should be admitted for treatment and to rule out cardiac ischemia.

7.1. C. Healthy young people often have infection with *Mycoplasma pneumoniae* in the absence of other risk factors, although risk factors need to be determined even in otherwise healthy patients. His chest x-ray film with the patchy infiltrates is consistent.

7.2. D. Intravenous drug users have a higher incidence of hematogenously spread and more dangerous pneumonias such as *Staphylococcus aureus*. A cavitary lesion can also appear, as can an empyema in these patients.

7.3. B. This patient is at risk for tuberculosis resulting from her homelessness and having grown up in a foreign country. She also has an apical lesion on her x-ray film that is suggestive of tuberculosis.

7.4. A. This woman has a common etiology of community-acquired pneumonia. She does not have risk factors for the other pathogens and her chest x-ray film has a *Streptococcus*-caused lobar infiltrate.

Back Pain

And when your back begins to smart,
It's like a penknife in your heart.

Mother Goose

INTRODUCTION
Eric Legome, MD
Section Editor

Back pain may be caused by myriad different organs and structures. The etiologies can be broken down into two major categories: primary and referred. Primary back pain arises from structures of the back proper, including the bones, ligaments, muscles, and nerves, and is discussed in detail in Chapter 15. Trauma, degeneration (e.g., osteoarthritis), and local pathological processes (e.g., tumor or infection) can cause pain in any of these structures.

Referred back pain is caused by organs or structures that are connected to the back either through anatomic proximity or through nervous connection. Examples include the abdominal aorta, the pancreas, the kidneys and ureters, and the gastrointestinal tract.

Referred back pain originates from structures that are not part of the back proper. Abdominal aortic aneurysm (AAA) is the most important cause of referred back pain and must be considered in all patients with lower back pain. The pain associated with AAA may be primarily abdominal in nature, but because the abdominal aorta lies in the retroperitoneum just anterior to the left side of the vertebral column, the pain may be felt in the back as well. Expansion of the aneurysm posteriorly may encroach on the vertebral bodies and nerve roots and thus produce many of the symptoms associated with primary back pain. Expansion of the aneurysm distally into the iliac arteries may produce pain in the groin.

The kidneys are retroperitoneal organs that are located at the T12 to L1 level and thus may be a cause of lower back pain as well. Pain afferents to the ureters arise from the lowest splanchnic nerve and enter the spinal cord at the T12 and L1 segments. Thus, the pain may be felt in the area of the kidney (the costovertebral angle), the flank, the ipsilateral lower quadrant, and/or the ipsilateral groin. In the emergency department, renal stones and pyelonephritis are the most common cause of back pain arising from the kidneys. Renal tumors or hematomas may also cause pain in the costovertebral region. There are many other causes of referred back pain including gallstones, pancreatitis, and ulcer disease. Although it is beyond the scope of this section to discuss them all, the differential of back pain is extraordinarily broad. A wide range of possibilities must be considered when evaluating the patient who presents with back pain.

CHAPTER **12**

Aortic Dissection

Todd W. Thomsen, MD

Clinical Scenario

A 65-year-old man presents to the emergency department (ED) by ambulance with a chief complaint of midback pain. The onset of pain was followed by a brief syncopal episode. He describes the pain as sharp and tearing, commencing midsternal and traveling to the interscapular area. The onset occurred over approximately 5 minutes. The pain is slightly improved now but still severe. He is unable to find any position that improves the pain. He has associated nausea but has not vomited. On review of symptoms, he denies any shortness of breath, abdominal pain, or neurological symptoms.

Past medical history is significant for a 20-year history of hypertension. He takes a diuretic but is poorly compliant with his medications. He denies cigarettes or illicit drug use. He admits to two to three alcoholic drinks per night.

Physical examination reveals an obese male in significant distress. He is pale and diaphoretic. He is clearly uncomfortable on the bed and is constantly changing his position. Vital signs are blood pressure of 180/110 mm Hg on the right arm and 130/90 mmHg on the left, a heart rate of 110 beats/minute, a respiratory rate of 18 breaths/minute, a temperature of 98.0°F, and oxygen saturation of 98% on room air. His skin is cool and diaphoretic. His jugular venous pulsation is elevated at 4 cm above the sternal angle. The pulmonary examination reveals bibasilar crackles. The cardiac examination reveals a regular rhythm and tachycardic rate. There is a high-pitched diastolic murmur best heard with the bell at the up-

per left sternal border and at the right sternal border. The right radial pulse is more prominent than the left radial pulse. The abdomen is soft and nontender without any masses appreciated. The back is nontender. There is no lower extremity edema and distal pulses in the feet are equal and strong bilaterally. The patient is unable to cooperate with a full neurological examination because of his distress, but it is grossly nonfocal.

The patient is placed on a cardiac monitor and high-flow oxygen. Two 16-gauge intravenous (IV) catheters are placed in the bilateral antecubital fossas.

An electrocardiogram (ECG) reveals a sinus tachycardia with 2 mm of ST-segment elevation in the inferior leads (II, III, and aVF).

A portable chest x-ray film reveals a slightly enlarged cardiac silhouette, cephalization of the pulmonary vasculature, and slight perihilar fluffy opacities consistent with mild pulmonary edema. There is obscuration of the aortic knob and a significantly widened mediastinum. The patient is given pain medication, placed on esmolol and nitroprusside drips to control his heart rate and then blood pressure, and sent for an immediate computed tomography (CT) scan. The scan reveals an aortic dissection from the aortic root to the midthoracic aorta. He is taken immediately to the operating room.

Clinical Evaluation

Introduction

One of the most lethal causes of chest and upper back pain is aortic dissection. An aortic dissection is caused by a tear in the intimal layer of the aorta with subsequent tracking of blood through the wall of the aorta. This creates a "false lumen," or a column of blood parallel to the true lumen of the aorta. The false lumen may obstruct the flow through major arterial tributaries or it may dissect retrograde into the coronary arteries, aortic valve, and pericardium. Other times it may dissect through the adventitial layer of the aorta and into the mediastinum or pleural space. This usually causes death, even with immediate diagnosis and treatment. The ED management of aortic dissection centers on rapid diagnosis and close attention to heart rate and blood pressure control. Surgical consultants should be notified as soon as the diagnosis is suspected because these patients may require rapid definitive care. The morbidity and mortality is significant, even with prompt diagnosis and treatment.

History

Patients with aortic dissection usually present to the ED with a complaint of chest and/or thoracic back pain. Because of the often-dramatic presentation, history taking is done concurrently with diagnostic and therapeutic measures. The pain of aortic dissection is classically sudden in onset, sharp, severe, tearing, and knifelike. The pain may have a pulsatile quality that correlates with heart rate. The location of the pain depends on the location of the dissection. It often migrates if the false lumen extends the course of the aorta. A dissection of the ascending aorta or proximal aortic arch causes anterior chest pain, similar in location to the pain of myocardial infarction. Dissection of the aortic arch may cause pain in the neck and jaw, and the pain of a descending aortic dissection is typically intrascapular upper back pain. Migration of pain is a distinguishing characteristic of aortic dissection when trying to differentiate it from myocardial infarction.

Associated signs and symptoms such as nausea, vomiting, diaphoresis, and light-headedness and, as in our patient, syncope are common. The patient may experience extreme apprehension or a feeling of impending doom. Neurological complaints such as numbness, tingling, weakness, or even paresis of the torso or lower extremities may occur because of spinal cord ischemia. Other important historical questions pertain to the risk factors associated with aortic dissection. The most common association is arterial hypertension. Patients with congenital heart anomalies, such as a bicuspid aortic valve or coarctation of the aorta, are at greater risk for aortic dissection. Persons with connective tissue disorders such as Marfan's or Ehlers-Danlos syndromes are also at risk. Pregnancy is also a risk factor. It is important to obtain a history of coronary artery disease or any other cardiovascular compromise, because these conditions may add to the patient's morbidity if present.

Physical Examination

As with our patient in the clinical scenario, the overall appearance of a patient with aortic dissection will often reveal apprehension, pallor, or general distress. Vital signs typically reveal tachycardia and hypertension. Hypotension in the setting of aortic dissection is an ominous sign. This means that either the dissection has propagated retrograde toward the heart, causing hemopericardium and cardiac tamponade, or it has dissected through the adventitia and is causing massive mediastinal hemorrhage. If the dissection occludes either the brachiocephalic or left subclavian arteries, there may be a different blood pressure between both arms. Likewise a pulse deficit may be appreciated in one arm; assessment includes evaluating the presence and strength of pulses in all extremities. A careful examination of the neck and cardiopulmonary examination should be performed. Evidence of pericardial tamponade such as engorged neck veins resulting from the lack of cardiac filling, distant heart sounds, and a pericardial friction rub may be present. Aortic valve involvement can be detected as a diastolic murmur over the apex of the heart suggestive of aortic insufficiency. The murmur is classically described as a high-pitched, blowing murmur best heard at the mid-left sternal border. It may help to have the patient lean forward with exhaled breath. A low, rumbling, apical diastolic murmur may also be appreciated. It is known as an Austin Flint murmur. Patients with acute aortic insufficiency may also be dyspneic and have rales on pulmonary examination resulting from congestive heart failure.

It is also useful to do a rapid neurological examination, including assessment of the patient's mental status. Global hypoperfusion causes decreased consciousness, and syncope occurs in 5% of patients with aortic dissection. A cranial nerve examination may reveal Horner's syndrome, caused by the compression of the superior cervical sympathetic ganglion by an expanding aortic hematoma. Findings would include unilateral mydriasis, ptosis, and possibly anhydrosis. Compression of the recurrent laryngeal nerve may cause hoarseness. Extremity examination may reveal sensory or motor deficits secondary to spinal cord ischemia.

Diagnostic Evaluation

Rapid diagnosis of aortic dissection is crucial so that early appropriate management can be instituted. An ECG should be performed. There are no findings pathognomonic for aortic dissection, so it may be more helpful to assess alternate causes of the symptoms. Ventricular hypertrophy may be present because of chronic hypertension. This would manifest as large QRS deflections in the precordial leads. Many patients with aortic dissection have ECG findings consistent with myocardial ischemia, such as mild ST-segment abnormalities or T-wave changes. Patients with a retrograde dissection may occlude coronary arteries, in particular the right coronary artery, and have ST-segment elevations that indicate myocardial infarction. These are usually seen in the inferior leads.

A portable upright anteroposterior (AP) chest x-ray film should be obtained as a screening study on any patient complaining of severe anterior chest or upper back pain. If possible, it should be followed by a posteroanterior (PA) chest and lateral film. The most common radiographic abnormality in aortic dissection is a widened mediastinum caused by a hematoma formed by the false lumen. These hematomas expand readily because of the lack of structural integrity of the adventitia. When evaluating the mediastinum on a chest radiograph, one should be able to follow the contour of the aorta as it ascends, traverses the arch, and descends out of the thorax. It should remain approximately the same diameter throughout its course. Other signs of an aortic anomaly include lateral displacement of the trachea and loss of the aortic knob, which is the angle produced by the descending portion of the aortic arch and the left pulmonary vessels. Although many patients with a dissection have an abnormal radiograph, a normal chest x-ray film does not rule out a dissection.

Traditionally, the gold standard for the diagnosis of aortic dissection was angiography, although this is being supplanted by newer modalities such as spiral CT scan, transesophageal echocardiography (TEE), and magnetic resonance imaging (MRI). Angiography involves arterial catheterization of the aorta, an invasive procedure that carries its own morbidity. It must be performed in an angiography suite by skilled operators, making it an expensive and time-consuming test. Its advantages are that it is very sensitive in detecting aortic dissection, and it is usually able to identify the exact location of the intimal tear or the defect in the intima that marks the origin of the dissection. It can also detect aortic regurgitation and the extent of branch artery occlusion that may exist. With the advent of newer technology, however, this modality is used less frequently in the ED.

CT scan is usually the first test performed after the chest radiograph for diagnosis of aortic dissection. However, the patient must be hemodynamically stable to travel to the radiology department and must be closely monitored during that time. Fortunately, the newer generation of CT scanners allows image acquisition within seconds, and a patient can be scanned in several minutes. The new-generation spiral CT allows rapid imaging of the aorta during peak contrast opacification. Through the use of volume averaging, motion artifact is eliminated and the images can be reformatted in multiple dimensions. This is referred to as CT angiography because the arterial images provide the three-dimensional quality obtained by conventional angiography.

Furthermore, CT is highly accurate for the detection of aortic dissection with values approaching 100% for both sensitivity and specificity. A disadvantage of the CT scan is that it provides no information about aortic insufficiency, which is helpful in determining appropriate surgical therapy.

Transthoracic echocardiography (TTE) has been used for the diagnosis of aortic dissection. However, its sensitivity and specificity are only approximately 80% and 90%, respectively. However, this modality is useful in determining the degree of aortic regurgitation and may be used in conjunction with positive CT scan results. TTE is limited by transmission through the sternum, ribs, and lungs. This hinders visualization of the posterior aortic arch and descending portion of the aorta. Because of these limitations, TTE is inadequate as a single modality in the diagnosis of aortic dissection.

TEE brings the ultrasound probe in much closer proximity to the aorta, allowing excellent visualization of the aortic arch and descending aorta. This increases the sensitivity to almost 100% for detecting the intimal flap and false lumen of aortic dissection. Color Doppler identifies the degree of flow through the intimal flap into the false lumen and allows evaluation of the degree of aortic regurgitation. It is also good for quantifying the amount of pericardial fluid and diagnosing cardiac tamponade. Its specificity for detecting aortic dissection is only 94% because of false-positive findings resulting from motion artifact. Furthermore, visualization of the ascending aorta is limited by the interposition of the right mainstem bronchus, although this site is uncommonly the origin of an intimal flap. Advantages of TEE are that it can be performed at the bedside in the ED, allowing for continuous monitoring, and that it does not require contrast. However, it requires an expert operator, typically a cardiologist; furthermore, the patient must be sedated for the procedure.

Differential Diagnosis

The differential diagnosis for aortic dissection is illustrated in Table 12.1.

Table 12.1.

Differential diagnosis of aortic dissection

Cardiac Conditions
Cardiac ischemia or myocardial infarction
Pericarditis or myocarditis

Vascular Conditions
Thoracic aortic aneurysm

Pulmonary Conditions
Pulmonary embolism
Pneumonia
Spontaneous pneumothorax

Gastrointestinal Conditions
Esophageal spasm or rupture
Pancreatitis
Peptic ulcer disease
Cholelithiasis/cholecystitis

Treatment

The primary objective of ED management of aortic dissection is preventing the progression of the dissection. This is best accomplished by reducing the mean arterial blood pressure and, more importantly, reducing the pressure gradient or the force of contraction (dP/dt), by controlling the heart rate (Table 12.2). By increasing the time of ejection of blood into the aorta, the relative stress on the aortic wall is decreased.

Table 12.2.

Treatment guidelines for aortic dissection

Supplemental oxygen
Two large-bore antecubital intravenous catheters
Cardiac monitoring
Consideration of an arterial line for pressure
    monitoring (ICU)
Blood pressure and arterial pressure gradient
    control: β-blocker (metoprolol, propanolol
    [Inderal] or esmolol) for rate control and
    sodium nitroprusside for blood pressure
    control *or* labetalol for combined pressure
    and rate control
Directly to operating room for Stanford type A
    dissections
Admission to ICU for Stanford type B dissections

ICU, intensive care unit.

Nitroprusside

Blood pressure control is usually maintained by IV infusion of sodium nitroprusside to keep the systolic blood pressure between 100 mm Hg and 120 mm Hg. Nitroprusside is a potent vasodilator that, when administered as an infusion, allows for very tight regulation of blood pressure. However, the resulting decrease in mean systolic pressure causes a reflex tachycardia via the baroreceptor response in the carotid sinus. The increased heart rate leads to an increase in the arterial pressure gradient or rate of rise of force of contraction (dP/dt).

β-blockers

A β-adrenergic blocking (β-blocking) agent is used in combination with nitroprusside to counteract this effect. The goal is to maintain a heart rate between 60 and 80 beats per minute. This can be attained with a steady infusion of esmolol, which is a short-acting β-blocker. Because of its short half-life, this agent can be titrated easily and shut off with a rapid reversal of its effect. Alternatively, propranolol or metoprolol can be used in intermittent IV boluses. Metoprolol has the advantage of being more specific to β-1 receptors. Labetalol, which has both α- and β-blocking properties, has been used as single agent in the management of aortic dissection. Its α-blockade results in peripheral vasodilation with reduced mean systolic blood pressure, and its β-blockade mitigates reflex tachycardia. If patients are unable to tolerate β-blockers because of allergy or pulmonary disease, a calcium channel blocker can be used. Arterial line blood pressure monitoring is recommended when these agents are used. These lines are placed in the intensive care unit (ICU).

Surgical Repair

Definitive therapy depends on the location and extent of the aortic dissection. The Stanford classification is the most commonly used system for defining aortic dissection. Stanford type A includes dissections that involve the ascending aorta, whether or not the arch or descending aorta is involved.

Stanford type B includes dissections of the descending aorta alone (Fig. 12.1). Up to 90% of patients with type A dissections will die within 3 months if not treated surgically. Conversely, the mortality rate is higher for patients with type B dissection who are treated surgically compared with medical management alone. Therefore, patients with type A dissections undergo immediate surgical repair with excision of the ascending aorta and placement of a synthetic graft. Aortic valve replacement is performed if the anatomy of the valve has been disrupted. Surgery is also indicated in patients with an intimal tear located in the aortic arch. For type B dissections, medical management is indicated. This includes tight control of blood pressure with oral agents and serial CT or MRI examinations to follow the progression of the dissection.

Disposition

Immediate operative repair is indicated for dissections involving the ascending aorta or aortic arch. The only contraindication to this is devastating neurological damage secondary to the dissection. If the dissection involves the descending aorta, then the patient is admitted to the ICU for antihypertensive therapy and observation for the development of complications. Complications of aortic dissection include progression of the false lumen, development of an aneurysm, and aortic rupture.

Pathophysiology

The aortic wall consists of three layers: the intima, media, and adventitia. An aortic dissection travels through the layers of the media. The media consists of concentric layers of elastic laminae that contain the protein elastin, which gives the aorta its resilience. Between these laminae are smooth muscle cells that contract in response to stretch that also adds to the aorta's elastic quality. Reticular fibers and glycoprotein ground substance contained in the media provide the structural integrity of the aorta. Degeneration of the

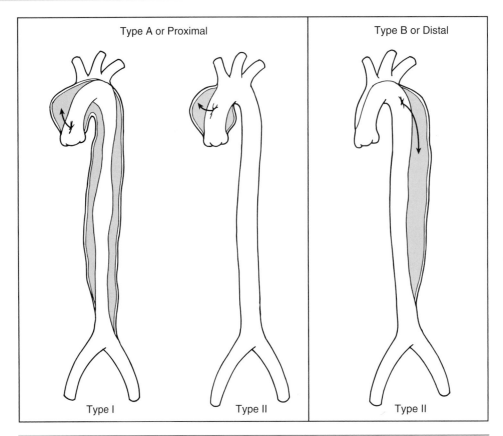

Figure 12.1
Stanford classification of aortic dissection types A and B. Type A includes dissections that involve
the ascending aorta, whether or not the arch or descending aorta is involved. Stanford type B
includes dissections of the descending aorta alone.

media occurs as a natural process of aging. However, there are disorders, such as Marfan's and Ehlers-Danlos syndrome, that result in a more rapid degeneration of the media and a higher prevalence of aortic dissection. Once a defect occurs in the innermost intimal layer, blood readily dissects through a track formed between two elastic laminae in the media.

Medial degeneration is believed to be accelerated by the oscillating hemodynamic forces exerted on the aortic wall during systole and diastole. Pressure gradients experienced during systemic hypertension result in large pressure fluctuations over time (dP/dt). This pressure translates to wall tension and repetitive stretch of the myofibers in the media because they provide structural in-

tegrity and elasticity in the aorta. Therefore, after years of repeated stretch and recoil, this layer begins to weaken.

An additional source of wall stress comes from the pendulum effect of the beating heart. The heart, ascending aorta, and aortic arch are suspended in the chest by the major arterial branches of the aortic arch. Its lack of restraint allows the heart to pump efficiently, aided in diastole by the recoil effect of the aorta. However, this enables the heart and aorta to shift laterally in the chest with each contraction. The aorta is fixed in the retroperitoneum just distal to the origin of the left subclavian artery. A stretching force is exerted at this point during each contraction, and over time medial degeneration occurs in this area. Subsequently, the proximal descending aorta is a common location for an intimal tear to occur.

Turbulent flow also contributes to local wall stress. By nature of the valve structure, the blood flow exiting the aortic valve is turbulent. A congenital bicuspid aortic valve further increases the downstream turbulence, which in turn increases wall stress. Aortic dissection is significantly greater in patients with congenital bicuspid aortic valve. Similarly, other congenital cardiac anomalies may increase turbulent flow, most commonly coarctation of the aorta. Finally, the hemodynamic changes that occur during pregnancy seem to account for a higher incidence of aortic dissection in young pregnant women. It is known that cardiac output increases by about 40% during pregnancy. This, coupled with the anemia of pregnancy, increases aortic turbulence and thus predisposes pregnant women to intimal tears and dissection.

Suggested Readings

Bourland MD. Aortic dissection. In: Rosen P, ed. *Emergency medicine—concepts and clinical practice*, 4th ed. St. Louis: Mosby-Year Book, 1998:2456–2478.

Junquiera LC, Carniero J, Kelly RO. *Basic histology*, 4th ed. East Norwalk, CT: Appleton & Lange, 1992:216–231.

Kouchoukos NT, Dougenis D. Surgery of the thoracic aorta. *N Engl J Med* 1997;336:1876–1888.

Moore KL. *Clinically oriented anatomy*, 3rd ed. Baltimore: Williams & Wilkins, 1992.

Sommer T, Fehske W, Holzknecht N, et al. Aortic dissection: a comparative study of diagnosis with spiral CT, multiplanar transesophageal echocardiography, and MR imaging. *Radiology* 1996;199:347–352.

Urban BA, Bluemke DA, Johnson KM, et al. Imaging of thoracic aortic disease. *Cardiol Clin North Am* 1999;17:659–682.

Wooley, CF, Sparks EH, Boudoulas H. Aortic pain. *Prog Cardiovasc Dis* 1998;40:563–589.

CHAPTER 13

Urolithiasis

Michael R. Filbin, MD

Clinical Scenario

A 26-year-old man is brought to the emergency department (ED) by ambulance. He complains of an acute onset of left flank pain. The pain is severe, sharp, and radiating toward the groin and testicles. It is intermittent with exacerbations every few minutes. The pain has moved slightly toward the left lower quadrant. He has not had this pain before; however, he had mild left flank discomfort in the morning on waking. He is nauseated and vomited once before arrival. He denies pain on urination but does have a sensation of urgency.

He denies any significant past medical history, including back pain, vascular disease, renal disease, or gastrointestinal problems. He does not smoke cigarettes. He drinks one to two beers each week. He denies any illicit drug use. The patient works as a construction worker. His family history is significant for a father with urolithiasis and hypertension.

The physical examination reveals a well-developed athletic man in significant discomfort. Vital signs show a blood pressure of 145/90 mm Hg, heart rate of 110 beats/minute, temperature of 98.6°F, respiratory rate of 18 breaths/minute, and oxygen saturation of 98% on room air. The patient is intermittently writhing on the bed and pacing the room. His skin is diaphoretic. His cardiopulmonary examination reveals tachycardia but is otherwise normal. He has mild back discomfort but no significant left costovertebral angle tenderness. The abdomen is soft, nontender, and without palpable masses. The genitourinary examination reveals normal male genitalia without masses or hernias. The testicles are descended bilaterally and are nontender. On rectal examination, the prostate is smooth and nontender.

An intravenous (IV) line is begun and normal saline is administered along with 5 mg of morphine, which is repeated once and provides adequate pain control. He also receives 12.5 mg of prochlorperazine (Phenergan) intravenously for his nausea with good results.

A urinalysis shows 3 to 5 red blood cells per high-powered field, 0 to 2 white blood cells per high-powered field, and concentrated urine. A noncontrast spiral computed tomography (CT) scan is obtained and shows a 3-mm radiopaque stone at the ureteral-vesical junction.

The patient feels significantly better when he returns from the CT scanner. He receives 500 mg of naproxen sodium by mouth that relieves the remaining discomfort. He is diagnosed with urolithiasis, or "renal" stones. He is discharged with a prescription for analgesics and a strainer for his urine and is told to follow up with his primary care doctor for further evaluation.

Clinical Evaluation

Introduction

Urolithiasis, also described as renal calculi or kidney stones, is one of the most common disorders of the urinary tract. The lay term "kidney stone" is a misnomer, because the stones may exist anywhere in the genitourinary tract. The clinical presentation of symptomatic urolithiasis is often quite striking. Patients have equated it to the pain of childbirth labor.

The primary goal of ED management is to rule out a more serious illness and to relieve the symptoms. In most patients, especially those with a first-time event and the elderly, radiological testing is performed to make a definitive diagnosis. Most patients with small calculi will eventually pass the stone, although those with large stones may require operative intervention. With adequate analgesia, hydration, and follow-up, they will have an excellent prognosis.

History

A thorough history is essential to differentiate between benign and life-threatening disorders that may present with back pain. The location, quality, radiation, and severity of the pain should be elicited. Associated symptoms should also be elicited and what was done to remedy the symptoms before arrival in the ED.

The pain is commonly described as abrupt in onset and originating in the flank or side of the abdomen. Severe, unremitting episodes lasting minutes to hours are typical but may vary. It is often termed "colicky," referring to a sharp waxing and waning pain resulting from hyperperistalsis of the smooth muscle of the ureter. Renal colic classically occurs during night or early morning, often waking the patient from sleep. The pain often radiates from the flank to the abdomen and into the groin. Referred pain may develop in the testicle or the labia majoris. Costovertebral angle pain is associated with a proximal stone near the origin of the ureter. Lower abdominal pain may indicate partial passage of the stone into the distal ureter or ureteral-vesicular junction. Changing body position or moving the bowels is sometimes attempted by patients to alleviate the pain. An inability to find a comfortable position is a common complaint ("renal colic").

Although no single factor predisposes a patient to urolithiasis, certain familial, lifestyle, seasonal, and occupational factors may provide clues to the diagnosis. The most common historical clue is that of patient's history of prior stone. Recurrence is generally the rule, and approximately 50% of patients will have a recurrence within 5 years of their first stone. There is a familial tendency to develop stones.

Factors that may precipitate renal colic include periods of immobilization, residence in a hot climate, history of urinary tract infection (UTI), dietary history, or use of certain drugs. Stone disease is most prevalent in white professional men with sedentary lifestyles.

Physical Examination

Simple observation of the patient often provides clues to the diagnosis. In the case of renal calculi, the patient usually is quite uncomfortable, moving around on the bed or pacing in the room. Patients with renal colic appear pale, diaphoretic, and clammy. Vomiting is common. Vital signs usually reflect the sympathetic response to pain. These include mild hypertension and tachycardia. Hypotension should raise concerns for possible sources of shock such as sepsis or hypovolemia. Fever is often but not always present, with concomitant urinary infection.

A thorough abdominal examination should be performed to exclude other serious etiologies. Palpation of the abdomen for aortic aneurysm is critical, especially in the elderly patient with known cardiovascular disease. Peritoneal signs such as rebound and involuntary guarding are unusual in renal colic. Their presence should prompt the physician to search for other causes of pain, such as ruptured appendix and ectopic pregnancy. Patients may complain of abdominal pain when examined but significant tenderness is infrequent. Bowel sounds may be hypoactive, representing an ileus. Costovertebral angle tenderness can be assessed but is not a reliable predictor of nephrolithiasis. Its presence should raise suspicion for pyelonephritis.

Diagnostic Evaluation

In the past, the urinalysis was the cornerstone of laboratory evaluation. With a classic history and presentation, this simple test can be helpful in both diagnosing ureteral obstructing stones and UTI. However, 10% to 20% of symptomatic stones do not result in microscopic hematuria, and patients with alternative serious diagnoses may also have hematuria. Furthermore, the presence of urine white blood cells may be the result of ureteral inflammation not acute infection. In the correct clinical scenario, the urinalysis may aid in the diagnosis of kidney stones and/or infection.

Routine serum white blood cell count determination is rarely helpful. Blood urea nitrogen and creatinine levels should be determined, especially in delayed presentations. Mild elevation may indicate dehydration resulting from vomiting. Acute renal insufficiency in the setting of acute obstruction usually takes at least 5 days to develop in healthy patients.

Stone protocol helical CT scanning of the abdomen without oral or IV contrast has become the study of choice to diagnose kidney stones in the ED. It is highly accurate, noninvasive, and rapid. It may provide alternative diagnoses if the patient does not have a kidney stone, such as abdominal aortic aneurysm or appendicitis. Ultrasound may detect hydronephrosis but has a much lower sensitivity for visualizing stones (64%), especially small ureteral calculi.

Intravenous pyelogram (IVP) uses contrast dye to detect renal or ureteral calculi. It is falling out of favor as the availability of helical CT becomes more widespread. Although accurate, IVP requires a significant increase in patient and staff time, along with an injection of IV contrast. The kidney/ureter/bladder (KUB) (i.e., abdominal) radiograph has a very low sensitivity for detecting stones and should not be ordered as a primary diagnostic test. Stones are often radiopaque; thus, a KUB might be a reasonable assessment in a patient presenting with a recurrent stone.

Differential Diagnosis

The differential diagnosis for nephrolithiasis is illustrated in Table 13.1.

Treatment

The goal of managing ureteral stones is pain control and diagnosis (Table 13.2). Often the results of a careful history, focused physical examination, and minimal laboratory data will lead to the correct diagnosis. Once life threats in the differential diagnosis are excluded, the clinician must move to rapid pain management. Patients with renal colic describe one of the most painful experiences of a lifetime. Timely administration of nonsteroidal antiinflammatory drugs (NSAIDs) (ibuprofen orally or ketorolac IV or intramuscular) or opioid agents (morphine) leads to enhanced patient comfort. Treatment

Table 13.1.

Differential diagnosis of urolithiasis

Urological Disease

Upper Urinary Tract
Renal infarct
Renal tumors
Pyelonephritis
Hemorrhage

Ureter
Urothelial tumors
Hemorrhage
Prior surgery scars
Metastatic tumors

Lower Urinary Tract
Urinary retention
Bladder tumors

Nonurological Disease

Abdominal Disease
Peritonitis
Biliary colic
Intestinal obstruction
Abdominal aortic aneurysm
Mesenteric ischemia

Retroperitoneal Disease
Lymphadenopathy
Tumor
Hemorrhage
Psoas abscess

Gynecological Disease
Endometriosis
Ovarian torsion
Tuboovarian abscess
Pregnancy
Ectopic pregnancy

Table 13.2.

Treatment summary for nephrolithiasis

Intravenous fluids: normal saline

Pain medication

Mild to moderate pain: acetaminophen, NSAIDs
(ibuprofen by mouth, ketorolac IV or IM)

Moderate to severe pain: narcotics: morphine IV
or subcutaneous, meperidine (Demerol) IV or IM

Antiemetics: prochlorperazine, droperidol (get
ECG, use with caution, currently FDA black
box drug), ondansetron

Antibiotics: if evidence of infection and stable,
oral antibiotics; if pyelonephritis suspected,
consideration of IV antibiotics and admission

ECG, electrocardiogram; FDA, Food and Drug
Administration; IM, intramuscular; IV, intravenous;
NSAIDs, nonsteroidal antiinflammatory drugs.

should not be withheld based on concern over masking an underlying abdominal lesion. The combination of a consistent history, lack of significant abdominal tenderness, and hematuria often is sufficient to establish the diagnosis. A diagnostic CT or IVP should be ordered if the etiology of the symptoms is in question. However, pain management can begin before more sophisticated imaging techniques begin.

IV fluids should be considered for patients who have been vomiting or are significantly dehydrated. Large volumes of IV fluids are not needed to "flush out" the stone as once believed. Normal saline infused at rates sufficient to correct minor dehydration is sufficient for most cases. Antiemetic medications help in controlling nausea and vomiting, which usually subside also with pain control. Antibiotics are not indicated for uncomplicated calculi.

Disposition

Indications for admission to the hospital are concomitant pyelonephritis, inability to control pain, single kidney, or very large obstructing stone. It takes many days for an obstruction and hydronephrosis to cause irreversible kidney damage; thus, a patient with an acutely obstructed stone whose pain is under control

with oral analgesics and who has rapid follow-up with an urologist, may potentially be discharged. Admission is not always warranted for UTI, but patients with a urinalysis consistent with infection should receive antibiotics. This is usually done in consultation with an urologist who can closely follow the patient.

Most stones less than 5 mm in diameter will pass spontaneously, whereas those greater than 8 mm generally will not. There are several treatment options for the urologist in the management of more difficult stones. The clinician should be aware of techniques such as extracorporeal shock wave lithotripsy (ECSWL), ureteroscopic manipulation, cutaneous nephrolithotomy, and surgery as possibilities during patient follow-up with the urologist.

Pathophysiology

An estimated 2% to 10% of the population will form urinary calculi at some time in their life. Many may be asymptomatic. The peak age of onset is between the ages of 20 to 30 years.

The emergency clinician will rarely need to identify the specific type of calculus present. However, a basic understanding of stone formation and excretion will help guide proper patient evaluation, management, and follow-up.

Urinary calculi may form at any level of the urinary tract but mainly arise within the kidney. Calcium oxalate, or a mixture of calcium oxalate with calcium phosphate, constitutes most stones (75%). Triple stones, or struvite stones, are composed of magnesium ammonium phosphate and represent approximately 15% of all stones. These stones occur almost exclusively in patients with urea-splitting bacteria in the urine and persistent UTI (e.g., *Proteus*, *Klebsiella* species). The remaining stones are made of uric acid (6% to 10%) and cystine (1% to 2%). An organic matrix of mucoprotein, making up 1% to 5% of the stone by weight, is present in all calculi. There are many causes for the initiation and propagation of stones. The main factor is supersaturation. Stones form in urine that is supersaturated with respect to the ionic components of the specific stone, and saturation is dependent on chemical free ion activities. An increase in the free ion activity will cause the urine to become supersaturated, a state that favors stone growth. Clinicians can determine a patient's potential for stone formation by measuring rates of urine solute excretion, in mass per unit time, of the principal components of stones. These studies are always left to the consultant urologist or primary care physician.

Calcium oxalate stones, as mentioned previously, are the most common types of stone. Hyperexcretion of calcium in the urine (hypercalciuria) is a major factor in stone formation. Certain bone diseases, sarcoidosis, or peptic ulcer disease may cause elevated serum calcium (hypercalcemia) and eventually lead to elevated urine calcium concentrations and stone formation. Increased absorption of calcium from the intestines, impaired renal tubular reabsorption of calcium, and increased uric acid excretion can also lead to hypercalciuria. The latter involves "nucleation" on calcium oxalate by the uric acid crystal leading to calcium oxalate stones with a uric acid core. In a variable proportion of patients with calcium stones, no cause can be found.

Oxalate constitutes the second component of calcium oxalate calculi. Crohn's disease, ulcerative colitis, radiation colitis, jejunal bypass surgery, ethylene glycol poisoning, and pyridoxine deficiency have all been associated with hyperoxaluria. Uric acid stones are common with gout and are also seen with certain leukemias. Only about half of these patients actually have elevated urine and/or serum uric acid levels. The mechanism likely responsible for stone formation is a tendency to excrete urine at a pH below 5.5, which favors uric acid stone formation.

Staghorn calculi, composed of magnesium ammonium phosphate, are formed after infections with bacteria such as *Proteus* and some types of staphylococci. As urea is converted to ammonia, the urine becomes more alkaline, predisposing to stone formation. These may be some of the largest stones.

Suggested Readings

Borghi L, Meschi T, Schianchi T, et al. Medical treatment of nephrolithiasis. *Endocrinol Metab Clin North Am* 2002;31:1051–1064.

Colussi G, De Ferraro ME, Brunati C, Civati G. Medical prevention and treatment of urinary stones. *J Nephrol* 2000;13(Suppl 3):S65–70.

Delvecchio FC, Preminger GM. Medical management of stone disease. *Curr Opin Urol* 2003; 13:229–233.

Manthey DE, Teichman J. Nephrolithiasis. *Emerg Med Clin North Am* 2001;19:633–654.

Shekarriz B, Stoller ML. Uric acid nephrolithiasis: current concepts and controversies. *J Urol* 2002;168(4 pt 1):1307–1314.

CHAPTER 14

Pyelonephritis

Robert E. Murray, MD

Clinical Scenario

A 32-year-old woman presents to the emergency department (ED) with a complaint of fever and back pain. She was well until approximately 4 days previously when she developed mild dysuria (pain with urination) and urgency. She made an appointment with her primary care doctor for the day of presentation, but early in the morning she awoke with moderate left back pain and a fever of 102°F. The pain is constant, dull, and throbbing without specific relieving or exacerbating factors. She took 1 g of acetaminophen with slight improvement in her pain and lessening of her fever. She has not had this pain in the past. Her urine appears cloudy. Her last menstrual period was 3 weeks before presentation and was normal for her.

She does not have any significant past medical or surgical history. She is sexually active with one male partner and uses oral contraceptives. She takes no other medications. She does not smoke cigarettes or use any illicit drugs. She reports drinking about two or three beers each week.

The physical examination reveals a well-developed young female in moderate discomfort. Vitals signs show a blood pressure of 130/85 mm Hg, heart rate 120 beats/minute, temperature 102.6°F, respiratory rate 18 breaths/minute, and oxygen saturation of 98% on room air. The patient is lying on the bed on her right side. Her skin is diaphoretic. The cardiopulmonary examination reveals tachycardia but is otherwise normal. She has significant left costovertebral angle (CVA) tenderness. The abdomen is soft, nontender, and without palpable masses. The genitourinary examination reveals normal female external genitalia without lesions or a hernia. The pelvic examination reveals a normal cervix without lesions or discharge or cervical motion tenderness.

Laboratory testing reveals a urinalysis with 20 to 30 red blood cells per high-powered field (hpf) and too numerous to count white blood cells (WBCs) per hpf with a positive leukocyte esterase (LE) and nitrite test. A β-human chorionic gonadotropin (β-HCG) qualitative pregnancy test is negative. The patient has an intravenous line begun and receives normal saline along with 5 mg of morphine sulfate, which provides adequate pain control. She also receives 1.25 mg of droperidol intravenously for nausea and 1 g of acetaminophen orally for her fever. A diagnosis of pyelonephritis is made based on the consistent historical, physical, and laboratory factors. She is given gentamicin 6 mg/kg intravenously.

Clinical Evaluation

Introduction

Pyelonephritis refers to a kidney infection. The clinical spectrum of acute pyelo-nephritis ranges from a cystitis-like illness with mild flank pain to gram-negative septicemia. The typical ED patient is a previously healthy woman with a few days' duration of urinary symptoms followed by more systemic signs of infection and back pain.

History

Pyelonephritis should be considered in any patient presenting with flank or back pain.

Most patients with this disease are women. The history should focus on an accurate description of the pain and associated factors. Onset, duration, localization, severity, radiation, and alleviating symptoms should be elicited.

Patients with acute upper urinary tract infection (UTI) will complain of flank pain or lower back pain. The pain is often described as aching or dull without radiation. The exception to this is a concurrent kidney stone, which may present more acutely (Chapter 13). The onset of a kidney infection is typically gradual. Patients describe urinary frequency, urgency, and burning for days before developing back pain. The pain is usually constant and mild. As the infection progresses, fever, nausea, and vomiting develop. The presentation may also be atypical; some patients may present only with fever, myalgias, and arthralgias. In elderly, debilitated, mentally ill, or pediatric patients, who may be unwilling or unable to give a classic history, there must be a high index of suspicion. In some patients, urinary calculi, prostate hypertrophy, congenital anomalies, and urinary retention from neurological disease should be also considered. UTIs in men begin to appear around age 50 when the incidence of benign prostate hypertrophy begins to rise. Other associated historical factors include recent hospitalization, surgery, pregnancy, sickle cell disease, or antibiotic use.

Physical Examination

A focused physical examination will aid in the diagnosis of pyelonephritis and the exclusion of more serious diseases.

Most young patients appear nontoxic. Vital signs may be normal. Tachycardia, orthostasis, tachypnea, or high fever may herald more advanced disease. Tachypnea is an early sign of systemic acidosis and should raise concern if present. Most patients will present with mild fever, but temperatures as high as 104°F are seen. Hypotension is uncommon, but in the elderly population should make urosepsis a diagnosis for exclusion. Flank pain in the older patient with a history of hypertension may be the presentation of expanding abdominal aortic aneurysm. Referred pain

from an inflamed gallbladder may be noted in the back, flank, or scapula, and patients with an inflamed gallbladder may also have fever and tachycardia. All women with abdominal or back pain need to be evaluated for intrauterine and ectopic pregnancy. Most healthy women with pyelonephritis will have CVA tenderness. The abdomen is usually nontender but may be sensitive to palpation from recurrent nausea and vomiting. A pelvic examination should be performed unless the diagnosis is clear, because pyuria may also be seen in sexually transmitted diseases. In men, a rectal examination should be performed to rule out prostatitis or benign prostatic hypertrophy. The bladder should be percussed and palpated to look for urinary retention, and a careful genitourinary examination to rule out epididymitis or sexually transmitted diseases.

Diagnostic Evaluation

The most useful diagnostic test is the urinalysis. In women, the pregnancy test is also important because management and potential complications may change. The urinalysis typically shows elevated leukocytes (usually greater than 10 WBC/mm^3) and bacteriuria. Although no accepted level of pyuria is diagnostic of infection in the urinary tract, the combination of bacteriuria and pyuria greatly improves the diagnostic yield.

Two of the most common screening tests are the LE test and the nitrite test. These can be measured by urine dipstick and together can improve overall diagnostic accuracy. Gram-negative bacteria possess an enzyme called nitrate reductase, which converts nitrate to nitrite. LE is found in neutrophils.

Urine collection is an important factor in analyzing urine specimens. The sterile catheterization is the quickest and most accurate method of obtaining specimens in young children and women. In women who are menstruating, it is the method of choice for obtaining a urinalysis. In adults, the clean catch specimen is a reasonable alternative and can be of diagnostic value if obtained correctly. This requires the patient to clean front to back with an enclosed wipe, to urinate a small amount first into the toilet, and then to collect the urine. Comparing the ratio of leukocytes to vaginal epithelial cells can be helpful. The lower the ratio, the more likely the leukocytes are vaginal contaminants.

Urine cultures are costly and rarely essential. In routine UTI and mild pyelonephritis in young, healthy women, urine culture is not required. Urine culture is required in certain groups at higher risk of complications, such as immunocompromised patients, diabetics, children, adult men, and pregnant women. Patients who require hospitalization should have a culture sent to the pathology laboratory.

Blood cultures have been shown to be positive in as many as 15% to 20% of hospitalized patients. Studies have shown that blood cultures rarely provide bacteriological diagnoses that are not present in the urine culture.

Imaging techniques are rarely needed but are appropriate for certain high-risk groups. Pyelonephritis in men is unusual and a search for obstructive uropathy should be undertaken. Refractory inpatient therapy or worsening clinical course should raise suspicion for perinephric abscess. Computed tomography (CT) and ultrasound are useful for assessing possible ureteral calculi or abscess.

Differential Diagnosis

The differential diagnosis for pyelonephritis is illustrated in Table 14.1.

Treatment

Most young, healthy women with pyelonephritis can be treated safely with oral antibiotics and analgesics. Nausea and vomiting or moderate to severe illness requires parenteral medication. If outpatient treatment for UTI has been instituted and the patient's condition worsened or failed to improve, a short course of intravenous antibiotics in the ED or in the inpatient setting will be necessary.

Oral treatment with a fluoroquinolone, such as ciprofloxacin or levofloxacin (Levaquin), is effective in a course of seven days. Trimethoprim-sulfamethoxazole (Bactrim DS) is also an effective and much less expensive alternative, although rates of allergic reactions and side effects are higher. Oral cephalosporins and amoxicillin/clavulanate

Table 14.1.

Differential diagnosis of pyelonephritis

Urological Disease

Upper urinary tract
Septic emboli
Renal tumors
Renal calculi
Perinephric abscess

Ureter
Urothelial tumors
Hemorrhage
Prior surgery scars
Metastatic tumors

Lower urinary track
Urinary retention
Tumors

Nonurological Disease

Chest/Abdomen
Peritonitis
Biliary colic
Intestinal obstruction
Abdominal/thoracic aortic aneurysm
Pneumonia

Gynecological Disease
Pregnancy/ectopic
Endometriosis
Tubo-ovarian abscess
Pelvic inflammatory disease
Ovarian torsion
Tumors

Retroperitoneal Disease
Hemorrhage
Tumor
Lymphadenopathy
Psoas abscess

may be used for 14-day treatment as well. Treatment for longer than 2 weeks has no apparent benefit.

Inpatient parenteral regimens include ampicillin and gentamicin, fluoroquinolones, and third-generation cephalosporins. Treatment is usually brief, with 24 to 48 hours of therapy until the patient is afebrile, followed by oral outpatient medication for 14 days total.

Table 14.2.

Treatment summary for pyelonephritis

Antibiotics

Inpatient Intravenous	*Outpatient Oral*
Ampicillin/gentamicin	A fluoroquinolone
A fluoroquinolone	Ampicillin/clavulanate
A third-generation cephalosporin	A second- or third-generation cephalosporin
Ampicillin/sulbactam	Trimethoprim/sulfamethoxazole

Intravenous Fluids
Normal saline or lactated Ringer's solution

Pain Management
Mild to moderate pain: nonsteroidal antiinflammatory medication, acetaminophen
Moderate to severe pain: oral opioids, oxycodone or hydrocodone preparations (Percocet, Vicodin); intravenous opioids: morphine, meperidine (Demerol), hydromorphone (Dilaudid)

Analgesia is usually required in the acute setting. If nausea and vomiting are absent, nonsteroidal antiinflammatory drugs or acetaminophen may relieve the discomfort. However, the patient will often require stronger medications such as oxycodone preparations. Frequently, intravenous opioids such as morphine will be needed for pain control. Antiemetics such as prochlorperazine (Compazine) and promethazine (Phenergan) will be useful for nausea and vomiting.

Treatment of pyelonephritis is summarized in Table 14.2.

Disposition

Most patients with uncomplicated pyelonephritis can be safely discharged home on antibiotics and analgesics. Indications for admission include failed outpatient management, sepsis, unilateral kidney, bilateral pyelonephritis, male patient, children, coexisting ureteral calculi, pregnancy, refractory pain or nausea and vomiting, and impaired renal function. ED stay is typically 4 to 6 hours and may be complicated by persistent vomiting, fever, and pain. Follow-up should always be arranged with the patient's primary care physician or urologist within 1 week. A urologist should evaluate all male patients and children in follow-up.

Pathophysiology

The microbiology of pyelonephritis is that of UTIs. Usually, the infecting organisms are derived from the patient's own fecal flora. Much less commonly, the origin of bacteria is from the bloodstream, termed hematogenous infection. Most cases of pyelonephritis seen in the ED will involve young, healthy, women. In this group, the source will almost invariably be an ascending infection from the lower urinary tract. The emergency clinician must keep in mind the groups of patients more susceptible to the hematogenous route and have a high suspicion in patients with certain comorbidities. Patients with immunocompromised states (human immunodeficiency virus, diabetes mellitus, immunosuppressive medication), chronic debilitation, and ureteral obstruction may be more susceptible to nonenteric organisms such as staphylococci and fungi. Refractory therapy and atypical presentations should alert the clinician to less common etiologies.

Gram-negative aerobic bacilli found in the gastrointestinal tract, with colonization extending to the perineal areas and genitalia, are the most common etiology of UTI and pyelonephritis. *Escherichia coli* is by far the most frequent cause of uncomplicated pyelonephritis. It is the dominant pathogen in more than 80% of cases of UTI in both men and women. *Proteus mirabilis, Klebsiella pneumoniae, Enterococcus* species, and *Staphylococcus saprophyticus* are responsible for the remainder of common organisms. Less common uropathogens such as resistant strains of *E. coli, Pseudomonas* species, *Mycobacterium tuberculosis*, and fungi may be found in hospitalized patients and in patients with complicated UTIs.

Several factors predispose individuals to the initiation and propagation of UTI. Any anatomic, functional, or foreign obstruction of urine flow will predispose patients to infection. Ordinarily, organisms introduced into the bladder are cleared by bladder evacuation. However, patients with prostatic hypertrophy, impacted renal calculi, and urethral catheters can have impaired urine flow and serve as a nidus for infection.

In the absence of instrumentation, UTI is much more common in women. The shorter urethra, lack of protective antibacterial properties of prostatic fluid, and urethral trauma during sexual intercourse make the female tract more susceptible to infection. Four percent to 6% of pregnant women also develop bacteriuria at some time during pregnancy, with a 20% to 40% incidence of pyelonephritis if untreated.

Certain bacterial properties also make infection more likely. The first step of ascending infection is colonization of the bacteria to the distal urethra by coliform bacteria. The ability of the bacteria to adhere to the mucosa is related to the organism's structure. *E. coli* carry chromosomally coded proteins for P-fimbria. These pili interact with receptors on the surface of uroepithelial cells, which leads to bacteria overgrowth.

Once bacteria gain entrance to the bladder, vesicoureteral orifice incompetence allows the organism to access the ureters and kidney. Usually, this orifice is a competent one-way valve. Infection, anatomic anomalies, and instrumentation may lead to an incompetent valve and reflux of infected urine into the ureters.

Acute pyelonephritis is a suppurative inflammation of the kidney caused by bacterial infection. The pathological hallmarks of infection are patchy interstitial inflammation and tubular necrosis. In the early stages, the neutrophilic infiltration is limited to interstitial tissue. Once infection extends into the tubules, rapid extension evolves from the involved nephron into the collecting tubules. Complications include papillary necrosis, pyonephrosis, and perinephric abscess. With uncomplicated infection, patients respond well to antibiotic therapy and pain control. In the presence of untreated obstruction, diabetes mellitus, or immunocompromised states, bacteriuria may persist for months to years. Recurrent pyelonephritis leading to systemic involvement, sepsis, and acute renal failure are serious long-term complications. Chronic pyelonephritis and renal scarring may damage the renal calyces and pelvis, leading to chronic renal failure requiring hemodialysis.

Suggested Readings

Cotran RS, Robbins SL, eds. *Pathologic basis for disease*, 6th ed. Philadelphia: WB Saunders, 1999.

Harwood-Nuss A, et al. Urologic emergencies. In: Rosen P et al., eds. *Emergency medicine: concepts and clinical practice*, 4th ed. St. Louis: Mosby, 1998:2227–2259.

Lingerman J. Calculous disease of the kidney and bladder. In: Harwood-Nuss A, ed. *The clinical practice of emergency medicine*, 2nd ed. Philadelphia: Lippincott, 1996:243–249.

Pearlman, MD, Tintinalli, JE, eds. *Emergency care of the woman*. New York: McGraw-Hill, 1998:306–307.

Roberts JA. Infections in urology. Management of pyelonephritis and upper urinary tract infections. *Urol Clin North Am* 1999;26:753–760.

Stamm WE, Hooton TM. Current concepts: management of urinary tract infections in adults. *N Engl J Med* 1993;329:1328–1334.

On-line medical dictionaries can be browsed at http://www.graylab.ac.uk/cgi-bin/omd?query=sepsis&action=Search+OMD
http://www.ncemi.org/

CHAPTER 15

Musculoskeletal Disorders

Eric Legome, MD

Clinical Scenario

A 45-year-old man presents to the emergency department (ED) with a chief complaint of severe back pain. The pain is located across his lumbosacral area. He awoke with the pain the morning of presentation, but he has experienced mild discomfort in the area since "working out" 72 hours ago at a health club. He has not felt this pain before. The pain is dull and "burning" with radiation into the right buttock. He denies weakness, numbness, or difficulty with urination.

Past medical history is significant for borderline hypertension. His family history is noncontributory. He smokes one pack of cigarettes per day. He denies alcohol or other drug use including any history of intravenous drug abuse. He takes no prescription medications.

On review of symptom, he denies chest pain, shortness of breath, fever or rigors, or any urinary complaints. He reports no weight loss.

Physical examination reveals a well-developed well-nourished male in obvious discomfort because of back pain. He is lying still on the bed. Vital signs show a heart rate of 90 beats/minute, a blood pressure of 165/90 mm Hg, a respiratory rate of 18 breaths/minute, and an oral temperature of 98.6°F. The lungs are clear; the cardiac examination reveals a regular rate and rhythm. The abdomen is soft and nontender without masses. The lower back is diffusely tender to palpation. No lesions or deformities are noted. The genital examination is within normal limits. The rectal examination reveals a prostate that is nontender and without masses. The rectal tone is normal. The stool guaiac is negative. The lower extremity examination shows well-perfused feet with equal distal dorsalis pedis and posterior tibial pulses. The ankle and knee deep tendon reflexes are 1+ and equal. The straight leg raise and crossed straight leg test leads to pain in the lower back without radiation. The patient has 5/5 strength with equal foot dorsiflexion, plantar flexion, and great toe dorsiflexion. Bilateral foot sensation is normal to light touch and pinprick.

His urinalysis is normal. He has no other laboratory tests or x-ray examinations performed.

Clinical Evaluation

Introduction

These historical and physical findings are consistent with a diagnosis of musculoskeletal back pain.

Back pain resulting from abnormalities of the lumbosacral spine is one of the most common presenting complaints in the ED. Most of the time, it is impossible to elucidate the exact source, because noxious stimuli from muscle, fascia, joint capsules, ligaments, and fibers of the annulus fibrosis are perceived similarly. Pain that is due to irritation of nerve roots is perceived differently and is usually characterized as sciatica. However, the initial treatment in uncomplicated cases is the same; thus, it is more important to rule out serious disease rather than find the exact etiology. The ED evaluation of back pain consists of a thorough history and targeted physical examination, with diagnostic testing reserved for a specific reason.

History

The examiner should direct the questioning toward several decision points: does the patient have serious systemic disease causing pain in or referred to the back, and, if not, is the pain musculoskeletal or radicular? Inquire if the patient has any urinary frequency or urgency or associated abdominal or pelvic pain, symptoms that could point to an alternative diagnosis with referred pain to the back. Ask about a previous history of cancer or recent systemic infection. These could predispose one to metastases, osteomyelitis, or abscess. Inquire about any recent use of intravenous drugs or any invasive surgical procedures, which are also risk factors for abscess or osteomyelitis. Check for medications that affect bones, such as steroids or heparin. Ask about systemic symptoms such as fever, rigors, nausea, vomiting, and weight loss. The time course of pain should also be inquired about, because pain that persists through the night and is not associated with movement should prompt a concern for neoplasia. Cancers that metastasize to bone are found frequently in the spine and present typically as persistent gnawing pain.

For patients with back pain resulting from the structures in the back, the character of the pain will point to the diagnoses as musculoskeletal or sciatic pain. Patients with musculoskeletal pain usually complain of poorly localized aching that is dull or burning. The pain is worse with movement and improved with rest. It may radiate, usually into the buttocks or thigh, but rarely below the knee. The patients may complain of weakness or the leg "giving out," but it should be due to pain rather than true weakness. Sciatica is pain that is sharp, well localized, and shooting. It is usually localized to a dermatomal distribution, and it may be more intense in the thigh and leg than in the back.

Most patients with sciatica have pain localized to the L4-L5 or L5-S1 discs, although a small number may have higher level herniation that radiate to the medial aspect of the thigh. The patient may complain of numbness or weakness in a specific distribution, mostly starting along the posterolateral aspect of the leg and traveling into the foot. Although it is usually due to irritation of the nerve root from a disc herniation, other causes include tumors, degenerative joint disease, or abscess compromising the nerve root or spinal canal. Inability to urinate or fecal incontinence in association with bilateral sciatica should prompt serious concern, because it is a sign of a massive herniated disc with compression of the cauda equina. Lesions that irritate or compress the posterior spinal roots will cause pain in the area of the skin and muscle innervated by that root. If the anterior root is involved, variable degrees of weakness, including paralysis, may ensue.

Physical Examination

Physical examination is focused toward ruling out neurological compromise or other systemic illness. The patient should be observed for his or her general demeanor. Most patients with musculoskeletal or sciatic pain will be relatively still because movement exacerbates symptoms. The patient who is writhing in pain should raise concern for a vascular or renal etiology. Visceral pain that radiates to the back is usually reproducible by abdominal palpation. Palpation of the spine and low back should be performed, concentrating on point tenderness or deformities. However, reproducibility for tenderness or spasm is variable. This probably signifies the multiple areas that may reproduce the symptoms. Because most significant disc herniations are at the lower lumbar levels, the examination should focus on secondary effects in the distal lower extremities. Pressure on the L5 nerve root (L4-L5 disc) causes weakness of dorsiflexion at the ankle and the great toe because the nerve innervates the extensor digitorum brevis and longus musculature, which allow these movements to occur. Associated numbness on the sole of the foot will be present. If the S1 root is affected, weakness of plantar flexion and eversion of the ankle ensue as this innervates the gastrocnemius, soleus, and peroneus muscles and provides sensation to the sole and lateral border of the foot. There may be an associated loss of the ankle jerk reflex. A small subset of patients has irritation of the L3-L4 that causes pain in the medial thigh. This may cause an abnormal knee jerk reflex. With sciatica, a rectal examination should be performed; if there is significant involvement of sacral fibers, as in cauda equina syndrome, abnormal perianal sensation and loss of sphincter tone may be present. The straight leg and crossed straight leg test should be performed. The straight leg test is best performed with the patient supine. The examiner grasps the heel with the knee completely extended. A positive test reproduces the symptoms of sciatica between 30 and 70 degrees of extension. The opposite leg is then similarly tested, looking for reproduction of the symptoms on the affected side.

Diagnostic Evaluation

In general, most patients require minimal or no testing. Lumbar spine radiographs rarely add value to the history and physical and are usually not indicated. Specific indications for x-ray films include history of significant trauma, constitutional symptoms, chronic use of steroids, pain persisting for several months, or advanced age. Although there are no absolute guidelines, a reasonable recommendation is that patients older than 50 years have lumbar radiographs taken on their first episode of low back pain. Indications for emergent magnetic resonance imaging (MRI) include signs and symptoms of a cauda equina syndrome (see the section on pathophysiology) with sciatica, perianal sensory loss and decreased rectal tone, concern for an epidural abscess or hematoma, or a rapidly progressive objective neurological abnormalities.

Differential Diagnosis

The differential diagnosis for musculoskeletal back pain is illustrated in Table 15.1.

Treatment

The treatment of back pain favors relief of pain with early mobilization and return to

Table 15.1.

Differential diagnosis of musculoskeletal and radicular low back pain

Vascular Conditions
Abdominal aortic aneurysm

Gynecological Conditions
Ovarian or uterine neoplasm
Ectopic pregnancy
Intrauterine pregnancy

Urological Conditions
Nephrolithiasis
Pyelonephritis
Urinary tract infection

Other Conditions
Bone neoplasm
Retroperitoneal hemorrhage
Tumor

usual activities (Table 15.2). In general, nonsteroidal antiinflammatory drugs (NSAIDs) are the initial treatment of choice in the patient with no contraindications. Although there is not extensive evidence of their benefit, many practitioners will use a short course of skeletal muscle relaxants as adjuvant treatment. Acetaminophen is also an acceptable treatment in patients with mild to moderate pain.

Severe pain is often unrelieved by the previously mentioned drugs, and a short course of opiates is a reasonable treatment

Table 15.2.

Treatment summary for low back pain

Acetaminophen
NSAIDs: ibuprofen by mouth, ketorolac IV or IM
Narcotics: morphine IV or SC, meperidine IV or IM
Other medications: muscle relaxants
  (cyclobenzaprine [Flexeril]) by mouth,
  methocarbamol by mouth
Activities: moderated activities, short-term rest
Consideration of physical therapy or chiropractor
  for musculoskeletal pain

IM, intramuscular; IV, intravenous; NSAIDs, nonsteroidal antiinflammatory drugs; SC, subcutaneous.

in the emergent setting. They are often given intravenously or intramuscularly in the ED with oral medication prescribed for several days afterward.

Prospective studies have shown that simple instructions for early resumption of moderated activity, no more than 1 to 2 days of bed rest (if needed), and pain control work as well as most physical therapy or chiropractic manipulation in the long run, although they may be minimally less effective initially.

Disposition

Most patients with low back pain will be discharged home. Indications for admission for musculoskeletal back pain are inability to control severe pain and/or inability to ambulate.

Most patients with sciatic pain can also be discharged, but along with the previous qualifications, they should not have any signs of a rapidly progressive neurological deficit or cauda equina syndrome.

Pathophysiology

Knowledge of the anatomy of lower back is crucial to understanding the pathophysiology of primary back pain. The lumbar spine is composed of the spinal cord and nerve roots, the vertebrae, the intervertebral discs, and multiple ligaments. The spinal cord in the adult ends near the L1-L2 vertebrae, but nerve roots extend distally to the sacrum as the cauda equina. Afferent sensory information from the local back structures travel through posterior rami of spinal nerves that exit the spinal canal via the intervertebral foramina. These nerves ascend ipsilaterally in the spinal cord for several segments and then cross anteriorly, continuing their path to the brain on the contralateral side of the cord.

The spinal cord and cauda equina are surrounded by the bony structures of the vertebral bodies and the intervertebral discs anteriorly, the pedicles anterolaterally, and by the laminae posterolaterally. Transverse processes extend laterally on either side from the junction of the pedicles and laminae, and a singular spinous process extends

posteriorly from the junction of the laminae. Adjacent vertebrae articulate via facet joints, which extend superiorly and inferiorly from the laminae.

Numerous ligaments—including the anterior longitudinal ligament along the anterior surface of the vertebral bodies; the posterior longitudinal ligament along the posterior surface; and the supraspinous ligament, which connects the spinous processes—connect the bones of the vertebral column. There are numerous muscles in the lower back; the erector spinae muscle has the most clinical importance. This large, thick muscle originates from the sacrum, iliac crest, and lumbar vertebrae and extends cephalad to insert on the posterior ribs and thoracic vertebrae.

Fractures can be classified as traumatic or pathological. Traumatic fractures may result from forces applied directly to the spine or from transmitted forces. For example, a person who falls from a height and lands on his heels may suffer from compression fractures of the vertebral bodies. Pathological fractures (i.e., fractures without traumatic etiology) most often are compression fractures of the vertebral bodies and usually occur in those with senile osteoporosis. Chronic steroid use may also produce osteopenia and lead to fracture. Pathological fracture can also be seen in patients with cancer that metastasizes to bone (e.g., breast, lung, and prostate cancer).

Metastatic lesions may also produce back pain by simple local invasion without fracture. Regardless of the etiology, back pain caused by bony lesions is commonly limited to a small focal region and is reproducible with direct palpation. Movement of the back may also exacerbate the pain.

Arthritis of the spine is a common cause of lower back pain. Osteophyte formation can occur anywhere in the bones and cause pain by compression of nerves as they exit the intervertebral foramen. Arthritis of the facet joints can cause back pain with movement. The degree of discomfort from arthritis does not always correlate with radiographical abnormalities, and patients with significant pain from vertebral arthritis may have relatively normal x-ray films.

Degeneration of the intervertebral discs may cause pain in the lower back. The discs are composed of a central gelatinous structure called the nucleus pulposus and an outer fibrocartilaginous structure called the annulus fibrosis. These are relatively elastic, but they become more brittle with age. Posterior herniation of the degenerated disc into the spinal canal, which can be spontaneous or associated with twisting or other movements of the back, is usually unilateral and can cause compression of spinal nerves. The resulting radicular pain is characterized by a sharp, shooting pain in the dermatomal distribution of the affected nerve that is exacerbated by stretching of the nerve. Most disc herniations occur at the L4-L5 or L5-S1 level and cause compression of the sciatic nerve. This clinical condition is referred to as sciatica and is associated with pain in the buttock, posterior thigh, lateral lower leg, and dorsum of the foot. Flexion of the hip with the knee extended reproduces the pain as the sciatic nerve is stretched. Dermatomal sensory loss and diminished reflexes may be present.

Spinal stenosis should be considered in all patients with lower back pain. This narrowing of the spinal canal may be caused by degeneration or herniation of an intervertebral disc, arthritis, tumor, or congenital abnormality. As the spinal cord or cauda equina becomes compressed, focal neurological findings distal to the level of compression may be found. Initial symptoms, such as focal leg weakness, sensory loss, or paresthesias, may be vague and can be induced by walking or standing. As the disease progresses, more profound neurological findings may arise, including bilateral leg paralysis, loss of deep tendon reflexes, urinary retention, and fecal incontinence.

Muscular strain, which is defined as microscopic stretching or tearing of muscle fibers, is one of the most common causes of back pain encountered in the ED. Strain is commonly seen after rigorous physical activity or motor vehicle accidents. These patients will have focal tenderness over the muscles and may have muscular spasm, which is palpable as a taut muscle group just lateral to the vertebral column.

The exact cause of most musculoskeletal low back pain is rarely found. Generally, a minor tear to the muscle or ligamentous fibers in the lower back leads to bleeding and inflammation. Subsequently, the posterior rami of the spinal nerve to the area are irritated, leading to the sensation of pain in the area. The rami provide afferent innervation to the muscles, ligaments, fibers of the annulus fibrosis, and facet joint capsules; thus, irritation to any of those may provide similar sensations.

Radicular pain is due to direct mechanical and inflammatory irritation of the nerve as it exits the spinal canal. There may be several causes, including a rupture of the annulus fibrosis with protrusion of the nucleus pulposus. It may press on the spinal nerve root or even the spinal cord. A large herniation may involve the anterior nerve root, leading to weakness and loss of reflexes. Other causes of direct irritation or compression include osteophytes, tumors, cysts, or abscesses. Extraspinal compression from retroperitoneal masses may also irritate a lumbar nerve root.

The cauda equina, or roots of the lumbar and sacral nerves in the spinal canal below the termination of the spinal cord, may be impinged on by a massive central disc herniation. This will lead to bilateral sciatica; urinary retention; and anesthesia of the perineum, buttocks, and upper posterior thighs (saddle anesthesia).

Suggesting Readings

Brody M. Low back pain. *Ann Emerg Med* 1996;27:454–456.

Deyo RA, Rainville J, Kent DL. What can the history and physical tell us about low back pain? *JAMA* 1992;268:760–765.

Frymoyer JW. Back pain and sciatica. *N Engl J Med* 1995;332:351–355.

Marriott A, Newman NM, Gracovetsky SA. Improving the evaluation of benign low back pain. *Spine* 1999;24:952–960.

Back Pain
Questions and Answers

Questions

1. A 58-year-old man presents to the emergency department (ED) with sudden onset of excruciating chest pain with radiation to the upper back. His electrocardiogram (ECG) shows no ST-segment abnormalities; a portable chest x-ray film reveals a wide mediastinum. On physical examination, his pulse is 114 beats/minute, blood pressure is 82/46 mm Hg, and oxygen saturation is 92% on room air. He is pale and diaphoretic; he has bibasilar crackles on pulmonary examination, and he has a III/VI diastolic murmur loudest at the apex. What is the next best step in the management of this patient?

   A. Computed tomography (CT) scan of the thorax with intravenous contrast to confirm the diagnosis of aortic dissection

   B. Transesophageal echocardiography at the bedside to confirm the diagnosis and evaluate the degree of aortic insufficiency to plan for surgery.

   C. Aortic angiography to precisely locate the intimal tear and assess the extent of aortic dissection and aortic valve involvement.

   D. Immediate ED thoracotomy.

2. A hemodynamically stable patient is sent for thoracic computed tomography (CT) scan because of tearing midscapular back pain and diaphoresis with a normal electrocardiogram (ECG) and chest x-ray film. The scan reveals an aortic dissection that originates just distal to the left subclavian artery and extends distally. What is the most appropriate management of this patient?

   A. Immediate transthoracic echocardiography to evaluate the degree of retrograde dissection and assess the competency of the aortic valve.

   B. Aortic angiography to precisely detail the extent of the aortic dissection in preparation for surgery.

   C. Immediate operative thoracotomy.

   D. Hemodynamic monitoring, administration of esmolol and sodium nitroprusside drips to reduce pulse and blood pressure to optimize the systolic pressure gradient (dP/dt), and admission to the intensive care unit.

3. Which of the following best characterizes the laboratory or diagnostic imaging findings for acute renal calculi?

   A. As many as 20% of symptomatic stones do not show microscopic hematuria on urinalysis.

   B. Blood urea nitrogen (BUN) and creatinine levels are markedly elevated in uncomplicated ureteral obstruction.

   C. Computed tomography (CT) scanning is a poor diagnostic test compared with renal ultrasound in diagnosing renal calculi.

   D. Kidneys, ureter, and bladder (KUB) plain radiography has a high sensitivity for detecting kidney stones.

4. Which of the following is characteristic of cauda equina syndrome?

   A. Pain isolated to the back and buttock

   B. Urinary frequency

   C. Hyperreflexia in the S1 distributions

   D. Bilateral sciatica

5. The most helpful laboratory test to order on a patient with a history of new back pain and recent intravenous drug use is:

A. An electrolyte panel

B. An estimated sedimentation rate

C. A blood culture

D. A urinalysis

6. Which of the following in an indication for admission for acute pyelonephritis?

A. Temperature greater than 102°F

B. Age greater than 30 years

C. Bacteriuria

D. Pregnancy

E. History of pyelonephritis

7. Which of the following best characterizes the presentation of pyelonephritis in young, healthy women?

A. Symptoms include severe abdominal pain and hypotension.

B. Fever is an uncommon finding.

C. Dysuria is seen only in severe cases.

D. Flank pain, urinary frequency, and urinary urgency are usually present.

E. Gross hematuria and renal failure are common.

8. Which of the following best describes the most common type of kidney stone?

A. Magnesium ammonium phosphate

B. Struvite (staghorn)

C. Uric acid

D. Cystine

E. Calcium oxalate

Directions: There are three sets of response options for the following scenario. You will be required to select one best answer from each question set.

9. A 34-year-old man presents by ambulance to the emergency department with severe right-sided back pain. He states the pain began 8 hours ago and has been getting steadily worse. He complains of pain that shoots down the back of the right leg and is exacerbated by certain positions. He feels unable to walk. He has no past medical history and takes no medications. He denies intravenous (IV) drug use. On physical examination, the patient appears very uncomfortable. His cardiovascular, pulmonary, and abdominal examinations are normal. He has no costovertebral angle tenderness. His back is nontender to palpation, but movement elicits pain. His motor examination is significant for weakness of the right great toe and foot with dorsiflexion. There is numbness of the dorsum of the foot. Rectal examination reveals good tone and sensation. Reflexes are intact.

9.1. Which of the following is the correct diagnostic maneuver?

A. Urinalysis

B. Computed tomography (CT) scan of the abdomen

C. Lumbar radiographs

D. Magnetic resonance imaging

9.2. Which of the following nerve roots is the origin of his symptoms?

A. L3

B. L4

C. L5

D. S1

Answers and Explanations

1. B. Although computed tomography (CT) and angiography are both used for diagnosis of dissection, the patient described is hemodynamically unstable. The safest management would be a diagnostic study at the bedside in which ongoing monitoring and treatment can be delivered. If the patient becomes too unstable, immediate operative exploration is warranted.

2. D. This patient has a Stanford type B dissection. This involves the descending aorta and usually begins distal to the left subclavian artery. The treatment is medical management to control blood pressure and pulse. Operative intervention is not indicated for this type of dissection, making angiography unnecessary. Transthoracic echocardiography might be done to assess cardiac function; however, the dissection begins at the subclavian and extends distally, away from the valves. Therefore, an emergent echocardiogram to assess valve competency is not indicated.

3. A. Although most patients with calculi have blood in the urine, 10% to 20% do not. Ureteral obstruction with renal failure is uncommon and suggests prolonged and/or bilateral obstruction. The blood urea nitrogen (BUN) and creatinine would not be expected to rise unless these conditions existed or the patient was profoundly dehydrated. Computed tomography (CT) scan is the diagnostic imaging modality of choice and has a high sensitivity. Kidneys, ureter, and bladder (KUB) x-ray film often misses calculi even in the presence of calcium-containing stones.

4. D. Cauda equina syndrome is characterized by bilateral or unilateral sciatica (pain down the legs), inability to urinate or new incontinence, perineal sensory deficits, and decreased reflexes not hyperreflexia or urinary frequency. It is due to a massively herniated central disc impinging on the cauda equina.

5. B. Although no laboratory test can completely rule out an infection, an estimated sedimentation rate is highly sensitive for epidural abscess and osteomyelitis, both concerns in a patient with intravenous drug abuse. Blood cultures may be helpful but takes several days for results; therefore, it would not be useful in the initial management of this patient. An electrolyte panel would offer no help in managing this patient, and a urinalysis, although useful in ruling out kidney stones or infection, does not help to make the diagnosis of the more likely diseases.

6. D. Any ill-appearing patient should be considered for admission regardless of objective criteria such as fever, but pregnancy always mandates admission given the risk of spontaneous abortion. Most patients have bacteriuria. Pyelonephritis is often recurrent in young, healthy women. There is

no specific age cutoff for admission; however, the elderly must be approached with more caution with the decision to treat as an outpatient. Fever is common in pyelonephritides and is not an isolated criterion for admission.

7. D. Pyelonephritis usually presents with fever and urinary symptoms or back pain. Any patient who presents with abdominal pain, hypotension, gross hematuria, and/or renal failure should prompt an aggressive and thorough investigation to other causes.

8. E. Calcium oxalate stones account for approximately 80% of renal calculi. Uric acid stones are also common but not nearly as common as calcium oxalate stones. These stones may be associated with acidic urine and may also precipitate in joints, causing gout. Struvite stones are made from magnesium, ammonium, and phosphate. They can be very large causing staghorn calculi. Cystine stones are uncommon and are caused by a hereditary genetic disorder.

9.1. A. This patient presents with musculoskeletal back pain. Although the diagnosis of sciatica or lumbar disc disease seems clear, a urinalysis should be done to rule out the possibility of either renal calculus or infection. Computed tomography (CT) scan is unnecessary in this patient because he is not at risk for vascular catastrophe and has no evidence of abdominal or retroperitoneal pathology. Plain x-ray films of the spine are not useful except in the elderly or patients with comorbidity such as cancer. The magnetic resonance imaging (MRI) would only be ordered if the patient were at risk for epidural abscess or cauda equina syndrome, which he is not.

9.2. C. The L5 nerve innervates extensor digitorum brevis and longus musculature, which is responsible for ankle dorsiflexion and dorsiflexion of the great toe. There are no reflexes involved and sensation is to the dorsum of the foot and lateral leg. Sensation of L3 is lower thigh, L4 is medial leg and medial foot, and S1 is lateral foot. Reflexes are L4 patellar and S1 Achilles, and motor is L3 quadriceps, L4 tibialis anterior, and S1 peronei (ankle eversion).

Abdominal Pain

He who does not mind his belly will hardly mind anything else.
Samuel Johnson

INTRODUCTION
Todd C. Rothenhaus, MD
Section Editor

Acute abdominal pain is one of the most frequent, and at times frustrating, chief complaints encountered by the emergency physician. Causes of abdominal pain range from benign to immediately life-threatening ones. Symptoms and signs are frequently nonspecific, and in as many as 40% of patients, despite meticulous investigation, a diagnosis may not be found.

There are two distinct types of abdominal pain: visceral pain and somatic pain. This results from the stimulation of sensory fibers along two separate neuroanatomic pathways. Visceral pain originates from hollow viscera that contain slow pain fibers in their walls that respond primarily to stretch. The fibers travel along the sympathetic nervous system to enter the spinal cord at multiple levels, resulting in a sensation of pain that is dull, crampy or colicky, and poorly localized. The anatomic location of the sympathetic chain along the midline results in visceral pain being localized in the midline. Pain from the liver, biliary tree, and small intestine is most commonly felt in the upper abdomen, whereas pain from the large intestine is most commonly felt in the lower abdomen. In distinction from visceral pain, the source for somatic pain is the abdominal wall and parietal peritoneum. They are innervated by myelinated fast pain fibers that travel along cutaneous dermatomes to enter the dorsal root ganglia then into the spinal cord, resulting in pain that is sharp and well localized.

This explains the common evolution and migration of pain in the acute abdomen. For example, the early visceral pain of appendicitis is caused by stretch of the hollow walls of the appendix causing a poorly localized, colicky, periumbilical pain felt nearer to the midline. As the parietal peritoneum becomes inflamed, the somatic sensory nerves become stimulated and the pain becomes localized to the right lower quadrant. This is extremely important to keep in mind when evaluating a patient with nonspecific midline abdominal complaints. He or she may be in the very early stages of an acute abdominal process, and the complaint must not be perfunctorily dismissed as benign.

Pain from visceral organs may also be referred to adjacent or distant structures innervated by common nerves. Pain from under the diaphragm may be referred to the shoulder, gallbladder and liver pain to the right shoulder, and splenic pain to the left shoulder. Pain from the kidney is often referred to the groin or testicle. The pain of inferior wall myocardial ischemia may present as epigastric pain because the heart rests on the diaphragm. Pneumonia of either lower lobe can be experienced as pain in the upper abdomen.

Management of acute pain through the administration of analgesia is an important and frequently unfulfilled responsibility of all physicians treating abdominal pain. Administration of analgesia in the modern day has never been shown to delay diagnosis or to increase complications. In fact, when patients are given analgesia, the abdominal musculature is relaxed, and the physical examination may more clearly localize the area of peritoneal inflammation.

This section focuses on developing an approach to common diseases of the abdomen.

Additional Reading

Silen W. Effect on diagnostic efficiency of analgesia for undifferentiated abdominal pain. *Br J Surg* 2003;90:5–9.

CHAPTER 16

Abdominal Aortic Aneurysm

Ami K. Davé, MD

Clinical Scenario

A 70-year-old man is brought to a local community emergency department (ED) by ambulance. He was in his usual state of health until 5 days ago when he developed a lower backache, which has become increasingly severe over the past 24 hours. Today, 30 minutes before calling 911, he developed an acute onset of abdominal pain, which he describes as throbbing and bandlike. The pain radiates to his left flank and lower back. His wife states that today he passed out immediately following the onset of pain. He denies any chest pain, nausea, vomiting, diarrhea, fever, chills, urinary symptoms, or recent trauma.

Past medical history reveals hypertension and hypercholesterolemia but no known history of diabetes, stroke, or cardiac disease. He has a 50-pack-year smoking history, and his family history is notable for his mother who died of a myocardial infarction at age 60.

Physical examination reveals a temperature of 97°F; blood pressure of 180/105 mm Hg; heart rate of 120 beats/minute; regular, respiratory rate of 16 breaths/minute; and oxygen saturation of 99% on room air. The patient is lying supine, comfortably on the stretcher, with no diaphoresis. He has good color and appears to be in no acute distress. Pertinent aspects of the examination include a tender, pulsatile mass in his upper abdomen, just left of the midline, with an audible abdominal bruit. Otherwise, his abdomen is soft, with no rebound or guarding. He has no flank or midline back tenderness or deformity. His peripheral pulses are palpable.

The patient is placed on a cardiac monitor and 100% oxygen via non-rebreather facemask. Two large-bore intravenous lines are inserted. Intravenous β-blockade is initiated to maintain a systolic blood pressure of 120 mm Hg. O-negative blood is ordered, and the vascular surgery service is notified of a patient with possible ruptured abdominal aortic aneurysm.

Laboratory examination includes a complete blood count (CBC), electrolytes, blood urea nitrogen, creatinine, urinalysis, and amylase, which are normal, except for a white blood cell count of 12,000 cells/mm^3 with a normal differential count. An electrocardiogram (ECG) reveals sinus tachycardia. The patient undergoes emergent computed tomography (CT) of the abdomen, which shows an infrarenal abdominal aortic aneurysm with an anterior-posterior diameter of 7 cm, with evidence of a contained rupture. The abdominal aortic aneurysm does not extend into the iliac arteries.

The patient is taken immediately to the operating room (OR) where the ruptured abdominal aortic aneurysm is repaired with a Dacron tube graft. The patient receives eight units of O-negative blood. He is transferred to the intensive care unit, remains intubated for 24 hours, and is discharged home on the tenth postoperative day. The patient remains well 8 months later.

Clinical Evaluation

Introduction

Abdominal aortic aneurysm is a relatively common and potentially life-threatening condition. It is the thirteenth leading cause of death in the United States, accounting for 0.8% of all deaths. Approximately 70%

of persons with ruptured abdominal aortic aneurysm will not survive long enough to reach a hospital; of those who do reach a hospital, fewer than 50% will survive to discharge.

Over the past few decades, the incidence of abdominal aortic aneurysm has increased. This is probably due to the increasing age of our population and improved diagnostic capabilities. With enhanced detection and improved surgical prognosis, most deaths are caused by rupture. Therefore, it is important for the emergency physician to be able to recognize this disease and begin proper management, before rupture occurs.

History

Approximately 75% of abdominal aortic aneurysms are asymptomatic and detected during routine physical examination. Aneurysm symptoms can be categorized as (1) none to mild resulting from a small, stable, or unruptured aneurysm; (2) moderate to severe from acute aneurysm expansion or rupture; or (3) secondary symptoms resulting from aneurysm impingement on adjacent structures, embolization, or thrombosis.

Patients may experience minor back or flank pain or abdominal pain. If abdominal pain is present, it is throbbing and pulsatile in nature. It is described as aching and bandlike and is located directly over the aneurysm, in the epigastrium, or the back (lumbar region). Pain may be present for 4 to 5 days before sudden rupture. Syncope, as opposed to pain, may be the patient's presentation. However, most abdominal aortic aneurysms are asymptomatic until they expand or rupture.

Expansion causes sudden, intense, and constant low back, flank, or abdominal pain. After rupture, radiation into the testicles, rectum, or groin is common. Patients with ruptured abdominal aortic aneurysm may present in shock. Look for signs of cyanosis, mottling, change in mental status, tachycardia, and hypotension. The diagnostic triad—hypovolemic shock, pulsatile abdominal mass, and abdominal or back pain—is not often seen. This is because most patients with rupture who make it to a hospital have a small posterolateral tear in the aortic wall, resulting in bleeding that is contained in the retroperitoneum. These patients arrive after the acute onset of pain and a possible syncopal event. Although pain persists, the patient remains relatively hemodynamically stable.

ED physicians are the first clinicians to evaluate these patients and must act quickly during this relatively stable period. Otherwise, frank intraperitoneal rupture and hemodynamic collapse will follow this sentinel bleed. Remember that the pain of an expanding aneurysm is similar to that of a ruptured aneurysm. The crucial difference is that symptomatic patients with unruptured aneurysms are hemodynamically stable.

The last category of symptoms includes those resulting from secondary complications. The expanding aneurysm may cause pressure on adjacent viscera and lead to bowel compression. Patients may present with early satiety, nausea, and vomiting. Sometimes the abdominal aortic aneurysm ruptures into the duodenum, with consequent hematemesis and melena. Isolated groin pain is a particularly deceiving presentation. This occurs with retroperitoneal expansion and pressure on a femoral nerve. Thrombus and atheromatous material may lead to distal embolization, and patients may present with acute limb ischemia.

Seventy-five percent of abdominal aortic aneurysms occur in patients older than 60 years, predominately in males, smokers, and patients with hypertension, chronic obstructive pulmonary disease (COPD), and high cholesterol. Abdominal aortic aneurysm is six times more common in men, specifically white men compared with black men. Racial differences in women are less prominent. Patients who have a first-degree relative with abdominal aortic aneurysm are also at increased risk. Other risks include a history of collagen vascular disease (i.e., Ehlers-Danlos syndrome, Marfan's syndrome) and α_1-antitrypsin deficiency. Diabetes alone is not an independent risk factor.

Physical Examination

The classic presentation of pain, hypotension, tachycardia, and a pulsatile abdominal mass is present in less than 30% to 50% of cases. Vital signs may be normal initially, even with a ruptured abdominal aortic aneurysm, because of retroperitoneal containment of the hematoma. Palpation may be difficult in an obese or uncooperative patient. Ascites, a tortuous aorta, and excessive lumbar lordosis further complicate the examination.

Have the patient lie on the stretcher with the knees slightly flexed. Palpate the aorta during exhalation. A tender, pulsatile mass left of the midline, between the xiphoid process and umbilicus, is diagnostic of an abdominal aortic aneurysm. This finding is more commonly seen with rupture. In thin individuals, a normal pulsatile aorta may be easily palpated. Gentle, deep palpation will not precipitate rupture.

Listen for an abdominal bruit or lateral propagation of an aortic pulse wave. This subtle sign may be more frequently found than the pulsatile mass. A bruit is present in fewer than 10% of patients with abdominal aortic aneurysm. Place the diaphragm of the stethoscope 2 inches above the umbilicus, in the midline. The presence of a bruit during systole is of little clinical value, but the presence of a systolic-diastolic bruit is suspicious.

The femoral pulses should be evaluated as well. The femoral artery runs obliquely right below the inguinal ligament and midway between the pubic symphysis and the anterosuperior iliac spine. Palpate for diminished pulses.

Diagnostic Evaluation

The time spent on diagnostic testing depends on the patient's condition. When a patient presents in shock with a pulsatile mass and a known history of abdominal aortic aneurysm, no further testing is necessary, and the patient should be taken immediately to the OR. If a patient is in shock and the diagnosis is in question, an ultrasound can be done in the ED. On the other hand, an obese patient with normal vital signs and severe abdominal, back, or flank pain should undergo emergent CT scan.

Plain radiographs, if performed before suspected aneurysm, may reveal aortic wall calcification. A lateral abdominal film may show a soft tissue bulge anterior to the lumbar spine. There is no role for plain films to look for an abdominal aortic aneurysm. It is insensitive and may delay definitive diagnosis and treatment.

For unstable patients, ultrasonography is a sensitive, noninvasive, and rapid test. It gives detailed visualization of the vessel wall and associated atherosclerotic plaques and allows accurate measurement of the aneurysm in two dimensions. It may be performed at the bedside, does not require ionizing radiation, and can detect free intraperitoneal blood. It is inexpensive and available in most hospitals. The biggest downside is its inability to detect leakage or rupture. It is also unreliable in defining the relationship between the proximal end of the aneurysm and the renal arteries and the distal extent of the aneurysm. For the surgeon, the visceral vessels are not imaged with enough detail to be useful in planning the operation. In addition, it is difficult to visualize the aorta in the presence of excessive bowel gas or obesity. Hence, ultrasonography is used mainly to screen patients at risk. It is helpful in assessing aneurysm size and in tracking its growth over time. It is commonly used to follow patients with aneurysms less than 4 centimeters in diameter.

CT scan with intravenous contrast is the most accurate test in the emergent setting for determining the size and location of an abdominal aortic aneurysm. It is approximately 80% sensitive and nearly 100% specific for detecting leakage or rupture. More specifically, helical or spiral CT scan offers three-dimensional views of the abdominal cavity and provides a detailed image of branch vessel and possible adjacent organ involvement. CT scan offers advantages over ultrasonography in defining aortic size and shape, involvement of visceral and renal arteries and extension into the suprarenal aorta and iliac arteries. It also displays the origin of the aneurysm and the character and thickness of the aortic wall. CT scan can detect as little as 10 mL of blood outside the lumen of the aorta. Obesity or bowel gas does not limit this test. Drawbacks include cost, long study time, exposure to intravenous contrast agents, use of ionizing radiation, and the need to send the patient out of the monitored ED setting. There are many instances of patients developing hypotension while being scanned. Therefore, its use in the emergent diagnosis of acute rupture is controversial, because it can delay definitive care. CT scan is the preferred initial test for patients with chronic, contained rupture.

Differential Diagnosis

The differential diagnosis for aortic aneurysm is illustrated in Table 16.1.

Treatment

Initial treatment should be directed at ensuring adequate oxygenation and ventilation and treating shock. Place the patient on 100% oxygen and begin continuous cardiac monitoring and pulse oximetry. At least two large-bore (preferably 14-gauge) intravenous lines should be inserted. (See Table 16.2.)

For hypertensive patients, acute blood pressure control should be achieved using anti-hypertensive agents and analgesics. The adrenoreceptor antagonists are particularly

Table 16.2.

Treatment guidelines for abdominal aortic aneurysm rupture

All Patients
IV access, 2 large-bore, minimum 18-gauge
    catheters
Supplemental oxygen
Continuous cardiac monitoring
Continuous pulse oximetry

Stable
Symptomatic (pain) and/or aneurysm >5 cm
Vascular surgery consultation
Admission to hospital
Hypertension: treat to maintain systolic BP
    100–120 mm Hg
IV β-blockers: esmolol, labetalol, metoprolol
IV nitroprusside
Pain management: IV opioids

Unstable/Shock
IV normal saline
Blood products for hypotension as soon as
    available
Intubation
Bedside ultrasound for diagnosis/CT if stabilized
Emergency vascular surgery consultation

BP, blood pressure; CT, computed tomography;
IV, intravenous.

Table 16.1.

Differential diagnosis of abdominal aortic aneurysm

Renal colic
Diverticulitis
Pancreatitis
Perforated ulcer
Musculoskeletal back pain
Intestinal ischemia
Inguinal hernia
Lumbosacral disc disease in the presence
    of shock and syncope
Myocardial infarction
Cerebrovascular disease
Cardiac arrhythmia

useful for lowering blood pressure. They include esmolol, labetalol, and metoprolol. Esmolol is a β_2-blocker with a short half-life and can be discontinued quickly if needed. Labetalol blocks both α- and β-adrenergic receptor sites. Finally, metoprolol is a selective β_1-adrenergic receptor blocker. These agents may induce bronchospasm and bradycardia and are contraindicated in patients with atrioventricular conduction abnormalities. Another intravenous agent is nitroprusside. It causes peripheral vasodilation by dilating both arteries and veins, resulting in decreased peripheral vascular resistance. Because of its rapid onset and short duration of action, it is easy to titrate. Side effects include reflex tachycardia, arrhythmia, and cyanide toxicity. When used, nitroprusside is frequently accompanied by a β-blocker to blunt the tachycardia. Pain control is important not only for patient comfort but also to treat tachycardia and hypertension. Opioid agents should be administered intravenously as needed.

Treating hypertension can slow aneurysm propagation and delay rupture. The goal is to maintain a systolic blood pressure of 90 to 100 mm Hg. The concern about the pressure is that it may force a tenuous clot to dislodge and cause even more bleeding. Patients with a leaking aneurysm, who are normotensive, do not require pharmacotherapy. If the patient is conscious and has adequate perfusion, fluids should be deferred until the rupture is controlled in the OR. Unnecessary volume resuscitation may raise the blood pressure, resulting in further hemorrhage.

Patients who are unstable require emergency surgical consultation. Operation should not be delayed to resuscitate a patient. Instead, the patient should be brought to the OR while rapid infusion of fluids is continued. Surgical treatment options include either conventional or endovascular repair. Conventional repair involves exposure of the aorta, aortic and iliac clamping, and replacement of the aneurysmal segment with a prosthetic graft. Endovascular repair delivers an endoprosthesis through the femoral artery and then secures the endograft using expandable stents.

Disposition

Presence of an asymptomatic abdominal aortic aneurysm is not an indication for admission. These patients should be referred for elective outpatient evaluation by a vascular surgeon. The treatment of the abdominal aortic aneurysm depends on its size and expansion rate. Current guidelines recommend elective repair for low-risk patients with an abdominal aortic aneurysm greater than 5 cm, or abdominal aortic aneurysm between 4 and 5 cm, with documented enlargement of more than 0.5 cm in less than 6 months. Patients who are symptomatic or unstable need prompt surgical consultation and evaluation for the possibility of operative repair, regardless of aneurysm size.

Pathophysiology

An aneurysm is a permanent, localized dilatation of an artery. Most aneurysms occur in the aorta, and most aortic aneurysms are infrarenal. True aneurysms result from dilatation of all three layers of the arterial wall: the intima (the innermost layer facing the lumen), the media (the middle layer), and the adventitia (the outermost layer). False aneurysms do not involve the dilatation of all three layers of the arterial wall but instead are due to disruption of the wall. A dissecting aneurysm is a type of false aneurysm that usually results from the degeneration of the arterial media, tearing of the intima, and subsequent development of a hematoma in the arterial wall.

True arterial aneurysms are defined as a 50% (1.5 times) increase in the normal diameter of the vessel. The normal diameter of the infrarenal aorta is 2 cm in men and 1.8 cm in women. Some abdominal aortic aneurysms remain stable in size, but their natural history generally involves slow expansion. Aneurysm diameter sizes range from 3 cm to those that reach up to 15 cm. The risk of rupture increases significantly once an abdominal aortic aneurysm exceeds 5 cm in diameter. Symptoms usually arise from complications that affect arterial aneurysms: rupture, thrombosis, or embolization.

The aorta is composed of three layers: an inner intima, with its endothelial lining; a medial layer, composed largely of elastic fibers; and an outer adventitia, which harbors the nerves and blood vessels that supply the aorta. Unlike smaller arteries, the aorta has very little smooth muscle. The aorta has to absorb repeated pressure waves from the heart and must be able to resist high pressures without rupture. The elasticity of the media allows it to dilate during systole. During diastole, the walls of the aorta relax and propel blood forward into the arterial branches. Local weakening of the aortic wall results in progressive dilatation and aneurysm formation. Wall tension is an important predictor of pending rupture, which occurs when the mechanical stress acting on the wall exceeds the strength of the wall tissue.

Wall tension can be calculated using Laplace's Law:

$$Wall\ Tension \sim PR/W$$

where P is mean arterial pressure, R is radius, and W is wall thickness. Hence, once the vessel diameter begins to widen, the wall stress is increased, resulting in further widening. The infrarenal location is a high-pressure zone because of reflected pressure waves from the aortic bifurcation. This may explain the why abdominal aortic aneurysm most commonly develop in this location.

The etiology of abdominal aortic aneurysm formation is mostly degenerative rather than atherosclerotic. An aneurysm develops when circumstances increase the forces exerted on the aortic wall or decrease the wall's ability to resist these forces.

The primary structural elements of the aortic wall are elastin and collagen. Any imbalance between the levels of elastase, collagenase, protease, and antiprotease may contribute to aneurysm formation. Cigarette smoking has been shown to cause protease-antiprotease imbalance, leading to degradation of elastic tissue in the lungs. This same process may also affect the aorta. Failure of elastin is the first step in aneurysm development, resulting in an increased mechanical load on the collagen. Elastin fibers are arranged in concentric lamellae in the aortic media, which forms the primary load bearing structure of the aortic wall. The half-life of elastin is approximately 70 years, and the adult aorta does not appear to produce functional elastin. This may explain why abdominal aortic aneurysm occurs primarily late in life. In addition, the number of lamellae falls dramatically on passing from the thoracic to the abdominal aorta, where aneurysm formation is most frequent. As elastolysis increases, collagen function becomes the important determinant of aneurysm growth.

The structural properties of elastin and collagen are complementary. Both must fail, if aneurysm dilatation and rupture are to occur.

Smoking is one of the most commonly cited risk factors for abdominal aortic aneurysm. Some of its effects are mediated through atherosclerosis. Atherosclerosis has conventionally been considered the most common cause of abdominal aortic aneurysm; however, it is only present in 25% of the patients. This process may cause medial weakening in a dilated aorta. The vasa vasorum are blood vessels that nourish the vascular walls. Because the infrarenal aorta lacks a vasa vasorum, the medial layer must get its oxygen and nutrition by diffusion through the lumen. Atherosclerotic plaques may interfere with oxygen delivery, resulting in ischemia of the media, weakening of the aortic wall, and ultimately dilatation. Inflammation may also contribute to aneurysm formation by weakening the aortic wall. Autoimmunity may play a role in this inflammatory process.

Suggested Readings

Blanchard JF. Epidemiology of abdominal aortic aneurysms. *Epidemiol Rev* 1999;21:207–221.

Ernst CB. Current concepts: abdominal aortic aneurysms. *N Engl J Med* 1993;328:1167–1172.

Henney AM, Adiseshiah M, Poulter N, et al. Abdominal aortic aneurysm: report of a meeting of physicians and scientists, University College London Medical School. *Lancet* 1993;341:214–220.

Santilli JD, Santilli SM. Diagnosis and treatment of abdominal aortic aneurysms. *AFP* 1997;56:1081–1090.

Thompson MM, Bell PRF. Arterial aneurysms. *BMJ* 2000;320:1193–1196.

Wilmink AB, Quick CRG. Epidemiology and potential for prevention of abdominal aortic aneurysm. *Br J Surg* 1998;85:155–162.

CHAPTER 17

Cholecystitis

Deborah R. Wong, MD

Clinical Scenario

A 40-year-old Native American woman presents to the emergency department (ED) with right upper quadrant pain. The pain began 2 weeks ago and is severe and intermittent in nature. The patient notes that symptoms seem to increase after meals and became excruciating today after eating some fried chicken. She states she has taken calcium carbonate (Rolaids) and cimetidine (Pepcid) without relief. She has had some nausea but no vomiting or diarrhea. Her last bowel movement was today and was normal in color. She has been experiencing fevers and some chills. She denies any jaundice, melena, recent travel, chest pain, shortness of breath or cough.

Past medical history reveals hypertension, obesity, and hypercholesterolemia. Her medications include simvastatin, oral contraceptives, and hydrochlorothiazide. Family history is significant for hypertension, hypercholesterolemia, and gallstones.

Physical examination reveals an obese female in moderate distress. Vital signs include a temperature of 101.3°F, heart rate of 110 beats/minute, blood pressure of 165/70 mm Hg, and a respiratory rate of 18 breaths/minute. Oxygen saturation is 100% on room air. Sclerae are anicteric. Cardiac examination is normal except for tachycardia. Lungs are clear to auscultation bilaterally. Abdominal examination reveals normal bowel sounds. There is moderate tenderness to palpation in the right upper quadrant and a Murphy's sign but no rebound tenderness. Digital rectal examination shows guaiac-negative, brown stool.

Intravenous access is established, and blood is sent for complete blood count, electrolytes, blood urea nitrogen (BUN), creatinine, liver function tests (LFTs), and amylase. The patient is administered intravenous morphine sulfate for pain, and a liter of normal saline is begun. She is sent to radiology for an upright chest x-ray and abdominal radiograph and a right upper quadrant ultrasound.

On return from radiology, the patient's vital signs have returned to normal with analgesia and fluid resuscitation. X-ray films reveal a nonspecific gas pattern, no free air, and normal lungs. Ultrasonography demonstrates multiple gallstones, the largest of which is 15 by 10 mm and impacted in the neck of a distended gallbladder. The gallbladder wall is thickened at 0.9 cm and there is a small pericholecystic fluid collection. Cystic and common bile ducts are within normal limits. Laboratory results are notable for a white blood cell count (WBC) of 13,600 cells/μL with a left shift, a total bilirubin of 2 mg/dL, an alkaline phosphatase of 120 U/L, amylase of 30 U/L, alanine aminotransferase (ALT) 70 U/L, and aspartate aminotransferase (AST) 75 U/L.

General surgery is consulted. The patient is admitted with a diagnosis of cholecystitis. Intravenous antibiotics are administered, and plans are made for cholecystectomy in the morning.

Clinical Evaluation

Introduction

Gallstones make up more than 95% of all biliary tract disease. In the United States, $6 to $8 billion per year are spent on the treatment of gallstones and their complications. Approximately 10% to 20% of the adult population will develop gallstones. Although 80% of patients with gallstones (cholelithiasis) are asymptomatic, many develop inflammation with or without infection of the gallbladder (cholecystitis). Right upper quadrant pain may be the presenting symptom for many diseases including abdominal, thoracic, cardiac, and renal sources. The emergency physician must be able to efficiently rule out the life threats and focus on the likely problem.

History

Patients with symptomatic cholelithiasis frequently describe their pain as intense and intermittent. The pain is located in the epigastrium or right upper quadrant and may radiate to the back. Symptoms may be worse after eating (postprandial) or may awaken the patient from sleep. Up to 75% of patients experience nausea and vomiting. Patients frequently complain of anorexia because they fear pain or nausea and vomiting after eating. A history of prior episodes of pain is frequently elicited. Patients may use antacids without relief of their symptoms.

Charcot's triad, consisting of fever, jaundice, and right upper quadrant pain, is the classic presentation of cholecystitis. If the gallstone is impacted in the cystic or bile ducts, patients may relate a history consistent with the obstruction of bile proximal to the stone. Stools may become clay-colored as transit of bile into the gut is disrupted. In turn, urine may be darker as renal excretion of conjugated bilirubin increases. Jaundice and icterus are often subtle and may only be noticed by the patient's family if they are noted at all. Ninety percent of cases of cholecystitis are secondary to obstruction of the gallbladder neck or cystic duct by a stone. Cholecystitis is distinct from biliary colic (symptomatic cholelithiasis) because there is an additional component of inflammation with or without infection. This subset of patients may note intermittent low-grade fevers and chills.

Risk factors for cholelithiasis include obesity, female sex, multiple births, age greater than 40 years, and white race. For years, students have remembered cholecystitis as the disease of Fs. Is the patient fat, female, fertile, flatulent, forty, or fair? Other risk factors include Native American heritage, rapid weight changes, hyperlipidemia, and a family history of gallstones.

Several other common gastrointestinal disorders such as pancreatitis, gastritis, peptic ulcer disease, and gastroesophageal reflux disease may present with similar symptoms. Additional history should include past medical history of any gastrointestinal pathology. Other important historical information includes risk factors for ischemic cardiac disease; pneumonia; or other symptoms of thoracic pathology, diabetes, and sickle cell disease.

Physical Examination

Physical examination begins with vital signs and general appearance. Just by looking at our patient, we can see that she has several risk factors for gallstones. She is overweight, female, within the peak age range, and in a high-risk ethnic group. Vital signs are notable for a low-grade fever and tachycardia, suggesting an inflammatory response as seen in cholecystitis and less suggestive of uncomplicated cholelithiasis. She has both borderline hypertension and tachycardia, which may be partially explained as a response to pain. More concerning would be a low blood pressure, which could indicate serious infection or sepsis.

On examination of the head and neck, the sclera should be assessed for icterus (yellowing of the sclera), which occurs when serum bilirubin concentrations exceed 2 to 3 mg/dL. Patients with cholelithiasis generally are nonicteric, although it may occur if the stone is preventing the flow of bile into the bowel. Patients may also exhibit jaundice (yellowing) of the skin, which may be noted in fair-skinned individuals when the serum bilirubin rises above 3 to 5 mg/dL.

The abdominal examination incorporates the general principles of inspection, auscultation, percussion, and palpation. Murphy's sign is elicited by having the patient take a deep breath while deeply palpating over the region of the gallbladder at the midpoint of the right subcostal margin. Patients with a Murphy's sign will stop inhaling midbreath secondary to pain. In less than 25% of patients, the gallbladder will also be palpable in this region. In some patients, percussion and palpation may also reveal a localized peritonitis in the right upper quadrant. Rectal examination will generally reveal brown guaiac-negative stool. However, as noted previously, stool may be clay-colored. In addition to the focused abdominal examination, careful examination of the lungs, heart, and back may help to rule out other pathology.

Diagnostic Evaluation

Blood tests may be helpful both in differentiating cholelithiasis from cholecystitis and in excluding other pathologies, but it should never be relied on to rule out the diagnosis. In patients with cholelithiasis, laboratory abnormalities are generally not present. An exception to this is mild to moderate bilirubinemia (<5 mg/dL), which may be associated with biliary colic. Elevations in bilirubin may also be detected in cholecystitis along with mild leukocytosis (12,000 to 15,000 cells/μL). LFTs may reveal increased transaminases (AST and ALT) up to four times normal and a doubling of alkaline phosphatase levels. Amylase, an enzyme normally secreted by the pancreas, may be mildly increased in cholecystitis, especially if obstruction to the common bile duct is present.

Ultrasonography is the most useful diagnostic test. Stones as small as 1 mm can be visualized. Sensitivity and specificity for detecting gallstones are greater than 95% in experienced hands. Gallstones appear as dense defects, and an echogenic shadow is cast distal to the defect. Although it can be difficult to image stones in the neck of the gallbladder and in the biliary and cystic ducts, obstruction to the normal flow of bile is suggested by examining the biliary system for dilatation. The diagnosis of cholecystitis is based on the combination of several additional criteria. One may see thickening (>3.5 mm) or sonolucency of the gallbladder wall, gallbladder distention, fluid around the gallbladder (pericholecystic fluid), or cystic echoes in the wall. A positive Murphy's sign during the ultrasonographic examination (sonographic Murphy's sign) also correlates with cholecystitis. A normal examination does not absolutely rule out cholecystitis, and repeat examination should be performed if clinical suspicion remains high.

Other less useful radiological tests include plain abdominal radiography and radionucleotide scintigraphy. Only 15% to 20% of symptomatic gallstones are calcified sufficiently to see on plain x-ray film. Despite this low sensitivity, a flat plate of the abdomen and upright abdominal film may be a relatively inexpensive starting point to rule out other etiologies.

Radionucleotide scintigraphy (also known as hepato-iminodiacetic acid [HIDA] scan) has sensitivity and specificity rates approaching that of ultrasound. In this test, the patient is administered radioactively labeled iminodiacetic acid (IDA) and uptake into the liver and biliary tree is imaged after 1 to 2 hours. A positive result would be the lack of filling in the gallbladder lumen. This test is most often used when the ultrasound is negative but cholecystitis is clinically still suspected. The obvious disadvantages of this study compared with ultrasound are the extra time involved, higher costs, and radiation exposure. These deficiencies render it less practical in the ED.

Differential Diagnosis

The differential diagnosis for cholecystitis is illustrated in Table 17.1.

Treatment

The treatment of patients with either symptomatic cholelithiasis or cholecystitis begins with pain control and volume resuscitation (Table 17.2). Patients are frequently volume depleted secondary to vomiting and decreased oral intake. Normal saline or lactated Ringer's solution should be infused at a rate sufficient to replace losses within a few hours. Electrolytes may need to be corrected as well.

Several agents may be administered for pain. Intravenous ketorolac (Toradol), a parenteral nonsteroidal antiinflammatory drug,

Table 17.1.

Differential diagnosis of cholecystitis

Abdominal Conditions
Peptic ulcer disease
Pancreatitis
Gastroesophageal reflux
Hepatitis
Hepatic abscess
Irritable bowel syndrome
Gastritis
Appendicitis

Genitourinary Conditions
Pelvic inflammatory disease
Pyelonephritis

Thoracic Conditions
Right lower lobe pneumonia
Pleuritis
Myocardial ischemia or infarction

is frequently used because it has few side effects. For severe pain, intravenous opiates such as morphine are generally indicated.

Operative treatment options for acute cholecystitis include laparoscopic cholecystectomy or standard (open) cholecystectomy. For gallstones, treatments include oral bile acid therapy (to dissolve stones), extracorporeal shock wave lithotripsy (to break up stones), or percutaneous gallstone removal. Laparoscopic cholecystectomy is currently the treatment of choice for most patients.

Although a bacterial infection is not invariably present, antibiotics are usually administered to cover the most commonly implicated bacteria including *Escherichia coli*, *Bacillus fragilis*, and *Clostridium perfringens*. Patients should not eat or drink (should be made "nothing by mouth" [NPO]), and a nasogastric tube may be required to drain gastric secretions if vomiting is severe. In those patients requiring admission, laparoscopic or open cholecystectomy is usually performed soon after admission if the patient is a surgical candidate. Other treatment options are similar to those discussed previously. It is interesting to note that 75% of patients with acute cholecystitis recover in 7 to 10 days

without treatment. However, 25% develop severe symptoms or complications such as cholangitis, sepsis, gallbladder rupture, cholecystenteric fistulae, or worsening of a preexisting medical condition.

Disposition

Patients with symptomatic cholelithiasis may be discharged from the ED if their pain can be well controlled. Close follow-up with a surgeon or internist is mandatory. Patients should be instructed to avoid fatty foods and to return for increasing pain, intractable vomiting, or fever. Cholecystitis generally requires admission to the hospital for administration of intravenous antibiotics. There is no benefit from delaying surgery. In fact, early operation may actually reduce complications. Patients can be admitted to a general surgical floor unless they show signs of sepsis or perforation. In those cases, an intensive care unit (ICU) or emergency surgery is more appropriate.

Pathophysiology

The normal gallbladder stores up to 50 mL of concentrated bile. This bile, which is created by the liver, is the major catabolic product of cholesterol and its primary route of elimination. Between meals, bile flows into the gallbladder because the resistances of the common bile duct and the sphincter of Oddi exceed that of the cystic duct and the distensible gallbladder. After a meal, hepatic bile secretion increases, the gallbladder contracts, and the sphincter of Oddi relaxes. The bile travels from the gallbladder lumen through the cystic and common bile ducts and into the gut via the ampulla of Vater and sphincter of Oddi. Most bile salts are recycled via enterohepatic circulation; however, approximately 5% are lost per day in feces.

The mechanisms of hormonal and neuronal control of gallbladder motility are complex and not fully understood. In 1928, Ivy and Oldberg extracted a substance that they called cholecystokinin (CCK) from the upper intestines of pigs. They injected CCK into dogs and noted that the gallbladder

Table 17.2.

Treatment of acute cholecystitis

Initial Treatment
Intravenous access
CBC, electrolytes, liver enzymes, amylase
Electrocardiogram
Volume resuscitate with normal saline
Pain control with intravenous ketorolac or opiates
Radiological studies: RUQ ultrasound +/− plain films
Nasogastric tube if indicated

Cholelithiasis
If asymptomatic in 4–6 hours, the patient may be discharged with close follow-up
    and low-fat diet.
If pain or vomiting is intractable or electrolyte abnormalities are severe, the
    patient should be admitted to surgery or medicine (NPO, intravenous, opiates,
    and antiemetics).

Acute Cholecystitis
Surgical consultation
Intravenous antibiotics
NPO, intravenous line, opiates, and antiemetics
Cholecystectomy +/− ERCP in 1–3 days

Complicated Cholecystitis (e.g., sepsis, suspected perforation)
Surgical consultation
Blood cultures (two sets)
Intravenous antibiotics
NPO, intravenous fluids, opiates, antiemetics, +/− vasopressors
Urgent surgery or admission to ICU

CBC, complete blood count; ERCP, endoscopic retrograde cholangiopancreatography;
ICU, intensive care unit; NPO, nothing by mouth; RUQ, right upper quadrant.

emptied in response. CCK is a linear polypeptide released by several areas of the gut in response to digestion products. It acts directly on the smooth muscle of the gallbladder possibly through a phosphodiesterase-induced reduction in intracellular cyclic adenosine monophosphate (AMP). Gastrin is a hormone related to CCK in structure; although less potent, it also promotes gallbladder contraction. Secretin enhances CCK's effect on motility, although alone it has no effects on the gallbladder. Vasoactive intestinal peptide (VIP) serves to inhibit contractions, as does adrenergic stimulation.

The mechanism of gallstone formation is poorly understood. Currently, it is believed that a combination of gallbladder stasis and alterations in the physiochemical properties of bile lead to a lithogenic state. Cholesterol gallstones form when cholesterol concentrations exceed the capacity of the bile salts to solubilize them (i.e., the bile becomes supersaturated with cholesterol). When this occurs, cholesterol monohydrate crystals are produced. Gallbladder stasis often precedes the formation of stones. Factors that promote the formation of stones are excess production of cholesterol, genetics, and disorders of bile acid metabolism. Risk factors are directly related to these mechanisms. For example, our patient has an increased estrogen level secondary to gender, oral contraceptive use, and obesity. This estrogenic state leads to an increase in 3-hydroxy-3-methylglutaryl coenzyme A (HMG-CoA) reductase activity, which in turn stimulates increased cholesterol uptake and synthesis.

Pigment stones, although less common in the United States, account for a large number of biliary calculi in the Asian population and in patients with hemolytic syndromes, such as sickle cell anemia. These stones are composed of insoluble calcium salts of unconjugated bilirubin. The pathogenesis of pigment stones is less clearly understood, but risk of development is related to high levels of unconjugated bilirubin in the biliary tree.

Gallstones lead to cholecystitis when a stone becomes impacted in the neck of the gallbladder or the cystic duct and leads to obstruction of normal bile flow. This is called calculous cholecystitis and accounts for 90% to 95% of cases. In the remaining cases of cholecystitis, no stones are found. This is called acalculous cholecystitis. In both, bile stasis (resulting from the obstruction of the stone or decreased gallbladder contractions) leads to degradation and inflammation of the gallbladder mucosa. Stasis also promotes bacterial seeding of the gallbladder. Patients who are on starvation diets or on total parenteral nutrition (TPN) are at increased risk because they do not have sufficient oral intake to trigger effective gallbladder contractions.

Acalculous cholecystitis is primarily seen in an ICU population in the setting of trauma, burns, sepsis, total parenteral nutrition (TPN), or multiple organ dysfunction syndrome (MODS). It is more insidious than calculous cholecystitis and has a mortality rate approaching 50%.

Suggested Readings

Chandler CF, Lane JS, Ferguson P, et al. Prospective evaluation of early versus delayed laparoscopic cholecystectomy for treatment of acute cholecystitis. *Am Surg* 2000;66:896–900.

Johnston DE, Kaplan M. Medical progress: pathogenesis and treatment of gallstones. *N Engl J Med* 1993;328:412–421.

Ryan JP. Motility of the gallbladder and biliary tree. In: Johnson LR, ed. *Physiology of the gastrointestinal tract.* New York: Raven Press, 1987:695–721.

Soper NJ, et al. Gallbladder stones. In: Pitt HA, Carr-Locke D, Ferrucci JT, eds. *Hepatobiliary and pancreatic disease: the team approach to management.* Boston: Little, Brown, and Company, 1995.

CHAPTER 18

Appendicitis

Karen Ann Casper, MD

Clinical Scenario

An 18-year-old man presents to the emergency department complaining of right lower abdominal pain. He states that he awoke this morning with an aching feeling in the middle of his abdomen. He had no appetite throughout the day. The patient describes the pain as initially dull and in the central abdomen. The pain seemed to move to the right lower part of his abdomen a few hours ago and has become more constant, sharp, and severe. He notes that during the drive to the hospital, the bumpy parts of the road seemed to make the pain worse. He felt mild nausea after he noticed the pain but did not vomit. He had a normal bowel movement in the morning, but he feels the urge to pass gas.

He states that he has no medical problems, takes no medications, and has no drug allergies.

Physical examination reveals a healthy appearing young man. Blood pressure is 130/85 mm Hg, pulse is 100 beats/minute, temperature is 100.6°F, and respiratory rate is 22 breaths/minute. The abdominal examination is notable for tenderness to palpation in the right lower quadrant (RLQ). There is also tenderness to percussion in the same quadrant. When the abdomen is deeply palpated and released, the patient notes significantly more pain on the release. When the bed is shaken, pain is noted in the RLQ. Rectal examination reveals no tenderness or blood and the prostate is nontender. Genitourinary (GU) examination is normal.

An intravenous (IV) line is placed and blood is drawn and sent for a complete blood count (CBC) and type and hold. A urinalysis

is normal. The patient receives IV morphine with relief of his pain. Surgery is consulted. They examine the patient and then contact the operating room to prepare for surgery. He is taken to the operating room for a presumed appendectomy.

Clinical Evaluation

Introduction

Appendicitis is a common abdominal emergency requiring a high index of suspicion for early and correct diagnosis. The appendectomy is the most common emergent surgical procedure. Appendicitis affects all age groups and presents with varied symptoms. Prompt recognition of the signs and symptoms of appendicitis are essential to early surgical intervention.

History

The classic presentation of acute appendicitis occurs in approximately 50% of cases. In this presentation, vague periumbilical or epigastric pain is followed by anorexia and nausea. This discomfort is present for several hours, progressing to more severe pain localized to the RLQ.

Other symptoms may be present in varying degrees. Vomiting may occur and usually follows the onset of the pain. The patient may complain of indigestion, gastritis, or flatulence. Either diarrhea or constipation may be noted. The examiner must be careful not to dismiss appendicitis as a diagnosis when these symptoms are present. Furthermore, the inflamed appendix may lie in close proximity to the ureter or bladder resulting in frequency, urgency, hematuria, and even

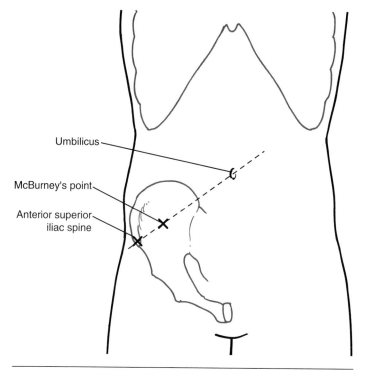

Umbilicus

McBurney's point

Anterior superior
iliac spine

Figure 18.1
This diagram illustrates the location of McBurney's point: the classic
location of tenderness in appendicitis.

pyuria. The patient may also be aware of a fever; however, it is not present in all cases of appendicitis.

Patients usually present within the first 24 to 48 hours after the onset of symptoms. Few patients report the presence of symptoms for longer periods or similar pain in the past.

Physical Examination

The examiner should keep in mind that the different locations of the appendix, the degree of inflammation of the appendix, age, and comorbidity of the patient all influence the presentation of appendicitis. Importantly, atypical presentations are more common in the young and the elderly. The vital signs are often within normal limits in cases of appendicitis. The temperature is frequently normal or may be only slightly elevated (38°C, 100°F). If perforation has occurred, the temperature may be higher. The pulse and blood pressure may be mildly elevated, if the patient is experiencing discomfort or is volume depleted from poor oral intake or vomiting. The degree and location of abdominal tenderness on physical examination is influenced by the location of the appendix and any appendiceal inflammation. RLQ tenderness at McBurney's point (see Fig. 18.1) is the classic location of tenderness. In this case, the appendix is anterior to the cecum.

Tenderness to percussion, guarding, and rebound tenderness reflect the degree of peritoneal inflammation. Voluntary guarding and rebound tenderness at McBurney's point is seen with early inflammation. As more of the peritoneal lining is involved, diffuse rebound tenderness, generalized pain on percussion and palpation, and involuntary guarding develop.

Other, less common, signs may be present on physical examination. Rovsing's sign is present when palpation of the left lower quadrant causes pain in the RLQ. The obturator sign is RLQ pain with internal rotation of the flexed right hip. The psoas sign is

RLQ pain with hyperextension of the right hip. Dunphy's sign is increased pain with coughing. The absence of any of these signs should never lead to the exclusion of appendicitis as a possible diagnosis.

The presence or absence of any of the classic findings or signs depends on the location of the inflamed appendix. An inflamed retrocecal appendix may present with flank tenderness. A digital rectal examination is an important component of the physical examination, because tenderness suggests peritoneal irritation by a retrocecal appendix. The physical examination should also include a GU examination in men and a pelvic examination in women. Testicular pathology and hernias may present with RLQ pain. Ectopic pregnancy, ruptured ovarian cyst, ovarian torsion, and pelvic inflammatory disease must be excluded from the differential in a woman presenting with RLQ pain.

Diagnostic Evaluation

Appendicitis is a clinical diagnosis. When the history and physical examination clearly suggest appendicitis, no further laboratory or radiographical studies are needed. In cases in which the diagnosis is unclear, further testing may be helpful. In appendicitis, the white blood count (WBC) is usually between 10,000 and 20,000 cells/μL. The differential tends to show more polymorphonuclear forms. In perforated appendicitis, the WBC may be higher (or lower in patients at the extremes of age). The urinalysis may show proteinuria, hematuria, or pyuria, if the inflamed appendix is near the ureter or bladder. In all women of childbearing age, a pregnancy test is mandatory.

Plain x-ray films of the abdomen are minimally helpful in establishing a diagnosis of appendicitis. An abnormal gas pattern may be seen on plain x-ray films, but it is a nonspecific finding. The presence of a RLQ fecalith (an opacity that represents calcified bile contents) is rare but when present strongly suggests appendicitis.

Atypical presentations of appendicitis can result in diagnostic delays. Further imaging studies may identify the presence of appendicitis. Over the last 2 decades, ultrasound and abdominal computed tomography (CT) scan have become accepted diagnostic studies. Institutional availability and expertise dictate which test is recommended.

Graded compression ultrasonography is a technique requiring a high degree of operator experience. Prospective studies of sonography show a sensitivity of 55% to 90% and specificity of 86% to 100%. A noncompressible appendix measuring 7 mm in the anteroposterior diameter constitutes a positive test. In indeterminate cases, the presence of increased appendiceal perfusion, or shadowing from a fecalith, increase the possibility of appendicitis. Gangrenous changes and periappendiceal abscesses may also be noted.

Ultrasonography is noninvasive, lacks radiation exposure, and can be performed in a timely fashion. It is particularly helpful in the pediatric population in which the patient is usually thin and without complicating pathology. In addition, unlike CT scan, sedation is rarely required. Limitations to this technique include operator experience; presence of perforation; overweight patients; severe abdominal pain preventing compression; and the possibility of a dilated, gas-filled appendix appearing as small bowel.

Abdominal CT is far more accurate than ultrasonography. Acquisition of 5-mm sections after the administration of IV, oral, and rectal contrast has led to increased sensitivity and specificity. In addition, abdominal CT is more likely to reveal an alternative diagnosis. Disadvantages include increased costs, radiation exposure, the potential for allergic reactions to contrast media, and longer imaging time.

Differential Diagnosis

The differential diagnosis for appendicitis is illustrated in Table 18.1.

Treatment

Once a diagnosis of appendicitis has been made, the importance of early appendectomy cannot be overemphasized. The surgeon may perform an open or laparoscopic

Table 18.1.

Differential diagnosis of appendicitis

Tubo-ovarian abscess
Pelvic inflammatory disease
Ovarian torsion
Ovarian cyst
Endometriosis
Ectopic pregnancy
Epididymitis
Testicular torsion
Diverticulitis
Crohn's disease
Colonic carcinoma
Constipation
Cholecystitis
Mesenteric adenitis
Gastroenteritis
Intussusception
Volvulus
Ureteral stones
Perforated viscus

procedure. Preoperative laboratory testing should be obtained according to the patient's underlying medical problems and the surgeon's discretion. In general, coagulation studies, a type and screen, a urinalysis, electrolytes, and CBC are acceptable. However, young healthy patients may require no laboratory testing.

While awaiting appendectomy, the patient should take nothing by mouth and have adequate hydration and analgesia. Electrolyte abnormalities should be corrected, and preexisting medical conditions should be addressed. The surgeon may also request preoperative antibiotics.

If the diagnosis of appendicitis is suspected but is not certain, patients should be admitted to the surgical service for serial examinations and observation. This scenario is particularly common in hospitals in which 24-hour CT scan is unavailable.

Disposition

All patients with appendicitis should be admitted. In addition, patients with an uncertain diagnosis of appendicitis, when radiological evaluation may be unavailable, should be admitted to a surgical service for observation and serial examination.

Pathophysiology

The appendix extends from the cecum. During embryological development the tip of the appendix can lie in many different locations: retrocecal, subcecal, preileal, pericolic, retrocolic, or pelvic. Accordingly, the position of the appendix can result in different clinical presentations of appendicitis.

The appendix is lined by colonic epithelium containing lymphoid follicles. These follicles are part of the gut-associated lymphoid tissue (GALT). The highest amount of lymphoid tissue is present between the first and second decades of life and decreases to a minimal level during the sixth decade.

Obstruction of the lumen of the appendix leads to the development of appendicitis. Obstruction is most frequently caused by hyperplasia of the lymphoid tissue (60%), followed by fecalith formation (35%). Other less common causes of obstruction include concretions, strictures, adhesions, and foreign bodies.

The autonomic nervous system supplies innervation of the appendix. There are no pain fibers in the appendix. The lack of pain fibers results in the vague presentation of early appendiceal inflammation. Pain fibers are present in the peritoneal lining of the abdominal cavity. Hence, when appendiceal inflammation involves the peritoneum, pain becomes more severe and well localized.

Obstruction of the lumen leads to stasis of mucus and bacteria. Ongoing mucus production and bacterial proliferation results in increased luminal pressure. As the pressure increases, arterial blood inflow is impeded, leading to localized infarction, gangrene, and, ultimately, necrosis. Eventually frank perforation through the appendiceal wall will occur. If localized adhesions are present, the contents of the appendix will form a contained abscess. If no adhesions are present, generalized peritoneal inflammation will result.

Suggested Readings

Balthazar EJ, Birnbaum BA, Yee J. Acute appendicitis: CT and US correlation in 100 patients. *Radiology* 1994;190:31–35.

Birnbaum BA, Jeffrey RB. CT and sonographic evaluation of acute right lower quadrant abdominal pain. *AJR Am J Roentgenol* 1998;170:361–371.

Brewer BJ, Golden GT, Hitch DC, et al. Abdominal pain. An analysis of 1,000 consecutive cases in a university hospital emergency room. *Am J Surg* 1976;131:219–223.

Franke R, Bohner H, Yang Q, et al., Acute Abdominal Pain Study Group. Ultrasonography for diagnosis of acute appendicitis: results of a prospective multicenter trial. *World J Surg* 1999;23:141–146.

Rao PM, Rhea JT, Novelline RA. Effect of computed tomography of the appendix on treatment of patients and use of hospital resources. *N Engl J Med* 1998;338:141–146.

19

Diverticulitis

Jeffrey A. Evans, MD

Clinical Scenario

A 67-year-old man presents to the emergency department with a chief complaint of abdominal pain. He was in his usual state of health until 2 days ago, when he experienced the gradual onset of dull, nonradiating, constant, left lower quadrant abdominal discomfort. The abdominal pain was associated with a subjective fever and was slightly worsened by eating. The patient denied recent weight loss, nausea, vomiting, diarrhea, hematochezia (blood in stool), melena (maroon stool), dysuria (pain with urination), or penile discharge. He frequently suffers from constipation, with his last normal bowel movement 6 hours before presentation.

Past medical history is noncontributory. There is no history of abdominal surgery. The patient states his diet is generally low in fiber and high in red meat. He takes no medications.

Physical examination reveals an overweight male with blood pressure of 147/88 mm Hg, heart rate of 75 beats/minute, respiratory rate of 16 breaths/minute, and temperature of 100.3°F. His abdomen is obese with hypoactive bowel sounds. There are no scars or hernias. There is moderate tenderness to palpation of the left lower quadrant. There is voluntary guarding but no involuntary guarding, rebound tenderness, Rovsing's sign, or palpable masses. Stool obtained by digital rectal examination is negative for occult blood. There is no jaundice, and the remainder of his physical examination is normal.

An intravenous line is established and blood is sent for complete blood count (CBC) and electrolytes. Morphine sulfate is administered intravenously to control pain. CBC shows white blood count 13,200/μL, hemoglobin 15.2 g/dL, hematocrit 45%, and platelets 272,000/μL. Electrolytes are normal.

Computed tomography (CT) of the abdomen and pelvis with oral, rectal, and intravenous contrast shows multiple diverticula of the sigmoid colon with adjacent increased soft tissue density and bowel wall thickening consistent with a diagnosis of diverticulitis. There is no pneumoperitoneum or intraperitoneal fluid collection.

The patient is admitted to the hospital for intravenous antibiotics and pain control. On the third hospital day, the patient's pain is improved, he tolerates oral intake well, and he is discharged on a 10-day course of broad-spectrum oral antibiotics and analgesics. The patient is counseled to observe a liquid diet until pain-free and a high-fiber diet thereafter. Primary care follow-up is arranged for screening colonoscopy.

Clinical Evaluation

Introduction

A colonic diverticulum is a herniation of mucosa and submucosa through the outer muscular layer of the large intestine. The presence of multiple diverticula is known as diverticulosis, a common condition found in 10% of people older than age 45 and in 50% to 60% of people older than 80 years. The incidence of diverticulosis follows a clear geographic distribution, with greater prevalence in Western and urbanized countries.

Diverticulosis alone is an overwhelmingly asymptomatic condition and should rarely be considered a diagnosis for a patient with abdominal pain. However, complications related to diverticula are a common cause of morbidity and mortality. Inflammation of one or more colonic diverticula is known as diverticulitis. Diverticulitis classically causes abdominal pain with fever and an elevated white blood count. In rare cases, bowel perforation, hemorrhage, obstruction, or fistula formation may be present.

History

The pain of diverticulitis may be colicky or constant with gradual or abrupt onset and is usually accompanied by a low-grade fever. Loss of appetite and vomiting may also occur. Diarrhea or constipation may be present. Bright red blood and melena are rare and suggest a colonic neoplasm or other diagnosis. Dysuria and urinary frequency are commonly associated complaints because of the proximity of the bladder and inflamed sigmoid colon.

Physical Examination

The vital signs may be noteable for fever and tachycardia.

Inspection of the abdomen is usually unremarkable. Auscultation may reveal decreased bowel sounds. Significant inflammation or perforation may result in completely absent bowel sounds. Palpation usually reveals localized tenderness, predominantly in the left lower abdominal quadrant. However, given the size and mobility of the colon, tenderness may be found anywhere throughout the abdomen. An inflamed sigmoid colon may be palpable in thin patients. Gentle percussion reveals rebound tenderness in most patients. If there is a perforation, the patient may have signs of peritonitis with exquisite diffuse tenderness and guarding. Approximately 50% of patients with diverticulitis have occult blood in their stool.

Diagnostic Evaluation

No blood test result can be used to reliably identify or exclude the diagnosis of diverticulitis. Although the white blood count is typically 10,000 to 15,000/μL, patients may have normal or significantly elevated counts. Patients may show evidence of dehydration on serum electrolytes, if oral intake has been severely diminished.

Suspected diverticulitis can usually be confirmed by CT of the abdomen and pelvis. CT scan should be performed after administration of oral, intravenous, and rectal contrast. Findings include the presence of diverticula with pericolic fat inflammation (wispy, streaky pericolic soft tissue densities) and bowel wall thickening with or without a peridiverticular abscess. Some institutions use ultrasound for the diagnosis of diverticulitis. Plain radiography with contrast enema was commonly used in the past but has fallen into disfavor. Barium enema is contraindicated in patients with suspected pneumoperitoneum. Although water-soluble contrast is safe for potential extravasation into the abdominal cavity, any enema can induce or exacerbate perforation by increasing intraluminal pressure. Contrast studies may show the presence of diverticula, luminal narrowing, and extracolonic leakage of contrast. All are nonspecific findings seen in diverticulosis, diverticulitis, Crohn's disease, and colon carcinoma.

Differential Diagnosis

The differential diagnosis for diverticulitis is illustrated in Table 19.1.

Table 19.1.
Differential diagnosis of diverticulitis
Appendicitis
Colon carcinoma
Irritable bowel syndrome
Inflammatory bowel disorder
Ovarian cyst/torsion
Ectopic pregnancy
Nephrolithiasis
Ischemic bowel
Abdominal aortic aneurysm
Pyelonephritis
Endometriosis
Adhesions
Psoas abscess
Bowel obstruction
Sigmoid volvulus

Treatment

Diverticulosis alone is often an incidental finding on abdominal imaging and requires no treatment. Treatment of diverticulitis is determined by the clinical status and general health of the patient. Patients without vomiting, and mild to moderate abdominal pain with no evidence of peritonitis, can sometimes be managed as an outpatient. Antibiotics should be initiated to cover Enterobacteriaceae, *Bacteroides,* and *Enterococcus* species. A quinolone and metronidazole or amoxicillin/clavulanate are currently recommended regimens. Patients should be advised to eat a liquid diet while symptomatic. The mainstay of preventing recurrent attacks is strict observance of a high-fiber diet.

Patients who present with any of the more serious complications of diverticulitis, including severe pain, peritonitis, fistula formation, overt bowel perforation, or hemorrhage, require admission to the hospital for intravenous antibiotics and possible surgical management (Table 19.2). Narcotic analgesia is frequently required. Antibiotics should cover gram-negative aerobic and anaerobic bacteria (Table 19.3). Multiple effective regimens are available. Surgical interventions range from percutaneous needle drainage of abscesses to total colectomy. Sigmoid resection is recommended for recurrent diverticulitis and fistulas. The long-standing recommendation of sigmoid resection for diverticulitis in any patient younger than 40 years is now controversial. Total colectomy, usually performed in two or three stages, is indicated for generalized peritonitis, sepsis, significant bowel perforation, and obstruction.

Table 19.2.

General treatment guidelines of diverticulitis

General Measures
Vital signs
Intravenous access
History and physical examination
CBC (include type and screen and PTT and INR if severe case)
CT scan

Mild to Moderate Pain, No Vomiting, No Evidence of Bowel Perforation
Discharge home
Outpatient PO antibiotics
Liquid diet
High-fiber diet once symptoms resolved
PMD follow-up
Outpatient colonoscopy to rule-out colon neoplasm

Severe Pain, No Orals, No Signs and Symptoms of Bowel Perforation
Admission to surgical or medical service with surgical consult
NPO
Intravenous fluids
Narcotic analgesia
Intravenous antibiotics

Generalized Peritonitis, Sepsis, Gastrointestinal Hemorrhage
Surgical consultation for emergency colonic resection
Send to operating room or admission to ICU
Intravenous antibiotics

CBC, complete blood count; CT, computed tomography; ICU, intensive care unit; INR, international normalized ratio; NPO, nothing by mouth; PMD, personal medical doctor; PO, by mouth; PTT, partial thromboplastin time.

Table 19.3.

Antibiotic treatment regimens

Inpatient Regimen

Metronidazole (Flagyl) for 10–14 days and fluoroquinolone (Levaquin) or gentamicin. May add ampicillin as well for 10–14 days. Medications are given intravenously as an inpatient.

Outpatient Regimen

1. Metronidazole and fluoroquinolone or trimethoprim/sulfamethoxazole for 7–10 days.
2. Amoxicillin/clavulanate for 7–10 days.

Disposition

The disposition of a patient with diverticulitis will fall into three categories that parallel the treatment options. Selected patients with first-time uncomplicated diverticulitis who can tolerate liquids and oral antibiotics can be treated as outpatients. Outpatient colonoscopy is recommended after resolution of symptoms to exclude a colonic neoplasm. Patients with more severe diverticulitis, who require parenteral antibiotics, analgesia, and fluid maintenance, qualify for conservative inpatient management. A regular medical floor with surgical consultation is generally appropriate. Patients exhibiting sepsis, hemodynamic instability, suspected or overt hemorrhage, fistula formation, or obstruction require intensive care admission and prompt surgical consultation for emergent or elective surgery.

Pathophysiology

The large intestine is a 90- to 125-cm tubular organ that incorporates the cecum, appendix, ascending colon, transverse colon, descending colon, sigmoid colon, and rectum. The sigmoid colon, which is shaped like the Greek letter sigma (Σ) is a portion of the descending colon that starts near the pelvic brim and ends at the rectum. The junction of the descending and sigmoid colon is not well defined, and sigmoid is more a descriptive than anatomical term. The ascending, transverse, and sigmoid sections of the colon are suspended by a mesentery.

The wall of the colon consists of four layers: mucosa, submucosa, muscularis, and serosa. The muscularis includes a circular inner layer and a longitudinal outer layer divided into three discrete bands called teniae coli. The teniae coli widen and become a confluent longitudinal layer at the rectosigmoid junction. There are frequent outpouchings of the colon wall called haustra, which give the colon its characteristic lumpy appearance. Each haustra is bordered by two semilunar folds, which incompletely traverse the diameter of the colon and are visible on plain radiographs.

The primary functions of the colon are water and sodium reabsorption and storage of feces until voluntary defecation. Feces are pushed from the cecum to the rectum by peristaltic segmented contractions of the colon. The diameter of the colon decreases from 8.5 cm proximally to 2.5 cm distally. The tapered lumen explains the predominance of certain pathological abnormalities in the proximal and distal colon. The walls of the colon experience a circumferential wall tension (T) and a radially directed transmural pressure (P). Tension and pressure are related by Laplace's law, which states that $P = T/r$ (where r is the radius of the vessel) in a cylindrical structure. Application of this law to the colon explains why wall tension is greater in the large-radius proximal colon. Conversely, outwardly directed transmural pressure is greater in the smaller radius distal colon. There is a greater transmural pressure in the narrow sigmoid colon. This explains the prevalence of diverticula in this area. In Western countries, 90% of patients with diverticulosis have involvement of the sigmoid colon. Only 15% have involvement of the ascending colon (for unclear reasons, the opposite distribution predominates in Asian countries). Like any herniation, diverticula are particularly prevalent in areas of preexisting weakness in the bowel wall. Diverticula are commonly found in two rows that border the colonic mesentery. The rows coincide with defects in the bowel wall where blood vessels penetrate the circular muscularis.

A diet low in fiber is one of the leading risk factors for diverticulosis. Low-fiber diets result in low stool bulk, prolonged transit times, and elevated colonic pressures that predispose to diverticular formation. This association explains the high incidence of diverticular disease among inhabitants of Western countries, who tend to eat low-fiber diets.

Diverticulosis alone is generally asymptomatic. When present, symptoms include intermittent lower abdominal pain or bloating and altered bowel habits. The clinical features of diverticulosis are indistinguishable from irritable bowel syndrome. Physicians should use caution in making either diagnosis until all serious abdominal pathology has been definitively excluded. Twenty percent of people with diverticulosis will develop symptomatic diverticulitis or other complications in their lifetime. Diverticulosis progresses to diverticulitis because of the formation of one or more closed abscesses. Stool impacted in a diverticulum obstructs its narrow opening to the bowel lumen. Mucus secretion and bacterial growth in the enclosed space cause distention and increased intraluminal pressure that impedes venous blood flow. Ultimately, localized mucosal ischemia leads to microperforation of the thin outer wall of the diverticulum. In most cases, the perforation is walled off by pericolic tissue. Infrequently, a large abscess or free perforation into the peritoneal cavity may occur.

Diverticula are rarely larger than 2 cm, but inflammation of one or more is sufficient to cause symptoms. Because diverticula predominate in the sigmoid colon—a structure usually found in the left iliac fossa—diverticulitis classically causes left lower quadrant abdominal pain. The differential diagnosis must include pathology of all the structures in the left lower quadrant. A focus of pain outside the left lower quadrant does not exclude diverticulitis. Diverticula can occur anywhere from the cecum to the rectum. Even sigmoid diverticula can cause pain outside the left lower quadrant. The sigmoid colon can have an unpredictable location because of its long mesentery. Right-sided abdominal pain is possible and is often misdiagnosed as appendicitis.

Not all diverticular disease presents with abdominal pain. Diverticula can rupture to create a large defect in the colon wall. These infrequent cases progress rapidly with stool contamination and generalized peritonitis. The term perforated diverticulitis has classically, and misleadingly, been reserved for these severe cases, even though all diverticulitis is the result of microperforation. Gastrointestinal hemorrhage is another potential complication of diverticula but rarely occurs in the setting of frank diverticulitis. Massive bleeding occurs in 5% of people with diverticulosis and is more common as a complication of right-sided diverticula. Fistulas may develop between the colon and bladder, small bowel, vagina, or abdominal wall. Small bowel obstruction may occur as a result of ileus or mechanical obstruction induced by adjacent colonic inflammation.

Suggested Readings

Ferzoco LB, Raptopoulos V, Silen W. Acute diverticulitis. *N Engl J Med* 1998;338:1521–1526.

Stollman NH, Raskin JB. Diverticular disease of the colon. *J Clin Gastroenterol* 1999;29:241–252.

Abdominal Pain
Questions and Answers

Questions

1. Which of the following is the *classic* triad of findings in patients with diverticulitis?

  A. Right lower quadrant abdominal pain, fever, and vomiting

  B. Right lower quadrant abdominal pain, fever, and diarrhea

  C. Fever, leukocytosis, and hematochezia

  D. Left lower quadrant abdominal pain, fever, and leukocytosis

  E. Left lower quadrant abdominal pain, fever, and hematochezia

2. Which of the following best describes the pathophysiology of diverticulitis?

  A. Increased intraluminal pressure leads to painful dissection of the colon wall.

  B. Mucus production in obstructed diverticula leads to wall necrosis, microperforation, and localized inflammation.

  C. Seeds and other nondigestible foods cause direct invagination of the colon wall with localized inflammation.

  D. Viral colonization of diverticula leads to localized inflammation.

  E. Normal gut flora colonizes congenitally acquired outpouchings of the colon wall.

3. A 22-year-old man presents with fever and right lower quadrant tenderness. Which of the following statements is most correct?

  A. Plain radiographs are frequently helpful in making the diagnosis of appendicitis.

  B. Ultrasound examination can be helpful in the diagnosis of appendicitis.

  C. Computed tomography (CT) findings of pericolic fat inflammation are pathognomonic for appendicitis.

  D. The administration of oral contrast can obscure the finding of appendicitis on CT scan.

4. A 35-year-old woman presents to the emergency department with right upper quadrant pain, fever, and vomiting. Her examination is unremarkable except for a Murphy's sign and epigastric tenderness. Laboratory studies include white blood cell (WBC) count of 14,000/μL, bilirubin 2.0 mg/dL, amylase 35 U/L, aspartate aminotransferase (AST) 70 U/L, and alanine aminotransferase (ALT) 85 U/L. The most appropriate radiographic study to order next is:

  A. Hepatobiliary iminodiacetic acid (HIDA) scan

  B. Abdominal computed tomography (CT) scan

  C. Right upper quadrant ultrasound examination

  D. Abdominal x-ray film

5. Factors that promote gallstone formation include which of the following:

  I. Gallbladder stasis

  II. Hemolytic anemia

  III. Multiple organ dysfunction syndrome

  IV. Pregnancy

    A. I and III

    B. II only

C. I, III, and IV

D. I, II, and IV

Directions: There are three sets of response options for the following scenario. You will be required to select one best answer from each question set.

6. A 75-year-old woman presents to the emergency department complaining of low abdominal pain radiating to her back. The pain began suddenly, was followed by one episode of vomiting, and has persisted for several hours. Past medical history includes hypertension, diabetes, and glaucoma. She had a hysterectomy 20 years earlier for fibroids. On physical examination, she is afebrile; vital signs are blood pressure of 102/88 mm Hg, and heart rate 98 beats/minute. She has right lower quadrant tenderness and mild guarding without rebound. No pulsatile mass is appreciated. Urinalysis is positive for microscopic blood.

6.1. Which statement is most correct?

A. The patient does not have an abdominal aortic aneurysm because the physical examination rules out a pulsatile mass.

B. The patient may be in early shock and should receive a large-bore intravenous catheter and fluids.

C. A urinalysis revealing hematuria rules out an aneurysm and appendicitis, making the most likely diagnosis a ureteral stone.

D. Basic laboratory studies and an ultrasound examination should be ordered.

E. Basic laboratory studies and a noncontrast ("renal") computed tomography (CT) should be ordered.

6.2. Her blood pressure suddenly drops to 65/40 mm Hg, her legs become cool, and her femoral pulses cannot be palpated. Which of the following assumptions is correct?

A. She should be intubated for airway control.

B. Immediate surgical consultation is required.

C. Uncrossmatched blood should be administered intravenously.

D. She is most likely suffering from a ruptured abdominal aortic aneurysm.

E. All of the above.

6.3. Assume instead that the patient in question 6 has a white blood cell count of 10,000/μL with a normal differential and an ultrasound examination that demonstrates no aortic aneurysm and no appendix visualized. Which statement about the patient is true?

A. The patient does not have appendicitis. She is afebrile, has a normal white blood cell count, and no appendicitis is seen on ultrasound examination.

B. Appendicitis should be ruled out with a contrast computed tomography (CT) of the abdomen.

C. The patient can be safely discharged with close follow-up.

D. The patient should be admitted for observation to the medical service with the diagnosis of undifferentiated abdominal pain.

E. The patient should be admitted for observation to the surgical service for serial abdominal examinations.

Answers and Explanations

1. D. In the *classic* case of diverticulitis, a patient will present with left lower quadrant abdominal pain, mild fever, and a white blood cell count greater than 10,000/μL. There is, of course, wide variation in presenting symptoms. Although diverticulitis causes left lower quadrant abdominal pain, in most cases, inflamed sigmoid colon may lie outside the left lower quadrant. Some individuals, especially those of East Asian ancestry, may develop symptomatic diverticula in the ascending colon. The presence and degree of fever and leukocytosis will depend on the severity of diverticulitis. Hematochezia is possible. Fecal occult blood is present in approximately 50% of cases. Frank rectal bleeding is rare.

2. B. Diverticulitis is localized inflammation secondary to microperforation of obstructed colonic diverticula. Diverticula become obstructed when food occludes its narrow opening into the colon lumen. Bacterial overgrowth and mucus secretion continues in this closed space, leading to increased wall pressures, decreased venous outflow, and necrosis. Microperforation occurs, and the symptoms of diverticulitis are caused by the ensuing inflammatory response. Seeds may be deposited in the diverticula but do not cause diverticula.

3. B. In a thin individual, an ultrasound examination may be used to diagnose appendicitis. It is technically difficult to find the appendix in many patients and is not the test of choice for acute appendicitis. Plain radiographs are frequently normal but rarely helpful in making the diagnosis of acute appendicitis. The finding of an appendicolith is a rare but highly specific finding in cases of acute appendicitis. Plain radiographs may help to rule out other significant causes of abdominal pain including bowel obstruction and perforated viscous. However, routine use of abdominal radiographs to determine the presence of appendicolith is not cost-effective. Oral contrast significantly enhances the bowel and hence the sensitivity of CT for appendicitis. Pericecal inflammation of fat is suggestive of appendicitis but is not diagnostic or pathognomonic of the entity.

4. C. Abdominal ultrasonography is the preferred radiographic study for patients with presumed cholecystitis and cholelithiasis. Hepatobiliary iminodiacetic acid (HIDA) scan has sensitivity and specificity rates approaching that of an ultrasound examination. However, the test is more expensive, involves ionizing radiation, and takes more time. Gallstones are rarely radiopaque. Hence plain abdominal x-ray films are rarely helpful at establishing the diagnosis An abdominal computed tomography (CT) scan is not as sensitive as an ultrasound examination for cholecystitis.

5. D. Gallstone formation is promoted by stasis leading to stone deposition from supersaturated bile and increased pigment production from hemoglobin breakdown products (as present in hemolytic anemia). Pregnancy increases the estrogen level in the blood, which promotes stone formation. The multiple organ dysfunction syndrome frequently results in bile stasis because of decreased gallbladder contractions, leading to inflammation of the gallbladder mucosa and bacterial

seeding of the gallbladder. Although stasis may be present, multiple organ dysfunction syndrome is more frequently associated with acalculous cholecystitis

6.1. B. A patient who is usually hypertensive may have relative hypotension, that is, although her blood pressure is greater than 100 mm Hg systolic, if her usual pressure is 140 mm Hg systolic or greater, she is actually hypotensive. A heart rate in an afebrile individual resting in a stretcher should not be in the 90 beats/minute range, which constitutes tachycardia. The patient may be entering early shock. Although a pulsatile mass on physical examination is suggestive of an aortic aneurysm, it is not always appreciated on physical examination. The ureter may be irritated by an aneurysm or the inflammation of appendicitis and cause microscopic hematuria. Therefore, urinalysis is not the most appropriate diagnostic procedure. The physical examination suggests an intraabdominal process; thus, a contrast computed tomography (CT) should be performed to look for appendicitis. An ultrasound examination is not as sensitive as CT for detecting appendicitis.

6.2. E. The clinical presentation, along with the suddenness of her decline, loss of distal pulses, and severe drop in pressure suggest shock resulting from volume loss, in this case blood loss from a ruptured abdominal aortic aneurysm. She must be emergently intubated and resuscitated with blood. A stat surgical consult is required for emergent operative intervention.

6.3. B. The elderly are particularly difficult to diagnose when presenting with abdominal pain. They do not necessarily have fever or elevated white blood cell counts nor do they always have focal guarding or rebound when presenting with surgical disease. In addition, the abdominal examination in the elderly is unreliable for surgical disease, and the most appropriate action is an emergent computed tomography (CT) of the abdomen, which could be performed after the patient reaches the ward or before that, providing there is minimal delay in either case. Although the ultrasound examination in experienced hands is quite sensitive for appendicitis, in general it is less reliable than CT. In addition, if the report does not specify that a normal appendix has been visualized, then appendicitis cannot be ruled out by that ultrasound examination. Discharging the patient home would be unsafe, given the answers provided previously. Serious abdominal pathology, including appendicitis, has not been ruled out. Admission to either an inpatient medical or surgical service, without the abdominal CT puts the patient at risk of increased morbidity. Diagnosing surgical illness in the elderly, by physical examination alone, is unreliable, and the patient could suffer a serious delay in diagnosis.

Vomiting

Everything is gratuitous ...When you suddenly realize it, it makes you feel sick ... that's nausea.

Jean Paul Sartre

INTRODUCTION
David A. Peak, MD
Section Editor

Vomiting or emesis is a complex activity with a broad range of causes. It is characterized by contraction of the abdominal muscles, descent of the diaphragm, and opening of the gastric cardia resulting in expulsion of stomach contents out of the mouth. Vomiting requires a cascade of efferent impulses to the respiratory, vasomotor, and salivary centers; cranial nerves VIII and X; abdominal muscles; diaphragm; stomach; and esophagus. Vomiting should be considered separately from nausea, retching, and reflux. Nausea is a subjective urge to vomit without a clear physical mechanism that may be associated with flushing and tachycardia. Retching involves spasmodic contractions of the diaphragm, thoracic, and abdominal musculature without the expulsion of gastric contents. Reflux involves transient relaxation of the lower esophageal sphincter, which allows stomach contents to effortlessly reenter the esophagus without musculature contraction.

Vomiting occurs after stimulation of the vomiting center. The vomiting center is a physiological rather than an anatomic entity, consisting of intertwined neural networks in the nucleus tractus solitarii of the medulla oblongata near the respiratory center. The vomiting center receives stimuli from the chemoreceptor trigger zone, the brain cortex, vestibular apparatus, and vagal and visceral nerves. Emetogenic substances from both the blood and cerebrospinal fluid (i.e., drugs, toxins, biochemical disorders) are mediated via the chemoreceptor trigger zone located in the area postrema on the floor of the fourth ventricle by dopamine-2 (D_2) neurotransmitters. Vomiting impulses from psychological stress (including anticipatory and learned vomiting), elevated intracranial pressure, or central nervous system tumors and infections are sent to the vomiting center through the cerebral cortex and limbic system via histamine-1 (H_1) neurotransmitters. Vomiting signals related to motion travels through the vestibular or vestibulocerebellar system to the vomiting center via muscarinic, cholinergic, and H_1 neurotransmitters. Finally, the vagal and visceral nerves send signals via H_1 neurotransmitters related to gastrointestinal irritation, delayed gastric emptying, or visceral distention or inflammation. Ongoing research focusing on the complex interaction between neurotransmitters (dopamine, opiate, histamine, acetylcholine, neurokinin 1, and serotonin) and receptors in the central and peripheral nervous systems has led to advances in prevention and treatment of emesis. Severe nausea and vomiting can result in dehydration, metabolic disturbances (metabolic alkalosis, hyponatremia, hypochloremia, hypokalemia), aspiration pneumonia, malnutrition, and esophageal injury and may have a substantial negative impact on quality of life, survival, and health care costs. Severe nausea and vomiting are among the most unpleasant of complaints even in patients with painful or debilitating diseases. Vomiting may be so distressing that patients may be unable to work, care for themselves, or take prescribed medications, and may lead patients to refuse treatments such as further cycles of chemotherapy for life-threatening malignancies. Even mild nausea and vomiting may have late sequelae, such as anticipatory vomiting—vomiting in anticipation of, or during, a recurrent noxious event, such as chemotherapy.

Vomiting may be a chief complaint or an associated symptom with a wide spectrum of pathologies including toxic-metabolic, gastrointestinal, neurological, psychological, and any disease or procedure that causes pain. A complete list of etiologies is beyond the scope of this section. The type of vomiting may present signs of a true emergency. Bloody emesis may require hemodynamic stabilization, and treatment before diagnostic intervention. Bilious vomiting suggests an obstruction or motility disorder distal to the ligament of Treitz and may signify a surgical emergency.

In the emergency department (ED), a patient with profound vomiting usually requires symptomatic and supportive therapy, simultaneously with, or before, determining the source of the stimulation of the vomiting center. Evidence suggests that prophylactic preventive therapy for vomiting is much more efficacious than treatment of ongoing symptoms. This is an additional consideration for the emergency physician who may need to use a medication or procedure that may induce vomiting. This section explores several pathological processes that lead to vomiting and the clinical approach to their diagnosis and treatment.

20

Gastrointestinal Bleeding

David A. Peak, MD, Diane B. Heller, MD, JD

Clinical Scenario

A 42-year-old man presents to the emergency department (ED) complaining of nausea, vomiting, and general malaise. He reports that he has not felt well for several weeks and that he began to have intermittent nausea and abdominal pain approximately 3 weeks ago. Shortly after, he noticed he had become more tired than usual. He reports feeling weak, which is much more profound when he exerts himself. Yesterday, he vomited blood three times.

His past medical history is remarkable for hepatitis, chronic low back pain from a prior motor vehicle accident, and alcohol abuse, although he states that he has not had a drink in almost a year.

He does not take any prescription medications, but he takes a lot of ibuprofen and aspirin for his back pain, and he has been using antacids for his nausea. He has no known drug allergies.

On physical examination, he is a pale, thin man who looks uncomfortable but is in no acute distress. Vital signs include temperature of 98.2°F, pulse of 104 beats/minute, blood pressure of 108/58 mm Hg, and respiratory rate of 20 breaths/minute with oxygen saturation of 97% on room air. He has dry mucous membranes, and his conjunctiva are pale. His lungs are clear to auscultation bilaterally, and the cardiac examination reveals tachycardia and normal rhythm, with no murmurs, rubs, or gallops. The abdomen is soft and nondistended, with normal bowel sounds and mild tenderness in the epigastric area. There is no rebound or guarding. Rectal examination is nontender with heme-positive black stool, no gross blood, no hemorrhoids or fissures, and a normal prostate. Skin examination shows multiple telangiectasias but no jaundice.

The patient is placed on a cardiac monitor with continuous blood pressure monitoring while two large-bore intravenous (IV) catheters are placed. Blood is sent for type and screen, complete blood count (CBC), and electrolytes. An upright chest x-ray film reveals no free air. A nasogastric tube is placed, and 250 mL of coffee-ground appearing stomach contents are aspirated. The stomach is lavaged with 500 mL of water, and the coffee-ground material clears. The patient's hematocrit is 29 mL/dL, a drop of five points since last recorded a few months before.

The patient is admitted to the floor for observation. His hematocrit remains stable. Upper endoscopy the next day reveals several areas of denuded epithelium of the gastric mucosa consistent with gastritis. No further bleeding is observed. He is discharged with close follow-up on acid-reducing medication, and is told to stop using nonsteroidal antiinflammatory medications and aspirin.

Clinical Evaluation

Introduction

Gastrointestinal (GI) bleeding may vary from life-threatening hemorrhage to subtle insidious bleeding that results only in anemia. Most GI bleeding is from an upper GI source. The annual incidence of upper GI bleeding is approximately 100 per 100,000, five times higher than the incidence of lower GI bleeding. The mortality from an acute upper GI bleed is between 8% and 10%. Although up to 80% of all GI bleeding stops spontaneously, every patient with a GI bleed must be treated as having a potentially life-threatening emergency until proven otherwise. Rapid assessment and resuscitation are the focus of care, with attempts to ensure hemodynamic stability before proceeding with definitive diagnosis and therapy.

History

The history of the present illness is crucial to diagnosis and treatment. If the patient has abdominal pain, the location, duration, and nature of the pain should be elicited. With gastritis or peptic ulcers, the patient will often describe an epigastric pain that is burning or gnawing and may radiate to the back. It is important to elicit any factors that alleviate or exacerbate the pain. With ulcer pain, the patient may report temporary relief with meals but an increase in the intensity of the pain several hours later. The patient may also describe postprandial bloating, distension, or nausea without abdominal pain.

If the patient has reported vomiting, the frequency of the vomiting and the appearance of the emesis should be elicited. The frequency of vomiting and the patient's ability to keep food and liquid down are important clues to whether the patient will be dehydrated. The appearance of the emesis is important to determine whether there is GI bleeding, and it can be a clue to the etiology of the bleeding. If the patient describes bright red blood in the emesis, as in the clinical scenario, the bleed is more likely to be brisk (e.g., an actively bleeding ulcer) or very proximal (e.g., a Mallory-Weiss tear or bleeding esophageal varices). If the patient describes a coffee-ground appearance to the emesis, the blood has been digested by gastric enzymes, changing its appearance to black. This is consistent with a past bleed.

Similarly, the appearance of the patient's stool can provide information about the source of bleeding. Melena, which is dark, tarry, malodorous stool, generally signifies an upper GI source or a very slow bleed in the right colon because it indicates that blood has had a significant amount of time to be degraded within the GI tract. In contrast, bright red blood from the rectum, also known as hematochezia, usually indicates a lower GI source. When hematochezia is a result of an upper GI bleed, it is likely to be a massive hemorrhage. There are confounding factors, however, when evaluating a patient's description of stool. Many substances that are ingested may alter the appearance of stool to mimic the presence of blood. For example, ingestion of iron supplements and bismuth-containing products can result in black stools, and the ingestion of certain foods such as beets can cause stool to turn red.

A variety of factors may make a patient more susceptible to GI bleeding. The use of nonsteroidal antiinflammatory agents and corticosteroids has been linked to increased frequency of GI bleeding. (You will recall that the patient in the clinical scenario had been taking a lot of aspirin and ibuprofen for his back pain.) Anticoagulants, such as warfarin (Coumadin), can also increase the likelihood of a GI bleed. You must inquire about a patient's history of alcohol and tobacco use, because each has been linked to an increased incidence of GI bleeding. In particular, a history of heavy alcohol use and cirrhosis should alert you to the potential presence of esophageal varices, a dangerous source of upper GI bleeding.

General questions about the way a patient feels can also provide valuable information. If a patient reports feeling weak and dizzy, it is more likely that the bleeding has progressed to the point of causing anemia or hypovolemia. Severe anemia can cause shortness of breath, chest pain, and even cardiac ischemia; thus, it is crucial to pursue this line of questioning, regardless of the age of the patient.

Physical Examination

As with any patient in the ED, it is important to pay close attention to the vital signs, which reflect the hemodynamic stability and may provide a clue to the degree of blood loss experienced by the patient.

The body may compensate for up to a 10% loss of blood volume with no alteration in vital signs. Between 10% and 20% total body blood loss, the heart rate may be elevated, and the patient may experience a drop in blood pressure or increase in heart rate when standing from a recumbent position. These postural changes in vital signs are known as orthostatic hypotension. It is often not until the patient loses greater than 20% of his or her blood volume that true hypotension will be present.

Several other physical findings may indicate blood loss. Pale skin and/or pale conjunctivae are an indication of anemia or blood loss. Extremities may be cool and capillary refill may be slow. Similarly, a patient may show signs of dehydration, such as dry mucous membranes and chapped lips, if there has been significant blood loss. Patients with underlying liver disease (a clue for concern about the presence of esophageal varices) often have telangiectasias, otherwise known as spider angiomas, and multiple bruises resulting from coagulopathy. They may also exhibit jaundice, scleral icterus, or palmar erythema.

Physical findings can vary greatly among patients with GI bleeding. Many patients with upper GI bleeding will experience epigastric tenderness, although it is not a universal finding. Severe tenderness with signs of peritoneal irritation such as rebound and guarding should raise suspicion for a perforated ulcer.

Another very important aspect of the physical examination is the rectal examination. Visual and tactile examination can identify hemorrhoids or anal fissures that are a potential source of bleeding. A stool sample should be obtained and examined for blood, either gross or occult. To look for occult blood, keep a sample of the stool for a heme test (Guaiac or Hemoccult test). If bright red blood is identified, an examination should be performed with an anoscope to look for internal sources of bleeding such as internal hemorrhoids or anal fissures.

Diagnostic Evaluation

The initial workup may proceed while therapy is being initiated and resuscitation is begun. A blood sample for type and cross should be sent to the blood bank in case transfusion of red cells or other blood products becomes necessary, and a CBC should be sent to obtain a baseline hematocrit. If the bleed is acute, however, the hematocrit will not show immediate changes because hematocrit is expressed in terms of red blood cell volume as a percent of total blood volume. It is not until the blood volume has been restored, either by the body's own repletion or by fluid resuscitation in the ED, that the hematocrit will accurately reflect blood loss. Therefore, serial hematocrits are more useful than a single data point. A platelet count is necessary to evaluate a patient's coagulation status and determine the need for platelet transfusion. A prothrombin time and partial thromboplastin time are also necessary to evaluate for a potential coagulopathy and serve as a clue to underlying liver disease because clotting factors are manufactured by the liver. This information may alter your resuscitative efforts as you evaluate the need for fresh frozen plasma to replace clotting factors.

An electrolyte panel may be helpful in select cases. Patients who have been repeatedly vomiting may demonstrate hypokalemia, hyponatremia, and metabolic alkalosis. A significant hemorrhage may result in a metabolic acidosis, either because of hypovolemia or because of the accumulation of lactic acid if the patient is in shock. Blood urea nitrogen (BUN) may be elevated because of hypovolemia and/or the resorption of blood from the GI tract. Liver function tests and serum amylase may be indicated because the differential diagnosis of epigastric pain and vomiting includes pancreatitis, hepatitis, and biliary disease. However, these diseases do not independently cause GI bleeding. Be aware that liver function tests may be chronically elevated with hepatitis or cirrhosis.

A stool heme test (placing a small amount of stool on a specially prepared card and adding developer) should be performed. A color change to blue indicates a positive test for occult blood in the stool. A positive test for occult blood requires only 20 mL/dL of blood in the stool. The test may be falsely positive after the ingestion of substances such as rare red meat, chlorophyll, iodide, and bromide. The test may be falsely negative after the ingestion of magnesium or ascorbic acid. You should also remember that a positive test is not necessarily an indication of active bleeding because the test may remain positive for up to 14 days after an episode of bleeding.

Upright posteroanterior (PA, or anteroposterior [AP] if portable) and lateral chest x-ray films are usually performed to look for free air under the diaphragm as evidence of perforation of a hollow viscus, such as the stomach in the case of a perforated peptic ulcer. Although perforation is a rare finding in a patient who presents with GI bleeding, it is an operative emergency and requires the immediate involvement of a surgical consultation.

An electrocardiogram (ECG) should be performed on all patients at risk for coronary artery disease, those with severe anemia, and any patient who has cardiac complaints such as chest pain or shortness of breath. Cardiac ischemia or injury may result from GI bleeding secondary to low blood flow or decreased oxygen delivery to the heart and may manifest as ECG changes.

An important diagnostic maneuver to identify an upper GI source of bleeding is the placement of a nasogastric tube. Gastric contents should be aspirated and inspected. The test is considered positive if the aspirate contains more than 10 mL of gross blood, more than 30 mL of pink fluid with greater than 25% visible blood, or more than 30 mL of dark fluid that is heme positive for occult blood. Nasal trauma with epistaxis may confuse a positive result, and a negative test does not exclude the possibility of an upper GI source of bleeding because bleeding may be intermittent. It is also possible that the source of bleeding is duodenal and that pyloric edema or spasm has prevented passage of blood from the duodenum into the stomach. If bright red blood is identified on aspiration, gentle nasogastric lavage with normal saline should be performed until the gastric contents are clear. Ice water should not be used because it alters the coagulation

function and can contribute to hypothermia. Active bleeding will fail to clear with lavage. However, it should be noted that large blood clots might cause the lavage to continue to return pink fluid, giving the false impression of ongoing bleeding.

In most cases, the gastroenterologist undertakes further diagnostic workup. The most common diagnostic modalities are endoscopy and colonoscopy, both of which can be used as therapeutic modalities. In less common situations, angiography, radionucleotide imaging, or other procedures may be undertaken to identify the patient's source of bleeding.

Differential Diagnosis

The differential diagnosis for GI bleeding is illustrated in Table 20.1.

Table 20.1.

Differential diagnosis for gastrointestinal (GI) bleeding

Upper GI Conditions
Duodenal ulcer
Gastric ulcer
Esophagitis
Gastritis
Mallory-Weiss tear
Esophageal varices
Arterial-venous (AV) malformation
Boerhaave's syndrome
Caustic ingestion
ENT causes (e.g., epistaxis [swallowed blood])

Lower GI Conditions
Hemorrhoids
Anal fissures
Diverticulosis
Ischemic bowel
Inflammatory bowel (colitis)
Meckel's diverticulum
Intussusception

Upper or Lower GI Conditions
Neoplasm
Vascular anomalies (angiodysplasia, AV malformations)
Vasculitis
Epistaxis

Treatment

Patients with GI bleeding may present a clinical spectrum ranging from stable to critically ill. The patient's hemodynamic stability and response to initial resuscitative efforts will guide initial treatment (Tables 20.2 and 20.3). Airway management may be an issue if the patient is persistently vomiting blood and cannot protect the airway, necessitating intubation.

The patient should be placed on oxygen and a monitor and, ideally, two large-bore IV catheters should be placed, with a normal saline infusion started. Fluid boluses of 10 to 20 mL/kg should be given in rapid succession to a hypotensive patient, and the patient should be continually reassessed. In unstable patients with persistent hypotension or tachycardia, a Foley catheter should be placed to monitor urine output. An adult should produce approximately 0.5 mL urine per kilogram of body weight per hour. Failure to meet this minimum urine output is a sign of persistent hypovolemia or renal failure. If the patient remains tachycardic or hypotensive after 40 to 60 mL/kg of normal saline have been infused, transfusion of blood should begin. In the unstable patient,

---

Table 20.2.

Treatment guidelines for gastrointestinal (GI) bleeding

Stable Patient
Check HCT level
Rectal examination
Consider NG tube if upper GI bleeding suspected
No evidence of active bleeding and stable HCT: discharge with follow-up
Evidence of active bleeding: admit for observation ± inpatient endoscopy

Unstable Patient
Two large-bore IV catheters, minimum 18 gauge
Supplemental O_2
Continuous cardiac monitor
Continuous pulse oximetry
NG tube
Consultation with gastroenterologist for emergent endoscopy/colonoscopy
Consultation with general surgery if lower GI source suspected with persistent bleeding that may require emergent colectomy
Bolus of 10–20 mL/kg normal saline IV, repeat for persistent hypotension and tachycardia
Cross-matched packed red blood cells (RBCs) for shock despite 40 mL/kg normal saline
Un-cross-matched packed RBCs for precipitously falling blood pressure or pressure not responding at all to IV fluids
Consideration of intubation for persistent shock state

Patient with Suspected Peptic Ulcer
H_2-blocker (e.g., cimetidine, ranitidine)
Proton pump inhibitor (e.g., omeprazole, pantoprazole)

Patient with Esophageal Varices
IV vasopressin or IV octreotide
IV propranolol for portal hypertension

H_2, histamine-2; HCT, hematocrit; IV, intravenous; NG, nasogastric.

Table 20.3.

Treatment options for patients with gastrointestinal (GI) bleeding

Treatment Option	Treatment Goal	Comment
Antacids	Neutralize gastric acid	Will not change morbidity or mortality from GI bleeding but may provide symptomatic relief for gastritis/ulcer disease
H_2 blockers	Inhibit acid secretion by blocking H_2 receptors in parietal cells of the stomach	Recommended for suspected or proven ulcer disease; proven to improve healing but no clear proof of decreased morbidity or mortality from acute GI bleeding
Proton pump inhibitors	Block H^+-K^+-ATPase pump, which is the terminal step in acid secretion in the stomach	Recommended for suspected or proven ulcer disease; proven to improve healing but no clear proof of decreased morbidity or mortality from acute GI bleeding
Vasopressin	Induces splanchnic artery vaso-constriction, therefore de-creasing splanchnic blood flow and portal pressure	Recommended for acute GI bleeding in patients with known or suspected esophageal varices; proven to decrease morbidity and mortality but has systemic vasoconstrictive effects as well
Octreotide	Induces splanchnic vasoconstric-tion, therefore decreasing splanchnic blood flow and portal pressure	Recommended for acute GI bleeding in patients with known or suspected esophageal varices; proven to decrease morbidity and mortality; benefit over vasopressin is increased selectivity for splanchnic circulation
IV fluids	Provides volume for treatment of hypotension	Recommended for all patients with GI bleeding even if not yet hypotensive
Blood	Treats anemia or hypotension	Recommended for patients whose hypotension is not responsive to 50–60 mL/kg IV fluids; also recommended for anemia at the discretion of the treating physician (as a rough guideline, HCT <30 mL/dL in elderly patients or patients with cardiac disease and HCT <20 mL/dL in young healthy patients
FFP	Corrects coagulopathy caused by decreased or altered produc-tion of clotting factors	Recommended for actively bleeding patients with elevated PT/PTT
Platelets	Corrects coagulopathy caused by thrombocytopenia	Recommended for actively bleeding patients with thrombocytopenia (rough guideline platelet count <50,000/mm^3)
Endoscopy	Vehicle for cautery, ligation, or sclerotherapy of actively bleed-ing vessels or banding of varices with potential to bleed; also an important diagnostic tool	Recommended urgently for all hemodynamically unstable patients with GI bleeding and nonurgently for stable patients; proven reduction in morbidity and mortality

FFP, fresh frozen plasma; H_2, histamine-2; HCT, hematocrit; IV, intravenous; PT/PTT, prothrombin time/partial thromboplastin time.

uncrossmatched blood, which is more quickly available, may be given until typed and crossmatched blood becomes available. Packed red blood cells are used most often in place of whole blood because of the ease of availability. The results of coagulation studies will determine the need for transfusion of platelets or fresh frozen plasma to correct thrombocytopenia or coagulopathy.

In the unstable patient who is actively bleeding, coincident to the initiation of resuscitative measures, a gastroenterologist should be consulted. The gastroenterologist's armamentarium will include such measures as endoscopy and colonoscopy, which have the potential to be therapeutic and diagnostic. These scope procedures can identify bleeding sources through direct visualization and use cautery, ligation, sclerotherapy, and local injection of octreotide or vasopressin to attempt to control bleeding. The use of IV vasopressin or octreotide has been shown to reduce mortality from GI bleeding with esophageal varices. Both vasopressin and octreotide work by decreasing portal venous inflow and portal pressure because of increasing splanchnic arteriolar flow. This decrease in hepatic flow relieves pressure in the varices and decreases the risk of bleeding until a definitive procedure, such as banding the vessels, can be accomplished. In the small percentage of patients with bleeding and hemodynamic instability refractory to these measures, surgical consultation for emergency surgery may be required.

In the hemodynamically stable patient, diagnosis and comfort measures take precedence. However, monitoring must continue to ensure that the patient remains stable while under your care. Initial symptomatic relief of epigastric discomfort (from gastritis or peptic ulcer disease) is often achieved by the use of antacids. In the ED, this is often combined with a viscous lidocaine solution to provide immediate local relief. Patients who may be candidates for urgent or emergent endoscopy or surgery should not receive oral medications, because this may increase the risk of aspiration during the procedure. IV administration of medications may be preferred in this subgroup of patients and in patients who have nausea.

Patients are also often given histamine (H_2) blockers or proton pump inhibitors to decrease gastric acid secretion. Outpatient treatment with these medications provides symptomatic relief and ulcer healing but may not provide acute relief of symptoms. Furthermore, the data have not conclusively proven that either medication has a statistically significant impact on morbidity or mortality from GI bleeding. Treatment of *Helicobacter pylori* infection with antibiotics is usually not begun in the ED because rapid and reliable testing is not readily accessible in most EDs.

Disposition

Patients with GI bleeding need to be evaluated to determine whether they may be safely discharged from the ED and to determine the level of care necessary for those patients requiring hospital admission. Patients with a history of GI bleeding without findings on physical examination consistent with bleeding (heme-negative brown stool, normal hematocrit, negative nasogastric lavage) may be discharged if they are hemodynamically stable (not tachycardic or hypotensive and without postural changes in vital signs). Patients with a minor rectal source of bleeding identified on physical examination, such as anal fissure or hemorrhoids, can also be discharged if they are hemodynamically stable.

Patients with heme-positive brown stool or coffee-ground emesis may be discharged if they are hemodynamically stable and have a normal hematocrit. These patients will often be observed in the ED and perhaps have a second hematocrit sent to ensure their stability before discharge. Patients in this category must have close follow-up and be seen again by a physician for reevaluation within 1 to 2 days. They must also be given detailed discharge instructions regarding symptoms and signs that would necessitate immediate return to the ED, such as recurrent bleeding, dizziness, shortness of breath, or chest pain. Patients in this category with comorbid disease, such as coronary artery disease or risk factors for massive GI bleeding such as known esophageal varices or anticoagulation therapy, may be admitted for observation.

Patients who are hemodynamically stable but have evidence of recent significant bleeding should be admitted to a general medical floor for observation. However, several criteria have been identified with increased morbidity and mortality from GI bleeding. These factors include unstable vital signs, active, persistent bleeding, age older than 75 years, large drop in hematocrit in the ED (>8%), initial hematocrit below 20 mL/dL, and unstable comorbid disease. Patients with any of these factors should be considered for intensive care monitoring.

Pathophysiology

The three major arteries supplying the stomach and intestines are the celiac, the superior mesenteric, and the inferior mesenteric arteries. The celiac artery, which branches into the common hepatic and splenic arteries, supplies the stomach and the first part of the duodenum and a portion of the pancreas, liver, and spleen. The superior mesenteric artery supplies the remainder of the pancreas and duodenum and the jejunum, the ileum, and the proximal two thirds of the colon. The inferior mesenteric arteries supply the distal third of the colon and the proximal rectum. The distal rectum is supplied by the rectal arteries, which branch off the internal iliac arteries. Along the mesenteric border of the intestines, there are also multiple arterial and venous arcades, which give rise to the vasa recta that encircle and penetrate the muscular layer of the intestines. Each part of the GI tract also contains a vast microcirculation composed of capillaries, venules, and arterioles, which anastomose and supply the submucosal and mucosal layers.

GI bleeding is caused primarily by two general mechanisms. First, there may be damage to the mucosal layer, which allows exposure of deeper vessels to the luminal side of the GI tract. An example would be peptic ulcer disease in which erosion through the mucosa or submucosa damages microvasculature. Alternatively, there may be acute rupture of a vessel into the lumen as a result of extrinsic factors such as vascular pressure instead of factors within the GI lumen. An example of this mechanism is when an increase in portal pressure results in bleeding from esophageal varices in a cirrhotic patient.

Peptic ulcer disease, the most common cause of upper GI bleeding, results from an imbalance between protective and injurious mucosal factors. Gastric mucosa is constantly exposed to endogenous and exogenous insults. The surface cells in the stomach and proximal duodenum secrete mucus and bicarbonate to neutralize the pH in the highly acidic environment and provide the first line of defense for the mucosal surface. Another protective mechanism is the remarkable ability of the mucosal surface to regenerate within 15 to 30 minutes of incurring injury. Prostaglandins protect the mucosa by stimulating the production of mucus and bicarbonate and by enhancing local blood flow and cell turnover.

Interference with these protective mechanisms can predispose a patient to peptic ulcer disease. Nonsteroidal antiinflammatory medications interfere with the production of prostaglandins. Alcohol, cigarette smoking, and corticosteroids have been found to be injurious to mucosal protective factors. A very important development in the past 10 years has been the recognition that infection with *H. pylori* can be a causative agent of peptic ulcer disease. This finding has significantly altered the outpatient evaluation and treatment of peptic ulcer disease.

Cirrhosis and subsequent development of portal hypertension are also significant risk factors for GI bleeding. A cirrhotic liver leads to increased resistance to blood flow and portal hypertension. This increased pressure, in turn, gives rise to the development of collateral vessels between the portal and systemic systems to divert blood flow from the liver. In many patients, these collaterals form in the esophageal submucosa or mucosa, making them prone to rupture from the high wall tension exerted by elevated portal pressures.

Diverticulosis or vascular anomalies such as angiodysplasia most commonly cause lower GI bleeds. Diverticula are herniations through the mucosal and submucosal layers of the colon at a site of weakness in the muscular layer. This point of weakness is usually at the site of penetration of mesenteric arterioles, and erosion of the vessel results in bleeding into the colonic lumen. With angiodysplasia, submucosal veins become dilated and tortuous, creating small arteriovenous communications. Normal wall tension within the colon can overcome these degenerative lesions and predispose them to rupture and bleeding. Tumors, both malignant and benign, are also common causes of lower GI bleeding because they may perforate blood vessels if they erode through the intestinal wall.

Suggested Readings

Andreoli TE, Bennett JC, Carpenter CCJ, et al. eds. *Cecil essentials of medicine*, 4th ed. Philadelphia: WB Saunders, 1991:258– 262.

Corley DA, Cello JP, Koch J, et al. Early indications of prognosis in upper gastrointestinal hemorrhage. *Am J Gastroenterol* 1998;93: 890–896.

Gora-Harper ML, Balmer C, Castellano FC, et. al. ASHP (American Society of Health System Pharmacists) therapeutic guidelines on the pharmacological management of nausea and vomiting in adult and pediatric patients receiving chemotherapy or radiation therapy or undergoing surgery. *Am J Health Syst Pharm* 1999;56:729–764.

Graber MA, Nugent A. Peptic ulcer disease: presentation, treatment and prevention. *Emerg Med* 1999; 31:66–78.

Haubrich WS, Kalser MH, Roth JLA, et. al. eds. *Bockus Gastroenterology*, 5th ed. Philadelphia: WB Saunders, 1995:61–86.

Henderson J. *Gastrointestinal pathophysiology.* Philadelphia: Lippincott-Raven, 1996:31–52, 213–234.

Lichter I. Pain and palliative care. Nausea and vomiting in patients with cancer. *Hematol Oncol Clin North Am* 1996;10:207–220.

Maton PN. Omeprazole. *N Engl J Med* 1991;324: 965–975.

Murray KF, Christie DL. Vomiting. *Pediatr Rev* 1998;19:337–341.

CHAPTER 21

Bowel Obstruction

Christopher E. Kabrhel, MD

Clinical Scenario

A 68-year-old woman presents to the emergency department with vomiting and abdominal pain. The vomiting was initially of food and then became clear or green. It began the previous night following a bout of severe pain that lasted several minutes and then dissipated. She has had recurrent episodes of this pain, which she describes as crampy, diffuse, and spasmodic with episodes coming about every 5 to 10 minutes and lasting 1 to 2 minutes. She also notes increased bowel sounds (borborygmi) and an episode of hiccups. Her last normal bowel movement was 2 days ago. She has not passed any stool or flatus in the past 12 hours. She has not noted any melena, fevers, diarrhea, or dysuria.

Past medical history is notable for hypothyroidism and type II diabetes that is controlled with diet alone. Past surgical history is notable for a total abdominal hysterectomy 5 years ago and an open cholecystectomy 20 years ago. She takes L-thyroxine, estrogen, and calcium supplements. She has no allergies and is a nonsmoker.

Physical examination reveals a middle-aged woman, sweating and in moderate distress. During the history, she experiences abdominal pain, and she grimaces and tightens her abdominal musculature. This lasts 2 minutes and then resolves over 30 seconds. Her vital signs are as follows: temperature 98.8°F, blood pressure 121/72 mm Hg, pulse 105 beats/minute, respiratory rate 18 breaths/minute, and oxygen saturation 98% on room air. The examination of the heart and lungs is normal. She has no costovertebral angle

tenderness. Her abdomen is mildly distended with a well-healed low transverse scar and a well-healed right subcostal scar. On auscultation, high-pitched musical bowel sounds are noted intermittently. Her abdomen is tender in the periumbilical region but she has no guarding, rebound, organomegaly, or masses. Rectal examination reveals normal tone and heme-negative brown stool. Pelvic examination shows postsurgical changes but is otherwise unremarkable.

The patient is placed on a cardiac monitor, and a 500-mL intravenous (IV) bolus of normal saline is started. nasogastric (NG) tube is placed, which removes normal stomach fluid and no blood. Chest radiographs are normal, but abdominal radiographs reveal multiple dilated loops of small bowel with air-fluid levels in a stepladder pattern on upright film. There is no gas filling the descending colon. Laboratory analysis reveals the following abnormal results: white blood count 13,700/mm^3, blood urea nitrogen 20 mg/dL, and creatinine 1.4 mg/dL. Serum amylase, lipase, bilirubin, and transaminase levels are normal. Urinalysis is normal.

The patient is admitted to the surgical service with the diagnosis of small bowel obstruction (SBO). Her symptoms resolve over 2 days in hospital, and she is discharged with regular followup.

Clinical Evaluation

Introduction

SBO is a disorder in which the small intestine fails to allow for regular passage of food and bowel contents. It is a common but serious problem. Patients with SBO make up approximately 20% of all hospital admissions for patients with abdominal complaints resulting in 300,000 operations annually. Surgical therapy for bowel obstruction was described as early as 350 BC when Praxagoras created a therapeutic enterocutaneous fistula. Despite this long history, the mortality of SBO was still 60% at the turn of the 20th century. This began to change in 1912, when Hartwell and Hoguet discovered that saline therapy prolonged the lives of experimental dogs. In addition, NG tube decompression and antibiotic therapy were advocated for cases of SBO. With such advances in diagnosis and surgical therapy, current mortality of this problem in the United States is down to approximately 3% to 5%.

History

Symptoms of SBO generally include recurrent spasms of poorly localized, crampy abdominal pain lasting from seconds to minutes. Waves of pain may rise and fall every 3 to 10 minutes depending on whether the obstruction is proximal or distal. With proximal obstruction, severe pain with bilious vomiting tends to bring patients to presentation within several hours. In these patients, abdominal distention is generally mild. With distal obstruction, vomitus may be feculent (orange-brown and malodorous), but pain and vomiting are generally less severe. This may delay presentation for a couple of days until distention becomes more pronounced. Obstipation, the inability to pass stool or flatus, is common in cases of complete obstruction, but only after bowel contents distal to the site of obstruction have passed.

The symptoms of adynamic ileus are slightly different. Distention is present but colicky waves of pain are absent. Patients generally note more constant discomfort from distention. Vomiting is common but is rarely profuse and is never feculent. Obstipation may be present.

If the patient's pain changes in character from spasmodic and diffuse to constant and focal, complications such as strangulation, ischemia, infarction, or perforation must be suspected.

A patient with an obstructing lesion may note more insidious symptoms such as a change in the character and quality of bowel movements or constitutional symptoms.

Physical Examination

The physical examination should begin with an assessment of the patient's distress and the circumstances, timing, and severity of the patient's pain. Early in SBO, vital signs are normal and the patient is afebrile. In time, however, pain, hypovolemia, and peritonitis lead to tachycardia and low-grade fever. Hydration status should be assessed, taking note of dry mucous membranes, poor urine output, and decreased skin turgor as evidence of hypovolemia.

Examination of the abdomen begins with inspection. Distention is the hallmark finding of obstruction. Patients with distal obstructions are typically more distended than those with proximal obstructions. The presence of surgical scars should also be noted. Borborygmi and hiccups (singultus) may be audible. Auscultation may reveal high-pitched musical sounds or "tinkles" with occasional "rushes." Percussion may elicit tympani. Diffuse tenderness to palpation is common, but focal tenderness, guarding, rebound tenderness, or the presence of a tender mass must alert the clinician to the presence of strangulation. It is notable, however, that various studies have shown that distinguishing strangulated from nonstrangulated obstructions is difficult even for experienced clinicians. Finally, a rectal examination should be performed to search for luminal masses and to document the presence or absence of stool in the vault. Blood in the stool is rare.

Diagnostic Evaluation

Laboratory test results are nonspecific, and no single test can reliably diagnose obstruction or distinguish strangulated from nonstrangulated bowel. Nonetheless, a complete blood count should be obtained and serum electrolytes should be measured. Leukocytosis with left shift is commonly present, but

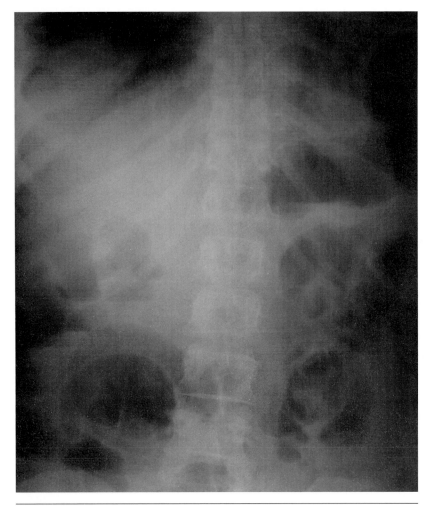

Figure 21.1
The upright abdominal x-ray film that shows air-fluid levels is demonstrating air trapped in the small bowel resulting from a distal point of obstruction. Mechanical obstruction (i.e., tumors, etc.) are most commonly found in large bowel obstruction, whereas adhesions are the number one cause for small bowel obstruction. It is standard of care to place a patient on continuous nasogastric (NG) suction to decompress the air-filled bowel and to remove the steady normal secretion of gastric fluid into the stomach.

a white blood cell count of 20,000/mm^3 or greater should alert the emergency physician to the possibility of gangrene or peritonitis. Hypovolemia may be reflected in an elevated hemoglobin and hematocrit. The blood urea nitrogen and serum creatinine will also rise with volume depletion, as seen in the clinical scenario. Electrolytes are generally normal until late in the course, but vomiting and volume loss can cause severe metabolic derangement, especially hypokalemia.

Sending preoperative lab specimens, such as a blood bank sample or prothrombin time and partial thromboplastin time, may also be indicated.

The first radiographical studies that should be ordered are supine and upright abdominal plain x-ray films, along with an upright chest radiograph. Plain x-ray films demonstrate the obstruction in 50% to 60% of cases, are suggestive in 20% to 30%, and are normal or misleading in the remainder.

Although useful for making the diagnosis, plain x-ray films rarely clarify the cause of the obstruction and are not helpful in diagnosing strangulated bowel.

In evaluating abdominal plain x-ray films for SBO, one must first identify the structures being imaged. Small bowel can be distinguished from large bowel by its smaller diameter, more central location, and its valvulae conniventes (linear densities that occupy the entire transverse diameter of the bowel image). In contrast, the large bowel is of greater diameter; lies peripherally; and has haustral markings, which are blunt, short densities occupying only part of the transverse diameter of the bowel image.

The typical plain x-ray film of an SBO shows dilated loops of small bowel with a large amount of gas proximal to the obstruction (Fig. 21.1). The number of dilated loops increases with more distal obstruction. There is generally minimal or no gas in the colon. On supine film these dilated loops of bowel may be arranged in a row or in a "stepladder" pattern. The upright or decubitus film is taken to demonstrate gas-fluid levels within the dilated loops of bowel. However, this finding may be absent when there is more liquid than gas in the bowel. In this case, gas may be trapped between the valvulae conniventes of the small bowel, resulting in the pathognomonic "string of pearls sign," an oblique series of radiolucencies on the upright x-ray film. A sentinel loop of U-shaped bowel whose lumen is thick and edematous is called the "coffee bean sign," and a fluid-filled loop resembling a mass is called the "pseudotumor sign." Both of these are rarely seen but can be diagnostic of a closed loop obstruction. If plain x-ray films indicate SBO, no other confirmatory examinations are necessary.

The most frequent diagnostic challenge is to distinguish SBO from paralytic ileus. In cases of adynamic ileus, gaseous distention is typically diffuse throughout the stomach, small intestine, and colon. Unfortunately, ileus is sometimes impossible to distinguish from mechanical obstruction based on plain x-ray films alone. When the diagnosis is in doubt, other imaging modalities may be required.

Computed tomography (CT) of the abdomen may be helpful in cases when standard radiographs are suggestive but not diagnostic. CT is also beneficial because it can clarify the cause of the obstruction. In fact, if CT shows the obstructed bowel but fails to demonstrate an obstructing lesion, adhesions are usually the culprit. Other modalities, such as ultrasonography and barium studies, also have been used effectively to diagnose SBO; however, these have been largely supplanted by CT scanning. It is worth mentioning that although barium by mouth is safe in the setting of SBO, it should never be given if large bowel obstruction is suspected because it can become inspissated in the colonic lumen as water is absorbed.

Differential Diagnosis

The differential diagnosis for SBO is illustrated in Table 21.1.

Treatment

Emergency department management must always begin with assessment of the stability of the patient and appropriate resuscitation. Management of SBO consists of aggressive fluid replacement, bowel decompression (with a NG tube placed to low suction), broad-spectrum antibiotics, and surgical consultation (Table 21.2). Operative planning depends on the severity of the fluid and electrolyte abnormalities, the opportunity to correct these abnormalities, and the risk of strangulation. If there are minimal metabolic disturbances and few comorbidities,

Table 21.1.

Differential diagnosis of bowel obstruction

Mechanical small bowel obstruction
Adynamic (paralytic) ileus
Large bowel obstruction
Spastic (dynamic) ileus–rare
Colonic pseudo-obstruction–rare
Acute gastroenteritis
Acute hemorrhagic pancreatitis
Acute mesenteric ischemia

Table 21.2.

Treatment guidelines for bowel obstruction

IV access and aggressive normal saline
  resuscitation
Blood draw for CBC and electrolytes
NG tube to low suction
Consideration of IV antibiotics
Surgical consultation
Operating room if emergent decompression
  required
Admission to floor for stable partial or complete
  obstruction without evidence of bowel
  strangulation/ischemia

CBC, complete blood count; IV, intravenous;
NG, nasogastric.

operative therapy can be undertaken immediately. If metabolic disturbances are more
severe, the patient may benefit from having
these corrected over several hours before
surgery. However, any patient with evidence
of strangulation, such as fever, tachycardia,
leukocytosis, localized abdominal tenderness, or radiographical evidence of necrosis
requires immediate surgery.

If the patient has none of the previously
mentioned findings, and strangulation is not
suspected, a trial of 1 to 2 days of conservative
management may be warranted. Studies have
shown that up to 75% of partial and 16% to
36% of complete obstructions will resolve
with nonoperative therapy alone. Early postoperative adhesive and Crohn's disease related
obstructions are most likely to respond to
conservative therapy, whereas obstruction resulting from intraluminal cancer or intussusception is better served with surgery. Most patients who respond to conservative therapy
will do so within 24 to 48 hours. There is
some evidence that patients with adhesive lesions treated nonoperatively may have a
higher incidence of recurrent obstructions;
however, most of these recurrences were also
amenable to nonoperative management.

Disposition

All patients with SBO should be admitted to
the hospital, usually to the general surgical
service. The plan for operative management
will depend on the condition of the patient
and the cause of the obstruction.

Pathophysiology

Bowel obstructions may be divided into two
general categories: mechanical obstructions
and nonmechanical obstructions. Nonmechanical obstruction, or adynamic ileus, is
the more common entity, and it is usually
self-limited. Mechanical obstruction, on the
other hand, frequently requires operative intervention. In the United States, the most
common cause of mechanical SBO is postoperative adhesions, causing 64% to 79% of
all cases. Hernias cause another 15%. Cancer
is the third most common cause, accounting
for 10% to 15% of cases. Rarely, intussusception, gallstones, inflammation, abscesses, or
bezoar may cause an SBO. Neoplasms usually cause large bowel obstructions, although
diverticulitis and sigmoid volvulus also can
be causative.

Nonmechanical obstruction, or paralytic
ileus, must also be considered in any patient
with obstructive symptoms. In this condition, bowel motility is decreased, leading to
circumstances mimicking obstruction. Ileus
can be caused by any peritoneal insult. Abdominal causes include surgery, intestinal
distention or ischemia, trauma, hemorrhage,
or peritonitis. Spillage of hydrochloric acid,
colonic contents, and pancreatic enzymes
into the peritoneal space are among the most
irritating events, whereas urine and blood are
less so. Retroperitoneal hematomas, especially when associated with vertebral fracture, frequently cause severe ileus. Thoracic
diseases such as lower lobe pneumonia, rib
fractures, and myocardial infarction can
cause ileus. Electrolyte abnormalities, especially hypokalemia, may also contribute to
decreasing gut motility.

In cases of mechanical SBO, the obstruction may be complete, blocking all
flow, or partial, allowing some fluid and gas
to pass. With complete SBO, there is significant disruption of secretory and absorptive
functions. The accumulation of secretions
and gas proximal to the obstruction leads to

intestinal distention. Up to 70% of intestinal gas results from swallowed air, primarily nitrogen, which is not absorbed by the intestine. The remainder is carbon dioxide from bacterial fermentation. In the first 24 hours, intestinal distention decreases absorption of sodium and thus water from the intestine. After 24 hours, secretion of sodium and water into the lumen occurs. This, of course, exacerbates the intestinal distention and the process becomes cyclical. There is loss of intravascular volume and electrolytes. In proximal obstruction especially, reflex vomiting exacerbates this volume loss and depletion of sodium, potassium, chloride, and hydrogen ions. Luminal pressure rises from normal, 2 to 4 cm H_2O, to 8 to 10 cm H_2O. In the setting of a closed-loop obstruction where back-flow is prevented, pressures can rise to 30 to 60 cm H_2O. High pressures cause small blood vessels to rupture as well as arterial insufficiency. Increased abdominal pressure can impair ventilation and the return of venous blood to the heart. Although the small intestine is normally almost sterile, the obstructed bowel is quickly overgrown by bacteria. These bacteria may translocate into the bloodstream. The culmination of this process if untreated is hypovolemia, sepsis, and shock. If patients progress this far, their mortality rate approaches 70%.

Strangulation occurs when the blood supply to the obstructed intestine is impaired. This happens when the intraluminal pressure exceeds the central venous pressure in the bowel wall or when constricting adhesive bands or hernial rings cut off venous flow and lymphatic drainage. Strangulation can lead to hemorrhage into the strangulated segment, gangrene, sepsis, or perforation of the bowel—any of which can be devastating.

Suggested Readings

Asbun HJ, Pempinello C, Halasz NA. Small bowel obstruction and its management. *Int Surg* 1989;74:23–27.

Balthazar EJ, Birnbaum BA, Megibow AJ, et al. CT of small bowel obstruction, *Am J Roentgenol* 1994;162:255–261.

Baker SR. Plain film radiology of the intestines and appendix. In: Baker SR, ed. *The abdominal plain film.* Norwalk, CT: Appleton & Lange, 1990.

Bizer LS, Liebling RW, Delaney HM, et al. Small bowel obstruction: the role of nonoperative treatment in simple intestinal obstruction and predictive criteria for strangulation obstruction. *Surgery* 1981;89:407–413.

Deitch EA, Bridges WM, Ma JW, et al. Obstructed intestine as a reservoir for systemic infection. *Am J Surg* 1990;159:394–401.

Fukuya T, Hawes, OR, Lu CC, et al. CT diagnosis of small-bowel obstruction: efficacy in 60 patients, *AJR Am J Roentgenol* 1992;158:765–769.

Gazelle GS, Goldberg MA, Wittenberg J, et al. Efficacy of CT in distinguishing small bowel obstruction from other causes of small bowel dilatation, *Am J Roentgenol* 1994;162:43–47.

Ko YT, Lim JH, Lee DH, et al. Small bowel obstruction: sonographic evaluation. *Radiology* 1993;188:649–653.

Megibow AJ, Balthazar EJ, Cho KC, et al. Bowel obstruction evaluation with CT. *Radiology* 1991;180:313–318.

Seror D, Fegin E, Szold A, et al. How conservatively can postoperative small bowel obstruction be treated? *Am J Surg* 1993;165:121–125.

Sosa J and Gardner B. Management of patients diagnosed as acute intestinal obstruction secondary to adhesions. *Am Surg* 1993;59:125–128.

CHAPTER 22

Hyperemesis

Vicki E. Noble, MD

Clinical Scenario

A 28-year-old gravida 2 para 1 (G2P1) woman presents to the emergency department (ED) at 12 weeks' gestation complaining of incessant vomiting. She reports having made four trips to the ED in the last 2 weeks for the same complaint. Despite temporary relief with hydration, she has been unable to keep down food or fluids for the last several days. She denies any vaginal bleeding, fever, chest pain, cough, or upper respiratory infection symptoms. She also denies any pain with urination (dysuria) or frequent urination (frequency). She notes that she has had a decided decrease in her urinary output and that it looks "very dark yellow." She describes her emesis as dark green or brown (bilious) "as I have nothing left in my stomach."

Her past medical history is significant for a similar presentation during her last pregnancy, although most of her symptoms had resolved by 12 weeks. She had a normal vaginal delivery at term.

Her only medications include multivitamins that she has not been able to keep down recently because of her vomiting. She has no known drug allergies. She denies using any alcohol or illicit drugs, although she had an occasional drink before she became pregnant. She has never been a smoker.

The patient appears listless and pale while lying on the stretcher as you walk into the examination room. She is very thin and reports that she has actually lost 4 pounds over the past 2 weeks. Her vital signs include a resting heart rate of 115 beats/minute, a

respiratory rate of 16 breaths/minute, blood pressure 105/70 mm Hg, and a temperature of 98°F. Her systolic blood pressure drops by 20 points when she changes position from lying to standing and her heart rate increases by 18 beats per minute. She has increased salivation and retches several times while you are examining her. Her eyes show anicteric sclera. Her oropharynx is clear, although she does have some posterior pharynx erythema. Her mucous membranes are dry. Her neck is supple with no lymphadenopathy and no thyroid tenderness, goiters, or bruits are observed. Her lungs are clear to auscultation bilaterally, and her heart is tachycardic with no murmurs or gallops heard. Her abdomen is soft with hyperactive bowel sounds and a mildly enlarged uterus. She has no flank tenderness on either side. Her lower extremities reveal no edema. Her skin turgor is decreased. Her pelvic examination is unremarkable with a closed cervical os and no cervical motion tenderness or adnexal masses. Her neurological examination including cranial nerves is unremarkable.

The patient's serum potassium is 2.8 mEq/L, and urinalysis reveals a large amount of ketones. Despite administration of 3 L of dextrose in normal saline and potassium intravenously, in addition to metaclopramide (Reglan) and ondansetron, the patient continues to retch and vomit and is admitted to the hospital with the diagnosis of hyperemesis gravidarum (HG). She is discharged the next day after an uneventful stay in the hospital with a prescription for oral antiemetics. She is to follow up in her obstetrician's office the next day.

Clinical Evaluation

Introduction

Nausea and vomiting in pregnancy (NVP) is common, affecting 50% to 90% of gravid women. It is more common in westernized countries, especially in urban settings. HG is the most severe form in the spectrum of NVP and refers to pathological vomiting to the extent that hydration and nutrition is impaired and electrolyte imbalance results. HG affects 0.3% to 2% of pregnancies with a peak incidence at 8 to 12 weeks' gestation. The term *hyperemesis* is usually used to refer to women during the first trimester of pregnancy; however, hyperemesis can develop in other clinical situations, including patients undergoing chemotherapy and women in the second or (rarely) third trimester. Symptoms usually resolve between 16 and 20 weeks of gestation.

History

It is essential to elicit the nature of the vomiting. The patient should be asked to comment on the number of episodes in a given time frame, the general volume of emesis, and the quality of the vomitus. NVP may exhibit the classic diurnal pattern with more pronounced symptoms generally in the morning compared to the evening or the symptoms may be constant. It is important to distinguish vomiting once after eating a large meal versus vomiting multiple times so that the emesis eventually becomes bilious (as in the patient described in the clinical scenario). Bloody vomitus may indicate a Mallory-Weiss tear, a complication of multiple or forceful episodes of vomiting. In addition, a lightheaded or dizzy feeling when standing can be a sign of severe dehydration (orthostatic hypotension) from vomiting (as in the patient in the clinical scenario) or from other conditions that would decrease a patient's intravascular blood volume. It is also important to determine if the patient has been able to hold down any liquids or solids, because that may mean the difference between hospitalization and outpatient treatment. Significant weight loss should be noted. Previous medical history, including gynecological history and risk factors for abnormal pregnancy, should be elicited. Several studies have indicated a higher risk of HG with nulliparity, multiple gestations, trophoblastic disease, and a history of HG with previous pregnancies. Vomiting beyond the twentieth week of gestation should prompt consideration for other disease states including peptic ulcer disease, gastroenteritis, appendicitis, biliary disease, hepatitis, pancreatitis, renal colic, pyelonephritis, gastroparesis, and severe esophageal reflux. Medications should be elicited including over-the-counter and herbal medications. Patients with a history of gastrointestinal intolerance to oral contraceptives have a higher incidence of both NVP and HG. A family history of endocrinopathies should be duly noted and considered in the differential diagnosis. The patient's social situation may influence the need for hospitalization because a strong support system may be necessary to help care for a patient at home. Finally, it is important to ask questions that will help you rule out other diagnoses. For example, painful urination (dysuria) is a symptom of a urinary tract infection, which should be treated in pregnancy either as an outpatient (uncomplicated cystitis) or as an inpatient (pyelonephritis in pregnancy). Other important historical questions include the presence of fever, difficulty breathing, chest pain or pain with breathing, significant abdominal pain, diarrhea, muscle spasms, or muscle weakness.

Physical Examination

The physical examination in hyperemesis centers on signs of dehydration, with careful attention to exclude complications and alternative or contributory diagnoses. Vital signs should be noted and repeated after therapy to determine if there is a change. Temperature in HG alone should be normal. The presence of fever should lead to an investigation to find a contributory or alternative diagnosis to account for the patient's condition. The respiratory rate should be normal, although a slight tachypnea may occur as respiratory compensation for lactic acidosis production seen in severely dehydrated or malnourished states. The pulse and blood pressure may be consistent with dehydration, as in the clinical scenario, with tachycardia, low blood pressure, or significant orthostatic changes. A patient is considered orthostatic when the systolic blood pressure drops by 20 mm Hg and heart rate increases by 15 to 20 beats/minute when the patient goes from lying to standing, allowing for 1 to 2 minutes for equilibration after changing position, and is consistent with decreased intravascular volume. Other signs of significant dehydration, including dry mucous membranes, decreased skin turgor (i.e., decreased elasticity), or high resting heart rates and low blood pressure, should be sought. Excessive salivation (ptyalism) may be observed.

In addition, it will be important to assess whether the patient has significant abdominal tenderness to rule out surgical diagnoses. Mild epigastric tenderness or very mild diffuse tenderness may be consistent with hyperemesis, but focal tenderness elsewhere and moderate to severe tenderness on examination should raise the suspicion of alternative diagnoses. Peritoneal signs, such as guarding, tenderness to percussion, and rebound, are not consistent with hyperemesis and should prompt a thorough evaluation for surgical pathology. Focal tenderness in the right lower quadrant should prompt the differential diagnosis of appendicitis. Focal tenderness in the right upper quadrant should prompt the differential diagnosis of biliary disease. Recall that the anatomy of the pelvic and abdominal contents change as pregnancy progresses (i.e., appendicitis may not present with right lower quadrant pain) and that pregnancy predisposes to certain types of abdominal pathology (i.e., biliary stasis, gastroparesis). In addition, you should note any signs consistent with infection. A thorough examination for focal signs of infection is mandatory including the oral pharynx (exudates consistent with strep throat), lungs (crackles indicating pneumonia), flank (costovertebral angle pain consistent with pyelonephritis), skin (any rash),

and lymph nodes. A thorough neurological examination should be normal. Abnormal reflexes should raise the suspicion for electrolyte abnormalities; ataxia, ocular abnormalities, and a global confusion are consistent with Wernicke's encephalopathy. Finally, a pelvic examination (including a rectal examination to check for blood) should be performed looking for cervical motion tenderness (signs of pelvic inflammatory disease), adnexal masses (signs of abscess, ectopic pregnancy or cysts), and signs of any discharge or blood. The uterus should be palpated to assess for size. An enlarged uterus may signal multiple gestations or molar pregnancy.

Diagnostic Evaluation

Laboratory tests that are essential for planning the treatment of HG include a chemistry panel including sodium, potassium, chloride, bicarbonate, blood urea nitrogen, and creatinine. Calcium, magnesium, and phosphorus levels should be included in an electrolyte panel because they can also be disrupted in dehydration and can cause significant morbidity. In addition, a urine sample is helpful to demonstrate ketosis and rule out a urinary tract infection. Thyroid function tests are occasionally indicated because a hyperthyroid state is among the differential diagnoses, especially for symptoms past 20 weeks' gestation. It should be noted that several studies have shown a transient increase in thyroid function associated with HG that usually resolves as the pregnancy progresses. Liver function tests may be helpful in certain cases if hepatitis is in the differential diagnosis, but it should be noted that mild increases (less than a fourfold rise) of transaminase levels are not uncommon in patients hospitalized with HG. A complete blood count (including white blood count) is obtained when infectious diseases are in the differential diagnosis for vomiting or when there is significant hematemesis. In addition, a large peripheral intravenous (IV) catheter will be necessary for fluid replacement. An electrocardiogram (ECG) should be considered when clinically indicated, to ensure that an underlying pericarditis or myocarditis is not responsible for the patient's symptoms. Finally, all women should have a quantitative β-human chorionic gonadotropin (β-hCG), if they are in their first trimester, to demonstrate pregnancy and the viability or normal growth patterns of that pregnancy.

It is important to keep in mind indications for pelvic ultrasound, because many of these patients will also meet them. A woman presenting to the ED with abdominal pain (with or without vomiting) should immediately prompt the differential diagnosis of ectopic pregnancy, if an ultrasound has not been performed to document intrauterine pregnancy. Ectopic pregnancy carries a significant morbidity and mortality risk if the presentation is missed. A pelvic ultrasound should be strongly considered in patients in whom the β-hCG levels are not increasing normally (during the first trimester the β-hCG should double every 48 hours) to document a viable pregnancy and rule out a missed or incomplete abortion or molar pregnancy. Finally, a pelvic ultrasound can help evaluate for a tubal abscess, ovarian torsion, a hemorrhagic ovarian cyst, and other gynecological pathology when the pelvic examination reveals an ovarian mass or severe unilateral adnexal tenderness. Some authors recommend a pelvic ultrasound for all HG patients because of the association with trophoblastic disease (molar pregnancy) and multiple gestations.

Differential Diagnosis

The differential diagnosis for hyperemesis is illustrated in Table 22.1.

Treatment

Table 22.2 outlines possible therapies for treating hyperemesis or refractory vomiting. The management of NVP and HG range from education and counseling with conservative dietary modifications for mild cases, to antiemetic drug therapy, and to total parenteral nutrition for severe cases. Termination of pregnancy for HG, once as high as 14%, is rare today.

Table 22.1.
Differential diagnosis of hyperemesis

Gynecological Conditions
Mole (molar pregnancy) hydatidiform
Ectopic or heterotopic pregnancy
Multiple gestations (may not be known at presentation)

Infectious Conditions
UTI, including pyelonephritis
Hepatitis
Pericarditis
Myocarditis

Metabolic Conditions
Diabetic ketoacidosis
Thyrotoxicosis
Addison's disease
Hypercalcemia
Iron-induced vomiting

GI Conditions
Gastroenteritis
Gastritis
Peptic ulcer disease
Pancreatitis
Small bowel obstruction
Cholecystitis (bile stasis secondary to increased progesterone in pregnancy)
Appendicitis

Neurological Conditions
CNS/vestibular abnormalities

Psychiatric Conditions
Conflicting feelings about pregnancy
Depression
Substance abuse
Physical or sexual abuse

CNS, central nervous system; GI, gastrointestinal; UTI, urinary tract infection.

Education and counsel for NVP should include reassurance that the symptoms are expected, common, and usually self-limited. Dietary modifications may alleviate symptoms; recommend frequent (every 2 to 3 hours) small meals, rich in easily digestible carbohydrates and low in fatty foods. Any foods or odors that precipitate symptoms should be avoided. Discuss with the patient

Table 22.2.

Treatment for hyperemesis

Treatment	Goal	Recommendation
Dietary modification	Goal is to work with the GI changes in pregnancy (decreased gastric emptying, lower esophageal pressure) and eat several small meals a day instead of fewer larger meals.	This treatment is only possible in the patient who is able to keep down oral liquids or solids and is part of an outpatient maintenance plan.
Thiamine (25–50 mg tid po or 100 mg IV weekly) Pyridoxine (30 mg po qd)	Thiamine should be given to every woman in whom malnutrition is considered. One of the main morbidities of this condition is Wernicke's encephalopathy, which may be precipitated by giving dextrose solution before giving thiamine in a malnourished patient.	Standard therapy for all office, inpatient, and emergency department visits
IV fluids	Treat the presumed dehydration and electrolyte imbalance (decreased bicarbonate). If the patient is hypokalemic, potassium may also be added to IV fluids judiciously.	Standard therapy for all office, inpatient, and emergency department visits
Metoclopramide (Reglan)	A promotility agent that has extensive data to show a lack of teratogenesis. Works primarily by dopamine antagonism. Class B (safe and efficacious in humans).	When fluids, thiamine, and pyridoxine fail to prevent nausea and vomiting, antiemetic pharmacological agents may be tried. Obviously in the first trimester, the concern is to not use any agents that may have teratogenic effects.
Prochlorperazine (Compazine)	Also a dopaminergic antagonist. Class C (clinically efficacious, but conflicting data on safety; does cross the placenta)	Can be administered as a rectal suppository if the patient is vomiting.
Promethazine (Phenergan)	Histamine 1 receptor blocker Class C	
Ondansetron (Zofran)	Serotonin receptor blocker Class B	
Diphenhydramine (Benadryl)	Antihistamine Class B	
Ginger	Has been studied in one trial and was shown to decrease nausea and vomiting; safety profile unknown	Used in conjunction with other therapies or when women are reluctant to take pharmacological antiemetic agents; ginger root may contain thromboxane synthetase inhibitor, which may affect testosterone receptor binding in fetus
Acupressure	Safe	No formal trials to prove efficacy but many anecdotal reports advocate its use in refractory cases
Steroids	Prednisolone given 16 mg tid × 3 days then tapered over 2 weeks	Recent prospective study that showed safety and efficacy versus Phenergan; not standard of care yet

GI, gastrointestinal; IV, intravenous; po, by mouth; qd, every day; tid, three times a day.

the risk-to-benefit ratio of iron pills, which are frequently prescribed, because they may contribute to nausea, vomiting, and epigastric pain.

The mainstay of emergency therapy for HG is correction of volume depletion and electrolyte abnormalities. Patients may require normal saline initially for severe volume depletion. This measure should be followed by administration of dextrose-containing solutions for severely malnourished states manifested by ketonuria without glucosuria, which represents breakdown of tissue for energy secondary to depleted glycogen stores. If HG is prolonged, parenteral multivitamins, including thiamine, should be given before glucose infusion to prevent vitamin deficiency-related complications in the severely malnourished patient. A small feeding may be attempted in the ED after volume depletion and electrolyte abnormalities are reversed.

Pharmacological therapy should be considered in patients who fail the conservative measures outlined previously. Obviously, in pregnant women care must be taken to not administer drugs with teratogenic properties. The classic teratogenic period is between day 31 and 71 after the last menstrual period, or the first 10 weeks of gestation, although drugs can still affect the fetus later in pregnancy. The risk-to-benefit ratio must justify the use of any drug during pregnancy, and a discussion and informed consent should precede use. As noted earlier, severe HG can cause depletion of maternal nutrient stores, resulting in adverse effects to the fetus. In one study, the mean dietary intake of patients with HG was less than 50% of the recommended daily allowances compared with controls. The overall incidence of fetal malformations in the general population is 1% to 3%. Drug exposures to teratogenic materials are thought to account for a similar number of birth defects. Because studies on pregnant women are unethical, there are no well-controlled trials regarding efficacy and little is known about the comparative efficacy of antiemetics. Furthermore, most of what is known about the teratogenic potential of medications was done in animal studies.

Disposition

Women who are unable to take any liquids by mouth after conservative treatment and women with dangerous electrolyte abnormalities or evidence of severe malnutrition (i.e., weight loss >5% total body weight) should be admitted to the hospital. Women with severe metabolic abnormalities (sodium level <120 mEq/L or mental status changes) may need intensive care unit (ICU) admission, although that is usually quite rare. In addition, if women do have evidence of severe malnutrition, total parenteral nutrition or tube feeds may need to be initiated to prevent further deterioration.

Pathophysiology

The exact mechanism or inciting disturbance that causes NVP and HG in the pregnant patient is still largely speculative. Serum β-hCG, progesterone, and estrogen levels all peak during the first trimester when the incidence of NVP and HG are highest. However, multiple studies have failed to show a relationship between β-hCG levels and the frequency or intensity of the NVP. Several studies have indicated that progesterone, possibly in conjunction with estrogen, contributes to relaxation of the lower esophageal sphincter, delayed gastric emptying, and prolonged small bowel transit time, all of which suggest a role in NVP and HG. In addition, serum hormone levels and frequency or intensity of symptoms have not directly correlated in scientific studies. A relation to thyroid hormone was also proposed. Because β-hCG binds to the same circulating plasma proteins as thyroid hormone, there was speculation that an increase in free thyroxine (T_4) or the active form of thyroid hormone displaced from plasma proteins could be responsible for some symptoms of HG. However, the correlation of these two values with clinical severity or even incidence of the disease has never been borne out in clinical studies. An association with pyridoxine deficiency has also been proposed. Increases in liver enzymes noted in HG have also been proposed as a contributing factor but never proven. Finally, psychological factors have been felt to play a role in NVP and HG; however, definitive scientific proof is lacking. It is probably fair to state that the mechanisms for NVP and HG are multifactorial with a strong suggestion that the altered hormone milieu associated with pregnancy plays a key role.

NVP is considered a favorable prognostic sign in pregnancy; NVP is associated with decreased risks of miscarriage, stillbirth, fetal mortality, preterm delivery, low birth weight, perinatal mortality, and growth retardation. Some authors consider the absence of some degree of NVP to be a potential manifestation of an abnormal pregnancy. HG was first recognized to be a potential cause of maternal death in the eighteenth century. However, since the 1940s, HG is a rare cause of maternal death because of the understanding about the associated fluid, nutritional, electrolyte, and metabolic abnormalities. In the modern era, in some studies, a relatively mild case of HG treated promptly and properly has conferred a similar favorable prognostic value. However, patients who manifest continued weight loss (>5% of prepregnancy weight) and electrolyte abnormalities may be at risk for decreased neonatal birth weight, growth retardation, and fetal anomalies, if symptoms are not controlled and electrolyte abnormalities are not corrected. HG is generally considered self-limited but has a slow recovery period with frequent relapses. Rare complications of HG include Wernicke's encephalopathy, pancreatitis, renal failure, and coagulopathies related to insufficient vitamin K intake.

Suggested Readings

Abell TL, Riely CA. Hyperemesis gravidarum. *Gastroenterol Clin North Am* 1992;21:835–849.

Bober SA, McGill AG, Tunbridge WM. Thyroid function in hyperemesis gravidarum. *Acta Endocrinol* 1986;111:404–410.

Brandes JM. First trimester nausea and vomiting as related to outcome of pregnancy. *Obstet Gynecol* 1967;30:427–431.

Broussard CN., Richter, JE. Nausea and vomiting of pregnancy, *Gastroenterol Clin North Am* 1998;27: 123–151.

Evans AJ, Li TC, Selby C, et al. Morning sickness and thyroid function. *Br J Obstet Gynaecol* 1986;93:520–522.

Gross S, Librach C, Cecutti A. Maternal weight loss associated with hyperemesis gravidarum: a predictor of fetal outcome. *Am J Obstet Gynecol* 1989;160:906–909.

Jarnfelt-Samsioe A, Samsioe G, Velinder G. Nausea and vomiting in pregnancy: a contribution to its epidemiology. *Gynecol Obstet Invest* 1983;16:221–223.

Kauppila A, Ylikorkala O, Jarvinen PA, et al. The function of the anterior pituitary-adrenal cortex axis in hyperemesis gravidarum *Br J Obstet Gynaecol* 1976;83:11–16.

Lacroix R, Eason E, Melzack R, et al. Nausea and vomiting during pregnancy: a prospective study of its frequency, intensity and patterns of change, *Am J Obstet Gynecol* 2000;182: 931–937.

Mendalie JH, Whitehead, SA, Andrews PL, et al. Relationships between nausea and/or vomiting in early pregnancy and abortion. *Lancet* 1957;2:117–119.

Nelson-Piercy C. Treatment of nausea and vomiting in pregnancy. *Drug Safety* 1998;19:155–164.

Robinson JN, Banerjee R, Thiet MP. Coagulopathy secondary to vitamin K deficiency in hyperemesis gravidarum. *Obstet Gynecol* 1998;92: 673–675.

Safari HR, Fassett MJ; Souter IC, et al. The efficacy of methylprednisolone in the treatment of hyperemesis gravidarum: a randomized, double-blind controlled study, *Am J Obstet Gynecol* 1998;179: 921–924.

Semmens JP. Female sexuality and life situations: an etiologic psycho-social-sexual profile of weight gain and nausea and vomiting in pregnancy. *Obstet Gynecol* 1971;38:555–563.

Van Stuijvenberg ME, Schabort I, Labadarios D, et al. The nutritional status and treatment of patients with hyperemesis gravidarum. *Am J Obstet Gynecol* 1995;172:1585–1591.

CHAPTER 23

Gastroenteritis

Melisa W. Lai, MD

Clinical Scenario

A 20-year-old man presents to the emergency department (ED) and reports frequent watery stools for the past 3 days and some nausea and vomiting after returning from a trip to Mexico. He has vomiting five to eight times per day and is unable to hold down food. He is a college student but has been unable to attend classes this week because of his symptoms. Three other friends who were on the same trip were also affected, although they all are nearly recovered. He denies fever, urinary complaints, or upper respiratory complaints.

He denies other past medical or surgical history except for an appendectomy at age 9. He has no allergies, takes no medicine, and drinks socially, but does not smoke or use illicit drugs. His family history is unremarkable except for lactose intolerance in his father and brother.

Physical examination reveals a well-developed, well-nourished young man who appears nontoxic. His vital signs while lying in the stretcher include a temperature of 97.9°F, pulse of 98 beats/ minute, blood pressure of 113/72 mm Hg, and respiratory rate of 20 breaths/minute with an oxygen saturation of 99% on room air. His pulse increases to 120 beats/minute and his blood pressure drops to 90/60 mm Hg after sitting up with his legs resting over the side of the stretcher. His mucus membranes appear dry. His neck is supple. Heart and lung sounds are unremarkable. His abdominal examination reveals a well-healed surgical scar in the right lower quadrant and a nontender, nondistended abdomen with normal bowel sounds.

Rectal examination reveals soft, watery, brown, heme-negative stool without mucus. His extremities are well perfused, and the skin is unremarkable.

Intravenous (IV) access is achieved and the patient receives a normal saline bolus of 500 mL over 15 minutes followed by 250 mL/hour along with an antiemetic medication. A stool sample is sent for analysis of ova and parasites, Gram stain, and culture. After 2 hours, the patient feels markedly better and is able to tolerate soup and crackers. The patient is discharged with a diagnosis of volume depletion and dehydration and nausea, vomiting, and diarrhea and instructed to return to the ED if he experiences severe abdominal pain, persistent nausea and vomiting, bloody stool, or fever. He is told to expect improvement over the next 3 to 5 days, to drink plenty of fluids, and that antibiotics do not seem appropriate in his management.

Clinical Evaluation

Introduction

Gastroenteritis is a nonspecific term applied to describe a variety of pathological states that cause acute diarrheal illness with nausea and vomiting. In fact, gastroenteritis is among the differential diagnosis for almost every type of abdominal pathology that may present to the ED. Most importantly, true gastroenteritis is a diagnosis of exclusion and one that many physicians prefer not to use as a discharge diagnosis.

The severity of illness for true gastroenteritis and diarrhea varies from mild to severe and is a common reason for patients to seek care. The United States alone has more than 100 million cases of acute diarrhea a year (representing one of the most common reasons for missing work), but only 10% of those affected seek medical attention and 1% to 2% require admission (usually along the extremes of the age spectrum). Even severe gastroenteritis, which is a leading cause of death in the developing world, can usually be managed with supportive care alone (including rehydration, intravenously or by mouth if tolerated, temperature control, and monitoring of vital signs).

Appropriate management requires an extensive history and physical examination, appropriate supportive measures, and often etiology-specific treatment while considering the myriad of illnesses that may initially masquerade as gastroenteritis.

History

The key parts of the history in any patient with diarrhea are the same as any other major symptom and constellation of symptoms. The PQRST mnemonic is particularly helpful when faced with an uncomfortable patient.

P—Provoking Factors or Palliation

Questions concerning provoking factors include the following:

What has the patient eaten recently?

Where has the patient traveled, if at all? (Recall our patient's travel to Mexico.)

Are there any sick contacts or people with similar symptoms in the patient's household or cadre of friends and peers?

Has the patient been on antibiotics?

Have they gone camping, been in a day care, or ingested raw fish or possibly spoiled food?

Questions concerning palliation refer to whether anything has made the symptoms better (antacid?) or worse (milk?).

Q—Quality or Quantity

Questions concerning the quality of the pain include the following:

Is the patient really having diarrhea (watery stools) or just loose bowel movements?

What is the quality of the stools (amount, color, consistency, odor, bloody, floating)?

Questions concerning quantity in this case refer to how many bowel movements the patient is having per day and the volume of stool and how much the patient is vomiting.

R—Region and Radiation

Questions concerning region and radiation would include the following:

Is there associated pain or cramping? Where?

Does it radiate (travel) to the back or groin or testicle/vulva?

S—Severity of Pain

On a scale of 1 to 10 or just in comparison with prior experiences:

What made this episode bad enough to seek medical attention?

What is the severity of pain (if present)?

T—Temporal Characteristics

Questions concerning temporal characteristics refer to the following:

How long has the illness been going on? Diarrhea for a month invokes a different spectrum of possibilities than several days.

Is there a distinct pattern?

Is it getting better or worse?

If the symptoms wax and wane, how long does the patient go between bouts?

What activities has the patient engaged in leading up to the diarrhea?

With women—when was her last menstrual period?

Is there a chance she could be pregnant?

Physical Examination

The key parts of a physical examination assess the patient's hydration status and attempt to exclude other causes of diarrhea and vomiting. Vital signs are usually consistent with volume depletion and may include tachycardia and low blood pressure. Recall our patient's tachycardia and blood pressure drop after sitting up signifying dehydration. A fever is common with infectious etiologies of gastroenteritis. A slight increase in respiratory rate may represent an anxious reflex or possibly a respiratory compensation for the bicarbonate dumping with frequent bowel movements. Dehydration may manifest as dry mucous membranes, chapped lips, delayed capillary refill, poor skin turgor, or as a sunken fontanel in infants. The abdominal examination is of paramount importance in a patient with suspected gastroenteritis to exclude causes of diarrhea and vomiting that may require surgical intervention. As seen in our patient, the abdomen should generally be nontender and nondistended without rebound or guarding and should not reveal any masses or hepatomegaly or splenomegaly. Focal tenderness, masses, or hepatosplenomegaly should provoke further workup. Rectal examination may be heme positive (indicating colonic mucosal disruption) or negative. The rectal examination should be otherwise unremarkable and should not reveal any abscesses, fistulas, fissures (which may represent inflammatory bowel disease), or obstructing tumors. Pelvic examination, if performed, should be normal.

Diagnostic Evaluation

Patients with gastroenteritis may not require any diagnostic testing. The need for diagnostic testing should be based on the need to further evaluate the seriousness of their dehydration and electrolyte status, to evaluate the patient for extracolonic etiologies, and, in certain cases, to determine the specific etiological agent. Generally, patients will require a workup if they have focal or severe abdominal pain, high fever, severe dehydration, or bloody stools; if they are immunocompromised; or when an epidemic diarrheal disease is suspected.

Stool studies and culture may be helpful to determine the nature of diarrhea and the specific etiological pathogen. Blood or leukocytes are considered a strong indicator of inflammatory diarrhea. This can be accomplished with a Wright stain or methylene blue examining for leukocytes and a Hemoccult test. Fecal leukocytes are present in greater than 75% of patients with *Salmonella* and *Shigella* but are less commonly seen with other invasive bacterial agents and may be positive in inflammatory bowel disease. Fecal leukocytes are usually absent in viral infections, giardiasis, and cases of enterogenic or toxigenic diarrhea. Routine stool culture tests for only *Campylobacter, Aeromonas, Salmonella, Shigella*, and *Yersinia* is not a useful or cost-effective test in most cases of diarrhea.

Testing for other pathogens, such as *Escherichia coli* 0157:H7, *Vibrio*, and *Shiga* toxin-producing bacteria require specific media and must be communicated to the laboratory. Specific indications for stool cultures include grossly bloody stools, stools that are positive for heme or leukocytes, prolonged course of diarrhea, or for epidemiological purposes (food handlers or illness associated with partially cooked hamburger).

Testing stool for ova and parasites should be reserved for those patients in whom parasitic disease is in the differential: the patient has recently traveled to an endemic region, has prolonged diarrheal disease, is immunocompromised, or has failed an antibiotic course. Enzyme-linked immunosorbent assays (ELISA) are available for *Giardia*, cryptosporidia, rotavirus, and *Clostridium difficile* toxin. These tests are expensive and only helpful in cases in which admission or follow up is ensured because the results will not be immediately available.

Routine laboratory tests are generally not indicated in mild to moderate disease. Severe diarrhea may be associated with hyponatremia or hypernatremia, hypokalemia, an elevated creatinine from decreased glomerular filtration rate, and decreased bicarbonate. Acidosis may be secondary to bicarbonate loss or from hypovolemia-induced lactic acidosis in severe disease. The white blood count (WBC) may be variable and is nonspecific. Eosinophilia may be present in parasitic infections. Finally, imaging studies such as plain abdominal radiographs (kidneys, ureter, bladder [KUB]) and upright x-ray films or computed tomography (CT) scan of the abdomen are

Table 23.1.

Differential diagnosis of gastroenteritis

Surgical abdomen (e.g., appendicitis, large or small bowel obstruction, intussusception)

"Food poisoning" (preformed toxins of *Clostridium perfringens, Bacillus cereus, Staphylococcus aureus*)

Shellfish poisoning (especially diarrheal shellfish poisoning from okadaic acid)

Histamine/scombroid poisoning

Hemolytic uremic syndrome

Botulism

Inflammatory bowel disease (ulcerative colitis and Crohn's disease)

Irritable bowel syndrome

Ischemic colitis

Radiation colitis

Carcinoid or VIP-secreting tumor

AIDS

Drug-associated diarrhea (laxatives, quinidine, colchicine, cholinergics)

Ciguatera poisoning

AIDS, acquired immunodeficiency syndrome; VIP, vasoactive intestinal peptide.

only helpful when bowel obstruction, perforation, toxic megacolon, or alternative diagnoses are entertained.

Differential Diagnosis

The differential diagnosis for gastroenteritis is illustrated in Table 23.1.

Treatment

The goals of emergency therapy while ruling out alternative diagnoses are supportive care (including rehydration and treatment of nausea, fever, and pain as needed), identification of any complications, and prevention of the spread of infection (Table 23.2). Certain etiologies of gastroenteritis may require definitive antibiotic therapy. In addition, the physician will want to identify any potential public health concerns that may prevent an epidemic (e.g., *E. coli* 0157:H7 contamination of fast-food hamburger in the Pacific Northwest in 1993).

Generally, treatment in the ED for true gastroenteritis (despite the nondiagnosis) is supportive care. Supportive care generally consists of rehydration and replacement of electrolytes. Electrolyte imbalances result from the rapid constant loss of water and absorptive properties of the gut during gastroenteritis. IV fluids should be used for severe dehydration, altered consciousness, and severe, intractable vomiting or diarrhea or if the time and environment are not conducive to oral rehydration therapy (ORT). Adults may require 1 to 2 L of normal saline (NS) or 5% dextrose normal saline (D5NS) or 5% dextrose with 0.5 normal saline (D5/halfNS) over the first 30 to 60 minutes. Severely dehydrated children require an initial bolus of 20 mL/kg.

Table 23.2.

Treatment of gastroenteritis for all patients

Rule out other causes

Rehydration: IV for patients with moderate to severe dehydration; oral if patient can tolerate fluids and has mild volume losses.

Treatment of complications: electrolyte abnormalities

Consideration of antiemetics

Consideration of antibiotics

IV, intravenous.

ORT uses iso-osmolar or hypo-osmolar agents to reverse dehydration and is largely responsible for the decrease in death rates for infectious diarrhea, such as cholera, in developing countries. The World Health Organization solution contains 90 mEq/L sodium, 20 mEq/L potassium, 80 mEq/L chloride, and 20 g/L glucose. The osmolarity is 310 mOsm/kg water. This therapy is based on coupled transport in which one glucose molecule is linked to one sodium molecule (and water) for entry at the intestinal brush border membrane. This coupled transport remains intact despite enterotoxigenic illnesses. Eight ounces (250 mL) is given every 15 minutes until fluid balance is restored, then 1.5 L of fluid is given per liter of stool produced. Other similar mixtures are commonly available (e.g., Pedialyte, Rehydralyte); however, the use of noncommercial iso-osmotic or hypo-osmotic liquids with balanced sodium and glucose contents can be equally effective. Oral rehydration has been shown to be as effective as IV therapy in situations in which patients can tolerate oral fluid.

Electrolyte repletion, especially potassium, should be guided by the degree of dehydration and laboratory values. For severely dehydrated patients, adding 20 mEq/L of potassium to IV fluids is reasonable. Potassium chloride may also be given orally in a 20- to 40-mEq dose. Sodium bicarbonate may be added to IV fluids but is usually not necessary.

Antiemetics should be considered for all patients with nausea or vomiting to facilitate toleration of oral fluid, which is a common goal for discharge. Common antiemetics used in the ED include droperidol (0.625 to 1.250 mg IV adult), prochlorperazine (5 to 10 mg IV adult), promethazine (12.5 to 25 mg IV adult), and ondansetron (4 to 8 mg IV adult). Droperidol was assigned a "black box" rating by the Food and Drug Administration (FDA) for its potential to cause arrhythmia in patients with a long QT interval. Some hospitals have taken the drug off formulary, whereas others permit the use of the drug only after an electrocardiogram (ECG) is performed to check the QT interval. Antiemetics are generally used less in the pediatric population.

Occasionally, emergency physicians may consider using outpatient antibiotics if they believe that the diarrhea is truly of infectious etiology and not solely toxin mediated. Empiric therapy for patients with heme-positive or leukocyte-positive stools has been an acceptable practice for years. Empiric therapy with fluoroquinolones or trimethoprim-sulfamethoxazole (TMP-SMX) has recently been questioned after an increase in hemolytic uremic syndrome was reported in antibiotic treated children with *E. coli* 0157:H7 infectious diarrhea versus controls. Several types of infectious diarrhea require antibiotic therapy (Table 23.3). Mild cases of *Yersinia* may be treated with TMP-SMX, whereas moderate to severe cases should receive

Table 23.3.

Antibiotic treatment for gastroenteritis

Infectious Agent	Treatment
Campylobacter	Erythromycin or azithromycin
Clostridium difficile	Metronidazole or vancomycin
Giardia	Metronidazole
Traveler's Escherichia coli or Shigella	Fluoroquinolone or TMP-SMX to reduce duration of symptoms
Yersinia	TMP-SMX or ceftriaxone IV if severe

IV, intravenous; TMP-SMX, trimethoprim-sulfamethoxazole.

ceftriaxone intravenously. Erythromycin or azithromycin are effective for *Campylobacter* infections. Metronidazole and vancomycin are effective in cases of *C. difficile* colitis. Metronidazole is also effective against parasitic infections with *Giardia* or entamoeba. Finally, the duration of travel's diarrhea caused by *E. coli* or *Shigella* may be halved with fluoroquinolones or TMP-SMX. Positive stool studies or ELISA studies will require definitive antibiotic therapy.

Disposition

Patient disposition from the ED should be based on the following:

1. Age (lower threshold to admit patients at extremes of age)
2. Presentation on admission (severely dehydrated, septic patients, severe electrolyte imbalance may require admission)
3. Improvement during at least a 2-hour observation (admit if inadequate improvement)
4. Home resources and social situation (further home improvement requires supportive resources)
5. Underlying etiology if the diagnosis is uncertain

The clinician may rely a fair amount on their own sense or "gestalt" about how a patient will fare at home before discharging them. If there is any question of a surgical abdomen evolving or a complicated infectious course, however, it is better to admit and watch for further improvement or wait for cultures.

If discharged, patients should be instructed to continue home oral rehydration. Early, age-appropriate refeeding should be initiated as soon as possible because complex carbohydrates provide additional coupled transport molecules. Instruct patients to consider rice, wheat, bread, potatoes, and lean meats. Hyperosmolar liquids should be avoided because they will facilitate osmotic losses. Lactose intolerance is uncommon; therefore, milk can usually be given safely and it is generally well tolerated even during diarrheal illness.

Antidiarrheal and antimotility agents probably have a safe role for the treatment of mild to moderate nonbloody gastroenteritis to decrease fluid losses. Their use in enteroinvasive forms of infectious diarrhea has been discouraged because of concern for causing increased bacterial numbers and bacteremia by slowing intestinal transport time.

Patients should be instructed on deterrence of spread with frequent hand washing, especially after bowel movements. Patients should be instructed to wash buttocks after each stool to avoid skin irritation from stool enzymes. Close contacts should be notified.

Most importantly, discharged patients should be instructed to return for bloody stools, worsening or changing abdominal pain, high fever, severe vomiting, or any concerns regarding rehydration. It is not unreasonable to explain to patients that appendicitis or other pathology may be initially misdiagnosed as gastroenteritis and that a deterioration or change in clinical status requires additional medical evaluation. Finally, patients should seek follow-up care if their diarrhea persists longer than 7 to 10 days.

Pathophysiology

In the gastrointestinal tract, the small intestine is the primary absorptive surface. A relatively liquid stool reaches the colon, where additional fluid is absorbed to produce a well-formed solid stool under normal conditions. Disorders that primarily affect the small intestine will result in greater amounts of diarrheal fluid, nutrition, and electrolyte losses.

The exact mechanism of vomiting associated with diarrheal disease is not well understood, but the vomiting center may be stimulated either by serotonin release or directly by certain preformed neurotoxins, as is the case with *Staphylococcus aureus* and *Bacillus cereus*.

Diarrhea is classified into five categories based on imbalances in fluid states and absorption:

1. Osmotic: secondary to increased fluid in the intestinal lumen or decreased absorption

2. Inflammatory: resulting from inflamed mucosal intestinal lining

3. Secretory: resulting from increased secretion

4. Motility: secondary to motility dysfunction

5. Decreased absorptive surface

Diarrhea may be produced merely by increased oral intake overwhelming the intestinal ability to absorb. Osmotic diarrhea is caused by the accumulation of nonabsorbable solutes, which draw liquid into the intestinal lumen. Examples include laxative, antacid, and sorbitol ingestion or disaccharidase deficiencies, steatorrhea, or other malabsorption processes, including those induced by manufactured products such as Olestra. Secretory mechanisms act at the cellular level to cause abnormalities of both absorption and secretion of electrolytes, many of which are associated with increases in intracellular cyclic adenosine monophosphate (cAMP) or cyclic guanosine monophosphate (cGMP). Examples include vasoactive intestinal polypeptide (VIP), serotonin, castor oil, bile salt or fatty acid enteropathy, and the toxins produced by *Salmonella, Shigella, Clostridium perfringens, Pseudomonas aeruginosa, Klebsiella pneumoniae, E. coli,* and *Vibrio cholera.* Infectious or noninfectious (e.g., inflammatory bowel disease) inflammatory processes cause destruction of intestinal mucosa, impairment of absorption, and an outpouring of blood and mucus. Any mechanism that increases motility (e.g., hyperthyroidism, irritable bowel syndrome, cholinergic agents, caffeine, and psychological stress) decreases the time for absorption. Finally, decreased bowel surface area after surgical resection leads to less absorptive surface area.

Infectious agents usually cause acute gastroenteritis, with viral infections (e.g., Norwalk, rotavirus, and adenovirus) accounting for approximately 50% to 75% of all cases, bacterial and protozoan etiologies 15% to 20%, and parasites 10% to 15% of cases. Infectious etiologies can be classified into four additional categories according to their primary pathological site of action:

1. Enterotoxin production

2. Cytotoxin production

3. Mucosal invasion

4. Adherence

Microorganisms such as *V. cholera, Salmonella,* and enterotoxigenic *E. coli* produce a toxin that primarily affects the small intestine and acts on the secretory mechanisms by elevating adenosine monophosphate (AMP) levels. This produces copious watery ("rice water") diarrhea without any mucosal invasion. Similarly, viral diarrhea is caused by viral replication in the intestinal mucosal cells of the small intestine that damages the transport mechanism and lead to nonbloody, noninflammatory diarrhea.

Cytotoxin-producing organism, such as *C. difficile, Shigella dysenteriae, Vibrio parahaemolyticus,* and enterohemorrhagic *E. coli,* cause mucosal cell destruction, which results in decreased absorption capability and bloody stools with inflammatory cells.

Enterocyte mucosal invasion by such organisms as *Campylobacter, Shigella,* and enteroinvasive *E. coli* cause cell destruction and bloody inflammatory diarrhea. Organisms such as *Salmonella* and *Yersinia* species invade cells but do not cause cell death and, therefore, do not cause frank dysentery (dysentery is diarrhea with blood, pus, and mucus in the stool).

Finally, some organisms cause diarrhea merely by overwhelming the normal host bacterial flora and thus impairing the normal physiological process. Some organisms, such as *V. cholera* and enterotoxigenic *E. coli,* produce proteins that aid in their adherence to the intestinal wall that may displace normal flora. Generally, diarrhea caused by this mechanism is dependent on inoculum size with approximately greater than 100,000 of *E. coli* required, but as little as 10 *Giardia* cysts or *Entameba* to overwhelm host defenses.

Ingestion of microorganisms coupled with certain host factors may lead to infection. Immunocompromised persons are at greater risk for infection. Alteration of normal bowel flora caused by antibiotics or in infants before normal colonization may lead to a void readily filled by pathogens. Achlorhydric states caused by antacids, histamine-2 (H_2) blockers, or gastric surgery alter the normal gastric pH, which is usually an effective antimicrobial defense. Finally, hypomotility, caused by diabetes mellitus, scleroderma, intestinal abnormalities, or antiperistaltic drugs (e.g., opiates, diphenoxylate, atropine, and loperamide) may result in pathogenic colonization, especially in the small intestine.

Suggested Readings

Bitterman RA. Acute gastroenteritis and constipation. In: Rosen P. ed., *Emergency medicine concepts and clinical practice*, 4th ed. St. Louis: Mosby-Year Book 1998:1917–1957.

Diskin A. Gastroenteritis. *emedicine.com Emergency medicine text*. Available at www.emedicine.com (accessed 6/10/04).

Gilbert DN, Noellering RC Jr, Sande MA. *The Sanford guide to antimicrobial therapy 2000.* Vienna, VA: Antimicrobial Therapy, 2000: 11–13.

Northrup RS, Flanigan TP. Gastroenteritis. *Pediatr Rev* 1994;15:461–471.

Seamens CM, Schwartz G. Food-borne illness: differential diagnosis and targeted management. *Emerg Med Rep* 1998;19:120–131.

Wong CS, Watkins SL, Tarr PL, et al. The risk of hemolytic-uremic syndrome after antibiotic treatment of Escherichia coli 0157:H7 infections. *N Engl J Med* 2000;342:1930–1936.

Vomiting
Questions and Answers

Questions

1. Choose the correct statement:

A. Mechanical forces are the most common cause of small bowel obstruction.

B. Nasogastric suction has never been demonstrated to improve patient outcome with bowel obstruction.

C. Multiple air-fluid levels on upright abdominal x-ray films are pathognomonic for bowel obstruction.

D. Adhesions are the most common cause of large bowel obstruction.

2. A 20-year-old pregnant woman presents with 2 days of nausea and vomiting. Which of the following answers regarding the cause for hyperemesis gravidarum is most appropriate?

A. Nulliparity

B. Multiple gestations

C. Trophoblastic disease

D. History of hyperemesis with prior pregnancy

E. All of the above

3. A 50-year-old male alcoholic patient presents to the emergency department complaining of dizziness. He notes black stools for several days. He appears pale but in no distress. His vital signs include a heart rate of 120 beats/minute, blood pressure of 100/60 mm Hg, and respiratory rate of 16 breaths/minute. His physical examination is significant for a soft abdomen with mild epigastric tenderness and black guaiac-positive stool. Which of the following is the appropriate first step in management?

A. Call the gastroenterologist for an emergent endoscopy.

B. Initiate two large-bore intravenous (IV) lines and bolus with normal saline.

C. Initiate two large-bore IV lines and begin uncross-matched blood.

D. Obtain stat portable upright chest x-ray film to look for free air and a surgical consultation.

E. Perform nasogastric lavage to look for acute gastric blood.

4. A 37-year-old woman just returned today from a trip to Mexico. She is complaining of several bouts of diarrhea and notes some blood in the last watery stool. Which of the following statements is true?

A. *Shigella, Campylobacter,* and enteroinvasive *Escherichia coli* produce bloody diarrhea by invading the mucosal enterocytes and killing them.

B. *Yersinia* and *Salmonella* species do not cause bloody diarrhea because they do not invade the mucosal cells.

C. *Clostridium difficile* and *Vibrio parahaemolyticus* also cause bloody diarrhea via mucosal invasion.

D. Definitive treatment for most gastroenteritis patients includes antibiotics and supportive care.

Directions: There are three sets of response options for the following scenario. You will be required to select one best answer from each question set.

5. A 22-year-old G_1P_1 woman presents to the emergency department complaining of crampy abdominal pain, nausea, and vomiting for several hours. She has a past medical history significant for endometriosis. She has had a cholecystectomy, an appendectomy, and an exploratory laparotomy to diagnose and remove tissue affected with endometriosis. She is currently on no medications, has no symptoms associated with a sexually transmitted disease (STD), has a single sexual partner, and always uses condoms. She has a healthy 2-year-old daughter. She has not eaten any poorly cooked meat and has had no ill contacts. Physical examination reveals an ill-appearing obese woman with a temperature of 100.0°F, blood pressure of 90/70 mm Hg, heart rate of 112 beats/minute, and respiratory rate of 14 breaths/minute, with a saturation of 99% on room air.

5.1. Assume that the physical examination reveals a tympanitic tender abdomen without focal guarding or rebound and negative rectal examination. The patient is not pregnant. What is the most appropriate sequence in caring for the patient?

A. Nasogastric tube, flat plate of the abdomen, surgical consultation, and admission to the surgical service for small bowel obstruction.

B. Analgesia, flat plate of the abdomen, intravenous (IV) hydration and laboratory tests, surgical consultation, and admission to the surgical service for small bowel obstruction.

C. IV placement for hydration and laboratory tests, analgesia, nasogastric tube, flat plate of the abdomen, surgical consultation, and admission to the surgical service for small bowel obstruction.

D. IV placement for hydration and laboratory tests, analgesia, nasogastric tube, flat plate of the abdomen, abdominal computed tomography (CT) scan, surgical consultation, and admission to the surgical service for small bowel obstruction.

5.2. The patient's urine b-human chorionic gonadotropin (β-hCG) is positive. How would you alter your management from question 5.1?

A. Management does not change.

B. A pelvic ultrasound should be performed once she is stabilized to determine if she has an intrauterine pregnancy.

C. The most likely diagnosis is hyperemesis. She should be hydrated with dextrose and normal saline.

D. X-ray films should be withheld because she is pregnant.

5.3. While in the emergency department, the patient receives a liter of intravenous (IV) normal saline. Before x-ray examination, the patient has several bouts of copious liquid stools. Her symptoms improve significantly. How does this change your management from 5.1?

A. No change in management.

B. The patient clearly has gastroenteritis. Hydrate her until her vital signs are stable. Reexamine her. If symptoms are somewhat better, discharge her with close follow-up.

C. Admit the patient to the medical service or gynecology service for observation for gastroenteritis with volume depletion.

D. Hydrate the patient, and check a flat plate of the abdomen. If there are signs of obstruction, obtain a surgical consultation and admit the patient to the hospital.

Answers and Explanations

1. C. Multiple air-fluid levels on upright abdominal x-ray films are pathognomonic for bowel obstruction. They illustrate fluid sitting in the bowel that is filled with air, which is able to pass through in the usual fashion. Mechanical obstruction caused by structural forces, including adhesions and tumors, are not the most common cause of bowel obstruction. Nonmechanical forces are usually caused by comorbid conditions such as bowel ischemia, postoperative ileus, and many other conditions leading to diminished motility. Nasogastric (NG) tube suction has been shown to improve outcome of bowel obstruction.

2. E. Nulliparity, multiple gestations, trophoblastic disease, and a history of prior hyperemesis are all historical or pathophysiological causes for hyperemesis. In a patient who presents with nausea and vomiting who is multiparous and does not have a history of hyperemesis, multiple gestations and trophoblastic disease should be kept in mind as possible causes, and appropriate workup should be obtained as needed.

3. B. Begin intravenous fluid resuscitation. This patient is showing signs of acute volume deficit by the tachycardia and low blood pressure. Blood products may be necessary, but unless his condition deteriorates, initial resuscitation with saline may be adequate and allow time for cross-matched blood and further workup. He will likely require endoscopy by a gastroenterologist during his admission; however, if he is easily stabilized with normal saline, this is not an emergent procedure. A nasogastric lavage is indicated once the patient is stabilized. If the lavage is positive for coffee grounds, then the bleeding is upper gastrointestinal (GI) in origin, and management would be by a gastroenterologist not a general surgeon. The surgical consultation is required for the unstable acute lower GI bleed, if an emergent colectomy is required.

4. A. *Yersinia* and *Salmonella* species do not cause a bloody diarrhea; however, they do invade mucosal cells without killing them. *Clostridium* and *Vibrio* species produce bloody diarrhea via toxin-mediated destruction not mucosal invasion. Most gastroenteritis patients will heal with supportive care only, usually by concerning themselves with maintaining good hydration and, therefore, do not require antibiotics.

5.1. C. This patient has a classic presentation for a small bowel obstruction. She has had several abdominal operations and is at risk for adhesions leading to obstruction. She is obese, which makes it likely that all her prior surgeries were open procedures because it is technically difficult to perform laparoscopic procedures on large patients. This patient is unstable and is in hypovolemic shock, albeit mild shock. She requires resuscitation first. The laboratory studies may be drawn off the intravenous (IV) catheter during IV placement. She should not leave the department for films until she is stable. There is no need to delay analgesia, and a nasogastric tube

may be placed before the x-ray films to relieve the intraabdominal pressure from the obstruction. The first two answers are incorrect, because resuscitation is either absent or mentioned too late in the sequence. Although a computed tomography (CT) scan of the abdomen will likely be needed, a surgical consultation team should see this patient early in her presentation, because she may require a trip to the operating room for lysis of adhesions emergently.

5.2. B. The simple answer to the treatment of the pregnant patient is "treat the patient, not the fetus." Once the patient is stabilized, an ultrasound examination is indicated to determine whether there is an intrauterine pregnancy. This may influence the surgeon's decision whether to operate or to observe the patient for resolution of symptoms. A computed tomography (CT) scan of the abdomen releases a significant amount of radiation, and decisions regarding its use in pregnant patients should be made with care. The fact that she is pregnant does not significantly alter the presumptive diagnosis of obstruction. That being said, prudence regarding x-ray exposure to the fetus should be exercised. However, x-rays and so forth must not be withheld from a pregnant patient just to protect the fetus. If the test is necessary for the pregnant patient, it must be done. Although unlikely, ectopic pregnancy can present. Thus, not performing an ultrasound examination would be incomplete management. Hyperemesis gravidarum is certainly possible, but patients do not classically present with distension, abdominal pain, and tenderness with a change in bowel habits.

5.3. D. Although diarrhea and liquid stools with vomiting are the hallmarks of gastroenteritis, the patient has had no ill contacts and does not give a history for food-borne illness. Her extensive surgical history puts her at risk for obstruction, and this diagnosis must be ruled out. It is comforting that she feels better, but she still may be partially obstructed, only allowing the liquid contents of the bowel to pass the obstruction. A surgical consultation is prudent. If all studies are negative, she may be admitted to a medical or gynecology service for observation with a surgical consultation to follow her on the wards.

Pelvic Complaints

Boy, you best pray that I bleed real soon.

Tori Amos

INTRODUCTION
Robert Dart, MD and Ron Medzon, MD
Section Editors

Knowledge of the anatomy of the pelvic structures, fascial planes, and nerve supply is requisite to understanding the signs and symptoms of pelvic pathology. These can be reviewed in detail in any good anatomy text. The bony pelvis forms a ring. Slung across this ring is the pelvic and urogenital diaphragm. The pelvic diaphragm forms a sling that provides support for the vagina and creates a sphincter for the rectum. The urogenital diaphragm provides support for the lower urethra and the anterior wall of the vagina. The presence of this sling allows mobility of the bladder and uterus, which is crucial during pregnancy to the normal functioning of the bowels and bladder. Numerous ligaments provide additional support and create fascial planes, which divide spaces between the rectum, uterus and vagina, and bladder into separate entities. These spaces become important in evaluating fluid related to infection and/or bleeding from pelvic organs.

The pelvic structures are innervated by both sympathetic and parasympathetic autonomic nerves. They control the bladder and urethra anteriorly and the uterus, vagina, cervix, rectosigmoid colon, and the anus posteriorly. The sympathetic supply originates from L1 to L3 levels of spinal cord, whereas the parasympathetic supply is derived from the sacral level S2 to S4.

Sensory innervation for the uterus and cervix differs. The uterus is innervated by fibers that follow the L2 to L4 sympathetic nerves. Because a major route of these fibers is from the abdominal sympathetic trunk, conditions causing pain in the uterus will create abdominal pain. In contrast, the cervix is innervated by sensory nerves that follow the sacral S2 to S4 parasympathetic paths. Thus, pain originating in the cervix is usually referred to the lumbosacral region.

It cannot be stressed too greatly that any woman of childbearing age with abdominal pain must have a thorough gynecological and obstetric history taken, requires a pelvic examination during physical examination, and requires a pregnancy test during diagnostic evaluation. She should also be questioned (in a nonthreatening manner) about domestic violence, and the emergency department should have a system in place to deal with a positive response. The following chapters discuss many of the most common complaints relating to the female reproductive system and their diagnosis, treatment, and pathophysiology.

CHAPTER 24

Abnormal Vaginal Bleeding in the Nonpregnant Patient

Laura J. Eliseo, MD, MPH

Clinical Scenario

A 23-year-old woman presents to the emergency department (ED) complaining of vaginal bleeding. The bleeding started 5 days ago and increased over the past 24 hours, saturating six maxi pads. She has mild midline crampy abdominal pain without nausea, vomiting, fever, or dysuria. She has had episodes like this in the past for which she was prescribed birth control pills, but she stopped these on her own 6 months ago. The patient denies significant past medical history, bleeding problems, or prior pregnancy. Her normal cycle length is 28 days and her last menstrual period occurred 6 weeks ago.

On physical examination, she is in no acute distress. Vital signs are blood pressure of 130/70 mm Hg, pulse of 72 beats/minute, respiratory rate of 16 breaths/minute, and temperature of 98.6°F. Orthostatic vital signs are normal. The abdomen is soft and nontender. Vaginal speculum examination reveals a small amount of blood without clots in the vaginal vault and a slow oozing of blood from the cervical os. No other discharge is noted. On bimanual examination, the uterus is normal size without cervical motion tenderness. No adnexal masses are appreciated.

A urine pregnancy test is negative, and the hematocrit is 40 mL/dL, which is the patient's baseline. It is determined that the patient is in no immediate danger from the bleeding. She is discharged with follow-up to see her gynecologist with the diagnosis of dysfunctional uterine bleeding (DUB).

Clinical Evaluation

Introduction

Abnormal vaginal bleeding in a nonpregnant patient is a common complaint for which women seek emergency care. Many women at some time will have an episode of bleeding that they perceive as abnormal. It is defined as vaginal bleeding at unusual or unexpected times or by excessive flow at the time of expected menses. The underlying etiologies of vaginal bleeding range from those resulting from normal female physiology to disorders that carry significant medical risk. This chapter discusses the spectrum of these disorders.

History

If vaginal bleeding is not severe and does not require emergent intervention, evaluation is started with a relevant history. (The following elements are the components of an excellent approach to any woman complaining of pelvic pain, and as such, will not be repeated in entirety in the next three chapters.) The history of present illness includes a description of the bleeding: time of onset, duration, volume (number of pads or tampons used), color, passage of clots, and frequency. Inquire about trauma (including abdominal trauma), pain, vaginal discharge, weakness, syncope, and near-syncope. In addition, solicit symptoms of coagulopathy: bleeding from multiple sites, easy bruising, or extensive bleeding. Recent weight gain, intolerance to cold, constipation, and other symptoms of hypothyroidism should be addressed and headache and vision changes indicative of a pituitary pathological condition.

A gynecological and obstetric history is an essential part of the evaluation. Elicit last menstrual period, gravida (total number of pregnancies including if presently pregnant), and para (list number of term infants, premature infants, abortions spontaneous or therapeutic, and living infants), current contraceptive methods, and use of hormone replacement therapy (HRT). Obtain a menstrual history: the patient's usual menstrual pattern (duration, cycle length, volume of flow), whether bleeding is cyclic or acyclic, and whether it is associated with pain or cramping. Symptoms and risk factors of infection should be addressed through questions about lower abdominal pain, pelvic pain, fever, chills, vaginal discharge, and sexual history. It is also important to ask about past episodes of abnormal bleeding, gynecological disease or surgery, past pregnancies, miscarriages, ectopic pregnancies, and symptoms of pregnancy (i.e., nausea and vomiting).

In the anovulatory patient, search for initiating events such as stress, eating disorders, or dramatic weight gain or loss. Suspicion of malignancy is heightened in patients older than 35 years who are obese or have a history of anovulation.

Inquire about past medical history, specifically for renal, hepatic, thyroid, endocrine, and coagulation disorders. Finally, past surgical history, use of medications (exposure to teratogens, anticoagulants, antiplatelet medications, hormones, birth control pills), allergies, social history, and family history (including history of blood dyscrasia) are part of the historical workup.

Physical Examination

A focused physical examination, including a careful pelvic examination, is essential for women with vaginal bleeding. Record vital signs assessing for orthostatic changes. Note the patient's general appearance. Pallor suggests the presence of anemia. Patients with a hematological pathological condition may have petechiae, purpura, or mucosal bleeding. Perform an abdominal examination assessing for tenderness, guarding, rigidity, evidence of peritoneal irritation, masses, organomegaly, and inguinal adenopathy. Assessment of visual fields should be performed if a pituitary pathological condition is suspected.

The pelvic examination includes inspection of the lower genital tract both externally and via speculum examination. Inspect for lacerations, foreign bodies, atrophic vaginitis, vulva or vaginal wall lesions, vaginal discharge, blood in the vaginal vault, cervical lesions, cervical polyps, cervical os (open or closed), and the presence of bleeding from the cervical os. On bimanual examination, assess uterine and adnexal size for enlargement, masses, irregular contour, and tenderness. Check for any cervical motion tenderness (infection). A rectal examination is also necessary to evaluate tenderness, masses, rectal bleeding, and presence of hemorrhoids.

If the patient is anovulatory, look for fatigue, constipation, hair loss, or edema, which are all evidence of hypothyroidism. A pituitary pathological condition often results in abnormal bleeding, and the patient may have associated breast discharge, loss of lateral visual fields, and headaches. Obesity and hirsutism may suggest polycystic ovarian syndrome.

Diagnostic Evaluation

Laboratory investigation includes pregnancy testing in all patients of reproductive age. Obtain cervical cultures if a sexually transmitted disease is suspected. A complete blood count provides an assessment of blood loss, infection, and platelet adequacy. If ecchymoses or petechiae are present, prothrombin time (PT), partial thromboplastin time (PTT), and international normalized ratio (INR) should be assessed. If bleeding is profuse and continuous, or associated with hypovolemia, the patient should be typed and cross-matched for possible transfusion.

If history and physical findings identify the individual at risk for liver disease, thyroid dysfunction, or a pituitary pathological condition, then appropriate testing may be initiated in the ED. Testing would include liver function, and levels of thyroid-stimulating hormone (TSH) and prolactin.

For patients with vaginal bleeding who have positive pregnancy tests, pelvic ultrasound examination is required to confirm a viable intrauterine pregnancy or to rule out ectopic pregnancy. Ultrasound examination should be performed to look for the presence of retained tissue when a patient has had an elective termination of a recent pregnancy. In addition, ultrasound scan may be helpful if uterine fibroids are suspected, an adnexal mass is identified, or a patient has focal adnexal tenderness and suspected pelvic inflammatory disease (PID) (tubo-ovarian abscess).

In women who are at increased risk for endometrial hyperplasia and carcinoma (>35 years old, postmenopausal, anovulatory, exposure to unopposed estrogen) with vaginal bleeding, either an endometrial biopsy or transvaginal ultrasound scan is part of the initial outpatient evaluation. Studies have shown that an endometrial stripe thickness greater than 5 mm is present in 96% of women with endometrial cancer and 92% of those with other endometrial disease, whether or not they used hormonal replacement therapy; thus, ultrasound examination is an excellent screening tool. Evaluation may be started in the ED or arranged in a follow-up setting with a gynecologist.

Differential Diagnosis

The differential diagnosis for vaginal bleeding in the nonpregnant patient is illustrated in Table 24.1.

Treatment

Most nonpregnant patients with abnormal vaginal bleeding do not require immediate intervention. In the hemodynamically unstable patient, assess airway, breathing, and circulation (ABCs), establish access with two large-bore intravenous (IV) lines, start fluid resuscitation, send type and screen, and place her on a cardiac monitor. Gynecological consultation is necessary and prompt

Table 24.1.

Differential diagnosis of abnormal vaginal bleeding

Complications of Pregnancy
Spontaneous miscarriage
Incomplete, threatened, or missed abortion
Ectopic pregnancy
Gestational trophoblastic disease
Placenta previa or abruption

Dysfunctional Uterine Bleeding
Estrogen withdrawal bleeding
Estrogen breakthrough bleeding
Progesterone breakthrough bleeding

Infection
Cervicitis
Vaginitis
Endometritis
Pelvic inflammatory disease
Sexually transmitted disease

Trauma
Laceration
Foreign body
Abdominal trauma

Pelvic Pathological Conditions
Cervix: polyp, dysplasia, carcinoma
Endometrium: endometrial polyp, leiomyoma, hyperplasia, carcinoma, endometriosis
Uterus: adenomyosis
Ovary: estrogen-producing tumors, cyst

Medications and Iatrogenic Causes
Oral contraceptives
Hormone replacement therapy
Steroids
Intrauterine devices
Tamoxifen therapy

Systemic Causes
Coagulation disorders
Thyroid disease
Pituitary pathology (hyperprolactinemia)
Hepatic disease
Renal disease
Polycystic ovarian syndrome
Excessive weight loss or gain
Stress

dilation and curettage is usually indicated. The woman with trauma-related vaginal bleeding that cannot be controlled by packing or conservative measures should be admitted for examination and repair under general anesthesia.

When fever is present, evaluate for pelvic infections, sexually transmitted diseases, and urinary tract infections. If PID is suspected, treatment is started in the ED.

The management of DUB includes both the management of hemorrhage if present and diagnosis of the underlying cause. Hormonal therapy is the preferred initial therapy for women with DUB. The specific treatment is dependent on whether it is used to control an acute heavy bleeding episode or whether it is used for control of recurrent bleeding episodes (Table 24.2).

Patients experiencing acute and heavy bleeding need consultation by a gynecologist. In younger patients (puberty and adolescence), treatment is generally initiated with nonsteroidal antiinflammatory agents that improve platelet aggregation and increase uterine vasoconstriction.

ED management of uterine fibroids is related to complications such as excessive blood loss or infection. Gynecological consultation is necessary for excessive bleeding that may require a dilation and curettage. Definitive treatment is a hysterectomy.

Patients with postmenopausal bleeding should be presumed to have endometrial carcinoma until proven otherwise. In such patients, referral to the gynecologist for further evaluation is essential even when the workup has been started in the ED.

Table 24.2.

Treatment options for dysfunctional uterine bleeding

Acute Dysfunctional Bleeding
Medical Treatment
Conjugated estrogens (Premarin) 25 mg q4–6 hours IV, until bleeding slows (maximum of four doses); po therapy may be initiated as an alternative—conjugated estrogen 2.5 mg qid.
Oral contraceptives should be initiated concurrently. Prescribe a 21-day package of oral contraceptives, containing 35 µg of estrogen, one pill tid for 7 days. Heavy cramping and withdrawal bleeding start 2–4 days after regimen is completed. On day 5 of withdrawal flow, begin daily-low dose combination BCP.
Alternatively, medroxyprogesterone (Provera), 10–20 mg/day for days 16–25 of each monthly cycle.

Surgical Treatment
Dilation and curettage
Endometrial ablation
Hysterectomy

Chronic Dysfunctional Bleeding
Medical Treatment
Cyclic oral contraception.
Medroxyprogesterone (Provera), 10–20 mg/day for days 16–25

Surgical Treatment
Endometrial ablation
Hysterectomy

Additional Therapy
Nonsteroidal antiinflammatory drugs: mefenamic acid 500 mg tid for 3 days during menstruation, or naproxen 250 mg tid for 3 days during menstruation, or ibuprofen 400–600 mg tid during menstruation

BCP, birth control pills; IV, intravenous; po, by mouth; qid, four times a daily; tid, three times daily.

Vaginal bleeding that is related to coagulopathy usually is secondary to von Willebrand's disease. Patients with von Willebrand's disease are initially treated with desmopressin (DDAVP). The usual dose is 0.3 µg/kg IV or subcutaneous (SQ) with a 30-µg maximum dose. Consultation with internal medicine or a hematologist is appropriate.

When an intrauterine device (IUD) has been identified as the cause of heavy vaginal bleeding, treatment is removal of the IUD. Patients taking oral contraceptives who experience breakthrough bleeding, but have a hematocrit within normal limits, should be reassured and referred for further evaluation by a gynecologist.

Disposition

Many treatments for abnormal vaginal bleeding are beyond the scope of the ED. Seek emergency gynecological consultation for patients requiring hemodynamic stabilization for admission to a surgical intensive care unit (ICU) and for those going directly to the operating room for a definitive procedure. In addition, a gynecologist should be consulted in most instances of medical management. Patients with PID who need IV antibiotic therapy are admitted. Most importantly, follow-up with a gynecologist or primary care physician must be arranged for all patients with abnormal vaginal bleeding.

Pathophysiology

An understanding of normal menstruation is necessary for evaluating the complaint of abnormal vaginal bleeding. Menstruation is usually established by age 13 and continues until approximately age 50. Once established at puberty, for most women the cycle will remain regular until menopause approaches. Normal menstrual cycles are defined as an interval between the first day of bleeding in one menstrual cycle and the first day of bleeding in the next menstrual cycle. A menstrual cycle is generally 28 days in length, with duration of flow lasting an average of 4 days; total menstrual blood loss on average is 40 mL per cycle. Table 24.3 displays the characteristics of the normal menstrual cycle. In the first part of the cycle, estrogen halts menstrual flow and promotes endometrial proliferation. After ovulation, progesterone stops endometrial growth, then promotes differentiation. If pregnancy does not occur, the corpus luteum regresses, and progesterone production falls, leading the endometrium to shed its lining with subsequent menstrual bleeding. Cycling is the result of a complex interaction of the hypothalamus, anterior pituitary gland, ovary, and endometrium. Dysfunction at any level can disrupt the menstrual cycle. Abnormal bleeding should be considered in terms of a deviation from an individual patient's established menstrual pattern.

In assessing these patients, it is helpful to place a woman in one of three categories: premenopausal (reproductive age), perimenopausal, or postmenopausal.

Premenopausal Bleeding

When evaluating the premenopausal woman with abnormal vaginal bleeding, the first step is assessment of the patient's pregnancy

Table 24.3.			
Qualities of normal menstrual cycle			
Characteristic	Average	Normal Range	Abnormal
Length	28 days	21–35 days	<21 or >35 days
Duration	4 days	1–8 days	>8 days
Total blood loss	40 mL	20–80 mL	>80 mL or <20mL

status. In the nonpregnant premenopausal woman, the most common cause of vaginal bleeding is DUB. DUB is abnormal bleeding not caused by pelvic pathological conditions, medications, systemic disease, or pregnancy; it is a diagnosis of exclusion. DUB is usually related to one of three hormonal imbalances: estrogen breakthrough bleeding, estrogen withdrawal bleeding, or progesterone breakthrough bleeding. Estrogen breakthrough bleeding occurs when excessive estrogen stimulates the endometrium to proliferate in an undifferentiated manner. Without sufficient progesterone to provide structural support, portions of the endometrial lining slough at irregular intervals. The usual progesterone-induced vasoconstriction does not take place, often resulting in profuse bleeding.

Estrogen withdrawal bleeding results from a sudden decrease in estrogen levels, whereas progesterone withdrawal bleeding is a result of a high progesterone-to-estrogen ratio. The endometrium becomes atrophic and ulcerated because of lack of estrogen and is susceptible to frequent, irregular bleeding. Ovulatory DUB is generally excessive bleeding associated with progesterone withdrawal, with a predictable cyclic menses.

Anovulatory DUB occurs in the absence of a cyclic production of progesterone and generally results in amenorrhea and intermittent bleeding that is irregular in timing and volume. Anovulation is the most common cause of DUB in women of reproductive age.

Perimenopausal Bleeding

Women approaching menopause experience shortened cycles with lighter flow and often become intermittently anovulatory. These changes are the result of a decline in the number of ovarian follicles and in estrogen levels. As follicles decrease in number, the level of follicle-stimulating hormone needed to stimulate ovulation increases. All perimenopausal women with persistent abnormal bleeding should be evaluated for the presence of endometrial hyperplasia or carcinoma.

Postmenopausal Bleeding

Five percent to 10% of all postmenopausal women with bleeding are found to have endometrial carcinoma. Women receiving HRT often present with abnormal bleeding, and 30% of these women have uterine pathological conditions. Women receiving sequential HRT may experience midcycle breakthrough bleeding as a result of missed pills, medication interactions, or malabsorption. If unscheduled bleeding occurs for two or more cycles, further evaluation is indicated. With continuous combined HRT, up to 40% of women will have irregular bleeding for 4 to 6 months after initiation of therapy.

Causes of Bleeding in Women of All Ages

Potential causes of bleeding related to pelvic pathological conditions are found in women of all ages. Cervical cancer, cervicitis (secondary to trichomonas or bacterial vaginosis), and cervical polyps may cause bleeding. Cervical polyps can cause light intermenstrual vaginal bleeding and postcoital bleeding. Polyps are generally small, red, friable, pedunculated tumors that protrude from the cervical canal. Other pelvic pathological conditions include endometrial atrophy, uterine leiomyomas, endometrial hyperplasia, adenomyosis, and endometrial polyps. Uterine leiomyomas (fibroids) are smooth muscle tumors that are the most common benign tumor of the female genital tract. Uterine fibroids occur in more than one fifth of white women older than 40 years; they occur more frequently and at an earlier age in black women. Abnormal bleeding related to uterine fibroids tends to be cyclic secondary to interference with endometrial shedding. Fibroids frequently cause excessive and prolonged menstrual periods (menorrhagia).

Vaginal bleeding secondary to endometriosis is characterized by the presence of proliferation of endometrial tissue outside of the uterus and is associated with pelvic pain. Ovarian pathological conditions such as tumors and cysts can be associated with menstrual irregularities. Associated symptoms may include pelvic pain, increase in pelvic or abdominal girth, or pressure in the pelvic region.

IUDs commonly cause abnormal vaginal bleeding. An IUD may perforate or erode in-to the endometrium or a blood vessel, resulting in heavy bleeding. Patients on oral contraceptives may experience breakthrough bleeding, particularly patients taking low-dose estrogen. Intermenstrual bleeding may occur as a result of missed pills or drug interactions. The most common interactions occur with phenobarbital, carbamazepine, some penicillins, tetracycline, and trimethoprimsulfamethoxazole. Progesterone-only means of contraception, such as time-released medroxyprogesterone injection, may prolong breakthrough bleeding because of anovulation.

Suggested Readings

American College of Emergency Physicians. Clinical policy for the initial approach to patients presenting with a chief complaint of vaginal bleeding. *Ann Emerg Med* 1997;29: 435–458.

Good AE. Diagnostic options for assessment of postmenopausal bleeding. *Mayo Clin Proc* 1997; 72:345–349.

Hochbaum S. Vaginal bleeding. *Emerg Med Clin North Am* 1987;5:429–441.

Jennings JC. Abnormal uterine bleeding. *Med Clin North Am* 1995;79:1357–1376.

Long CA. Evaluation of patients with abnormal uterine bleeding. *Am J Obstet Gynecol* 1996; 175:784–786.

Munro MG. Medical management of abnormal uterine bleeding. *Obstet Gynecol Clin North Am* 2000;27:287–304.

Shwayder JM. Pathophysiology of abnormal uterine bleeding. *Obstet Gynecol Clin North Am* 2000;27:219–234.

Spencer CP, Cooper AJ, Whitehead MI. Management of abnormal bleeding in women receiving hormone replacement therapy. *BMJ* 1997;315:37–42.

Weber A, Belinson JL, Bradley LD, Piedmonte MR. Vaginal ultrasound versus endometrial biopsy in women with postmenopausal bleeding. *Am J Obstet Gynecol* 1997;177:924–929.

CHAPTER 25

Complications of First Trimester Pregnancy

Robert Dart, MD, Janet Simmons Young, MD

Clinical Scenario

A 28-year-old woman presents with a 3-day history of vaginal bleeding and crampy abdominal pain. The pain is in the suprapubic area. It was mild initially but has increased in intensity. The bleeding started as spotting but over the last few hours has become heavy with clots. She has saturated three pads over the last 2 hours. The patient denies passing any tissue. Her last menstrual period (LMP) was 10 weeks ago and was normal. She had a positive urine home pregnancy test 3 weeks ago but has yet to have her first prenatal visit. This is her third pregnancy. Her two prior pregnancies were uncomplicated, and she has two healthy children.

Past medical history is otherwise negative. She takes no medications and has no drug allergies. She is a nonsmoker, is refraining from alcohol, and does not use any illicit drugs.

On examination, she appears uncomfortable secondary to pain. Vital signs reveal a blood pressure of 130/80 mm Hg, heart rate of 105 beats/minute, respiratory rate of 16 breaths/minute, and a temperature of 98.6°F.

Her abdomen is mildly tender in the suprapubic region without guarding or rebound. On pelvic examination, there is a moderate amount of clotted blood in the vagina without tissue evident. The cervical os is open to palpation. No cervical motion tenderness is present. The uterus is 8 weeks' size and mildly tender. No adnexal mass or tenderness is evident.

The patient's hematocrit is 33 mL/dL. The blood type is A positive. A transvaginal ultrasound scan reveals a low-lying gestational sac containing a 1.5-cm fetal pole without a fetal heart beat. The cervical os is open by ultrasound scan. The patient is seen by the gynecology consultant, who agrees that the patient has a nonviable pregnancy, and elects to perform an electrical dilation and evacuation (D & E) procedure. Postprocedure, the patient is discharged to home in stable condition.

Clinical Evaluation

Introduction

Abdominal pain or vaginal bleeding in the first trimester of pregnancy is a common occurrence and represents approximately 1% of all adult emergency department (ED) visits. The clinician is faced with two main questions: Is the pregnancy intrauterine, and if so, is the pregnancy viable? This chapter discusses the approach taken to answer these important questions.

History

For a complete general obstetric and gynecological history, refer to Chapter 24. In addition to the general history, it is of paramount importance to assess the patient's risks for ectopic pregnancy (EP). These include a prior EP, pelvic inflammatory disease (PID), infertility, intrauterine device (IUD) use, and tubal ligation. In fact, any patient with a history of a tubal ligation who becomes pregnant should be considered to have an EP until proven otherwise.

Nausea and vomiting are common in early pregnancy, affecting more than 50% of women. In most cases, symptoms are mild and do not require specific treatment. However, in 0.5% of pregnancies, symptoms are more severe, leading to dehydration, weight loss, and ketosis, a condition referred to as hyperemesis gravidarum (Chapter 22).

Patients with molar pregnancies most commonly present with vaginal bleeding. The bleeding ranges from mild to profuse and can be intermittent. Symptoms of hyperemesis commonly occur in molar pregnancies. In addition, these patients are at increased risk for pregnancy-induced hypertension or preeclampsia. In fact, the occurrence of preeclampsia before 24 weeks is highly suggestive of a molar pregnancy.

Physical Examination

A thorough approach to the general gynecological examination is covered in Chapter 24 An open internal cervical os is suggestive of spontaneous abortion, either in process or already completed.

Other than visualization of products of conception at the cervical os or identification of a fetal heart beat using a stethoscope or handheld Doppler, no physical examination finding can confirm or exclude EP with certainty. Table 25.1 lists physical examination findings suggestive of this diagnosis.

In patients with molar pregnancy, physical examination may reveal a uterine size that is greater than expected by dates or the absence of fetal heart activity with a uterus that is palpable well above the pubic symphysis.

Diagnostic Evaluation

Laboratory investigation includes a complete blood cell (CBC) count and electrolytes. A dramatic drop in the hemoglobin and hematocrit levels signifies significant blood loss and may alert the clinician to more severe bleeding than initially anticipated. Electrolyte abnormalities, in particular potassium

---

Table 25.1.

History and physical examination findings predictive of ectopic pregnancy (EP)

Variable Name	Odds Ratio (95% CI)
Findings that increase risk of EP	
Pain intensity moderate to severe	3.4 (1.6–7.1)
Pain location lateral	2.2 (1.2–4.0)
Pain quality sharp	2.0 (1.0–4.0)
Presence of CMT	3.3 (1.6–6.6)
Lateral or bilateral abdominal tenderness	2.0 (1.1–3.7)
Lateral or bilateral pelvic tenderness	2.4 (1.3–4.4)
Positive peritoneal signs	7.9 (3.1–20.0)
IUD use within past year	5.0 (1.1–28.0)
History of infertility	5.0 (1.1–28.0)
History of pelvic surgery	2.0 (1.0–4.3)
History of tubal ligation	18.0 (3.0–139)
Findings that decrease risk of EP	
Pain midline	.31 (.14–.66)
Uterine size on examination > 8 weeks	.42 (.19–.96)

CI, confidence interval; CMT, cervical motion tenderness; IUD, intrauterine device.
From Dart R, Kaplan B, Varaklis K. Predictive value of history and physical exam in patients with suspected ectopic pregnancy. *Ann Emerg Med* 1999;33:283–290. Printed with permission.

level, glucose level, and renal function, are especially important in the vomiting patient. If the patient's blood type is not on file, you must send a sample to confirm that she is not Rh negative (Rh⁻) and thus at risk for fetal hemolysis. In addition, having the blood type on file is important should a surgical emergency arise requiring rapidly available type-specific blood.

Ultrasound has become the study of choice for evaluation of the symptomatic pregnancy. Ultrasound findings can be divided into several categories: diagnostic of an intrauterine pregnancy (IUP); suggestive or diagnostic of an EP; indeterminate for EP; or diagnostic for other conditions in pregnancy including fetal demise, retained products of conception (spontaneous abortion), or gestational trophoblastic disease. Indeterminate ultrasound scan can be further divided into five classes that are helpful in predicting the likelihood of EP and a viable IUP.

During pregnancy, trophoblastic cells produce β-human chorionic gonadotropin (β-hCG). Therefore, in gestational trophoblastic disease, β-hCG levels are often higher than expected based on the expected gestational age of the pregnancy. The characteristic appearance of a molar pregnancy at ultrasound is a grapelike cluster of material within the endometrial cavity. In other cases, molar pregnancy appears less defined and is visible on ultrasound scan as a collection of echogenic material within the endometrial cavity (similar to the presence of retained products of conception after a spontaneous abortion). The performance of a D&E is both diagnostic and therapeutic. Persistently elevated or rising β-hCG values after the procedure suggests the presence of a gestational trophoblastic tumor. In addition, because the lung is one of the primary metastatic sites of this disease, a chest x-ray examination is often used as an initial screening test for choriocarcinoma. Determining levels of β-hCG is also useful in early diagnosis of EP. Modern urine assays can reliably detect β-hCG at levels of 50 mIU/mL. Therefore, as an initial screening test, the accuracy of urine assays approaches that of serum. The urine assay for β-hCG has a small false-negative rate; thus, it is prudent to send a serum assay in

any patient for whom you have a high index of suspicion of having an EP.

Overall, β-hCG values tend to be lower with EP compared with IUP. Studies have found the risk of EP to be up to four times greater in women with β-hCG values less than 1,000 mIU/mL compared with those with β-hCG values above this threshold. Serial β-hCG values can be useful in differentiating EP from IUP in patients with nondiagnostic ultrasound examinations. Patients with β-hCG values that rise by less than 66% are at highest risk for EP. Those with β-hCG values that fall by more than 50% at 48 hours are at low risk. Finally, interpreting the β-hCG rate of change in concert with whether or not the endometrial cavity is empty at transvaginal ultrasound scan further increases diagnostic accuracy (Table 25.2).

Progesterone is produced by the corpus luteum in early pregnancy. Progesterone levels initially rise at the time of ovulation. Progesterone values tend to be higher with a viable IUP compared with a nonviable IUP or an EP. Some centers use progesterone as the initial screening test for EP. Pregnancies with progesterone values greater than 25 ng/mL have a good overall prognosis and a low rate of EP. When the progesterone value is less than 5.0 ng/mL. greater than 99% of pregnancies are nonviable. A low progesterone level does not differentiate between a nonviable IUP and an EP.

Differential Diagnosis

The differential diagnosis for complications of the first trimester of pregnancy are illustrated in Table 25.3.

Treatment

Treatment of bleeding during the first trimester is as varied as the diagnoses. Treatment guidelines are summarized in Table 25.4. All Rh⁻ pregnant women with vaginal bleeding should be given anti-Rh negative immunoglobulin (RhoGAM) to prevent potential fetal hemolysis.

D & E of the uterus, by either vacuum aspiration or curettage, can be particularly useful to differentiate between EP and intrauterine products of conception, especially

Table 25.2.

Predicting ectopic pregnancy[a]

Category	Criteria	Odds Ratio (95% Confidence Intervals)
High risk	β-hCG increase, <66% uterus empty β-hCG decrease, <50% uterus empty β-hCG increase, >66% uterus empty	24.8 (8.9–69.1) 3.7 (1.5–9.1) 2.6 (1.0–7.0)
Intermediate risk	β-hCG increase, <66% uterus not empty	0.8 (0.3–2.5)
Low risk	β-hCG decrease, >50% uterus not empty β-hCG decrease, <50% uterus not empty β-hCG increase, >66% uterus not empty β-hCG decrease, >50% uterus empty	0.0 (0.0–0.9) 0.0 (0.0–0.6) 0.0 (0.0–1.5) 0.2 (0.1–0.9)

β-hCG, β-human chorionic gonadotropin.
[a]Predictions are based on the β-hCG rate of change in concert with whether or not the uterus is empty at ultrasound scan.
From Dart R, Mitterando J, Dart L. Rate of change of serial β-human chorionic gonadotropin values as a predictor of ectopic pregnancy in patients with indeterminate transvaginal ultrasound findings. *Ann Emerg Med* 1999;34:703–710. Printed with permission.

when the possibility of a viable IUP has been excluded or the pregnancy is unwanted. Identification of chorionic villi in the pathological specimen confirms the presence of an

Table 25.3.

Differential diagnosis of bleeding or pain during first trimester

Pregnancy-Related Conditions
Ectopic pregnancy
Molar pregnancy
Isoimmunization (hydrops fetalis)
Abortion: threatened, complete, or incomplete

Gynecological, but Nonpregnancy-Related Conditions
Leiomyomata uteri (fibroids)
Cervical polyps
Cervicitis
Endometriosis
Ruptured corpus luteum or follicular cyst
Salpingitis: acute or chronic
Adnexal torsion

Nongynecological Conditions
Appendicitis
Gastroenteritis
Urinary tract infection
Urolithiasis
Inguinal hernia

IUP. However, absence of chorionic villi is consistent with both EP and a completed abortion. In these cases, a repeat β-hCG test usually clarifies the diagnosis. With a complete abortion, over time, the β-hCG should rapidly fall to zero. With an EP, over time, the β-hCG value falls slowly or continues to rise.

Traditional D & E is performed using an appropriately sized cannula connected to a collecting apparatus and a vacuum pump. It is the procedure of choice when the age of gestation on ultrasound examination is 8 weeks or greater, but it can also be used with a smaller volume of endometrial contents. Because cervical dilation is often required, this procedure is typically performed using a paracervical block along with intravenous and/or inhalation anesthesia.

Ectopic Pregnancy

The two most common therapeutic interventions for EP are surgical management or medical treatment with methotrexate. Surgery can be performed via laparotomy or laparoscopy. If future fertility is not desired or if tubal rupture has occurred, then the affected tube is typically removed (salpingectomy). Alternatively, salpingotomy can be performed whereby the tube is incised, the

Table 25.4.

Treatment guidelines for bleeding and pain during first trimester pregnancy

Stable
Laboratory studies: hematocrit level, blood type, quantitative β-hCG
Ultrasound scan: if no prior IUP documented
Anti-Rh⁻ immunoglobulin by 72 hours if bleeding and Rh⁻
D & E: unwanted pregnancy or nonviable IUP

> Look for chorionic villi in tissue sample to rule out ectopic pregnancy
>
> If no chorionic villi, repeat β-hCG in 48 hours to confirm value is falling
>
> Stable or rising, repeat β-hCG, consider ectopic pregnancy

Suspected/Confirmed Ectopic Pregnancy
Consideration of methotrexate
Consideration of salpingectomy

Nonviable IUP
Expectant management
Consideration of D & E
Consideration of intravaginal misoprostol

Molar Pregnancy
Serial β-hCG assays for 1 year
No further pregnancy desired and nonmetastatic, then hysterectomy
Desired future pregnancy or metastatic, consideration of chemotherapy
  (methotrexate, actinomycin D)

Unstable
Documented ruptured ectopic with free fluid (blood) in pelvis, low BP, tachycardia

> Two large-bore IV catheters
>
> Normal saline running "wide open" IV to keep BP >100 mm Hg
>
> Continuous cardiac monitor and vital signs monitor
>
> Type and cross-match blood (2 units typically)
>
> Complete blood count and electrolyte levels
>
> Emergent gynecology consultation
>
> Emergent salpingectomy in operating room

β-hCG, β-human chorionic gonadotropin; BP, blood pressure; D & E, dilation and evacuation; IUP, intrauterine pregnancy; IV, intravenous.

EP is expressed out, and the affected tube left in place.

Methotrexate is the agent most commonly used for medical treatment of EP. It is a structural analogue of folic acid, which inhibits the formation of nucleotides that are necessary for DNA and RNA synthesis. Rapidly dividing cells are particularly susceptible. Studies find the success rate to be 95% in patients with β-hCG values less than 5,000 mIU/mL but only 76% in patients with β-hCG values above this level.

Nonviable Intrauterine Pregnancy

Several options are available for managing patients with a nonviable IUP. These include expectant management, manual aspiration, vacuum evacuation, and medical management. The choice depends on the amount of bleeding, the volume of intrauterine contents visualized by ultrasound, and the patient's hemodynamic status and personal preference. Patients with persistent heavy bleeding or hemodynamic instability should undergo urgent uterine evacuation. In the remaining patients, the timing of uterine evacuation depends on the availability of resources to perform this procedure, and it could be done on a semielective basis.

Medical management of the nonviable pregnancy has developed as an offshoot of research using chemotherapeutic agents to induce therapeutic abortions. To be eligible, the gestation must be less than 8 weeks old by ultrasound scan. Intravaginal misoprostol, a prostaglandin analogue, is most commonly used for this indication. Misoprostol works by speeding cervical dilatation and initiating uterine contractions, thereby leading to expulsion of the products of conception.

Expectantly managed patients are followed without intervention, with the assumption that the body will naturally expel the remaining products of conception. Manual vacuum aspiration is performed with a vacuum-locked syringe attached to a plastic cannula. The vacuum in the syringe provides the necessary suction to evacuate the uterus. Vacuum evacuation is performed using a cannula attached to a vacuum pump. Some clinicians use the term *electrical evacuation* to distinguish vacuum aspiration using a pump from manual evacuation using a syringe.

Molar Pregnancy

Patients in whom β-hCG levels fall to zero do not require further treatment; however, their β-hCG levels should be followed serially and they should practice pregnancy prophylaxis for 1 year. Patients with persistently elevated β-hCG levels, no evidence of metastatic disease, and no desire for future fertility are best managed by hysterectomy. Patients with a desire for future fertility or with evidence of metastatic disease can be managed with chemotherapy. Methotrexate

and actinomycin D are the two most commonly used chemotherapeutic agents.

Disposition

Patients who are diagnosed with EP are admitted to a gynecology service. Identified ruptured EP is a surgical emergency, because the patient is at risk for life-threatening hemorrhage, and the patient should be taken to the operating room (OR) immediately.

Patients with suspected EP who are managed expectantly should be scheduled for follow-up in 72 hours with a repeat ultrasound scan and quantitative β-hCG assay. If the sac has passed at follow-up imaging, no further workup is required. If the sac persists, then alternative management options should be considered.

Patients with impending or incomplete abortions who do not have definitive therapy in the hospital should be instructed to return if, after several hours, they are saturating more than one pad an hour with blood or have persistent severe pain.

Pathophysiology

Early Pregnancy Development

Egg fertilization takes place in the fallopian tube approximately 48 hours after ovulation. The fertilized egg continues down the fallopian tube and into the endometrial cavity, undergoing several cell divisions along the way. Approximately 7 days after fertilization, the zygote implants into the endometrial cavity of the uterus. It is at this point that β-hCG production starts. About 21 to 24 days after fertilization, a gestational sac can be identified within the endometrial cavity; at 28 to 35 days, a fetal pole with a fetal heartbeat can be visualized by transvaginal ultrasound scan.

Complications in the first trimester of pregnancy are common. Overall, 50% of all conceptions are lost. In some cases, the fertilized ovum fails to undergo normal cleavage and never implants, whereas others achieve implantation but undergo early abortion before being clinically recognized. In addition, approximately 10% to 20% of clinically recognized pregnancies end in spontaneous abortion.

Ectopic Pregnancy

An EP is a fertilized ovum that implants at a site other than the endometrial cavity of the uterus. Approximately 95% of EPs implant in the fallopian tube, most commonly in the ampullary portion. Other implantation sites include the ovary, abdominal cavity, and cervix. Interstitial EPs implant at the junction of the uterus and the fallopian tube. This area is highly vascular, and interstitial EPs are often large and grow rapidly, with a high propensity to rupture.

Molar Pregnancy

Trophoblasts are embryonic cells that give rise to a large part of the placenta. The remaining maternal portion of the placenta is derived from the endometrial lining of the uterus. Gestational trophoblastic disease involves a spectrum of pregnancy-related trophoblastic abnormalities including hydatidiform mole and gestational trophoblastic tumors. The incidence is approximately 1 in 1,000 pregnancies. Women older than 45 years have a 10-fold higher relative risk compared with women in the 20- to 40-year age range.

If a fetus or an embryo is present, the hydatidiform mole is classified as partial; if an embryo is absent, the mole is classified as complete. The two major types of gestational trophoblastic tumors are invasive moles and choriocarcinomas. Both conditions tend to be locally invasive with penetration by trophoblastic elements into the myometrium of the uterus. The distinguishing feature of choriocarcinoma is the propensity of this condition to metastasize. Gestational trophoblastic tumors invariably develop after a molar pregnancy, a normal IUP, or an abortion or EP.

Although histological features have been used to characterize these disorders, these features have not been shown to directly correlate with malignant potential. Risk factors that suggest a poor prognosis include a pretherapy β-hCG level greater than 40,000 mIU/mL, persistence of lesions greater than 4 months, brain or liver metastases, prior chemotherapeutic failure, or a prior antecedent term pregnancy.

Rh Incompatibility

Some transfer of fetal red blood cells into the maternal circulation often occurs during pregnancy. The potential for transfer is higher in mothers with vaginal bleeding, EP, or molar pregnancy. An Rh⁻ mother who is carrying an Rh⁺ fetus develops antibodies to the fetus's red blood cells, recognizing the Rh⁺ factor as a foreign antigen. If the mother then has a subsequent pregnancy with another Rh⁺ fetus, the anti-Rh⁺ antibodies can cross into the fetal circulation, leading to severe fetal hemolysis (hydrops fetalis). Women with first trimester bleeding, EP, or molar pregnancy must have their blood type checked, and all who are Rh⁻ must be administered anti-Rh immunoglobulin (RhoGAM). This has been demonstrated to decrease the likelihood of maternal isoimmunization to fetal red blood cells.

Suggested Readings

Bashiri A, Neumann L, Maymon E, Katz M. Hyperemesis gravidarum: epidemiologic features, complications and outcome. *Eur J Obstet Gynecol* 1995;63:135–138.

Dart R, Mitterando J, Dart L. Rate of change of serial β-human chorionic gonadotropin values as a predictor of ectopic pregnancy in patients with indeterminate transvaginal ultrasound findings. *Ann Emerg Med* 1999;34:703–710.

Dart R, Howard K. Subclassification of indeterminate pelvic ultrasonograms: stratifying the risk of ectopic pregnancy. *Acad Emerg Med* 1998;5:313–319.

Dart R, Kaplan B, Varaklis K. Predictive value of history and physical exam in patients with suspected ectopic pregnancy. *Ann Emerg Med* 1999;33:283–290.

Herabutya Y, Prasertsawat P. Misoprostol in the management of missed abortion. *Int J Gynecol Obstet* 1997;56:263–266.

Hammond CB, Borchert I, Tyrey I, et al. Treatment of metastatic gestational trophoblastic disease: good and poor prognosis. *Am J Obstet Gynecol* 1973;451:1973–1978.

Lipscomb GH, McCord ML, Stovall TG, et al. Predictors of success of methotrexate treatment in women with tubal ectopic pregnancies. *N Engl J Med* 2000;341:1974–1978.

McCord M, Muram D, Buster J, et al. Single serum progesterone as a screen for ectopic pregnancy: exchanging specificity and sensitivity to obtain optimal test performance. *Fertil Steril* 1996;66:513–516.

Pelvic Infections

Robert Dart, MD, Rebecca Steinberg, MD

Clinical Scenario

A 20-year-old woman, $G_2P_0Ab_2$, presents to the emergency department complaining of lower abdominal pain and fever for 2 days. Her symptoms actually started several days earlier with a greenish vaginal discharge and midline low pelvic pain. She has had sexually transmitted diseases (STDs) in the past, has two male sexual partners, and does not use any contraception. She tested negative for human immunodeficiency virus (HIV) 3 months ago and denies alcohol or drug use. Her appetite is normal, as are her urinary and bowel habits. She has no other past medical history, is on no medications, and has no medication allergies.

Physical examination reveals a temperature of 101.1°F, pulse of 98 beats/minute, respiratory rate of 12 breaths/minute, blood pressure of 110/67 mm Hg, and O_2 saturation of 98% on room air. Her lungs are clear; heart sounds normal; and she has no pharyngeal exudates, redness, or skin rashes. Abdominal examination reveals suprapubic tenderness and bilateral low pelvic tenderness. There is mild bilateral guarding without rebound. Pelvic speculum examination reveals a green exudate at the cervical os; there is cervical motion tenderness and bilateral adnexal tenderness on bimanual examination, left more so than right. The complete blood cell (CBC) count is 15,000/mm^3 with a predominance of neutrophils. The serum pregnancy test is negative, and an ultrasound scan shows a small amount of free fluid in the pelvis, thickened fluid-filled tubes, and no evidence of adnexal masses to suggest an abscess. A glass slide cervical smear reveals gram-negative diplococci. The patient is admitted for observation and intravenous antibiotics with a presumptive diagnosis of gonococcal pelvic inflammatory disease (PID). She is released the next day on oral antibiotics and pain medications without fever and with improving symptoms.

Clinical Evaluation

Introduction

PID is commonly encountered in the United States. More than 1 million women are treated each year. This number probably underestimates the disease's true prevalence, because many women with acute PID are asymptomatic, or experience mild or atypical symptoms, and are not diagnosed unless they have advanced disease. Therefore, one fourth of women with PID will develop chronic pelvic pain, suffer from infertility, or will go on to have an ectopic pregnancy. PID and its sequelae account for as much as $1.6 to $1.9 billion of direct medical costs in the United States.

History

Pelvic Inflammatory Disease

As in all women patients with pelvic complaints, the history includes a detailed gynecological history (Chapter 24). Symptoms of PID include abdominal pain, vaginal discharge, fever, postcoital pain or bleeding, and intermenstrual bleeding. On occasion, upper abdominal pain may develop if the infection has spread to the perihepatic spaces. Women with periurethral involvement may develop urinary urgency, frequency, or dysuria. Women are most susceptible to development of PID in the first 7 days after onset of menstruation, because the onset of menstruation provides an opportunity for a cervical infection to spread into the endometrial cavity.

Pay special attention to PID risk factors when obtaining the history. Multiple sexual partners, frequent intercourse, and a recent new sexual partner put the patient at increased risk. A patient is at three times greater risk to develop PID if her first sexual intercourse was before the age of 15. Contraceptive practices also affect the risk of developing PID. Barrier contraceptive methods protect against STDs and are protective against PID. Oral contraceptive use does not clearly show a protective effect; however, some studies support this view. Use of an intrauterine device (IUD) increases the incidence of PID during the first 4 months after insertion but returns to baseline by 5 months and beyond. Use of douching products increases PID risk, particularly if the product is used more than three times per month. Finally, a prior history of any STD increases a patient's future risk of having PID.

Vulvovaginitis

Infectious causes of vulvovaginitis include bacterial vaginosis, candidiasis, and trichomoniasis. Patients with bacterial vaginosis typically report a malodorous vaginal discharge. Symptoms of vaginal irritation or pain typically are not prominent. Symptoms of candidal vaginitis include vaginal itching, irritation or pain, burning with urination, pain with intercourse, and increased vaginal discharge. Symptoms of trichomonal infection range from an asymptomatic carrier state in up to 50% of women to severe acute inflammatory disease. A malodorous discharge is noted in about 50% to 75% of patients and about 25% to 50% report severe pruritus. About 50% of women report pain with intercourse. Women often report urinary frequency or dysuria because this organism often resides in the urethra and the adjacent Skene's glands.

Causes of noninfectious vaginitis include a hypersensitivity reaction from skin irritants and atrophic vaginitis. Hypersensitivity vaginitis typically occurs as an allergic reaction to a vaginal cream being used for another condition. Management should be directed at eliminating the offending agent. Irritant vaginitis often occurs in the young or elderly secondary to prolonged contact of urine against the perineal skin. Often the findings in these cases are more prominent on the external genitalia than on the vaginal mucosa. Atrophic vaginitis typically occurs in postmenopausal women. Because of reduced endogenous estrogen, the epithelium becomes thin and lacking in glycogen. This results in reduced lactic acid production and an increase in vaginal pH, encouraging bacterial overgrowth.

Genital Ulcers

Sexually transmitted organisms cause most genital ulcers. In the United States, the most common causes of genital ulcers are herpes simplex, syphilis, and chancroid. Although not common in the United States, lymphogranuloma venereum (LGV) and granuloma inguinale occur frequently in developing countries and should be considered in patients who have recently resided in an endemic area.

Approximately 22% of the U.S. population is infected with genital herpes. Of these, 75% are asymptomatic. Symptoms include labial burning or pain and pain from enlarged lymph nodes. Patients often have recurrent outbreaks and, therefore, may give a history of prior episodes. Patients with primary syphilis typically present with a complaint of a solitary painless genital ulcer. Chancroid is caused by the organism *Haemophilus ducreyi*, an unencapsulated gram-negative rod. An inflammatory papule initially develops at the inoculation site. It then erodes into a deep ulcer with ragged margins and a yellowish gray exudate. Granuloma inguinale is caused by *Calymmatobacterium granulomatis*, a gram-negative rod. The lesions are often multiple, painless, and irregular with a clean base. Often the borders of the ulcers are rolled up. The lesion is highly vascular, which gives the ulcer base a beefy red appearance. LGV is caused by *Chlamydia trachomatis*. The primary lesion starts with a small pustule that rapidly ulcerates. One or several ulcers may be seen and may go unnoticed because they are small. The second stage is characterized by the development of unilateral or bilateral bubo formation. A bubo is caused by a number of lymph nodes that coalesce to form a tender mass, several centimeters in diameter.

Physical Examination

Pelvic Inflammatory Disease

Patients with PID typically have bilateral lower abdominal tenderness unless an associated tubo-ovarian abscess (TOA) has developed, in which case a unilateral mass or focal tenderness is present. Peritoneal signs of guarding or rebound are present in approximately 60% of patients and are related to the spread of pus from the fallopian tubes into the peritoneal cavity. Cervical motion tenderness is present in 80% of patients. Vaginal or cervical discharge is identified on speculum examination 70% of the time. Fever is present in approximately 30% of patients. An adnexal mass is identified in 20% of patients and should raise concern for the possibility of a TOA.

Vulvovaginitis

Patients with bacterial vaginosis have a thin gray to white vaginal discharge noted on pelvic examination. The vaginal mucosa otherwise appears normal. Findings with candida vaginitis include vaginal erythema, edema, excoriations, pustule formation, and labial fissures. The discharge often has a cheeselike consistency and does not have a distinctive odor. Trichomonal vulvar findings may be absent but typically include vaginal erythema, edema, and a copious profuse malodorous discharge. The discharge may either be yellow-green or grayish white. A strawberry-like appearance to the cervix is noted in a minority of patients.

Genital Ulcers

On examination, genital herpes appear as clusters of vesicles 2 to 4 mm wide on an erythematous base and may be noted on the labia, cervix, inner thighs, or in the perianal area. Within a few days, these vesicles progress to erosions. In addition, inguinal lymph nodes may be enlarged and tender to palpation. In syphilis, the ulcer is indurated, is nontender, and typically has a clean base. Without treatment, the ulcer typically resolves in 2 to 3 weeks. In some patients, a macular rash involving the trunk, palms, and soles of the feet is also present. This signifies the occurrence of secondary syphilis. Chancroid lesions are tender to palpation. Multiple lesions may be present as the infectious exudate autoinoculates other areas. Tender lymphadenopathy is present in about 30% to 60% of cases. Untreated cases may develop lymphatic obstruction with resulting peripheral and scrotal edema. Granuloma inguinale ulcers are painless and beefy red with rolled up borders. Associated granulomas that may simulate lymph nodes may appear in the skin. Actual lymph node enlargement does not occur unless the lesion becomes secondarily infected. In LGV, a small number of pustules, sometimes ulcerated, may be observed. If they have coalesced around a lymph node, large, fluctuant, tender lymph nodes (buboes) may be observed. If nodes above and below Poupart's ligament are involved, a groove sign typical of this condition may be present. A minority of patients may be systemically ill from hematogenous spread. Lymphatic obstruction develops in a minority of cases. In addition, with rectal involvement, rectal strictures and perianal fistulas may be observed.

Diagnostic Evaluation

Pelvic Inflammatory Disease

No single laboratory test confirms or excludes the diagnosis of PID. Some tests raise the likelihood of the presence of PID if they are positive but do not confirm the diagnosis or need to be present for the patient to have PID. CBC counts greater than $10,000/mm^3$, erythrocyte sedimentation rate greater than

15 mm/hour, a C-reactive protein greater than 5 mg/dL, and/or a vaginal smear with more than three white blood cells (WBC)/high-power field are suggestive of infection and may be used with a physical examination indicative of PID to make the diagnosis.

In women with PID, cervical specimens are positive for either *C. trachomatis* or *Neisseria gonorrhoeae* in up to 70% of patients. Endometrial biopsy or laparoscopy should be considered in patients with an uncertain diagnosis or in patients with suspected PID who fail to improve with 48 to 72 hours of antibiotic therapy. Ultrasound examination may reveal thickened fluid-filled tubes or a TOA. It can also reveal ovarian torsion, ruptured ovarian cysts, ectopic pregnancy, and other nonpelvic pathological conditions. Any of these modalities definitively make the diagnosis of PID. In cases in which the diagnosis remains unclear, and especially with focal tenderness on examination, a computed tomography (CT) scan of the abdomen may be useful. Appendicitis, urolithiasis, and diverticulitis are among the nongynecological diseases that may be found on CT.

Vulvovaginitis

Three criteria can be used to diagnose bacterial vaginosis. First, the pH of the vaginal discharge should be greater than 4.5. Second, the discharge, when mixed with potassium hydroxide, emits a pungent fishy odor. This is termed a positive sniff test. Finally, when the discharge is mixed with saline and viewed under microscopy, clue cells can be identified. Clue cells are epithelial cells that have a fuzzy or moth-eaten appearance and are typically surrounded by a preponderance of bacteria. *Candida* can be diagnosed using routine microscopy of the vaginal discharge dissolved in 10% potassium hydroxide (KOH). Pseudohyphae are found in most cases. However, in about 10% to 30% of cases, microscopic findings are negative for *Candida*. In patients with symptoms and signs consistent with candidal vaginitis but with negative findings on microscopy, the diagnosis can usually be confirmed by vaginal culture. The vaginal pH should be in the 4 to 4.5 range and the sniff test should be negative, unless the patient is coinfected with a second organism. However, these diagnostic tests are mostly academic, because most physicians empirically treat women who present with the characteristic clinical symptoms and signs of candidiasis. With trichomonas, vaginal pH is typically elevated and the sniff test is often positive. Saline wet-mount examination reveals a preponderance of WBCs. In addition, motile trichomonads are directly visualized in approximately 50% to 70% of cases. Cultures of this organism are positive in approximately 95% of cases and should be considered in patients with suggestive findings but a negative wet-mount examination.

Genital Ulcers

Genital herpes are identified using the Tzank preparation on scrapings from genital lesions, which often reveals multinucleated giant cells. In addition, the organism can be cultured using viral media. It is particularly important to make this diagnosis in pregnant patients because the virus may be transmitted to the infant during delivery. *Treponema pallidum* is the spirochete that causes syphilis. A dark-field examination of ulcer scrapings often allows visualization of the offending organism. Serological tests for syphilis such as the rapid plasma reagin (RPR) test and Venereal Disease Research Laboratory (VDRL) test should also be drawn, although these tests are often negative within the first 2 weeks after the ulcer appears. Chancroid is difficult to identify because this organism is hard to culture. Cytological examination of the exudate may reveal the classically described "school of fish," which consists of parallel chains of pleomorphic gram-negative rods. However, this method is neither sensitive nor specific for this condition. Detection of *H. ducreyi* DNA in the ulcer specimen by polymerase chain reaction (PCR) is currently the best method for confirming this diagnosis. There are no routine culture techniques for the organism that causes granuloma inguinale. Cytological diagnosis is difficult and is dependent on visualizing intracytoplasmic inclusion bodies (Donovan bodies) within histiocytes. In LGV, culture of the aspirate from an involved lymph node is the most specific test for confirming this diagnosis.

Differential Diagnosis

The differential diagnosis for pelvic infections is illustrated in Table 26.1.

Treatment

All pelvic infections are treated with antibiotics. Treatment guidelines for PID are listed in Table 26.2. Cervicitis is treated with a single dose regimen of ceftriaxone 125 mg intramuscular (IM) and 1 g of oral azithromycin.

Ceftriaxone can be replaced by oral ciprofloxacin 500 mg once or ofloxacin 400 mg once, and the azithromycin can be substituted by doxycycline 100 mg twice a day for 7 days. Single-dose regimens are preferred to ensure compliance. Administration of 2 g of azithromycin is also an effective single-agent treatment, but it can have poorly tolerated gastrointestinal effects and is not usually prescribed. Uncomplicated PID may be treated with outpatient antibiotics; however, there should be a low threshold to admit these patients because of the risk of future sterility. Medical management occasionally fails, and an abdominal hysterectomy and bilateral salpingo-oophorectomy is required. A ruptured TOA is a surgical emergency. All patients

Table 26.1.

Differential diagnosis for pelvic infections

Pelvic	Nonpelvic
Cervicitis/PID/TOA	*GI*
Gonorrheal infection	Appendicitis
Chlamydial infection	Diverticulitis
Vulvovaginitis	Mesenteric lymphadenitis
Candidal infection	Perforation of hollow viscus
Trichomonas	*GU*
Bacterial vaginosis	Urinary tract infection
Hypersensitivity	Pyelonephritis
Atrophic vaginitis	Urolithiasis
Condyloma acuminatum	
Genital Ulcers	
Herpes simplex	
Syphilis	
Chancroid	
Lymphogranuloma venereum	
Granuloma inguinale	

GI, gastrointestinal; GU, genitourinary; PID, pelvic inflammatory disease; TOA, tubo-ovarian abscess.

Table 26.2.

CDC guidelines for the treatment of PID

Recommended
Oral
Ofloxacin 400 mg bid for 14 days PLUS Metronidazole 500 mg bid for 14 days

IV
Cefotetan 2 g every 12 hours or cefoxitin 2 g every 6 hours PLUS doxycycline
   100 mg every 12 hours

Alternative
Oral
Doxycycline 100 mg twice daily for 14 days PLUS a single dose of one of the
   following: ceftriaxone 250 mg IM, cefoxitin 2 gm IM with probenecid 1 g
   po, or other third-generation cephalosporin IM

IV
Clindamycin 900 mg every 8 hours PLUS gentamicin 2 mg/kg load, then
   1.5 mg/kg every 8 hours

bid, twice daily; CDC, Centers for Disease Control and Prevention; IM, intramuscular; IV, intravenous; PID, pelvic inflammatory disease; po, by mouth.
From Centers for Disease Control and Prevention. 1998 Treatment guidelines for treatment of sexually transmitted diseases. *MMWR Morb Mortal Wkly Rep* 1998;47.

with STDs must be instructed to have their partner evaluated and treated as well.

Treatment guidelines for vulvovaginitis are listed in Table 26.3. A single dose of

Table 26.3.

Treatment of infectious vaginitis[a]

Bacterial vaginosis
Metronidazole 500 mg orally bid for 7 days
Clindamycin cream 2%, 5 g intravaginally at
   bedtime for 7 days
Metronidazole cream 0.75% 5 g intravaginally
   bid for 5 days

Candida vaginitis
Fluconazole 150 mg po for 1 dose
Miconazole 200 mg vaginal suppositories at
   bedtime for 3 days
Butoconazole 2% intravaginally at bedtime for
   3 days

Trichomoniasis
Metronidazole 2 g po as a single dose

bid, twice daily; po, by mouth
[a]A single drug should be used to treat each condition.

150 mg of fluconazole is often as effective as several intravaginal insertions of antifungal cream. Metronidazole comes in an intravaginal cream and in an oral preparation for bacterial vaginosis. For treatment of noninfectious vaginitis, vaginal estrogen cream is used at bedtime.

Treatment guidelines for genital ulcers are listed in Table 26.4. Failure to recognize, diagnose, and treat a syphilitic chancre will lead to the patient developing secondary syphilis, which may be more difficult to discern, because the only sign may be a mild maculopapular rash. Although two thirds of patients will not progress, tertiary syphilis manifests as either gumma or granulomatous degeneration of the large arteries; the most catastrophic manifestation is involvement of the vasa vasorum of the aorta, which can lead to dissection. If vessels in the central nervous system are involved, severe neurological damage may result.

Disposition

Indications for hospital admission for patients with PID include uncertain diagnosis,

Table 26.4.

Treatment of genital ulcers[a]

Herpes Simplex: Primary Infection
Acyclovir 400 mg po tid for 7–10 days
Famciclovir 250 mg po tid for 7–10 days
Valacyclovir 1 g po bid for 7–10 days

Herpes Simplex: Episodic Recurrences
Acyclovir 400 mg po tid for 5 days
Famciclovir 250 mg po bid for 5 days
Valacyclovir 1 g po bid for 5 days

Syphilis
Benzathine penicillin G 2.4 million units IM for
   1 dose
Doxycycline 100 mg po twice daily for 14 days
   (penicillin-allergic patient)

Chancroid
Azithramycin 1 g po
Ceftriaxone 250 mg IM for 1 dose

Lymphogranuloma Venereum
Doxycycline 100 mg po bid for 21 days

Granuloma Inguinale
Trimethoprim-sulfamethoxazole double strength
   po bid for minimum of 3 weeks
Doxycycline 100 mg po bid for a minimum of
   3 weeks

bid, twice daily; IM, intramuscular; po, by mouth; tid,
three times daily.
[a]A single drug should be used to treat each condition.

pregnancy, failure to respond to outpatient therapy within 48 hours, presence of an IUD, evidence of a TOA, or an immunocompromised or poorly compliant patient. In addition, inpatient therapy should be considered in patients who are unable to tolerate oral fluids, have a high temperature, or exhibit upper peritoneal signs. Bacterial vaginosis and infectious ulcers can all be treated with outpatient therapy. Patients must be instructed on safe sexual practices until treatment is completed, and beyond, for prevention of HIV and hepatitis and recurrent STDs or PID, which can cause sterility by scarring the fallopian tubes.

Pathophysiology

Pelvic Inflammatory Disease

PID is the result of an ascending infection, which begins in the cervix and vagina and then extends into the upper reproductive tract, including the uterus and its ligaments, the uterine tubes, and the ovaries.

Most cases of PID are sexually transmitted and start with a cervical infection that ascends into the endometrial cavity. Studies show that young women have a lower prevalence of protective antibodies against the bacteria that cause PID. Young women also have more penetrable cervical mucus and have larger areas of the ectocervix in which columnar epithelia dominate. Endometritis or infection of the endometrial cavity is diagnosed histopathologically by identification of plasma cells in the endometrial stroma. Later, salpingitis, or inflammation of the uterine tubes, proceeds. Acute complications of salpingitis include pyosalpinx, a collection of pus in the oviduct, or a TOA. Ultimately, a perihepatic infection may develop as a result of the continuous ascending infection. Significant scarring of the fallopian tubes can cause sterility and put the woman at higher risk for future ectopic pregnancy.

The most predominant organisms in PID are *N. gonorrhoeae* and *C. trachomatis.* Although *N. gonorrhoeae* and *Chlamydia* are believed to be the inciting organisms in most cases, the infection is polymicrobial. Other organisms involved in the infectious process are *Mycoplasma hominis; Ureaplasma urealyticum;* genital *Mycoplasma* organisms; facultative aerobic bacteria such as *E. coli,* group *B. streptococcus, Gardnerella vaginalis,* and *Haemophilus influenza;* and anaerobic bacteria such as *Peptostreptococcus* and *Bacteroides* species. In approximately 15% of women with PID, no identifiable organism is isolated from the upper genital tract.

Bacterial Vaginosis

Bacterial vaginosis is the cause of approximately 40% to 50% of the cases of infectious vulvovaginitis. Organisms associated with this infection include *Gardnerella vaginalis,* *M. hominis,* and *Mobiluncus* species and other anaerobic gram-positive cocci. The pH of the healthy vagina is less than 4.5 because of the production of lactic acid by *Lactobacillus* species. *Lactobacillus* species are present in the vaginal flora of 96% of normal women but are found in only 6% of women with bacterial vaginosis. It is thought that the rise of vaginal pH secondary to the absence of *Lactobacillus* contributes to the bacterial overgrowth found with this condition. Although high rates of bacterial vaginosis have been reported from STD clinics, it is unclear whether sexual transmission plays a role in this condition.

Bacterial vaginosis is a risk factor for miscarriage and premature birth in the pregnant patient and increased infectious morbidity following cesarean section or gynecological surgery. In addition, it may predispose women to acquire sexually transmitted infections, including HIV.

Candidiasis

Candidal vaginitis accounts for approximately 20% to 25% of cases of infectious vaginitis. *Candida albicans* is responsible for 80% to 95% of candidal vaginitis. *Candida glabrata* is the second most common candidal species. Candidal species are present in the vaginal flora of 10% to 15% of asymptomatic women at any given time. It is postulated that overgrowth of this organism leads to the development of symptoms. Factors contributing to overgrowth of this fungus include use of broad-spectrum antibiotics, oral contraceptives, and corticosteroids and pregnancy, diabetes, and other factors that affect the immune response. Sexual transmission is not believed to be a causative factor.

Candidal species adhere to vaginal epithelial cells and, therefore, cause more vaginal inflammation than other organisms.

Trichomoniasis

Trichomonas is a flagellated protozoan organism that accounts for approximately 15% to 20% of cases of infectious vaginitis.

Trichomonas is almost always sexually transmitted. It frequently occurs concurrently with gonococcal infection and bacterial vaginosis. Trichomonas produces hydrogen ions, which combine with oxygen, thus removing oxygen from the environment. This is believed to promote growth of anaerobic organisms. In addition, the flagellar action of trichomonads is thought to help push pathogenic bacteria into the upper genital tract, increasing the risk for a patient to develop PID. As with bacterial vaginosis, this condition is associated with an increased risk of premature rupture of membranes in pregnant women and postoperative infections in women undergoing gynecological surgery.

Genital Ulcers

All conditions causing genital ulcers are a result of direct transmission through sexual intercourse. The organism C. *granulomatis* causes granuloma inguinale. Syphilis is due to the spirochetal organism *T. pallidum.* Chancroid is caused by the bacteria *H. ducreyi.* LGV is caused by C. *trachomatis.* Although herpes simplex type 2 is the primary virus causing genital ulcers, herpes simplex type 1 can also be found in individuals who practice orogenital intercourse. It is thought that congential herpes infections are passed to the fetus during actual vulvar-fetal contact during delivery rather than via the placenta.

Suggested Readings

Centers for Disease Control and Prevention. 1998 guidelines for treatment of sexually transmitted diseases. *MMWR* 1998;47(RR-1): 1–118.

Eschenbach D, Wolner-Hanssen P, Hawes S, et al. Acute pelvic inflammatory disease: associations of clinical and laboratory findings with laparoscopic findings. *Obstet Gynecol* 1997;89: 184–192.

Jacobson L, Westrom L. Objectivized diagnosis of acute pelvic inflammatory disease. *Am J Obstet Gynecol* 1969;105:1088–1098.

Peipert J, Boardman L, Hogan J, et al. Laboratory evaluation of acute upper genital tract infection. *Obstet Gynecol* 1996;87:730–736.

Quan, M. Pelvic inflammatory disease: diagnosis and management. *JABFP* 1994;7:110–123.

Rosen T, Brown T. Genital ulcers. Evaluation and treatment. *Dermatol Clin* 1998;16:673–685.

Schaaf V, Perez-Stable E, Borchardt K. The limited value of symptoms and signs in the diagnosis of vaginal infections. *Arch Intern Med* 1990; 150:1929–1933.

Sobel J. Vulvovaginitis in healthy women. *Comp Ther* 1999;25:335–346.

Pelvic Pain

Robert Dart, MD

Clinical Scenario

A 35-year-old woman comes to the emergency department (ED) with a complaint of abdominal pain and vaginal bleeding. Her last menstrual period was 6 weeks ago. She missed her expected period but has been having vaginal bleeding at a rate of three pads per day over the last few days. Her pain is a dull ache in her left lower quadrant. It has become more severe over the last 24 hours, and she has now developed pain and pressure in her rectal area. In the past she has had one pregnancy that ended in a miscarriage at 7 weeks' gestation. She has been trying to get pregnant over the last 3 years without success. She has no other past medical history, is not taking any medications, and has no drug allergies.

On physical examination her vital signs are a blood pressure of 120/80 mm Hg, a heart rate of 90 beats/minute, a respiratory rate of 16 breaths/minute, and a temperature of 98.6° F. Her lungs are clear and her heart sounds are regular without murmurs. Her abdomen is soft, with bilateral lower quadrant tenderness, left greater than right. On pelvic examination, a small amount of blood without clots is in the vaginal vault, and the cervical os is closed to palpation. There is cervical motion tenderness and bilateral adnexal tenderness, left greater than right.

The urine pregnancy test is positive, and her hematocrit is 37 mL/dL. On ultrasound examination, the uterus is empty, and there is a 3-cm complex adnexal mass on the left, discrete from the ovary with a moderate volume of echogenic fluid in the

cul de sac. She is taken to the operating room with a presumptive diagnosis of a bleeding ectopic pregnancy. Laparotomy reveals a leaking left ampullary ectopic pregnancy with 300 mL of blood in the cul de sac. The patient does well and is discharged on the second postoperative day.

Clinical Evaluation

Introduction

Pelvic pain is a common complaint, particularly in young women, and can be secondary to a variety of different etiologies. Many causes of pelvic pain do not require definitive diagnosis and treatment on an emergent basis. However, a number of etiologies can lead to significant complications if diagnosis and treatment are delayed. Differentiating urgent from nonurgent causes of pelvic pain is the main challenge faced by the emergency physician.

History

A complete gynecological history is described in Chapter 24 and must be elicited from every woman with pelvic or abdominal pain. In addition, the time course of the pain should be elicited, including the duration, whether the pain was constant or intermittent, and whether it was abrupt in onset. Most patients with appendicitis or ovarian torsion present within 48 hours of symptom onset. Abrupt onset of pain suggests hemorrhage from a ruptured ovarian cyst or ectopic pregnancy, perforation of a hollow viscus, or an obstructing ureteral stone. The severity, location, and pain character should also be elicited. Lateral pelvic pain is often related to a process in the tube or ovary. Crampy midline pain is often related to a uterine process. Ask the patient if she has had episodes of similar pain in the past. Chronic recurrent pain is consistent with endometriosis, recurrent ovarian cysts, or a persistent ovarian mass. Important associated symptoms include the presence of fever, nausea, vomiting, anorexia, diarrhea, vaginal discharge, vaginal bleeding, abdominal distension, back pain, or urinary symptoms. Fever suggests an infectious process. Vomiting and anorexia are more common with a gastrointestinal process than with a pelvic process. Abdominal distension suggests obstruction of a hollow viscus or an enlarging tumor. Urinary symptoms suggest a urinary tract infection (UTI). However, urinary symptoms are sometimes present with processes that cause irritation of the urethra, such as vaginitis or pelvic inflammatory disease (PID). The quantity and duration of vaginal bleeding should be determined. In the nonpregnant patient, bleeding may occur with dysmenorrhea, PID, dysfunctional uterine bleeding, and cervical or uterine cancer. In the pregnant patient, bleeding may be associated with a nonviable intrauterine pregnancy (IUP), an ectopic pregnancy, or with a viable IUP.

A sexual history should be obtained, which includes the last menstrual period date, prior pregnancy history, and most recent sexual contact. Past medical history should include prior pelvic or abdominal surgery. In addition, any history of chronic pelvic pathological conditions such as recurrent ovarian cysts, fibroids, endometriosis, PID, or benign or malignant pelvic tumors should be described.

Physical Examination

The vital signs should be checked first. Tachycardia or hypotension suggests significant volume loss from a gastrointestinal source, external hemorrhage from uterine bleeding, intraabdominal hemorrhage from a ruptured ovarian cyst or ectopic pregnancy, or septic shock from a process causing pelvic or intraabdominal peritonitis. Fever suggests

an infectious process. The remainder of the physical examination should be directed toward the pelvis and abdomen.

When examining the abdomen, pay particular attention to the presence of diffuse or localized tenderness, guarding, rebound, abdominal distension, or masses. Localized lateral peritoneal signs may be present with appendicitis, ovarian torsion, diverticulitis, or tubo-ovarian abscess (TOA). Diffuse peritonitis suggests a ruptured hollow viscous, PID, or intraabdominal hemorrhage from either an ectopic pregnancy or ruptured ovarian cyst. A lower abdominal mass may be an enlarged uterus from an IUP, a uterine fibroid, a distended bladder from urinary retention, or an ovarian tumor. Smaller masses detected primarily on the bimanual pelvic examination may be an ovarian cyst, ovarian tumor, ovarian torsion, or TOA. Check for the presence or absence of cervical motion tenderness, and whether any blood, pus, or products of conception are coming from the cervical os. In the pregnant patient, determine whether the internal cervical os is open or closed.

Diagnostic Evaluation

The level of human chorionic gonadotropin (hCG) should be ascertained for any patient of childbearing age with pelvic pain, including those who have had a tubal ligation. Although pregnancy is uncommon after tubal ligation, when it does occur it has a high likelihood of being in the fallopian tube. A urinalysis should be obtained on any patient with symptoms suggestive of a UTI. In addition, approximately 90% of patients with a ureteral stone have hematuria on urinalysis, making this a good initial screening test. Obtaining a complete blood cell (CBC) count, erythrocyte sedimentation rate (ESR), or C-reactive protein level may be helpful in differentiating infectious from noninfectious causes of pelvic pain. The hematocrit level is also helpful in assessing the degree of blood loss. Identifying large amounts of white blood cells obtained from a wet preparation of cervical discharge is suggestive of the diagnosis of PID or cervicitis. Cervical cultures are used to confirm the diagnosis and for epidemiological data.

Ultrasound and computed tomography (CT) scans are the imaging modalities of choice in patients with pelvic pain. If the differential diagnosis primarily includes appendicitis, diverticulitis, or a ureteral stone, then CT scan is the best study. No oral or intravenous contrast is needed for a stone study. Ultrasound examination is best in patients with suspected ectopic pregnancy, PID or TOA, an ovarian cyst or tumor, or ovarian torsion. Laparoscopy is the gold standard for evaluating patients with pelvic pain. It should be considered in any patient with acute pelvic pain in whom the diagnosis is uncertain after CT or ultrasound scan and in whom the possibility of an intraabdominal or pelvic pathological condition remains a significant concern. In addition, laparoscopy is also useful in identifying causes of unexplained chronic pelvic pain.

Differential Diagnosis

Table 27.1 describes the differential diagnosis of pelvic pain. Ectopic pregnancy should be the primary concern with patients in the first trimester of pregnancy unless the diagnosis of a viable IUP has been confirmed by ultrasound scan. In the stable nonpregnant patient, the initial focus should be in differentiating gastrointestinal from pelvic causes of abdominal pain. Nausea and vomiting more commonly occur with a gastrointestinal cause. The presence of cervical motion tenderness suggests pain originating from the pelvic organs. The next step is differentiating infectious from noninfectious causes of abdominal pain. The presence of fever or an elevated white blood count (WBC), ESR, or C-reactive protein level suggest the diagnosis of PID/TOA, appendicitis, diverticulitis, or a UTI. In those with fever and an elevated WBC count, the presence of cervical motion tenderness, particularly when associated with the identification of pus from the cervical os, suggests the diagnosis of PID.

Table 27.1.

Differential diagnosis of pelvic pain

Ovarian Conditions
Ectopic pregnancy
Cyst: follicular, corpus luteum, theca luteum
Trophoblastic disease
Torsion
Endometrioma: "chocolate cyst"
Tumor: adenoma, carcinoma, benign cystic teratoma
Infection: abscess

Uterine Conditions
Sexual assault or abuse
Placenta previa
Abruptio placentae
Abortion: threatened, spontaneous
Infection: PID, toxic shock
Periodic pain
Endometriosis
Synechiae: scar tissue, Asherman's syndrome
Hyperplasia
Polyps
Leiomyomas (fibroids)
Malignancy

Nongynecological Pain
Appendicitis
Urolithiasis
Diverticulitis
UTI/Pyelonephritis

PID, pelvic inflammatory disease; UTI, urinary tract infection.

Treatment

The management of appendicitis, ruptured ectopic pregnancy, and ovarian torsion is surgical. Patients with PID are managed with antibiotics. In TOA, surgery is reserved for those with a TOA that has ruptured or that fails to improve after a trial of antibiotics. Patients with an ovarian cyst without rupture are managed with analgesia alone. Nonsteroidal antiinflammatory drugs are usually sufficient, although some women experience pain that requires narcotic analgesics. Those with frequent recurrent symptoms can use oral contraceptives to suppress the generation of new cysts. The management of patients with hemorrhagic ovarian cysts depends on the degree of blood loss. Those with evidence of mild bleeding by ultrasound scan, stable vital signs, stable hematocrit, and reliable follow-up can often be managed as outpatients. Patients with evidence of more severe bleeding should be resuscitated with crystalloid and blood products as needed and should be admitted for observation. Those with evidence of continued ongoing blood loss are candidates for operative therapy.

The primary focus of acute treatment for patients with endometriosis is to ensure adequate analgesia. The patient's gynecologist best directs specific medical therapy for this condition.

Disposition

Most patients with pelvic pain can be managed as outpatients as long as surgical causes of pain have been excluded, even if a specific etiology has not been identified. However, it is important to arrange adequate follow-up, because laparoscopic studies have demonstrated that a specific etiology can be identified in up to 75% of patients.

Pathophysiology

Ovarian Cysts

After ovulation, the follicle can accumulate fluid or blood and can reach sizes of many centimeters. The distension of the ovary causes lower abdominal pain in these patients. The normal corpus luteum resorbs by 14 days. If it persists beyond this time, still producing progesterone, the woman will likely experience amenorrhea and subsequent vaginal bleeding and lower abdominal pain. In contrast, if the corpus luteum fails to produce adequate progesterone, vaginal bleeding may occur early in the woman's cycle.

Ovarian Torsion

Torsion is usually a direct result of abnormal pelvic anatomy, either an abnormally long tube or ovary or excessive tortuosity of the veins of the fallopian tube. Sudden changes in movement may cause the ovary to flip over the vessels, causing obstruction of blood flow. There are theories that the fallopian tube may spasm, causing torsion of the ovary, even in women with normal pelvic anatomy. Interruption of the fallopian tube from tubal ligation may also free the ovary, increasing the risk of torsion.

Endometriosis

Endometriosis is the presence of ectopic endometrial tissue. It can be spread contiguously from the uterus to adjacent tissues (adenomyosis), which results most often in menorrhagia (excessive bleeding) and dysmenorrhea (painful menses). Alternatively, endometrial tissue can be found outside the uterus in the peritoneal cavity. The reason for the appearance of endometrial tissue outside the uterus is not known. Theories include the spread of desquamated endometrial cells through the fallopian tubes into the peritoneal cavity and metaplastic changes in the celomic epithelium of the peritoneal cavity. Women experience pelvic pain that does not have to be related to the menstrual cycle. Pain can be manifested as a backache or as pain during intercourse. Endometriosis causes infertility in approximately 30% of patients.

Suggested Readings

Bongard F, Landers D, Lewis F. Differential diagnosis of appendicitis and pelvic inflammatory disease. A prospective study. *Am J Surg* 1985;150:90–96.

Buckley R, King K, Gorman J, Klausen J. History and physical exam to estimate the risk of ectopic pregnancy: validation of a clinical prediction model. *Ann Emerg Med* 1999;34: 664–667.

Cacciatore B, Leminen A, Ingman-Friberg S, et al. Transvaginal sonographic findings in ambulatory patients with suspected pelvic inflammatory disease. *Obstet Gynecol* 1992;80:912–916.

Cunanan R, Courey N, Lippes J. Laparoscopic findings in patients with pelvic pain. *Am J Obstet Gynecol* 1983;146:589–561.

Dart R. Role of pelvic ultrasonography in the evaluation of the symptomatic first trimester pregnancy. *Ann Emerg Med* 1999;33:310–320.

Dart R, Kaplan B, Varaklis K. Predictive value of history and physical examination in patients with suspected ectopic pregnancy. *Ann Emerg Med* 1999;33:283–290.

Eschenbach D, Wolner-Hanssen P, Hawes S, et al. Acute pelvic inflammatory disease: associations of clinical and laboratory findings with laparoscopic findings. *Obstet Gynecol* 1997;89:184–192.

Lee E, Kwon H, Suh J, Fleischer A. Diagnosis of ovarian torsion with color Doppler sonography: depiction of twisted vascular pedicle. *J Ultrasound Med* 1998;17:83–89.

Liu W, Esler S, Kenny B, et al. Low dose nonenhanced helical CT of renal colic: assessment of ureteric stone detection and measurement of effective dose equivalent. *Radiology* 2000;215:51–54.

Morcos R, Frost N, Hnat M, et al. Laparoscopic versus clinical diagnosis of acute pelvic inflammatory disease. *J Reprod Med* 1993;38:53–56.

Styrud J, Josephson T, Eriksson S. Reducing negative appendectomy: evaluation of ultrasonography and computer tomography in acute appendicitis. *Int J Qual Health Care* 2000;12:65–68.

Pelvic Complaints
Questions and Answers

Questions

1. Which of the following statements is true?

  A. Regression of the corpus luteum and a drop in estrogen causes the sloughing of the endometrium of menstruation.

  B. Dysfunctional uterine bleeding in a young woman who is not pregnant is most often a direct result of pelvic pathological conditions or medication side effects.

  C. Most perimenopausal women with persistent vaginal bleeding have endometrial carcinoma.

  D. Vaginal bleeding secondary to uterine fibroids is usually cyclical with menses.

2. Choose the correct statements:

  I. All Rh$^-$ pregnant women with vaginal bleeding require administration of Rh immunoglobulin (RhoGAM).

  II. Molar pregnancies present with vaginal bleeding and low β-human chorionic gonadotropin (β-hCG) levels and are seen as grapelike clusters on pelvic ultrasound examination.

  III. Patients with a β-hCG level less than 1,000 IU/mL are more likely to have an ectopic pregnancy.

  A. Only I and II are correct.

  B. Only I and III are correct.

  C. Only II and III are correct.

  D. All are correct.

3. A 22-year-old G_2P_0 woman presents with 1 day of fever and right lower quadrant pain. She has no appetite and has vomited once. She has no prior medical problems and has never had abdominal surgery. She is sexually active with one partner and uses condoms. On physical examination, she is febrile to 101.2°F and is tender in the right lower quadrant, with guarding and rebound at McBurney's point. Her white blood count (WBC) is 14,000/μL and urinalysis is normal, including a negative pregnancy test.

What is the most appropriate next step?

  A. The patient has a classic presentation of appendicitis. She needs a surgical consultation and a computed tomography (CT) scan of the abdomen without further physical evaluation.

  B. Only if pelvic examination reveals right adnexal tenderness, a pelvic ultrasound examination should be done to look for a tubo-ovarian abscess.

  C. If pelvic examination reveals cervical motion tenderness and bilateral adnexal tenderness, the patient should be admitted for intravenous (IV) antibiotics for pelvic inflammatory disease (PID) without further evaluation.

  D. Despite a normal pelvic examination and a negative CT of the abdomen, the patient should have a pelvic ultrasound examination.

4. A 19-year-old G_0P_0 woman presents to the emergency department complaining of sudden onset severe left lower quadrant pain. She has no medical problems, no prior surgery, and is not pregnant. She is afebrile. Her abdomen is tender

to deep palpation in the left lower quadrant with mild guarding and no rebound tenderness.

Which statement is correct?

A. If the pain resolves with pain medication and observation in the emergency department, the patient may be followed up as an outpatient.

B. If a pelvic ultrasound examination reveals an ovarian cyst and little free fluid in the pelvis, and her pain is well controlled, she can always be safely discharged home.

C. Ultrasound examination can only detect an ovarian torsion while the ovary is still in torsion.

D. Evidence of an ovarian cyst and free fluid in the pelvis may require that the patient be admitted for observation.

Directions: There are three sets of response options for the following scenario. You will be required to select one best answer from each question set.

5. A 23-year-old woman G_2P_2 presents to the emergency department complaining of abdominal pain and vaginal bleeding. Her last menstrual period was 10 weeks ago. She is sexually active and does not use contraceptives. She has never had a sexually transmitted disease and has a single sexual partner, her husband. On physical examination, she is afebrile, has normal vital signs, and has mild diffuse lower abdominal tenderness without guarding or rebound. Pelvic examination reveals a small amount of dried blood in the vaginal vault and mild left adnexal tenderness.

5.1. If the patient has a positive pregnancy test, what is the next step in caring for this patient?

A. Give her detailed instructions on the risks of threatened miscarriage and discharge her with gynecology follow-up.

B. Order a pelvic ultrasound examination to rule out ovarian torsion.

C. Order a quantitative β-human chorionic gonadotropin (β-hCG). If it is over 1,000 IU/mL, get an ultrasound examination to rule out ectopic pregnancy.

D. Order a pelvic ultrasound examination to rule out ectopic pregnancy.

5.2. You have ordered a pelvic ultrasound examination for this patient. The ultrasound examination results show no ectopic pregnancy but are indeterminate for intrauterine pregnancy. What is the appropriate next step?

A. Discharge the patient with the diagnosis of early pregnancy with appropriate follow-up.

B. Admit the patient for observation for ectopic pregnancy.

C. Inform the patient that she does not have a viable pregnancy and may have an ectopic pregnancy. Treat with methotrexate to eliminate a possible ectopic pregnancy.

D. Discharge the patient with the diagnosis of early intrauterine pregnancy versus ectopic versus miscarriage. Have her follow up for a serial quantitative β-human chorionic gonadotropin (β-hCG) in 2 days.

5.3. The patient informs you that she performed a home pregnancy test 2 weeks ago, which was positive. Your laboratory reports that the urine β-human chorionic gonadotropin (β-hCG) assay results are negative. A serum quantitative β-hCG assay also returns as negative. Which of the following is correct?

A. If the patient's pain resolves and her examination improves and she is stable, she can be safely discharged without an ultrasound examination, with the diagnosis of threatened abortion.

B. The patient requires an ultrasound examination to rule out an intrauterine pregnancy.

C. The patient requires a blood type screen and should receive anti-Rh antibody if she is Rh negative.

D. The patient must get an ultrasound examination to rule out adnexal pathology and can be discharged safely if it demonstrates a spontaneous abortion is in progress.

Answers and Explanations

1. D. Fibroids tend to cause excessive menstrual bleeding that is cyclical with the menstrual cycle. Regression of the corpus luteum is associated with a drop in the plasma concentration of progesterone, not a drop in estrogen, which leads to menstrual bleeding. Dysfunctional uterine bleeding is usually due to hormonal imbalances and is a diagnosis of exclusion once pelvic pathological conditions, medication side effects, and the like have been ruled out. Endometrial carcinoma occurs in 5% to 10% of perimenopausal women with abnormal vaginal bleeding.

2. B. Rh$^-$ women with vaginal bleeding who have Rh$^+$ partners are at risk for fetal hemolysis. It is prudent to administer Rh immunoglobulin to all Rh$^-$ patients with bleeding. There is an increased incidence of ectopic pregnancy in women with low β-*human chorionic gonadotropin* (β-hCG) levels. Molar pregnancies typically cause *higher* β-hCG levels than expected for the woman's estimated date of conception.

3. D. This patient does have a classic presentation for appendicitis; however, it cannot be stressed too often that every woman of childbearing age with abdominal pain MUST have a pelvic examination. Adnexal pathology can cause right lower quadrant tenderness that mimics appendicitis. Patients may present with right lower quadrant pain and tenderness without adnexal tenderness by physical examination, and yet prove to have a tubo-ovarian abscess. The ultrasound examination should be performed despite the lack of findings on the bimanual examination. A computed tomography (CT) scan may be an appropriate first test, but an ultrasound examination should be done if the scan is negative and the pain and tenderness persist. Because of the localizing symptoms and signs to the right lower quadrant, despite bilateral adnexal tenderness an ultrasound examination is prudent to evaluate for an abscess.

4. D. Ovarian cysts with little free fluid in the pelvis and well-controlled pain are not correct discharge criteria because they do not indicate that the patient has been adequately observed and assessed for ongoing blood loss. Thus, patients are not "always" stable for discharge. If her

vital signs and hematocrit level remain stable, then she may be discharged. Otherwise, if the hematocrit level is dropping, her blood pressure is low, or her heart rate is persistently tachycardic, she is showing signs of persistent bleeding and should be admitted. The key operative is "ongoing blood loss." The question refers to bleeding cysts. Fluid on ultrasound examination may be blood or other fluid. This patient may be experiencing acute ovarian torsion. If her pain resolves, she should still have an ultrasound examination to look at blood flow to the ovary. Despite detorsing, an ultrasound examination can still reveal characteristic changes in the ovary that suggest torsion has occurred, and it may be prudent to admit the patient for observation.

5.1. D. Although some pain is normal in pregnancy, any focal pain must be taken seriously. In the pregnant patient, ectopic pregnancy is the critical diagnosis to make or rule out. If the patient has already had an ultrasound examination by her obstetrician documenting an intrauterine pregnancy (IUP), a repeat ultrasound examination may not be necessary. Heterotopic pregnancy, a rare condition that is an ectopic pregnancy in addition to an IUP, is remotely possible. Ovarian torsion is part of the differential but much lower on the differential diagnosis than ectopic pregnancy in a pregnant woman. β-human chorionic gonadotropin (β-hCG) levels of less than 1,000 IU/mL have been demonstrated to increase the risk of ectopic pregnancy.

5.2. D. An indeterminate ultrasound examination is precisely what the label implies. Early in pregnancy, a viable intrauterine pregnancy (IUP) may not yet show the signs that an ultrasound machine is sensitive enough to pick up. Therefore, the diagnosis remains ectopic versus IUP versus spontaneous abortion (miscarriage). A patient whose condition is stable and who wants to keep the pregnancy may be followed up in 48 hours. An IUP that is viable will double its β-hCG value approximately every 2 to 3 days. If the pregnancy is unwanted, methotrexate is a treatment option to terminate an undetected ectopic pregnancy. An unstable patient, or one with severe unremitting pain, may be admitted for observation and may require exploratory laparotomy.

5.3. A. Assuming that the home pregnancy test result was not a false positive, and that she was truly pregnant, then she is now no longer pregnant and is miscarrying (spontaneously aborting). Provided that she is stable, no further testing is absolutely necessary in the emergency department. The decay of the β-human chorionic gonadotropin (β-hCG) occurs over time; thus, the fetus must have died some time ago for the quantitative β-hCG to be negative. An ultrasound examination would most likely show fetal demise or debris within the uterine cavity indicating a lost pregnancy. Rh immunity is not required because she is not pregnant. If her pain resolves and her examination has improved, there is no absolute need for an ultrasound examination, because it is evident from history that she is miscarrying. Although some obstetrics and gynecological physicians might offer a dilation and extraction procedure, it is not required in an otherwise stable patient.

Headache

"Talking of axes," said the Duchess, "chop off her head!"

Lewis Carroll 1865

INTRODUCTION
Ron Medzon, MD
Section Editor

Headache is a common presenting complaint to the emergency department (ED), representing 3% to 5% of all ED visits. Patients commonly present because they are experiencing a headache that is new to them or is more severe than anything they have suffered in the past. Alternatively, they present to the ED as a last resort, having put up with their headache for years but never having sought medical attention. The actual incidence of life-threatening causes for headache is quite low. Headaches are common and frequently benign in late childhood and adolescence. However, they are uncommon in the young child and a more exhaustive search for an underlying cause may be warranted in this group.

Headache symptoms may be caused by any pain-sensitive structure in the head. These include the skin and associated soft tissues; the periosteum of the skull; the tissues of the eye, ear, and oral, nasal, and sinus cavities; the cranial nerves (V, IX, and X), the first three cervical nerves, parts of the meninges, or the intracranial blood vessels. The bones of the skull and the tissue of the brain are insensate. The varied nature of these structures gives rise to a large number of headache syndromes.

Headaches are generally divided into three categories: tension type, vascular, and traction and inflammatory.

Tension headaches result from a constriction of the muscles of the neck and scalp. Typical causes for this constriction are psychological stress, cervical arthritis, or a defensive reaction of muscles to a nearby injury.

Vascular headaches are thought to arise from abnormal activity in the neurons of the trigeminal nerve's path. This triggers a complex cascade of events including the release of vasoactive peptides; the most prominent is serotonin. The vasodilation causes neurogenic inflammation, which is a process of extravasation of plasma proteins. The strongest evidence supporting these mechanisms is the effectiveness of ergot and triptan medications in migraines, which block neuropeptide release and in turn cure the headache. Interestingly, it is postulated that the process of neurogenic inflammation can be initiated by many internal and external stimuli, including infectious material or blood irritating the meninges. This would mean that subarachnoid hemorrhage and meningitis, among other causes for headache, share a common pathophysiological pathway. This may explain why patients with subarachnoid hemorrhage and headache get similar relief with some of the migraine-related pain medications. Hypertensive headaches are also considered vascular. It should be noted that not until the diastolic pressure rises above approximately 120 mm Hg is it thought to significantly contribute to headache pain.

Traction headaches are caused by mechanical forces on the intracranial structures; examples are tumors, edema, and large amounts of blood. Also, consider diseases of the eyes, ears, nose, and teeth. Inflammatory causes include temporal arteritis, phlebitis, and cranial neuralgias.

Although a reasonable attempt to break the pain cycle should be made, complete pain relief is often not achieved in the ED. Realistic expectations should be discussed with the patient and a good aftercare plan should be made. The patient should be given an explanation of the most likely etiology of his or her headache, including the processes that have been ruled out during the ED visit. Discharge instructions for benign causes of headache, should include a plan for continued pain control, directed follow-up, and a discussion about the signs and symptoms that should bring them back to the ED.

CHAPTER **28**

Subarachnoid Hemorrhage

Fred N. Jones, MD

Clinical Scenario

A 33-year-old woman presents to the emergency department (ED) complaining of severe headache, vomiting, and blurred vision. She states that the headache came on suddenly after dinner while watching television. She vomited twice shortly after the onset of the headache. The headache was so severe she thought she might black out from the pain. On review of systems, she states that she feels tightness in the back of her neck and that the bright fluorescent lights are irritating to her eyes. She denies fevers, weakness, or numbness. She denies trauma or domestic violence. She has a strong family history of migraine and has had prior headaches; this headache is unlike any previous headache.

Past medical history is unremarkable. She takes oral contraceptives and has no known drug allergies. She does not smoke, use drugs, or consume alcohol. Her last menstrual period was 2 weeks ago.

Physical examination reveals an alert, oriented woman in moderate distress. Vital signs reveal a blood pressure of 190/108 mm Hg, pulse of 108 beats/minute, respiratory rate of 20 breaths/minute, and a temperature of 98.9°F. Her oropharynx and tympanic membranes are normal. Cardiac, lung, and abdominal examination are normal. On neurological examination, she complains of blurred vision but cannot be more specific; her visual acuity is 20/25 in both eyes. The eyes have equal and reactive pupils, extraocular movements are intact, and funduscopic examination is normal. There is mild photophobia when shining the

light in the patient's eyes. Cranial nerves II through XII are otherwise normal. Strength is preserved in all extremities with normal and equal reflexes. Sensation is intact to light touch, pinprick, and proprioception bilaterally. Balance and gait are normal.

The patient is treated with prochlorperazine intravenously for vomiting and undergoes a noncontrast computed tomography (CT) scan of her head. She tolerates the procedure well, but on return to the ED complains of persistent severe headache and blurred vision. She is given meperidine for analgesia. The CT scan is normal, with no mass or intracranial blood. The lumbar puncture (LP) yields clearly bloody fluid the color of Hawaiian Punch. The color remains consistent through the collection of four sample tubes. Cell count analysis shows 624,000 red blood cells (RBCs)/mL in tube 1 and 580,000 RBCs/mL in tube 4.

The patient is admitted to the intensive care unit (ICU) with the diagnosis of subarachnoid hemorrhage (SAH) from presumed rupture of a berry aneurysm. She is scheduled for cerebral angiography, and neurosurgery is consulted. The patient is monitored with frequent neurological examinations and blood pressure control with intravenous nitroprusside. The patient has a successful operative clipping of the aneurysm and is discharged home on the third hospital day in good condition.

Clinical Evaluation

Introduction

Despite advances in diagnostic and treatment modalities, SAH still carries a case mortality rate of 35% to 40%, only slightly decreased from the 50% case fatality rate of 30 years ago. Survivors are often left with persistent neurological deficits, often making them unable to return to their prebleed lives. Unfortunately, more than 25% of patients who are eventually diagnosed with SAH were misdiagnosed on their first presentation. Because of its high morbidity and mortality, SAH must be expeditiously diagnosed and treated.

History

The classic history of a SAH is of an explosive onset, debilitating headache. The headache is often associated with vomiting, and blurred or double vision. The patient (or a family member) may report doubling-over or even passing out at the initial attack of the pain. SAH has many subtle presentations and is often missed. The physician must be meticulous in extracting details about the onset, course, and quality of the pain; any neurological symptoms; systemic accompaniments; prior risk factors; or preceding headache.

As with the evaluation of any pain, the history must elicit the onset, duration, quality, and location of the pain. The pain from SAH is characterized as explosive or like a thunderclap; the patient can frequently tell you to the minute when it started. The pain may last for days without significant improvement. The pain may have resolved, either spontaneously or with over-the-counter or prescription medications. Two thirds of patients with SAH report onset during vigorous activity. Quality and location are less helpful in the diagnosis because they are more subjective and less specific. The pain is more often referred to as sharp and constant, but patients with SAH have reported throbbing, tight, and dull pain. Location of the pain does not aid the diagnosis but may help localize the lesion. A bilateral headache is more common in anterior cerebral artery aneurysms. A unilateral headache is more common in posterior communicating or middle cerebral artery aneurysms.

Associated symptoms also provide important clues. Neurological symptoms of a posterior communicating artery aneurysm adjacent to the third cranial nerve most commonly include visual changes such as recent onset ptosis (drooping eyelid), ipsilateral dilated pupil, and sometimes diplopia (double vision). Motor signs may include weakness and hemiparesis. Aphasia (inability to produce coherent speech), and mood alterations such as profound disinterest in routine life are rare symptoms.

Neurological findings on history are dependent on location of the SAH and may be entirely absent. Neck and back rigidity arising from meningeal irritation by blood are also part of the classic SAH. This stiffness is more common in posterior or basilar hemorrhage but may be entirely absent. Convulsions (seizures) are occasionally a component of SAH; if they occur, they are likely due to an underlying seizure disorder. Other systemic complaints include nausea, vomiting, back pain, or chest pain. A patient may also be confused so that he or she cannot give a history or may not even complain of pain. The emergency physician must be wary of attributing such behavior to dementia or drug use.

As with all patients, physicians must ask about the past. Has this happened before? Is it different than past headaches? These answers may reassure you or help confirm your diagnosis. A "first and worst" presentation is more likely to be SAH than other presentations. Ask about risk factors such as smoking or hypertension. In addition, be sure to inquire about systemic diseases such as atherosclerosis or inherited high-risk conditions.

Physical Examination

The physical examination is often less useful than the history because many patients have normal or only subtle findings that may be overlooked in an emergency screening neurological examination. Many patients are often quite uncomfortable and may prefer darkened rooms. Their behavior can range from highly agitated, to normal cooperative, to drowsy, to unresponsive. The most common findings on examination are ocular. You may find evidence of third nerve involvement such as dilated pupil or decreased medial gaze. One may see the absence of lateral gaze, demonstrating involvement of the sixth cranial nerve. A funduscopic examination may show subhyaloid hemorrhage.

These are generally associated with large bleeds and other signs may be there as well. This finding may be a very important clue to the diagnosis in the patient who is found comatose with no witnesses.

Nuchal rigidity can be assessed by a patient's unwillingness to flex the neck or in the less responsive patient by absence of hyperextension when the shoulders are lifted from the bed. Focal neurological signs such as ptosis, a nonreactive pupil (particularly with an ipsilateral eye that is significantly deviated laterally), facial and or extremity weakness, or aphasia often heighten the suspicion of a ruptured berry aneurysm.

Diagnostic Evaluation

The mainstay of clinical diagnosis is an approach using CT scan and LP. Given the variability with which SAH can present and the poor specificity of history and physical examination, it is imperative to pursue diagnostic testing in any patient in whom the diagnosis is considered.

The CT scan should be the first test used to evaluate for SAH. It is generally readily available, fast, and well tolerated by patients. It is also excellent for detecting other causes of headache, such as tumors or epidural hematoma. As scanner technology has improved, so has sensitivity to subarachnoid blood, although it is not perfect. The limitations of CT stem from the nature of blood in the subarachnoid space. The increased density from the RBCs differentiates the collection of blood from the surrounding brain tissue (Fig. 28.1). Unfortunately this can appear similar to bone and can be misread as bony artifact. CT performance diminishes with decreased hematocrit and with the passage of time. A scan done within

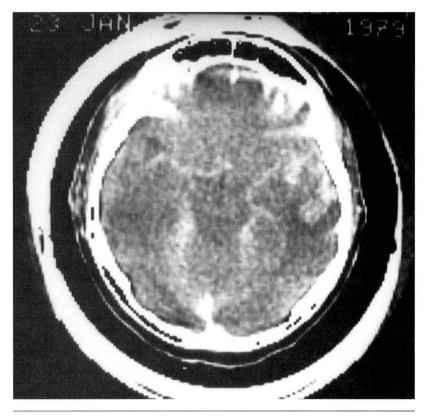

Figure 28.1
Computed tomography (CT) scan showing acute subarachnoid hemorrhage. Blood appears bright white, and in this example is seen extensively in the subarachnoid space.

the first 12 to 24 hours has a sensitivity of 93% to 98% depending on the size of the bleed and the skill of the reader. After 2 days, the sensitivity drops to approximately 85%, and by 5 days approaches 55%. Although 93% may at first appear reassuring, the high morbidity and mortality of SAH requires further testing to ensure that the scan is not falsely negative. A positive CT scan should be considered diagnostic and the patient treated accordingly.

LP allows for a direct evaluation of the contents of the subarachnoid space. There is a theoretical risk of brainstem herniation if an LP is performed in a patient who has increased intracranial pressure (ICP). Therefore, the LP should be done after a CT scan has ruled out obvious hemorrhage or increased ICP. Opening pressure should be measured, because it is elevated in cerebral venous stenosis and pseudotumor cerebri, two SAH mimickers. A typical positive tap has copious RBCs in both the first and last tubes drawn, usually in the hundreds of thousands. However, occasionally some LPs are "traumatic taps" in which blood is introduced into the cerebrospinal fluid (CSF) by the procedure itself when the needle passes through a vein. Traditionally, it was taught that, if there was a large decrease in RBC counts from first to last tube, the tap was traumatic and there was not SAH. Unfortunately, differentiating a traumatic versus a positive tap is not that simple. To confirm SAH, a second tap can be done one interspace above the first; if that is clear, then the first tap was traumatic. The second option is to spin the bloody CSF in a centrifuge and examine the supernatant for a yellow tint as compared to water. This xanthochromia is caused by accumulation of bilirubin from the breakdown of RBCs. It should not be present in a traumatic tap. The human eye may miss a large fraction of xanthochromic CSF so the supernatant should be evaluated for absorption via spectrophotometry. A positive LP with xanthochromia should be considered diagnostic for SAH.

If CT scan and LP are negative but clinical suspicion is still extremely high, consult neurology and consider further testing.

The gold standard test for SAH is cerebral angiography. This clearly locates the aneurysm, shows its size and morphology, identifies continued bleeding, and helps determine the specific treatment. Given the invasiveness and risks of this procedure, it should be used only for those with a high likelihood of disease and is not effective for the initial evaluation.

Magnetic resonance imaging (MRI) has not shown benefit over CT scan in detecting SAH. Magnetic resonance angiography may demonstrate very small aneurysms, but time and patient intolerance have made this test unwieldy for ED use.

Differential Diagnosis

The differential diagnosis for SAH is illustrated in Table 28.1.

Treatment

The patient diagnosed with a SAH requires urgent consultation with neurosurgery and sometimes expedited cerebral angiography. The patient will be evaluated for either intraarterial embolization or surgical clipping of the aneurysm. In the interim, the patient will require symptomatic care. If the patient is obtunded (Glasgow coma

---

Table 28.1.

Differential diagnosis for subarachnoid hemorrhage

Stroke
Migraine
Meningitis
Encephalitis
Arterial dissection
Temporal arteritis
Acute angle closure glaucoma
Cerebral venous and dural sinus thrombosis
Tumor
Pseudotumor cerebri (benign intracranial
   hypertension)
Stroke
Trauma
Coital headache

Table 28.2.

Treatment guidelines for subarachnoid hemorrhage

Head CT scan
LP, if CT scan negative
Confirmed blood in CSF
IV catheter placement
Complete blood count and electrolytes
Continuous cardiac and vital signs monitoring
Emergent neurosurgery consultation
MRI or MR angiogram
Consideration of cerebral angiogram
Emergent surgery or admission to surgical
    intensive care unit
Declining mental status: consideration of
    intubation
Management of hypertension to keep mean
    arterial BP >130 mm Hg
IV labetalol
IV nitroprusside
IV narcotics for pain
Consideration of nimodipine

BP, blood pressure; CSF, cerebrospinal fluid; CT, computed tomography; IV, intravenous; LP, lumbar puncture; MR, magnetic resonance; MRI, magnetic resonance imaging.

score [GCS] 10 or less), he or she must be intubated for airway control and to decrease risk of aspiration.

Treatment guidelines for SAH are summarized in Table 28.2.

Blood pressure should be monitored, and if extremely elevated it should be treated. The most commonly used agents are labetalol and nitroprusside. The mean arterial pressure should not drop below 130 mm Hg, because that will result in decreased cerebral perfusion pressure.

The patient's pain may require treatment with narcotics. Treat any vomiting with antiemetics. The patient must be monitored closely for signs of rebleeding or elevated ICP. This is best done in an ICU or neurological ICU where available.

Recent trials have evaluated the calcium channel blocking agent nimodipine to reduce posthemorrhage vasospasm. Evidence shows that when started within 3 to 4 days of the bleed, it decreased the incidence of and morbidity from vasospasm. It has yet to be determined whether or not it is necessary to begin treatment in the ED.

Disposition

All patients who are diagnosed within the first 24 hours of a SAH should be admitted to an ICU for close neurological monitoring. Any deterioration in the patient's status may prompt a repeat CT scan to determine progression of the bleeding or whether there is new or increasing ICP requiring urgent neurosurgical intervention.

The patient with negative CT scan and LP may usually be symptomatically treated and safely discharged with close follow-up with primary care and/or neurology to further evaluate the cause of headache.

Pathophysiology

Bleeding into the subarachnoid space is most commonly due to a leaking or ruptured berry aneurysm. These outpouchings of the cerebral arteries can be found in approximately 2% of the general population. They are thin-walled, with defects in the artery's muscular and/or elastic lamina. They range in size from a few millimeters to 3 cm. They can frequently be found at or near arterial bifurcations, primarily near the circle of Willis. Ninety percent are in the anterior cerebral circulation. Bacterial endocarditis can cause mycotic aneurysms, which can lead to SAH. However, these are generally found in the distal cerebral circulation. Other causes of SAH include trauma, arteriovenous malformations, coagulopathies, and extension of an intraparenchymal bleed into the subarachnoid space.

Rupture of berry aneurysms frequently occurs during activities that elevate ICP, such as heavy lifting, straining, or sexual intercourse. SAH also occurs in people at rest and even asleep. SAH is more common in women than in men and is more common in

African Americans than in Caucasians. Although rare during the first 3 decades of life, the incidence of SAH increases with age (the median age is 50 years). Risk is increased by smoking and hypertension and by such hereditary disorders as Marfan's syndrome, Ehlers-Danlos disease, neurofibromatosis, and autosomal dominant polycystic kidney disease.

The intense pain of SAH is due to meningeal irritation and increased ICP. Localizing symptoms are caused by increased pressure on adjacent structures and by diffuse damage from elevated ICP resulting from edema or obstructing hydrocephalus. A phenomenon of diffuse vasospasm can occur 3 to 5 days later that compounds the damage from the initial bleed. This can lead to ischemia remote from the site of initial hemorrhage.

Suggested Readings

Edlow J, Caplan LR. Primary care: avoiding pitfalls in the diagnosis of subarachnoid hemorrhage. *N Engl J Med* 2000;342:29–36.

Goetz CG. *Textbook of clinical neurology.* Philadelphia: WB Saunders, 1999.

Johnston SC, Selvin S, Gress D. The burden, trends, and demographics of mortality from subarachnoid hemorrhage. *Neurology* 1988 May;50(5): 1413–1418.

Newman LC, Lipton RB. Emergency department evaluation of headache. *Neurol Clin* 1998;16: 285–303.

Rinkle G, Dijibuti M, Algra A, et al. Prevalence and risk of rupture of intracranial aneurysms: a systematic review. *Stroke* 1998;29:251–256.

Wijdicks EF. *Neurologic catastrophes in the emergency department.* Boston: Butterworth Heinemann, 2000.

CHAPTER 29

Migraine

Thomas Perera, MD

Clinical Scenario

A 37-year-old woman presents to the emergency department (ED) complaining of a headache. The pain started at 11 a.m. with a rapid, but not instantaneous, onset. A few minutes before the headache, she had noticed some wavy lines in her vision. The pain was intense, located on the left side, and throbbing. The patient felt nauseous and somewhat lightheaded. She had vomited twice. She noted that the pain was made worse by loud noises, bright lights, and physical activity. She has had similar headaches in the past, often in periods of stress, but she has not gone to see a doctor about them. She denies neck pain, recent upper respiratory symptoms, weakness, or numbness.

Past medical history is noncontributory. She lives with her husband and child. She denies tobacco use and drinks alcohol only occasionally. She uses no drugs and takes birth control pills as her only medication.

On review of systems, she denies vision changes or watery eyes, sinus pain or congestion, fever, numbness or tingling, night sweats, or weight loss.

Physical examination reveals a normal appearing, well-developed woman in obvious discomfort. She is lying in bed with her arm over her eyes and has asked that the lights be turned down low. Vital signs are heart rate of 80 beats/minute, blood pressure of 150/80 mm Hg, temperature of 98°F, and respiratory rate of 16 breaths/minute. There is no evidence of any head trauma. She has no sinus, scalp, or temporal tenderness. Pupils are 5 mm, equal size, round, and reactive to light and accommodation. She has

normal optic fundi and her extraocular muscles are intact. Her vision is tested at 20/30 right eye (OD) 20/20 left eye (OS). She has normal dentition with moist mucous membranes. The tympanic membranes are normal. The neck is supple and moves easily through a full range of motion. There are no nodes palpable, and there are no bruits in the neck. The chest is clear to auscultation. The cardiac examination shows a regular rhythm and rate with no murmurs, rubs, or gallops. The abdomen is soft and nontender with normal bowel sounds and no masses. Neurological examination is normal. This examination includes testing for cranial nerves, strength, sensation, gait, and mental status. The patient also has no Kernig's or Brudzinski's sign.

The presumptive diagnosis of migraine headache is made. The patient has a negative urine pregnancy test. The patient receives 25 mg of intravenous (IV) promethazine (Phenergan) and 15 mg of IV ketorolac (Toradol) with minor relief of her headache. Administration of 6 mg of subcutaneous sumatriptan completely relieves the headache, and she is discharged with follow-up for further evaluation.

Clinical Evaluation

Introduction

Headache is one of the most common presenting complaints in EDs, representing 1% to 6% of all visits. Patients come to the ED to get relief from their pain and to be reassured that the headache does not represent a life-threatening medical problem. There are 13 broad categories of headaches and

128 distinct headache syndromes. Migraine headaches represent some of the most common varieties. As with many things in emergency medicine, the role of the clinician in evaluating headache is twofold. The first and most important role is to exclude more dangerous diagnoses. The most important of these include subarachnoid hemorrhage, meningitis, and tumor. The second role of the clinician is to make the diagnosis of migraine headache. This second step is important because treatment varies considerably for different types of headache. The ED diagnosis of migraine is based on a thorough history and physical examination. Diagnostic testing is usually only necessary to rule out a more serious diagnosis that could not be excluded by other means.

History

The most common historical features of migraines include unilateral moderately intense headaches that are pulsating or throbbing in nature and are made worse by physical activity. The pain generally lasts 4 to 72 hours and is accompanied by nausea, vomiting, photophobia, and phonophobia (sensitivity to loud sounds). The patient interview should be aimed at these points and at excluding pathological causes of headache.

Begin by inquiring about the time and rate of onset. This should include what activity the patient was doing when the headache started and was the headache slowly progressive (tension or migraine) or sudden and severe (subarachnoid). Ask whether the patient noticed anything odd before the headache began, including changes in vision or odd smells. This premonitory symptom is called the "aura." Migraines may occur with or without aura. Ask about the duration of the headache. Tension headaches and tumors may give prolonged headaches or daily headaches. Ask the patient about the type and location of pain and have him or her quantify the intensity of the pain. This can often guide you to important alternative causes of headache.

Migraine headaches are usually one sided but can be bilateral. Inquire about activities that make the pain better or worse. Include specifically whether bright lights, loud noises, or neck and head motion affect the headache. Neck pain and stiffness alone can be a cause of headaches and can be an important clue to the diagnosis of meningitis. Ask about whether the patient has had a recent change in vision. This can be an important focal neurological finding or a common cause for headache. Intense pain located behind one eye with associated tearing and congestion can represent a cluster headache. Ask what other symptoms the patient may be experiencing besides the headache. Specifically inquire about cold symptoms; congestion; and green, bad-tasting sputum. Fever is a particularly important finding. Although fever can trigger a migraine, it is often associated with other types of headache. Nausea and vomiting are common with migraine, but focal abdominal pain is rare. Also ask about weight loss, night sweats, and other symptoms suggestive of neoplastic processes.

It is important to inquire about the patient's past history of headaches. Does the patient have headaches often or is this episode the first memorable headache that he or she experienced? Does the patient get headaches once a month, only when he or she does not get a cup of coffee, or when he or she does not wear glasses? Any change in the patient's usual pattern of headache can represent a pathological cause of headache. Even patients who get migraines regularly can have meningitis or subarachnoid hemorrhage.

Also inquire what medication the patient may have taken in an attempt to eliminate the pain and what effect these medications had. This will help guide your therapy and occasionally will reveal an accidental acetaminophen or aspirin overdose.

Inquire about the past medical history of the patient. Hypertension, atherosclerotic heart disease, connective tissue disorders, and polycystic kidney disease all can be clues to other types of headaches. Also ask about the family history of headaches. Migraines can run in the family.

Physical Examination

The physical examination of patients with migraine headaches should be predominantly normal. The examination is aimed at excluding the physical findings of the pathological causes of headaches. Always review the vital signs of patients with headache. Fever may indicate an infections process. Blood pressure and pulse may be elevated in patients in severe pain. Patients who have been vomiting are at risk for tachycardia or low blood pressure. The general appearance of patients with migraine can be normal, or they can look like they are in considerable discomfort. They often want the light in the room off and the door closed against loud noises.

The head and neck examination is particularly important with migraine headaches. Examine the skin for rashes. Feel the scalp for tender points. Palpate the temporal artery on both sides. Palpate the muscles of mastication and the temporomandibular joint. Palpate and percuss the sinuses. Feel for preauricular nodes and examine the tympanic membranes. Examine the eyes for irritation, tearing, and limitation to or pain with ocular motion. Although photophobia may limit the examination, check the pupils for size and reactivity to light. Examine the fundi for papilledema and venous pulsations. If other points in the history and examination suggest glaucoma, measure an ocular pressure. Examine the teeth and gums for signs of trauma or infection. Palpate the neck for lymphadenopathy. Listen for bruits. Examine the spine and the paraspinal muscles for tenderness and spasm. Have the patient move the neck through a full range of motion.

Perform the Kernig's and the Brudzinski's test. Kernig's test is performed by passively extending the knee with the patient lying supine and the hip and the knee flexed to 90 degrees and eliciting pain in the hamstring. Brudzinski's sign is elicited by passively flexing the neck, attempting to bring the chin within a few finger-breadths of the chest (patients with irritated meninges will reflexively flex one or both knees) and finding that the patient flexes the hip reflexively.

Complete the usual pulmonary and cardiovascular examinations. The abdominal examination should focus on discovering pathological reasons for vomiting. Examination of the extremities may reveal evidence of vasculitis or peripheral vascular disease. Finally, the most important part of the examination is the neurological examination. Perform a full neurological examination, including mini mental status, motor and sensory, and cerebellar examinations, and check the patient's gait. These tests are important to exclude hemorrhagic stroke and intracranial bleeds. Some atypical migraine headaches have associated focal neurological signs, but these are diagnoses of exclusion.

Diagnostic Evaluation

Most patients with their typical migraine headache require no diagnostic tests in the ED. If the history or physical examination has suggested a pathological alternative cause for the headache, then this should be pursued with the appropriate tests. If it is the patient's first severe headache or if this headache represents a change in the usual pattern of headaches, then the patient may require a head computed tomography (CT) scan and a lumbar puncture to rule out infection, tumor, or bleed. The head CT scan may suggest a cause for the headache, and it will help exclude causes of increased intracranial pressure, which may affect your decision to perform the lumbar puncture. At this point, the head CT scan is not sensitive enough to exclude subarachnoid bleeding; thus, a lumbar puncture must be performed.

There is rarely a need for an emergent magnetic resonance imaging (MRI) scan, and the decision to obtain one should be guided by the patient's presentation. Many of the treatments for migraine cannot be used if the patient is pregnant; thus, perform a pregnancy test on all women of childbearing potential. It is important to treat the pain that the patient is experiencing as you get your testing completed.

Differential Diagnosis

The differential diagnosis for headache is illustrated in Table 29.1.

Table 29.1.

Differential diagnosis of headache

Acute Conditions
Subarachnoid hemorrhage
Meningitis
Hypertension
Acute angle closure glaucoma
Posttraumatic
Cerebral ischemia
Substance withdrawal (caffeine, drug of abuse)
Migraine
Cluster
Trigeminal neuralgia
Tension-type
Coital
Carotid dissection

Subacute Conditions
Brain tumor
Intracranial abscess
Chronic subdural hematoma
Postconcussive

Treatment

After pathological causes of headache have been ruled out, a myriad of effective treatment options are available (Table 29.2). The U.S. Headache Consortium identified several goals for treatment of the migraine sufferer: reduce the attack frequency and severity, reduce disability, improve the quality of life, prevent headaches, avoid headache medication escalation, and educate and enable patients to manage their disease. Obviously, in the ED your objective is to provide relief while trying to avoid escalating the use of pain medications.

Migraine headaches are often self-limited. The ED environment is often not conducive to treating a patient suffering from a migraine headache. Placing the patient in a quiet, comfortable, dark room is optimal but often impossible. IV fluids may help with the mild dehydration that the nausea and vomiting can cause. Nonsteroidal antiinflammatory agents are a good first option. Usually the patient has already tried ibuprofen or naproxen before presenting to the ED and is still in pain. Prochlorperazine or metoclopramide is probably the most commonly used treatment for migraine in EDs.

Other neuroleptics such as haloperidol, thiothixene, chlorpromazine, and droperidol have also been shown to be effective. (Care must be taken when using droperidol, because the U.S. Food and Drug Administration labeled it a "black box" drug in 2002.) One should always watch for the side effects of these medications, including akathisia, and extrapyramidal symptoms. Ergotamines and triptans are probably more effective in aborting migraine headaches, especially if given early in the course. These can be given alone or in combination with prochlorperazine or metoclopramide to help with the nausea.

Many clinicians also use prednisone and sometimes diazepam, in addition to one or more of the previous medications, but there are no studies to confirm their efficacy. Because of their addictive potential and the availability of other options, opiates are often avoided for treatment of migraine headaches. They can be effective both in the ED and as therapy at home. Intranasal lidocaine has also been shown to be effective in those patients who can tolerate it, although it is suggested that there is a higher rate of headache recurrence when it is used. There are no randomized studies that look at barbiturate-containing medications and migraine. However, they have been widely used in the past but have fallen out of favor because of more migraine-specific medications that are not addictive.

Preventive medications used in migraines are too numerous to mention. The most effective ones include amitriptyline, divalproex sodium, propranolol, and timolol.

Disposition

Most patients with migraine headaches can safely be discharged with follow-up. Complete pain relief should not be the determining factor in the disposition. Only about 65% of patients get full relief from their ED visit. The rest get resolution of pain over the next day or so. Pain that is so severe that it cannot be adequately treated at home does require admission. Intractable nausea leading

Table 29.2.

Treatment options for migraine headache[a]

Drug	Dose	Adverse Effects
Antiemetics		
Prochlorperazine	25 mg PR 10 mg IM or IV	Extrapyramidal symptoms, sedation Sedation and dystonia rare
Metoclopramide	10 mg IM or IV 20 mg PR	
Chlorpromazine	0.1–1.0 mg IM 12.5–37.5 mg IV	
NSAIDs, Combination Analgesics		
Ibuprofen	400–800 mg po (up to 2,400 mg tested)	Gastric upset, nausea, vomiting
Naproxen	750–1250 mg po	Gastric upset, nausea, vomiting
Acetaminophen	650 mg (up to 4,000 mg tested)	Well tolerated
Ketorolac	30–60 mg IM tested (often used as 15–30 mg IV)	Gastric upset, nausea, vomiting
Acetaminophen + ASA + caffeine	500 mg + 500 mg + 130 mg (2 tabs) po	Insomnia
Ergot Alkaloids and Derivatives		
Dihydro-ergotamine (DHE)	1 mg SC or IM 1–2 mg IV	Nausea, vomiting, flushing, anxiety, contraindicated if cardiac disease
Triptans		
Sumatriptan	Nasal spray 5–20 mg 6 mg SC 25–50 mg po	Contraindicated for patients with cardiac disease, rare MI and stroke, flushing
Rizatriptan	5–10 mg po	
Zolmitriptan	2.5–5.0 mg po	
Opiates		
Morphine Sulfate Acetaminophen + codeine	2–4 mg IV 1–2 tabs po	Sedation, nausea, dizziness
Corticosteroids		
Dexamethasone	6 mg IV for rescue status migrainosus	
Other Medications		
Lidocaine intranasal	4% solution 1–4 drops	Intranasal irritation, possible headache recurrence
Isometheptene	2–5 capsules (Midrin) po 2–6 capsules (Midrid) po	Drowsiness, dizziness, nausea
Butalbital + ASA + caffeine + codeine	50 mg + 325 mg + 40 mg + 30 mg po	Sedation, risk for barbiturate overuse, rebound headache

ASA, acetylsalicylic acid; IM, intramuscular; IV, intravenous; MI, myocardial infarction; po, by mouth; PR, rectally; SC, subcutaneous.

[a]This list is not exhaustive. Only representative drugs from each class of medications have been included.

to the inability to take in fluid or medication also requires admission.

The discharge instructions should include information about what should be done for increasing and unremitting pain or nausea. Have the patient follow up with his or her regular physician to discuss abortive and preventive treatment options. As always, include the symptoms for which they should return to the ED.

Pathophysiology

The pathophysiology of migraine is not yet fully understood. Current theories on the etiology of migraine headache suggest that it is a neurovascular disorder. The neurovascular theory takes the view that vascular change is secondary to neural activation. The exact location and type of the originating neuronal stimulus has not been found, but a hypoperfusion of moderate intensity appears in the posterior cortex and spreads anteriorly. This mirrors the migrainous march of the neurological deficit that has been demonstrated and is similar to the phenomenon of cortical spreading depression. The hypoperfusion is followed by a phase of long-lasting hyperperfusion, which seems to be a result of vasodilation and inflammation. This process stimulates the surrounding trigeminal sensory nerve pain pathway, which is a key mechanism underlying the generation of headache pain associated with migraine. The complexity of this process explains why so many different classes of drugs, from nonsteroidal antiinflammatory drugs to neuroleptics, can be effective treatments for migraine headaches.

The exact mechanism of some of the effective treatments remains in question.

Suggested Readings

Baron JC. [The pathophysiology of migraine: insights from functional neuroimaging]. *Rev Neurol* 2000;156(Suppl 4):4S15–23.

Bartleson JD. Treatment of migraine headaches. *Mayo Clin Proc* 1999;74:702–708.

Goadsby PJ. Advances in the pharmacotherapy of migraine. How knowledge of pathophysiology is guiding drug development. *Drugs Res Dev* 1999;2:361–374.

Hargreaves RJ, Shepheard SL. Pathophysiology of migraine—new insights. *Can J Neurol Sci* 1999; 26(Suppl 3):S12–19.

Matchar DB, Young WB, Rosenberg JH, et al. *Evidence-based guidelines for migraine headache in the primary care setting: pharmacological management of acute attacks.* US Headache Consortium (endorsed by American College of Emergency Physicians), American Academy of Neurology, 2002.

Sanchez del Rio M, Reuter U, Moskowitz MA, et al. Central and peripheral mechanisms of migraine. *Funct Neurol* 2000;15 (Suppl 3):157–162.

Smetana GW. The diagnostic value of historical features in primary headache syndromes: a comprehensive review. *Arch Intern Med* 2000; 160:2729–2737.

Welch KMA. Drug therapy: drug therapy of migraine. *N Engl J Med* 1993;329: 1476–1483.

CHAPTER **30**

Central Nervous System Infections

J. David Walsh, MD

Clinical Scenario

A 42-year-old African American man walks into the emergency department (ED) complaining of severe headache, photophobia, nausea, and vomiting. His symptoms gradually worsened today since waking from sleep with a dull headache. He notes a productive cough for 1 week and complains of neck and back pain and chills and sweats. He denies any weakness, difficulty speaking, or trouble with his gait. Review of systems is otherwise unremarkable.

Past medical history is significant for sickle cell disease and adult-onset diabetes. He takes glyburide, and Percocet (oxycodone) as needed for sickle-cell related pain. He smokes a pack a day of cigarettes, drinks occasional alcohol, and uses intravenous (IV) heroin, but denies cocaine or other drug use. He currently resides in a local shelter.

Physical examination reveals a tired man vomiting stomach contents. Vital signs are temperature of 103°F, blood pressure of 130/75 mm Hg, a pulse of 125 beats/minute, respiratory rate of 26 breaths/minute, and room air oxygen saturation of 100%. Other than photophobia, the results of examination of his head, eyes, ears, nose, and throat are normal. There is shotty cervical lymphadenopathy. His neck gives stiff resistance when passively flexed toward his chest.

Cardiovascular examination is normal except for tachycardia. Lung examination reveals crackles at the right base. On neurological examination, he is an alert, confused man, oriented to place and self but not to time. Rapid head movements worsen his headache. Cranial nerves III to XII are

grossly intact. There is no evidence of papilledema on funduscopic examination, but there is photophobia. General strength and sensation examinations are normal.

This patient is at high risk for a bacterial infection, and his symptoms and signs are consistent with meningitis. He has two blood cultures drawn simultaneously and a urinalysis. Two grams of ceftriaxone and 1 g of vancomycin are administered empirically before lumbar puncture (LP) is performed. After a normal head CT an LP is done. LP results include a white blood cell count of 1200, with 92% polymorphonuclear cells and only 50 red blood cells (RBCs) in tube 4. Urinalysis results are negative, and chest x-ray film shows a right lower lobe infiltrate. The patient is admitted to an intensive care unit (ICU) bed with isolation precautions with the presumptive diagnosis of bacterial meningitis and pneumonia. Blood cultures eventually grow out *Streptococcus pneumoniae*, and despite a prolonged hospital stay, he recovers and is discharged with a referral to a detoxification center.

Clinical Evaluation

Introduction

This patient's symptoms, physical examination, and multiple risk factors make his presentation suggestive of meningitis (viral or bacterial), by far the most common of the central nervous system (CNS) infections. However, many factors of his presentation are suggestive of encephalitis, abscess, empyema, or septic thrombophlebitis of a dural venous sinus. All of these entities (with the exception of viral meningitis) are potentially lethal and warrant aggressive workup and treatment. The onus lies on the emergency physician to highly prioritize patients with possible meningitis and to know when to pursue the diagnosis of other less common, but not rare, CNS infections.

History

Meningitis

The complaints associated with meningitis correlate with the pathophysiology of the infection and include symptoms and signs of systemic infection, meningeal inflammation, cerebral vasculitis, and increased intracranial pressure.

Patients have systemic complaints, much as the patient in the clinical scenario, of fevers, chills, and myalgias. In addition, patients with bacterial meningitis may complain of a rash. Patients may have experienced a recent respiratory illness; this is often seen in either viral or bacterial meningitis. Patients with viral meningitis may have a history of preceding gastrointestinal (GI) or genitourinary (GU) illness.

Neck stiffness is a common symptom of meningeal inflammation, and the patient in the clinical scenario experienced this. Complaints such as hearing loss, difficulty swallowing, double vision, facial droop, or facial sensation loss may also be seen as symptoms of meningeal inflammation. Cerebral vasculitis manifests itself as focal neurological abnormalities or seizures. Signs of elevated intracranial pressure include headache and altered mental status in the form of confusion and disorientation. Other symptoms of elevated intracranial pressure include cranial nerve palsies and seizures.

Encephalitis

Encephalitis viruses have a tropism for specific anatomic locations within the brain parenchyma, leading to neurological deficits correlating with the brain area affected. Headache, fever, and myalgias may be the patient's only complaint, and physical examination is sometimes necessary to elicit associated neurological deficits. Patients often present with altered mental status and sometimes with personality changes. Patients with encephalitis may report time spent outdoors, recent insect bites, or animal bites in the past few months.

Central Nervous System Abscess and Empyema

Headache, fever, seizures, and/or focal neurological complaints are the classic triad accompanying all of the intracranial suppurations. Of these, only focal neurological complaints separate the focal CNS suppurations from meningitis. Otalgia or facial pain correlating with sinusitis may raise the suspicion level for a nonmeningitic CNS infection.

Physical Examination

Meningitis

Patients with meningitis tend to appear ill. Viral meningitis or early bacterial meningitis may have a more benign presentation. Patients with severe meningeal inflammation may assume the "tripod" position (also called Amoss sign or Hoyne sign) in which the knees and hips are flexed, the back arches lordotically, the neck extends, and the arms are brought back to support the thorax. Vital signs will show fever and possibly tachycardia, hypotension, and tachypnea.

When suspecting meningitis, neck stiffness should be tested for by passive flexion of the patient's neck, looking for rigidity. The Brudzinski sign is present if passive neck flexion with the patient in the supine position causes flexion of the knees and hips. Kernig's sign is tested in the sitting patient with legs dangling and is present if passive flexion of the knee elicits spasm of the knee flexors. Jolt accentuation of headache is an excellent test for meningeal inflammation with one small study showing it to have a sensitivity of 97% to 100% for meningitis. It is elicited by having the patient rotate the head back and forth in the horizontal plane at a frequency of two to three rotations per second.

None of the individual signs of meningeal inflammation have been studied significantly to draw meaningful conclusions about their sensitivity and specificity. However, 99% to 100% of patients with meningitis have at least one sign or symptom of fever, neck stiffness, or change in mental status. The patient in the clinical scenario exhibits classic physical examination findings of a patient with meningitis, including neck stiffness, Kernig's and Brudzinski signs, jolt accentuation of his headache, fever, and mental status change.

After looking for signs of meningeal inflammation, examine for signs of papilledema (blurring of the optic disc borders) on funduscopic examination, signs of preceding respiratory or otorhinogenic illness (pharyngeal inflammation, otitis media, or auscultatory findings consistent with pneumonia), or petechial rash (present in 73% of patients with meningococcemia). A complete neurological inspection concludes the examination.

Encephalitis

Focal neurological deficits predominate in encephalitis and can be accompanied by fever. Neurological deficits tend to correlate with the anatomic location affected by each virus. For example, herpes simplex virus (HSV) goes to limbic structures of temporal and frontal lobes, presenting clinically as psychiatric disturbance, memory difficulty, dysphagia, ataxia, hemiparesis, or seizures. Arboviruses go to the basal ganglia, leading to choreoathetosis and parkinsonism. Rabies tends to affect the brainstem nuclei, leading to cranial nerve X deficits in swallowing and possibly choking. None of these findings are sensitive or specific for encephalitis but raise suspicions if present.

Central Nervous System Abscess and Empyema

Fever, mental status changes, and focal neurological deficits necessitate a search for focal CNS suppuration. Bulging or ruptured tympanic membranes, sinus tenderness, dental infection, facial cellulitis, proptosis, and papilledema all should be sought after as nonspecific, nonsensitive signs of focal CNS infection. Griesinger's sign (posterior auricular swelling resulting from mastoid emissary vein obstruction) is seen in half the cases of

septic lateral transverse sinus thrombosis. Gradenigo's syndrome of facial pain and lateral rectus muscle weakness can be seen with cranial epidural abscess or septic lateral transverse sinus thrombosis.

Diagnostic Evaluation

Meningitis

If the history and physical examination are suggestive of meningitis, urgent LP is indicated, preferably before or concurrent with antibiotic administration but certainly not delaying antibiotic administration by more than several minutes. CT scan is indicated prior to LP in any patient with altered mental status, focal neurological findings, HIV, the elderly, and patients with a coagulopathy. In patients who do require CT scan, empiric antibiotics should be given before CT scan.

When performing LP, the opening pressure should be measured (with the patient in a lateral recumbent position). Cerebrospinal fluid (CSF) is then collected sequentially into tubes 1 to 4. Tubes 1 and 4 are sent for cell count and differential. Tube 4 is also sent for culture and Gram stain. Tube 2 is sent for protein and glucose measurements. Tube 3 can be held for other studies such as *Borrelia* antibody, India ink stain, latex agglutination for fungal antigen and cryptococcus, acid-fast stain for tuberculosis, or counterimmune electrophoresis for partially treated bacterial meningitis (Chapter 72) (Table 30.1).

Encephalitis

Because most patients with encephalitis present with focal neurological deficits and/or altered mentation, a CT scan of the head is usually the first diagnostic test done. CT scan is not very sensitive for encephalitis, showing changes in only about 50% of patients with early disease. Magnetic resonance imaging (MRI) is much more sensitive and may be performed to look for other etiologies such as stroke.

Neither viral assays nor antibody assays are sensitive for detection of viral pathogens,

Table 30.1.

Analysis of lumber puncture results in infections of the central nervous system

Tube	Laboratory Test	Results
1	RBCs WBCs *Differential*	Usually none unless traumatic NL: <5/mm^3, elevated in all types of meningitis *Predominance of PMNs suggests* *bacterial infection*
2	Glucose Protein	NL: Ratio of CSF to serum glucose is 0.6:1 Depressed in bacterial meningitis NL: 15–45mg/dL Elevated in infection and many other central pathological conditions
3	Gram stain	NL: No organisms. Organisms identified in bacterial meningitis if untreated 80%, if prior antibiotics up to 60%
4	RBCs	NL: None. If traumatic RBC count in tube 1, RBCs should be significantly reduced in tube 4. If SAH is suspected and RBC count does not change from tube 1 to tube 4 or the patient has xanthochromia, suggests SAH.

CSF, cerebrospinal fluid; NL, normal limit; PMN, polymorphonuclear; RBC, red blood cell; SAH, subarachnoid hemorrhage; WBC, white blood cell.

necessitating the use of CSF polymerase chain reaction (PCR) tests to identify specific pathogens. Of the encephalitides, HSV is the only treatable entity. Therefore, it is imperative to rule this in or out (with CSF PCR) in all patients in whom encephalitis is suspected. With the advent of CSF PCR, brain biopsy is no longer used as a means of identifying HSV encephalitis. CSF findings in any of the encephalitides can include lymphocytic pleocytosis, elevated CSF protein, and presence of RBCs. Low levels of CSF glucose are uncommon and should suggest searching for a different diagnosis. Attempts to identify non-HSV encephalitis pathogens are an esoteric pursuit, except perhaps in the case of their use as biological warfare agents.

Central Nervous System Abscess and Empyema

All patients presenting with altered mentation, focal neurological findings, or papilledema should have a CT scan of the head before LP.

CT findings of brain abscess (Fig. 30.1) or subdural or epidural empyema are absolute contraindications to LP.

Differential Diagnosis

The differential diagnosis of CNS infections is illustrated in Table 30.2.

Treatment

Meningitis

Empiric therapy for meningitis targets the most likely pathogens. *S. pneumoniae* affects all ages except for infants younger than 1 month old, and drug resistance to *S. pneumoniae* has climbed in recent years, necessitating double coverage in age groups likely to be infected with it. Meningococcus affects ages 1 month to 50 years. *Haemophilus influenzae* (H. flu), previously a common pathogen, has been all but eradicated by the advent of the *H. influenzae* vaccine. The young (<1 month) and old (>50 years) are targets of *Listeria monocytogenes*. Group B

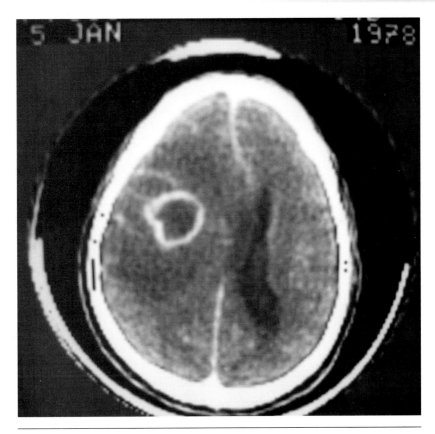

Figure 30.1
Computed tomography (CT) scan of central nervous system (CNS) abscess.
Findings include a ring-enhancing lesion, surrounding edema, and midline shift
with loss of the right lateral ventricle.

streptococci are responsible for 49% of bacterial meningitis in patients younger than 1 month old, but it is not a significant pathogen in other age groups.

Patients who are younger than 1 month should receive ampicillin and either cefotaxime or gentamicin as empiric therapy. Ampicillin provides good empiric coverage for group B streptococci and *Listeria* species. Cefotaxime also covers group B streptococci and adds broad-spectrum gram-negative coverage. Gentamicin, if used instead of cefotaxime, has a synergistic effect with ampicillin versus *Listeria* species, while providing broad-spectrum gram-negative coverage.

Patients who are 1 to 3 months of age should receive either cefotaxime or ceftriaxone with either vancomycin or ampicillin as empiric antibiotic therapy. Cefotaxime and ceftriaxone both have excellent CNS penetration and provide good coverage for *S. pneumoniae* and *Neisseria meningitidis*. The addition of ampicillin provides double coverage for both *S. pneumoniae* and *N. meningitidis*. Vancomycin provides double coverage for *S. pneumoniae* but does not cover *N. meningitidis*. Because of low and erratic CNS penetration, there is some evidence that vancomycin should be double dosed (15 mg/kg q 6 hours). IV dexamethasone should also be given to reduce tumor necrosis factor (TNF) production associated with bacteriolysis.

Patients aged 3 months to 50 years should receive ceftriaxone, ceftazidime, or meropenem, in addition to vancomycin and dexamethasone. Meropenem, like the third-generation cephalosporins, provides excellent coverage for both *S. pneumoniae* and *N. meningitidis*.

Table 30.2.

Differential diagnosis of infections of the central nervous system

Infectious Conditions
Normal Host
Bacterial meningitis
Viral meningitis
Abscess
Encephalitis
Cysticercosis (from endemic areas)
Septic cavernous sinus thrombosis

Immunocompromised (transplant patient, AIDS, chemotherapy)
Toxoplasmosis
Cryptococcus meningitis
Listeria meningitis
Cytomegalovirus encephalitis
Herpes simplex encephalitis
Tuberculous meningitis
CNS syphilis

Noninfectious Conditions
CNS lymphoma
CNS tumors
Stroke
CNS hemorrhage
Uremic or hepatic encephalopathy

AIDS, acquired immunodeficiency syndrome; CNS, central nervous system.

Patients older than 50 years, or patients who are alcoholic, should receive the same regimen as those 1 to 3 months old: ampicillin with ceftriaxone or cefotaxime and dexamethasone. Meropenem can be substituted for ampicillin and the cephalosporin.

Encephalitis

Herpes encephalitis is the only encephalitis pathogen for which more than supportive care is possible. Patients with fever and neurological deficit who do not have evidence of meningitis or a CNS abscess may be treated presumptively for herpes encephalitis with IV acyclovir (10 mg/kg every 8 hours). Duration of therapy is still debated, but 3 weeks of therapy may reduce the 10% relapse rate commonly seen with the more commonly studied 10 days of therapy.

Central Nervous System Abscess and Empyema

Empiric antibiotic therapy should be geared toward the likely source of infection. In general, a third-generation cephalosporin and metronidazole are recommended. Special consideration should be given to trauma cases for streptococcal and staphylococcal infections and to contiguous otitis media infections for *Pseudomonas aeruginosa*.

Steroid use is controversial but use with cerebral edema or with midline shift seems advisable.

Neurosurgical drainage is indicated for many focal CNS infections; therefore, a neurosurgeon should be consulted for all focal CNS infections.

Disposition

All patients with CNS infections should be admitted to the hospital, with the exception of stable, minimally ill-appearing patients with viral meningitis. Those with waxing and waning mental status or apparently rapidly progressing and worsening symptoms should be admitted to the ICU. All of the focal CNS suppurations (brain abscess, epidural abscess, subdural empyema, and septic thrombophlebitis of dural venous sinuses) require neurosurgical consultation for possible trephination and drainage.

Pathophysiology

Meningitis

Meningitis usually arises when an airway pathogen enters the blood and then crosses the blood–brain barrier into the subarachnoid space. Direct contiguous spread from adjacent abscess, sinus, or middle ear is an uncommon, but occasional, route of entry into the CNS. Traumatic or neurosurgical penetration into the arachnoid space is another less common avenue of bacterial entry. Once the blood–brain barrier is violated, the body's inflammatory response to bacteria in the meninges amplifies the effect of bacterial proliferation, leading to swollen meninges. There is CSF volume expansion secondary to decreased CSF circulation, and a resultant decrease in CSF absorption. Vasogenic edema combines with the previously mentioned inflammatory responses to increase intracranial pressure. This not only destroys brain matter by direct pressure effects but also threatens adequate perfusion.

Up to 80% of viral meningitis cases are caused by enteroviruses, including echovirus, coxsackievirus, and nonparalytic poliomyelitis. Other precipitants of viral meningitis include mumps, HSV type 2, lymphocytic choriomeningitis, adenoviruses, and acute human immunodeficiency virus (HIV) infection. Viruses cause a milder inflammatory response than their bacterial counterparts, and the disease is usually self-limited.

Encephalitis

Encephalitis is inflammation of the brain parenchyma. Numerous arthropod-borne adenoviruses cause encephalitis, including tick-borne viruses and mosquito-borne viruses such as Eastern equine encephalitis (EEE), Western equine encephalitis (WEE), and Venezuelan equine virus (VEE). EEE, WEE, and VEE are also potential weapons of biological warfare or terrorism because they are inexpensive and simple to produce and because they are stable during storage and dissemination.

Rabies virus (after introduction by animal bite), herpes zoster, and HSV-1 invade the brain parenchyma by retrograde travel through neuronal axons.

Central Nervous System Abscess and Empyema

Approximately 75% of brain abscesses and nearly all cranial epidural abscesses, subdural empyemas, and septic thrombophlebitis of dural venous sinuses originate in direct spread from trauma or neurosurgical procedures or from adjacent sinus, otic, or (less frequently) skin or dental infections. Most often, contiguous spread is facilitated by diploic (valveless) veins draining the CNS and adjacent sinuses, allowing infection to travel down a pressure gradient. Less often, contiguous spread is facilitated by os-

teomyelitic breakdown of bone and/or meningeal layers.

Epidural spinal abscesses, in contrast to epidural cranial abscesses, most often originate via hematogenous spread of bacteria, from literally any source of infection. Epidural spinal abscess can be caused by contiguous spread as well. One common scenario is seen in IV drug users with bloodborne infections resulting from unsterile injection techniques. The bacteria can enter the bone via the bloodstream, causing osteomyelitis of a vertebral body, and an epidural abscess can form if there is contiguous spread from the bone to the epidural space. Pathogens for any of the intracranial infections correlate with the pathogens most frequently seen in the original infection site. All intracranial infections of otorhinogenic (ears, nose, and throat) origin favor aerobic, microaerophilic, and anaerobic streptococci (particularly *Streptococcus milleri*) as their pathogens. In brain abscesses of otorhinogenic or sinus origin, non-streptococcal anaerobes such as *Bacteroides* are frequently seen. *Staphylococcus* organisms are the most common pathogens in posttraumatic and postoperative intracranial suppurations and in septic cavernous sinus thrombosis, which usually result from the spread of facial skin infections. *S. pneumoniae*, *Escherichia coli*, and *H. influenzae* must be considered as possible pathogens in cases in which the source of infection is pneumonia or meningitis.

Suggested Readings

Attia J, Hatala R, Cook DJ, et al. Does this adult patient have acute meningitis? *JAMA* 1999; 282:175–181.

Barry B, Delattre J, Vie F, et al. Otogenic intracranial infections in adults. *Laryngoscope* 1999; 109:483–487.

Ferre C, Ariza PF, Viladrich JJ, et al. Brain abscess rupturing into the ventricles or subarachnoid space. *Am J Med* 1999; 106:254–257.

Fitzpatrick MO, Gan P. Lesson of the week: contrast enhanced computed tomography in the early diagnosis of cerebral abscess. *BMJ* 1999;319: 239–240.

Gopal AK, Whitehorse, JD, Simel DL, Corey GR, et al. Cranial computed tomography before lumbar puncture: a prospective clinical evaluation. *Arch Intern Med* 1999;159(22): 2681–2685.

Heilper KL, Lorber B. Focal intracranial infections. *Infect Dis Clin North Am* 1996;10: 879–898.

Levitz RE. Herpes simplex encephalitis: a review. *Heart Lung* 1998;27:209–212.

Talan DA. New concepts in antimicrobial therapy for emergency department infections (state of the art). *Ann Emerg Med* 1999;34: 503–516.

Central Nervous System Neoplasms

Michelle Fischer Keane, MD

Clinical Scenario

A 48-year-old woman presents to the emergency department (ED) complaining of a severe headache. On further questioning, she describes a dull, aching headache that she has had for the past 2 weeks. She also states that her headache is worse in the morning and is associated with nausea and vomiting. Her headache feels better after the vomiting. She has never suffered with headaches in the past. acetaminophen (Tylenol) "takes the edge off" of the pain but never completely alleviates her headache. She also describes unsteadiness when walking, feeling as though "she has had too much to drink." She denies fevers, photophobia, visual symptoms, or recent travel.

Past medical and surgical history are significant for breast cancer and a right mastectomy 5 years ago with no subsequent chemotherapy or radiation therapy. She also suffers from hypertension, for which she takes metoprolol. She has no known drug allergies and does not drink or smoke. There is a family history of coronary artery disease and breast cancer.

Physical examination reveals a white woman in no obvious distress. Vital signs include blood pressure of 212/110 mm Hg, a pulse of 65 beats/minute, respiratory rate of 12 breaths/minute, and an oxygen saturation of 99% on room air. Pupils are 4 mm bilaterally, round, and reactive to light. There is horizontal nystagmus bilaterally. Extraocular muscles are intact and tympanic membranes are clear bilaterally; the pharynx is clear without exudates, and there is no lymphadenopathy. The cardiac, respiratory, and abdominal

examinations are unremarkable. Examination of the chest shows evidence of a healed right mastectomy scar and no obvious deformity. Extremities are without evidence of clubbing or cyanosis. There is trace pedal edema. Neurological examination demonstrates cranial nerves III through XII intact. There is no evidence of papilledema, afferent pupillary defect, or visual field deficit (cranial nerve II). Strength is 5/5 in all extremities. There is no evidence of pronator drift. Light touch and proprioception are normal in all limbs. There is slight dysmetria with finger to nose testing with the right upper extremity. Gait is wide-based and unsteady and there is a Romberg sign (ataxia, or loss of balance when standing upright with eyes closed). Reflexes are 2+ throughout with toes down going bilaterally.

The patient receives a noncontrast computed tomography (CT) scan of the brain, which demonstrates a 2 × 2-cm mass in the right cerebellum. There is surrounding edema but no evidence of hemorrhage or infarct. These findings are consistent with a central nervous system (CNS) neoplasm. The patient is admitted to the neurosurgical service.

Clinical Evaluation

Introduction

In the United States, approximately 17,500 patients are diagnosed with a primary CNS neoplasm and another 66,000 with symptomatic brain metastases each year. The most common metastatic culprits are small cell carcinoma of the lung (38%), breast cancer (22%), melanoma (8%), and genitourinary and gastrointestinal system cancers. Primary CNS neoplasms account for 5% to 10% of all neoplasms and occur mainly in younger adults (age <50 years). Metastatic lesions are seen principally in older patients. Of the primary brain tumors, intraparenchymal tumors such as astrocytoma, oligodendrog-lioma, ependymoma, and medulloblastoma occur more commonly than extra-parenchymal tumors such as meningioma, neurofibroma, and craniopharyngioma. Most intracranial tumors diagnosed in the ED, perhaps secondary to the rapid growth producing acute symptomatology, are high-grade astrocytomas, also called glioblastoma multiforme (GBM).

History

In 54% of patients with CNS neoplasms, headache is the primary complaint, and 26% present primarily with seizures. The most common presentation of CNS neoplasms is progressive neurological deficit (68%)—usually motor weakness (45%). The incidence of headaches is identical in primary and metastatic CNS neoplasms. Lesions most likely to produce headache are aggressive, rapidly growing tumors such as GBM. The presence of headache is related to increased intracranial pressure (ICP), tumor size, and the amount of midline shift. Brain tumors cause headache because of traction or displacement of pain-sensitive intracranial structures such as dura mater, cranial nerves, and venous sinuses.

The classic headache of CNS neoplasm is mild and subacute at onset, occurs predominantly in the morning on awakening (possibly because of hypoventilation during sleep), and improves after rising. There is usually a dull, non-throbbing headache, worsened by Valsalva's maneuver—coughing or straining and bending forward—that gradually increases in severity and duration. Headaches are usually frontotemporal and often are misdiagnosed as tension headaches or sinusitis. The headache may be associated with other symptoms of increased ICP such as impaired consciousness, nausea, and vomiting. The vomiting is characteristically projectile, occurs in the early morning hours, and is not preceded by nausea. Unfortunately, this classic pattern occurs in only 8% of patients with CNS neoplasms.

Physical Examination

Signs and symptoms associated with a CNS neoplasm depend on the location of the tumor, and the major distinction is between supratentorial and infratentorial or posterior fossa tumors.

Supratentorial signs and symptoms include (a) those resulting from increased ICP from mass effect of tumor or edema or from obstruction of cerebrospinal fluid (CSF) drainage (hydrocephalus, less common in supratentorial tumors); (b) focal deficits resulting from destruction of brain parenchyma by tumor invasion, compression of parenchyma by the mass or edema, or compression of cranial nerves; (c) headache; (d) seizures—rare with posterior fossa tumors; (e) mental status changes—depression, lethargy, apathy, and confusion; (f) symptoms suggestive of a transient ischemic attack (TIA) or stroke that may be due to occlusion of a vessel by tumor cells or hemorrhage into the tumor; and (g) possibly in pituitary tumors, symptoms resulting from endocrine disturbances, CSF leak, or pituitary apoplexy.

Posterior fossa tumors present with signs and symptoms of increased ICP resulting from hydrocephalus and include (a) headache; (b) nausea and vomiting; (c) papilledema, 50% to 90% incidence; (d) gait disturbance and ataxia; (e) vertigo; and (f) diplopia, especially sixth nerve (abducens) palsy. Cerebellar hemisphere lesions in the posterior fossa may cause ataxia of extremities, dysmetria, and intention tremor. Lesions of the cerebellar vermis may cause broad-based gait, truncal ataxia, and titubation. Brainstem lesions usually result in multiple cranial nerve and long tract abnormalities in addition to nystagmus (especially rotatory or vertical).

Diagnostic Evaluation

The preferred diagnostic tools include CT scan with contrast and magnetic resonance imaging (MRI) with and without gadolinium. Contrast-enhanced CT scan has a 95% accuracy rate in detecting and localizing CNS neoplasms. Noncontrast CT scan, the first-line method in the ED, is only 85% accurate;

however, it is used first because it is an excellent study to detect intracranial blood. A contrast-enhanced CT scan may obscure a clinically relevant bleed. Therefore, noncontrast CT scan alone cannot be used to exclude the presence of intracranial neoplasms. Findings on noncontrast CT scan include hyperdense lesions that displace surrounding structures and edema, seen as a hypodense halo surrounding the suspicious mass. With the addition of intravenous (IV) contrast, better definition of the lesion is made possible by highlighting the peripheral area of increased tumor vascularity. Morphological features of the mass on CT scan can also aid in diagnosing the lesion as malignant (irregular, inhomogeneous borders) versus benign (smooth borders).

Differential Diagnosis

The differential diagnosis for CNS neoplasms is illustrated in Table 31.1.

Treatment

Management of CNS neoplasms consists of referral to a neurosurgeon and oncologist. Obviously acute management depends on the degree of associated symptoms. For example, seizures are managed via standard practice guidelines. As always, evidence of acutely elevated ICP is a neurosurgical emergency for fear of tonsillar herniation.

Table 31.1.

Differential diagnosis of neoplasm of the central nervous system

Migraine
Cluster headache
Tension headache
Subarachnoid hemorrhage
Cerebrovascular accident
Epidural and subdural hematoma
Meningitis
Temporal arteritis
Carotid and vertebral artery dissection
Cerebral venous thrombosis
Encephalitis
Acute closed angle glaucoma
Benign intracranial hypertension

Methods of Lowering Intracranial Pressure

Normal ICP is less than 20 mm Hg. Permanent brain damage occurs with pressures greater than 30 mm Hg. Cerebral perfusion pressure (CPP) is the pressure at which blood must be pumped into the brain in order that it receives sufficient oxygen and glucose. CPP is calculated by subtracting the ICP from the mean arterial pressure (CPP = MAP – ICP). The ICP is a reading obtained from an intracranial bolt, which is placed by a neurosurgeon and is a relatively minor procedure. There are several methods available to acutely lower ICP. The first is elevating the head of the patient's bed 30 to 45 degrees. This maneuver reduces ICP by enhancing venous outflow and promoting displacement of CSF from the intracranial compartment to the spinal compartment. Mean arterial pressure (MAP) is also reduced (and thus CPP is reduced) at the level of the carotid arteries. The onset of action is immediate. This method has become controversial, because it is not sufficient to lower the ICP without knowing the CPP. The CPP may be optimal even with the head at 0 degrees of elevation in a patient with systemic arterial hypertension, depending on the ICP, as discussed in the previous equation.

Hyperventilation, once considered a first-line measure against elevated ICP, must now be regarded as a method to be used in moderation only. It is primarily used in obtunded patients who are intubated. When indicated, hyperventilation should only be used to keep the partial pressure of carbon dioxide (pCO_2) 30 to 35 mm Hg. Hyperventilation lowers ICP by reducing pCO_2, which causes cerebral vasoconstriction, thus reducing the intracranial blood volume. Vasoconstriction also lowers cerebral blood flow (CBF), which may produce focal ischemia in areas with preserved autoregulation caused by shunting. Reducing pCO_2 from 35 to 29 mm Hg lowers ICP 25% to 30%. The onset of action is less than 30 seconds with a peak effect in 8 minutes. Duration of effect is usually 24 hours, after which it is difficult to return to normocarbia without rebound elevation of ICP. Because of this, hyperventilation must be weaned slowly.

Mannitol, an osmotic agent, lowers ICP by several mechanisms. The first is via immediate plasma expansion, which reduces the hematocrit, and blood viscosity, which increases CBF and O_2 delivery. This reduces ICP within a few minutes. The second mechanism is via its osmotic effect. Increased tonicity draws edema fluid from the cerebral parenchyma. This takes up to 30 minutes to establish a gradient with an effect lasting 1.5 to 6 hours. When urgent ICP reduction is needed, an initial dose of 50 to 100 g IV (15% to 25% solution) should be given over 30 minutes. Keep in mind that a large previous dose of mannitol will reduce the effectiveness of subsequent doses; therefore, always use the smallest effective dose. The timing of administering mannitol should be discussed with the neurosurgeon.

Furosemide, a loop diuretic, may reduce ICP by reducing cerebral edema and may also slow the production of CSF. It also acts synergistically with mannitol. Administer 10 to 20 mg IV every 6 hours.

Steroids, specifically the glucocorticoids, reduce vasogenic cerebral edema surrounding brain tumors, thereby lowering ICP. They have little effect on cytotoxic cerebral edema or the derangements commonly seen following trauma. High-dose dexamethasone (Decadron) has a loading dose of 0.5 to 1.5 mg/kg intravenous push (IVP) with maintenance of 0.2 to 0.5 mg/kg every 6 hours.

Disposition

Most patients with a newly diagnosed CNS neoplasm should be admitted to the hospital for a complete workup and diagnosis. Any patient with evidence of increased ICP warrants an intensive care unit (ICU) admission. Obtunded patients, or those whose neurological examination is rapidly deteriorating, may require intubation and an ICU admission. Neurology and neurosurgery should both be involved in the evaluation, because some tumors are amenable to surgery, whereas others require radiation or other palliative measures.

Pathophysiology

The brain is not pain sensitive. Headache in the presence of brain tumor may be due to any combination of the following: increased ICP, invasion or compression of pain-sensitive structures, secondary to difficulty with vision, extreme hypertension resulting from increased ICP, or psychogenic cause. Elevated ICP may be due to tumor mass effect, hydrocephalus, mass effect from associated edema, or hemorrhage. The pain-sensitive CNS structures are the dura, blood vessels, and periosteum. Vision difficulties can include diplopia resulting from cranial nerve dysfunction (specifically III, IV, or VI from direct compression and abducens palsy from increased ICP), which disrupts conjugate gaze. The patient may have difficulty focusing because of optic nerve dysfunction. Optic nerve compression from a superior source can compress the sympathetic fibers leading to Mueller's muscle in the upper eyelid, causing it to droop (ptosis).

Suggested Readings

Evans RW. Diagnostic testing for the evaluation of headaches. *Neurol Clin* 1996;14:1–30.

Field AG, Wang E. Evaluation of the patient with nontraumatic headache: an evidence based approach. *Emerg Med Clin North Am* 1999;17: 127–151.

Greenberg MS. *Handbook of neurosurgery*, 4th ed. Lakeland, FL: Greenberg Graphics, 1997.

Harwood-Nuss AL. *The clinical practice of emergency medicine*, 2nd ed. Philadelphia: Lippincott-Raven, 1996.

Pfund Z. Headache in intracranial tumors. *Cephalalgia* 1999;19:787–790.

Pousada L, Levy DB, Osborn HH. *Case studies in emergency medicine*. Baltimore: Williams & Wilkins, 1993.

Schiff D, Batchelor T, Wen PY. Neurologic emergencies in cancer patients. *Neurol Clin* 1998; 16:449–487.

Sztajnkrycer M, Jauch EC. Unusual headaches. *Emerg Med Clin North Am* 1998;16:741–758.

Headache
Questions and Answers

Questions

1. A 45-year-old woman presents to the emergency department (ED). She is diagnosed with an intracranial mass. Which symptom in the following list is likely to have been her complaint in the ED?

A. Acute neurological deficit

B. Generalized seizure

C. Headache worse in the morning, better during the day

D. Sudden severe headache

E. Photophobia and neck stiffness

2. Which of the following symptoms is typical of migraine headache?

A. Photophobia and neck stiffness

B. Watery eyes and nose

C. Flashing lights

D. Vise-like pain in the head

3. A 23-year-old woman presents to the emergency department complaining of severe headache for 3 days, fever, and stiff neck. She had a cold 1 week ago but has otherwise been in excellent health. Results of her physical examination are normal other than a low-grade fever, tachycardia, and pain upon flexion of the neck. A lumbar puncture is performed and is significant for normal levels of glucose and protein in cerebrospinal fluid (CSF), a white blood count (WBC) of $400/mm^3$ in tube 1 and $450/mm^3$ in tube 4, with a differential of 95% lymphocytes and 5% polymorphonuclear cells; there were no red blood cells. She most likely has:

A. Bacterial meningitis

B. Herpes meningitis

C. Viral meningitis

D. An abscess

4. A patient arrives at the emergency department (ED) complaining of the precipitous onset of a severe thunderclap right-sided headache, neck stiffness, and blurred vision. On examination, you discover ptosis, an ipsilateral dilated, poorly reactive pupil, with decreased medial and vertical gaze of the right eye and marked meningismus. Where is the aneurysm?

A. The right posterior communicating artery

B. The left posterior communicating artery

C. The right middle cerebral artery

D. The left anterior communicating artery

Directions: There are three sets of response options for the following scenario. You will be required to select one best answer from each question set.

5. A 46-year-old woman presents to the emergency department (ED) complaining of a severe headache with blurred vision, photophobia, nausea, and vomiting. She has a history of severe headaches, which are usually relieved by ibuprofen and acetaminophen. This headache is not relieved by these medications. The headache has been continuous for 24 hours and is somewhat better than when it first began. She does not complain of neck stiffness or fever. Physical examination reveals a woman in moderate distress with mild photophobia, supple neck, and an otherwise unremarkable neurological examination. Vital signs are normal except for a heart rate of 103 beats/minute.

5.1. Choose the correct statement:

A. The patient should be treated presumptively with antibiotics for bacterial meningitis, and a computed tomography (CT) scan of the head and a lumbar puncture (LP) should be obtained.

B. The patient should be treated with ceftriaxone and ketorolac for presumptive migraine.

C. The patient requires a head CT scan and lumbar puncture to rule out subarachnoid hemorrhage.

D. The patient should be treated for migraine. If the pain is relieved, she may be safely discharged.

5.2. A head computed tomography (CT) scan and lumbar puncture (LP) are both normal. What is the next appropriate step in caring for this patient?

A. Discharge with the diagnosis of probable migraine.

B. Treat her headache. If pain is not completely resolved, admit for pain control and further evaluation.

C. Treat her headache. If she shows some improvement, discharge her with follow-up for further evaluation.

D. The nature of the headache and the negative CT have ruled out a central nervous system (CNS) mass. Treat her headache, and then discharge her with primary care follow-up.

5.3. Further investigation into her records reveals that she has acquired immunodeficiency syndrome (AIDS). How does this change your management of this patient?

A. There is no change in management. She is afebrile, and can proceed with a computed tomography (CT) scan and lumbar puncture (LP) without antibiotics.

B. Potential etiologies for her headache now include central nervous system (CNS) toxoplasmosis, CNS lymphoma, and glioblastoma multiforme.

C. If CT and LP are negative, an emergent magnetic resonance imaging (MRI) scan of her brain should be performed, or she

should be admitted to the hospital for further evaluation.

D. If CT and LP are negative, she can be treated for migraine and discharged with follow up.

Answers and Explanations

1. B. Seizure, both generalized and focal, occurs in 26% of patients. Sudden severe headache or "worst headache of my life" is classically associated with subarachnoid hemorrhage. The headache associated with an intracranial neoplasm is usually mild in nature, described as dull and nonthrobbing with a subacute onset and worse in the morning. It occurs with approximately 54% of all intracranial masses. The most common presentation of an intracranial mass is progressive, not acute, neurological deficit and occurs in 68% of patients. Photophobia and neck stiffness are typical complaints for subarachnoid hemorrhage or meningitis.

2. C. Migraines have a myriad of presenting symptoms including photophobia, visual disturbances, and nausea and vomiting. The visual symptoms vary from wavy lines in the field of vision, to seeing flashing lights (scotomata), which are classic findings in migraine. Neck stiffness is not a common complaint, and in conjunction with photophobia is more likely a subarachnoid bleed or meningitis. Some complicated migraines even manifest with weakness in an extremity. A vise-like pain in the head is most typical of a tension-type headache, where the scalp muscles are physically squeezing against the skull, creating severe pain. Patients who suffer from cluster headaches frequently also have runny noses and watery eyes.

3. C. This patient has no significant past history and is unlikely to have an unusual pathogen. Therefore, she most likely has either bacterial or viral meningitis. With a relatively low white blood count (WBC), predominantly lymphocytes, and a normal glucose level, viral infection is almost certainly the etiology. With a nonfocal examination, it is unlikely to be herpes meningitis. In addition, she had a precedent viral illness and after 3 days of symptoms is not toxic appearing. If this were an acute bacterial infection, she would be much sicker after 3 days of infection, and her lumbar puncture should have shown a predominantly polymorphonuclear cell differential.

4. A. An aneurysm on the right posterior communicating artery would put pressure on the right third cranial nerve, causing ipsilateral weakness or paralysis of the lateral rectus muscle. A left posterior communicating artery lesion would cause the above symptoms to occur on the left side of the face. An aneurysm of the right middle cerebral artery may cause a right-sided headache but is more likely to cause language difficulties or contralateral hemiparesis. An aneurysm of the anterior communicating artery will cause a bilateral frontal headache and sometimes alteration of level of consciousness.

5.1. C. Although the patient gives a history of headaches, this is clearly a departure from her usual headache. She has no fever or infectious symptoms consistent with meningitis. Computed tomography (CT) scan may be negative for subarachnoid blood, but lumbar puncture (LP) would reveal xanthochromia, a yellow color significant for hemolyzed red blood cells in the cerebrospinal fluid (CSF), indicating a subarachnoid bleed. The most common diagnosis is migraine, and the patient should be treated for her pain immediately. Ceftriaxone is an antibiotic not an analgesic. Promethazine and ketorolac are appropriate first-line agents for migraine. Resolution of pain does NOT rule out an intracranial bleed; therefore, the patient cannot be safely discharged without being treated for the pain, and if the pain goes away, the patient should not be discharged until a subarachnoid hemorrhage has been ruled out.

5.2. C. The normal computed tomography (CT) scan and lumbar puncture (LP) rule out a subarachnoid bleed. Although it is satisfying to make patients completely pain free, patients with migraines frequently take hours or days before complete resolution of their pain. A patient with moderate relief of pain, therefore, does not warrant admission. However, a patient with very severe unremitting pain, without any response to analgesics, may require an admission for pain control. Although the diagnosis of migraine is probable, she should receive analgesia and be observed for improvement before discharge. CT technology is not sufficient to rule out a mass lesion, especially without intravenous (IV) contrast.

5.3. C. She should have a magnetic resonance imaging (MRI) scan of the brain to look for central nervous system (CNS) lymphoma or other pathology. Because she is stable, she could be admitted to the hospital and have the studies done urgently. The patient is immunocompromised. The absence of fever does not rule out an infectious process. She should receive prophylactic antibiotics before computed tomography (CT) and lumbar puncture (LP) to cover bacterial pathogens. Although a negative CT and LP are good signs, a persistent headache with photophobia in an acquired immunodeficiency syndrome (AIDS) patient is a concerning constellation. There are no data to suggest that AIDS patients are at increased risk for astrocytoma or glioblastoma multiforme.

Change in Mental Status

It is a far, far better thing to have a firm anchor in nonsense than to put out on the troubled seas of thought.

John Kenneth Galbraith, 1958

INTRODUCTION
Elizabeth L. Mitchell, MD
Section Editor

Patients who present with alterations in mental status are some of the most challenging cases in emergency medicine. Etiologies can include life-threatening overdoses, stroke, sepsis, intracranial bleed, metabolic abnormalities, environmental disorders, dementia, and psychiatric disorders. These can be grouped into three major categories: systemic disorders, substance-related disorders, and diseases of the central nervous system.

In most of these patients, the difficulty we have as physicians lies in the presentation, with the inability to give an accurate history. These patients have alterations in cognitive ability (content/awareness), level of consciousness (wakefulness), or both. This implies dysfunction of the cerebral cortex, for thought, or the reticular activating system, for level of consciousness. Patients may present with a range of symptoms including confusion, unresponsiveness, emotional lability, hallucinations, or agitation, which may wax and wane or even change during their hospital stay. Coincident with the patient's mental status are clinical systemic signs, which help point the physician in a particular direction. These may include fever, tachycardia, depressed respiration, diaphoresis, cool or clammy skin, and other clinical signs. Findings may necessitate emergent or urgent resuscitative measures including airway protection and fluid resuscitation. Therapies such as glucose administration and naloxone may be used as both diagnostic and therapeutic tools, particularly when no information is available or when information includes a history of diabetes or a history of narcotics. When possible, we must seek information from any potential source: family, paramedics, old records, and witnesses.

Outcomes may be immensely satisfying for the practitioner (a simple intervention can bring about dramatic improvement in a matter of seconds), or they may be complex diagnostic puzzles (requiring emergent treatment concurrent with skillful acquisition of information to determine the underlying etiology and appropriate therapy). In some cases, there is no obvious answer, and we have to institute a broad treatment plan to cover numerous possibilities. The mnemonic "I Watch Death" can be used to differentiate causes of mental status changes:

I = infectious

W = withdrawal (e.g., benzodiazepines, alcohol)

A = acute metabolic,

T = trauma

C = central nervous system (CNS) disease

H = hypoxia

D = deficiencies (e.g., B_{12}, thiamine)

E = environmental

A = acute vascular

T = toxins/drugs

H = heavy metals

The following four chapters cover just a few of the many causes of mental status changes. Throughout this text, however, you will encounter many more of the causes of this very common emergency department complaint.

CHAPTER **32**

Acute and Chronic Alcohol Intoxication

Merle A. Carter, MD, Edward Bernstein, MD

Clinical Scenario

A 50-year-old homeless white woman is brought into the resuscitation room of the local trauma center by emergency medical services (EMS) after having been found down and agitated at the scene. She had been evaluated in the emergency department (ED) several days prior for diffuse abdominal pain and alcohol intoxication, was medically cleared for detoxification, and subsequently was discharged to a nearby alcohol treatment facility.

From prior records, her past medical history includes cirrhosis and alcohol-related hepatitis, chronic pancreatitis, hypertension, seizure disorder, and cerebrovascular accident without residual deficit. Past surgical history is unremarkable. She has denied taking any medications regularly and has no known drug allergies. She smokes 1 to 2 packs of cigarettes a day and admits to drinking daily but denies use of cocaine, heroin, or other drugs of abuse. Family medical history is largely unknown.

Physical examination reveals a disoriented, agitated, and ill-appearing woman without obvious signs of trauma. Vital signs include an axillary temperature of 96.8°F, blood pressure of 110/70 mm Hg, heart rate of 130 beats/minute, respiratory rate of 40 breaths/minute, and a room air oxygen saturation of 98%. She is placed on a cardiac monitor with continuous pulse oximetry and intermittent blood pressure monitoring. Blood alcohol concentration by Breathalyzer is 180 mg/dL and the patient's glucose level by beside glucometer is 30 mg/dL.

Head and neck examination reveals icteric (yellow) sclera, dry mucous membranes, and no jugular venous distension. Pupils are equally reactive to light; extraocular movements cannot be tested because of her mental status. Cardiopulmonary examination is without abnormality. Her abdomen is soft with active bowel sounds, diffusely tender to palpation in all quadrants with voluntary guarding, but without rebound tenderness or palpable masses appreciated. Rectal examination reveals occult blood-positive brown stool, without evidence of hemorrhoids, fissures, or masses. Extremities are without vascular deficit or Babinski sign. Deep tendon reflexes and sensation are symmetric. The patient is oriented only to herself. Her neurological examination is noted only for symmetric use of all extremities, intact reflexes, and intact gag.

Intravenous (IV) access is established and the patient is given 2 amps (50 grams) of $D_{50}W$ (high-concentration dextrose in water). Serum studies and an arterial blood gas are obtained, and an electrocardiogram (ECG) is performed.

Notable abnormalities on laboratory test values include serum glucose of 29 mg/dL, pH of 7.11, and bicarbonate level of 6.5 mEq/L, magnesium of 1.4 mg/dL, and a platelet count of 81,000/mm³. Coagulation indices and liver function values are moderately elevated. Urinalysis (UA) is positive for ketones but otherwise without signs of infection. Urinary and serum toxicology screens are negative, except for an ethanol level of 189 mg/dL.

ECG reveals sinus tachycardia but is otherwise normal. Chest and abdominal kidneys, ureter, and bladder (KUB) x-ray films demonstrate no active disease or focal infiltrates, no dilated loops of bowel, air-fluid levels, or subdiaphragmatic free air. Visible edema of small bowel and cirrhosis were subsequently seen on abdominal computed tomography (CT) scan, but no evidence of intraperitoneal free fluid or masses are noted. CT scan of the head is essentially negative, with the exception of diffuse cortical atrophy consistent with chronic alcohol use.

The patient is admitted to the medical intensive care unit (MICU) for management of withdrawal syndrome and alcohol-related ketoacidosis as a cause for her agitation and disorientation. In the subsequent 2 days, her status improved with aggressive IV hydration, benzodiazepines, and vitamin replacement. She left the hospital against medical advice 3 days later and has since been lost to follow-up.

Clinical Evaluation

Introduction

Alcohol is consumed regularly by nearly half of the adult U.S. population and is the most abused drug worldwide. The cost of substance abuse (SA) to our society—in lost productivity, medical and legal expenses, and social and interventional services—is close to $300 billion annually. Alcohol abuse and its consequences alone accounted for more than 60% of this disturbing figure.

EDs continue to shoulder the burden in intervening in crises precipitated by alcohol use. Annually, more than 100,000 deaths are related to alcohol use and as many as 40% of all ED patients are acutely intoxicated or are considered problem drinkers at the time of presentation.

The goal of this chapter is threefold: to review alcohol intoxication, abuse, and withdrawal as a common cause of altered mentation; to provide the framework with which the student can approach the evaluation and management of an acutely intoxicated or withdrawing patient; and to assist the student in recognizing some of the subtleties, challenges, and pitfalls associated with treating these patients in the emergency setting.

History

In few other patient encounters will your bedside manner be tested more than with an acutely intoxicated or withdrawing patient. In your interactions, be careful not to appear critical, which can precipitate a volatile eruption in an already potentially precarious situation. The rapport with which you initiate contact will determine how smoothly the remainder of your interaction will proceed and how cooperative your patient will be with your questioning, examination, and subsequent management.

The structure and content of each patient encounter varies greatly. For example, the history and physical of a patient who is awake and alert, but acutely intoxicated, is markedly different from that of a patient who is obtunded. Frequently, critical information must be obtained from family, friends, coworkers, witnesses, ambulance personnel, and prior medical records, if the patient is unable to provide that information. In some cases, it may be reasonable to wait until the patient becomes sober and then elicit a more thorough history and physical examination. In the patient who can attend to questions, it is critical to find out what brought the patient to the hospital and what events they recall surrounding this visit. In addition, a careful and complete review of systems must be obtained to search for health issues that may not be apparent even to the patient.

If the patient is able to answer questions, it is helpful to gather information about not only what has brought him or her to the ED but also history pertaining to habits of drinking (how much does he or she generally consume in a day, what type of alcohol does he or she drink, and when was his or her last drink). In addition, obtain information about prior problems related to alcohol: prior withdrawal symptoms, seizures, cirrhosis, pancreatitis, and/or gastrointestinal (GI) bleeding.

Once the patient's chief or presenting complaint has been established, ascertain the details concerning the events leading up to arrival at the ED. This should include how the patient arrived (e.g., ambulance, family member or friend, or self), where the patient was found and in what condition, whether there were any witnesses, and why help was summoned. These details provide important information about the patient's physical condition and mental status before arrival.

Do not forget to ask about current prescribed and over-the-counter medications, including oral contraceptives, and medications he or she should be taking but is not. This provides information about medical history and compliance and the likelihood of compliance with proposed treatments following this visit.

Physical Examination

In the alcohol-intoxicated patient, it is important to do a complete and thorough physical examination. The physical examination may uncover one of the many alcohol-related health problems common to the chronic alcoholic, of which the patient may be unaware.

Acute and chronic alcohol use can lead to many physical problems. One of the most common is trauma and its sequelae. A thorough search for traumatic injuries may uncover signs suggestive of head trauma (hemotympanum, scalp lacerations, or hematomas), neck pain suggestive of cervical trauma, or extremity pain or deformity suggestive of fracture. A careful chest examination may elicit abnormal breath sounds suggestive of pneumonia, aspiration, hemothorax, or pneumothorax. An abdominal examination may be significant for ascites (suggesting cirrhosis) or pain (suggesting pancreatitis, hepatitis, or internal injury). A rectal examination may reveal occult heme-positive stool. Skin findings may reveal jaundice (suggesting hepatitis or cirrhosis) or numerous bruises (suggestive of trauma, bleeding diathesis, or domestic violence). Finally, although all patients should be completely undressed in their ED visit, this is particularly important for the intoxicated patient who may have occult injuries or disease processes. If a patient is uncooperative, shows no sign of trauma, and is hemodynamically stable, time may be taken to allow the patient to become sober, at which point he or she

may refuse further medical attention or may be more prepared to complete the workup.

Diagnostic Evaluation

Generally speaking, a patient who presents to the ED for acute intoxication as a cause of change in mental status, without evidence of traumatic injury; other drug use; or respiratory, cardiovascular, or metabolic derangement, will not require a complete set of laboratory evaluations. These patients should be placed on a monitor and observed regularly for signs of clinical or neurological deterioration.

Serum glucose and blood alcohol concentrations are two pieces of information that are of paramount importance when an apparently intoxicated patient arrives at the ED. Do not assume that if a person behaves or *appears* drunk that he or she actually *is* drunk. Changes in mentation, speech, or gait may be the result of other more subtle causes (e.g., endocrine, metabolic, cerebral, cardiac, infectious, or traumatic). Each should be ruled out before settling on "intoxication" or "withdrawal" as the presenting diagnosis.

Alcohols diffuse easily across cell membranes of alveoli, are exhaled in gas form with CO_2, and are detectable in expired air. The Breathalyzer, a handheld device into which a patient blows through an aperture or a straw, is used to determine the approximate blood alcohol concentration (BAC) of a patient you suspect has been using ethanol. Concentrations are expressed on the Breathalyzer in milligrams per deciliter (mg/dL) of blood. Hence, a BAC of 80 mg/dL corresponds to 0.08%, the legal limit in many states. Breathalyzer results are most reliable when used within 15 to 30 minutes of the last drink and are compromised if the patient gives a poor expiratory effort, has chronic lung disease, or is vomiting or belching during expiration or if the apparatus has been improperly calibrated.

Ethanol undergoes hepatic enzymatic oxidation and follows zero- or first-order elimination determined by the concentration in the system. It follows zero-order elimination if the BAC is 20 to 300 mg/dL and first-order elimination for concentrations less than 20 mg/dL or greater than 300 mg/dL. Therefore, a tolerant drinker can expect to have a reduction in BAC between 30–40 mg/dL per hour. A nontolerant drinker metabolizes more slowly and less efficiently, and BAC levels for this patient fall between 15 to 20 mg/dL per hour. The patient's clinical status, the BAC, and knowledge of ethanol's kinetics are important considerations when planning the amount of observation time required before it is safe to consider discharge.

Glucose is also metabolized differently in alcoholic patients than in nondrinkers. Even in the context of malnutrition, the metabolism of alcohol increases the ratio of reduced nicotinamide adenine dinucleotide to oxidized nicotinamide adenine dinucleotide ($NADH/NAD^+$ ratio), inhibiting gluconeogenesis and increasing the production of CO_2 and lactate from pyruvate through the Krebs-tricarboxylic acid (TCA) cycle. Therefore, hypoglycemia is a frequent consequence of acute or chronic alcohol use and is often the cause of altered mentation, particularly in an already malnourished alcoholic patient. A bedside glucometer is a quick and simple method for determining approximate serum glucose level and is an invaluable tool to implicate or absolve hypoglycemia as the mechanism for disordered mentation.

The decision to pursue other diagnostic tests depends on the condition of the patient and any findings on physical examination. If the patient's mental status does not seem appropriate for the level of intoxication, a more extensive workup may be indicated and may include one or more of the following tests: cranial CT scan, toxicological screening, arterial blood gas, or electrolytes. When considering one of the other alcohols (isopropyl, ethylene glycol, and methanol), diagnostic evaluation should include arterial blood gas sample, serum osmolality, urine for crystals, and alcohol levels. Ethylene glycol and methanol can cause significant morbidity and mortality and should be considered in any patient with an altered mental status of unclear etiology. Patients who may have coingested ethanol will have a persistent acidosis and altered mentation. Early treatment is essential to avoid such sequelae as renal failure (ethylene glycol), blindness (methanol), and death.

Other diagnostic considerations should include a chest x-ray film if the patient has respiratory problems or fever. Signs of trauma may suggest the need for cervical spine x-ray films, chest and extremity x-ray films, and in some instances abdominal or head CT scan. Other conditions associated with alcoholism that may prompt evaluation include pancreatitis, hepatitis, cirrhosis (liver function tests), GI bleeding (complete blood cell [CBC] count, nasogastric tube), subacute bacterial peritonitis (SBP) (paracentesis) alcoholic ketoacidosis (AKA), hypokalemia, hypomagnesemia (electrolytes), and infections (CBC count, UA, chest x-ray film). Any patient who takes medications, such as phenytoin, should have drug levels sent if indicated. The decision to pursue any or all of these tests is determined by the presentation and clinical status of the patient.

Differential Diagnosis

The differential diagnosis for alcohol intoxication is illustrated in Table 32.1.

Treatment

Acute Intoxication

Clinical status dictates therapy (Table 32.2). As mentioned previously, each patient requires a workup that is directed toward his or her particular presentation, complaints, or

Table 32.1.

Differential diagnosis for alcohol intoxication

Ethylene glycol ingestion
Methanol ingestion
Isopropyl alcohol ingestion
Opiate and sedative ingestion
Hepatic encephalopathy
Hypoglycemia
Trauma: subdural hemorrhage, subarachnoid hemorrhage
Other inhalation or ingestion (e.g., carbon monoxide)

Table 32.2.

Treatment guidelines for alcohol intoxication and withdrawal

Stable Intoxication
IV fluids if signs of dehydration
Breathalyzer alcohol level useful
Check glucose level, replete if necessary
Observation and assessment at intervals
Offer detoxification on discharge

Stable Withdrawal (tremulous, mild hypertension, and tachycardia but oriented)
IV normal saline
Electrolytes (include calcium, magnesium, phosphorus), serum alcohol level
Check glucose level, replete if necessary
Continuous cardiac and blood pressure monitoring
Electrolyte repletion if indicated
Oral benzodiazepine usually sufficient (diazepam 10 mg)
IV benzodiazepine (lorazepam 1–2 mg, diazepam 5–10 mg) may be necessary
Observation and assessment at frequent intervals
Consistently stable: discharge to a detoxification program optimal

Unstable Intoxication
May require physical restraints if behavior is out of control
IV normal saline
Check glucose level, replete if necessary
Electrolytes (including calcium, magnesium, phosphorus), serum ethanol level,
    consider serum and urine toxicological screens
Head CT scan if obvious significant trauma (large laceration and hematoma of scalp)
IV benzodiazepine (lorazepam 1–2 mg, diazepam 5–10 mg)
Consider neuroleptic (e.g., haloperidol 2.5–5 mg IM or IV)
Electrolyte repletion if indicated
Thiamine 100 mg IV if Wernicke's encephalopathy suspected

Unstable Withdrawal
Continuous cardiac and blood pressure monitoring
IV normal saline
Check glucose and replete
Electrolytes (including calcium, magnesium, phosphorus), replete as needed
Thiamine 100 mg IV
Multivitamins IV
IV benzodiazepine (lorazepam 1–2 mg, diazepam 10 mg) repeated frequently as
    needed
Consider neuroleptic (e.g., haloperidol 2.5–5 mg IV or IM)
Consider barbiturate IV
Consider IV β-blocker
If out of control, consider intubation
Admission to intensive care unit

CT, computed tomography; IM, intramuscular; IV, intravenous.

symptoms. For some patients, treatment may consist of no more than a period of observation. Others may need IV fluid hydration and repletion of potassium and/or magnesium. In addition, patients should receive thiamine and multivitamins. In the IV preparation, this is commonly referred to as a "banana bag" because IV fluid with multivitamins and thiamine takes on a yellow color.

Wernicke-Korsakoff syndrome and beriberi are the result of chronic thiamine deficiency. The most severe of these is the Wernicke-Korsakoff syndrome, which includes global confusion, psychosis, ataxia, ocular dysfunction, hypothermia, hypotension, and coma. Wernicke's encephalopathy is a potentially fatal outcome of poorly managed alcohol abuse if thiamine is not included in routine care. Thiamine is necessary before any administration of glucose in alcohol-abusing patients. Failure to give thiamine before glucose can quickly precipitate a dangerous encephalopathy.

Ethylene Glycol and Methanol

Although this chapter focuses entirely on ethanol, it would be incomplete without a brief mention of other potentially fatal alcohol poisonings. Both ethylene glycol and methanol, when consumed in even small quantities, can have significant morbidity and mortality including profound acidosis, renal failure, and blindness. They should be included in the differential of any patient with altered mentation and acidosis.

Alcohol Withdrawal

The management of patients in withdrawal is initially similar to that of the acutely intoxicated patient; however, active withdrawal frequently requires additional intervention including symptom-reducing oral or IV medications. The most widely used medications in the treatment of withdrawal syndromes are the sedative-hypnotic benzodiazepines, including lorazepam (Ativan) and diazepam (Valium).

Benzodiazepines augment g-aminobutyric acid (GABA) activity and mimic the effects of ethanol at the receptor site, thus diminishing the dysphoric consequence of abrupt cessation. Currently, there is no consensus regarding which one of the benzodiazepines is most useful in the setting of withdrawal, and use of any particular one of these is based on practitioner preference. The dose required to treat withdrawal symptoms is variable and depends on the individual patient and the degree of agitation and accompanying symptoms.

In general, lorazepam and diazepam are the most popular, are easily titrated, and can be given orally or intravenously in patients unable to swallow or who are otherwise uncooperative. Be cautious when using this class of medications. High doses of these medications increase the risk of respiratory depression and therefore the potential for intubation.

Occasionally, therapy with benzodiazepines alone is not sufficient. For patients whose symptoms are refractory to high doses of benzodiazepines, the neuroleptic butyrophenones (e.g., haloperidol) are common adjuncts to withdrawal management. These are dopamine-selective antagonists and are useful in reducing many of the common effects of withdrawal, such as disorientation and hallucinations. These drugs should not be used as monotherapy, particularly because of their potential to lower the seizure threshold. This poses a danger to patients in withdrawal from alcohol, who are already at risk for seizures. Combinations of haloperidol and lorazepam, for example, are safe and easily titrated to the patient's level of symptomatic relief.

Because of ethanol's effect on β-adrenergic and α-adrenergic neurotransmitter systems (see the section on pathophysiology), β-adrenergic blocking and α-adrenergic agonist medications are also considered in the autonomic manifestations of withdrawal, such as tachycardia, diaphoresis, and hypertension. However, these medications are infrequently used in the routine emergency management of alcohol intoxication or withdrawal and should be used with caution, particularly in patients with known contraindications to their use.

Although relatively rare, delirium tremens (DTs) presents a particular challenge to the ED. The DTs are more common in patients with chronic, long-term ethanol use and include altered mental status, marked confusion and disorientation, frightening hallucinations, tremors (known as "the shakes"), and severe agitation. These symptoms usually begin 48 hours to several days following the last drink and are generally accompanied by tachycardia, hyperthermia, tachypnea, and hypertension.

Approximately 5% of patients presenting to the ED in alcohol withdrawal develop DTs. Mortality in patients undergoing aggressive management for DTs can be as high as 10% to 15%, even higher for those patients who do not respond to treatment or are unable to seek treatment.

Patients with the DTs often require chemical and/or physical restraint in addition to close one-to-one monitoring. Management of this complication of withdrawal is similar to that already mentioned. However, given the severity of these symptoms and the mortality associated with DTs, early and aggressive management is paramount.

Higher doses, or several combinations of the medications mentioned thus far, may be necessary to gain control of this frightening constellation of signs and symptoms. Consider adding a high dose of a long-acting barbiturate to DT management as symptoms dictate or if agitation is refractory to the most common methods of treatment with benzodiazepines or neuroleptics.

Barbiturates are useful because they augment GABA's inhibitory effects by opening GABA-mediated chloride channels without binding the neurotransmitter directly. Phenobarbital also blocks a subclass of receptors that bind the excitatory neurotransmitter glutamate. The net result of these actions is an overall decrease in dysphoric symptoms and a smoother withdrawal.

Disposition

Disposition of patients treated for acute uncomplicated alcohol intoxication is generally straightforward, and hospital admission is rarely indicated. However, plans for discharge of the intoxicated patient should proceed only when the patient is visibly and functionally recovered from the effects of alcohol use. Under the appropriate supervision, you should be comfortable that alcohol alone is responsible for the patient's mental status. Before discharge, be certain that intoxication has not obscured other potentially dangerous coingestions or other medical, surgical, traumatic, or psychiatric disorders requiring intervention.

To safely discharge the patient with changes in mental status relating to alcohol (or the intoxicated patient when sober), be sure the patient has stable vital signs; is able to tolerate food or a beverage without vomiting; and is conversant, oriented, and ambulatory. Patients should be carefully screened for suicidal ideation, coingestions, serious infections, or traumatic injury requiring hospitalization. Hypoxia and metabolic abnormalities such as hypoglycemia must be corrected before discharge. Appropriate prescriptions, follow-up appointments, and referrals for SA treatment are important components of the discharge process.

Patients with ongoing signs or symptoms of alcohol withdrawal syndrome (AWS) require admission for close observation and further management. The number and severity of these symptoms dictates whether an intensive care unit setting is advisable. Where withdrawal is extremely mild, it can be managed in the ED, requiring straightforward medical management and a prolonged period of observation.

Disposition to Detoxification

Advice given to patients to stop or to reduce their consumption or to seek an inpatient or outpatient detoxification program may often be rejected. Factors including the patient's readiness to change, the approach of the health care provider, and the availability of treatment facilities have all been implicated in this failure. Patients may not seek treatment because of a lack of information about their options, lack of motivation or realization that they need help, or the perception that treatment is simply not effective.

Some providers may believe that referring patients to SA treatment is not within the realm of their clinical responsibility. Others may feel uncomfortable or inadequately trained to make appropriate treatment plans and necessary referrals. Still others may be skeptical about the effectiveness of SA treatment. No one would argue that failure to arrange appropriate follow-up for an asthma exacerbation is an unacceptable practice. However, many practitioners fail to arrange appropriate aftercare or follow-up for drug- or alcohol-dependent patients. Recent evidence supports the claim that alcohol treatment outcomes are comparable to that of other chronic conditions (e.g., hypertension, asthma, and diabetes) and that medication compliance and relapse rates are similar across these illnesses.

Several strategies have proven useful in assessing the degree to which alcohol use is a problem and in aligning patients with aftercare in an effort to ensure a safe discharge. Using National Institute on Alcohol Abuse and Alcoholism (NIAAA) information, begin by assessing the extent of the problem:

- On average, how many days per week do you drink alcohol (beer, wine, and liquor)?
- On a typical day when you drink, how many drinks do you have?
- What is the maximum number of drinks you had on any given occasion during the last month.

Once this has been assessed, the problem can be further explored with the aid of an appropriate interviewing strategy.

The Cut-Annoyed-Guilty-Eye-opener (CAGE) questionnaire and the brief negotiation interview (BNI) are two such strategies. The CAGE is a brief questionnaire to assess the level of alcoholism and was designed to be nonconfrontational in its approach. Found on the National Institute on Alcohol Abuse and Alcoholism Web site (www.niaaa.nih.gov), the questionnaire contains the following questions:

C: Have you ever felt you should cut down on your drinking?

A: Have people annoyed you by criticizing your drinking?

G: Have you ever felt bad or guilty about your drinking?

E: Have you ever had a drink first thing in the morning as an "eye-opener" to steady your nerves or to get rid of a hangover?

Each question is scored with a 0 or 1. A total score of 2 or greater indicates a clinically significant problem.

The BNI has had considerable success for more than 7 years at Boston Medical Center, and now at Yale New Haven Hospital and in other ED programs and involves the following steps:

1. Establish rapport and ask permission to raise subject.
2. Provide feedback comparing quantity and frequency,
3. Ask, "What connection do you see between your drinking and this ED visit today?"
4. Assess readiness to change on scale of 1 to 10, ask, "why not less?"
5. Explore pros and cons if not ready or if resisting.
6. Explore options and negotiate a feasible plan.

Ideally, every ED should have a list of referral sites available for treatment programs for drugs and alcohol.

Other sources for this information include the local yellow pages, local Alcoholics Anonymous community service phone numbers, or the following web sites: the Center for Substance Abuse Treatment Internet facility locator (http://www.samhsa.gov/centers/csat/csat.html), http://findtreatment.samhsa.gov/facilitylocatordoc.htm (a direct facility locator), the NIAAA URL for screening and intervention (http://www.niaaa.nih.gov/publications/Practitioner/HelpingPatients.htm#step1a). Information about the BNI can be accessed at the Web site (http://www.ed.bmc.org/sbirt).

If a patient is unsure of his or her readiness for treatment, ask what would it take for him or her to be ready. Finally, if the patient is not ready, accept the fact and offer information, support, and the opportunity to return for help. In either case, ask permission to give feedback about your concerns for his or her health and safety. A clinician's role is also that of a teacher. It is important to provide information concerning the effects of alcohol on the patient's health or alcohol-related injury.

Pathophysiology

In our society, many of us use the term *alcohol* loosely when referring to ethanol. In reality, the alcohols comprise a wide range of compounds, including intoxicants and poisons, some of which are more deleterious than others.

Intoxication may take many forms, even for the same individual within different contexts involving alcohol. However, in the presence of chronic use, the body adjusts to alcohol and other drugs of abuse such that a constellation of well-known and well-studied symptoms result when the alcohol or drug is stopped abruptly or reduced following prolonged use.

Ethanol diffuses easily across cell membranes by virtue of its solubility in lipids and in water. Hence, it is able to reach all areas of the body easily, which contributes to its profile of resulting and comorbid diseases. Absorption of ethanol is rapid and takes place primarily within the stomach and small intestines. Its metabolism, on the other hand, requires a longer period.

Ethanol metabolism involves an oxidation reaction of ethanol to acetate, its corresponding acid, by means of a rate-limited step catalyzed by alcohol dehydrogenase and occurs primarily within the liver, rendering the liver particularly vulnerable to the consequences of chronic alcohol use. The remaining ethanol is left unmetabolized and is detectable in the expired air of breathing and in the urine. In general, the liver is able to metabolize a specific amount of ethanol per hour, a rate that is primarily constrained by the concentration of catalytic enzymes available for this process, which can vary between individuals.

Although many think of ethanol as a stimulant, it primarily exerts its effects as a central nervous system (CNS) depressant. The precise mechanism by which this occurs remains controversial. In the past, ethanol was thought to affect the CNS via GABA-mediated inhibitory synaptic transmission, given its effect profile similar to that of benzodiazepines and barbiturates. More recently, however, the focus has shifted away from GABA-mediated mechanisms as the only target for ethanol. Now, α- and β-adrenergic systems and the excitatory glutamate-N-methyl-D-aspartate (NMDA) receptor complex are thought to be additional targets for these ethanol-mediated effects.

NMDA-mediated glutamate transmission has historically been implicated in memory and learning. This transmission is known to inhibit dopamine release from the nucleus accumbens and mesolimbic pleasure and reinforcement centers of the CNS. Acutely, ethanol inhibits NMDA-receptor function, and chronically it appears to be responsible for upregulation of these catecholamine receptors. Inhibition of NMDA increases dopamine release, a mechanism that is thought to be responsible for the cognitive and memory impairments associated with alcohol use and with reinforcing this behavior.

The pathophysiology of alcohol withdrawal is complicated by the fact that ethanol influences several neurotransmitter systems simultaneously (GABA, glutamate-NMDA transmission, and dopamine) and that abrupt cessation severely disrupts these already abnormal interactions. Cessation of ethanol diminishes GABA's inhibitory activity, affects central adrenergic activity, reverses NMDA inhibition, and increases glutamate and dopaminergic excitatory transmission. The overall consequence of this sudden CNS excitation is seen in the common presentations of AWS (including disorientation, hallucinations, tachycardia, tremors, anxiety, insomnia, and withdrawal seizures) and explains why benzodiazepines are so effective in the treatment of alcohol withdrawal.

The AWS results from the abrupt discontinuation of ethanol following a period of chronic exposure. Most develop these symptoms within 6 to 48 hours of the last drink, and the syndrome can last from 2 to 3 days to as many as 10 days. You should acquaint yourself with other disorders that can be mistaken for alcohol withdrawal, including acute schizophrenia, encephalitis, drug-induced psychosis, thyrotoxicosis, anticholinergic poisoning, and withdrawal from other substances of abuse.

In addition to AWS and the DTs, other common and potentially dangerous consequences of alcohol use are alcohol withdrawal seizures (considered in Chapter 34) and AKA.

AKA is another complication of alcohol use often accompanied by poor nutrition. Chronic malnourished ethanol abusers and binge drinkers with periods of fasting can easily develop hypoglycemia. Prolonged periods of relative starvation can precipitate ketoacidosis. Volume depletion in these patients only intensifies the acidosis through decreased renal excretion, particularly that of the ketoacids acetoacetate and β-hydroxybutyrate.

Suggested Readings

Benet LZ, Kroetz DL, Sheiner LB. Pharmacokinetics: the dynamics of drug absorption, distribution, and elimination. In: Molinoff PB, Ruddon RW, eds. *Goodman and Gilman's the pharmacological basis of therapeutics*, 9th ed. New York: McGraw-Hill, 1996:3–27.

Bernstein E, Bernstein J, Levenson S. Project ASSERT: an ED-based intervention to increase access to primary care, preventative services, and the substance abuse treatment system. *Ann Emerg Med* 1997;30:181–189.

Bosron WF, Ehrig T, Li T. Genetic factors in alcohol metabolism and alcoholism. *Semin Liver Dis* 1993;13:126–135.

Cherpital CJ. Screening for alcohol problems in the emergency department. *Ann Emerg Med* 1995;26:158–166.

Charness ME, Simon RP, Greenberg DA. Ethanol and the nervous system. *N Engl J Med* 1989; 321:442–450.

D'Onofrio G, Bernstein E, Bernstein J, et al. for the SAEM Substance Abuse Task Force. Patients with alcohol problems in the emergency department. Part 2: intervention and referral. *Acad Emerg Med* 1998;5:1210–1217.

Harwood H. *Economic costs of alcohol and drug abuse*. Fairfax, VA: Lewin Group, 1998.

Lieber CS. Seminars in medicine of the Beth Israel Hospital, Boston: medical disorders of alcoholism [review]. *N Engl J Med* 1995;333: 1058–1065.

Mayo-Smith MF. Pharmacological management of alcohol withdrawal. A meta-analysis and evidence-based practice guideline. *JAMA* 1997;278:144–151.

McMicken DB. Alcohol withdrawal syndromes. *Emerg Med Clin North Am* 1990;8:805–819.

Tabakoff B, Cornell N, Hoffman PL. Alcohol tolerance. *Ann Emerg Med* 1986;15:1005–1010.

Tabakoff B, Hoffman PL. Ethanol and glutamate receptors. In: Deithrich RA, Erwin VG, eds. *Pharmacological effects of ethanol on the nervous system*. Boca Raton, FL: CRC Press, 1996: 73–93.

Metabolic Disorders

Robert Lowenstein, MD

Clinical Scenario

A 27-year-old African American man, with a past medical history of type 1 diabetes mellitus, is brought to the emergency department by his family for episodes of lethargy and changes in level of consciousness during the past 24 hours. The family notes a 4-day history of vomiting, excessive voiding, and a need to drink large quantities of fluids. His symptoms progressively worsened with increasing weakness, fatigue, and a complaint of blurred vision. These physical complaints were at first attributed to the flu, from which a household member had recently recovered. His family reports that he is not very compliant with his insulin administration and that he stopped taking the medicine a few days ago because he had not felt well enough to refill his prescription.

His past medical history includes type 1 diabetes mellitus. He has had no hospitalizations or surgeries. He is a social drinker and does not smoke or use illicit drugs. His only medication is insulin, and he has no drug allergies.

On physical examination he is thin, pale, ill appearing, and breathing quickly with short rapid breaths. His temperature is 98.7°F, blood pressure is 100/70 mm Hg, pulse is 115 beats/minute, respiratory rate is 34 breaths/minute, and oxygen saturation on room air is 98%.

He has dry mucous membranes and a fruity odor on his breath. His neck veins are flat. His lungs are clear to auscultation without wheezes. His heart rate is rapid, with a regular rhythm and no murmurs. On abdominal examination, he has hypoactive bowel sounds with mild distention and is diffusely tender without focal guarding or rebound. On neurological evaluation he is lethargic and somnolent but arousable and oriented to person.

The patient is placed on 2 L of oxygen (O_2) by nasal cannula with continuous pulse oximetry and cardiac monitoring. An intravenous (IV) line is established, and a finger-stick glucose measurement reads too high to quantify on the glucometer. A complete blood cell (CBC) count with differential, electrolytes, ketones, arterial blood gas (ABG), electrocardiogram (ECG), and urinalysis (UA) are ordered.

The ABG results reveal that he is acidotic with an arterial pH of 7.20. Abnormal chemistry results include an elevated potassium (K^+) level of 6.0 mEq/dL, a bicarbonate level of 10 mmol/L, and an elevated glucose level of 450 mg/dL. The calculated anion gap (AG) is elevated at 30 mEq/L. UA reveals ketones and glucose. ECG shows a normal sinus rhythm with peaked T waves consistent with the high K^+ level.

The patient is diagnosed with diabetic ketoacidosis (DKA). Two liters of IV normal saline are infused, followed by 7 units of IV insulin and an ampule of IV calcium chloride. An IV insulin drip is started, and the patient is admitted to the intensive care unit (ICU). He has an uncomplicated course in the hospital and is discharged on his second hospital day after having extensive diabetic teaching and counseling.

Clinical Evaluation

Introduction

There are numerous metabolic abnormalities that cause changes in mental status. This chapter focuses on hyperosmolar states, which include two entities: DKA and hyperglycemic hyperosmolar nonketotic syndrome (HHNS), also referred to as HONC (hyperosmolar nonketotic coma). Both contribute to severe metabolic derangements that can impair consciousness.

DKA and HHNS are two of the most serious life-threatening acute complications of diabetes, with a mortality rate of 1% to 2%. Clinically, these entities are similar, but they differ in a variety of ways. DKA occurs most often in persons with type 1 diabetes, but persons with type 2 diabetes are also susceptible. By definition, DKA is a triad consisting of hyperglycemia, ketones (acetoacetate and β-hydroxybutyrate), and metabolic acidosis. The precipitating factors associated with DKA include infection, inadequate insulin (commonly from noncompliance), initial presentation of new onset diabetes, and other unknown factors.

HHNS, on the other hand, typically occurs in elderly persons with type 2 diabetes. HHNS is characterized by extreme hyperglycemia, hyperosmolar state, and prolonged dehydration in the absence of significant ketoacidosis.

It is important to characterize the differences between type 1 and type 2 diabetes. People with type 1 diabetes constitute only 10% to 20% of diabetes cases, are usually diagnosed before the age of 30, experience autoimmune destruction of islet cells of the pancreas and therefore require exogenous insulin, have no associated obesity, and have a propensity to develop ketoacidosis. People with type 2 diabetes constitute 80% to 90% of diabetes cases, are usually diagnosed after the age of 50, are commonly obese, experience endogenous insulin resistance, and have a propensity toward HHNS.

History

Patients presenting to the ED with a change in mental status are unable to provide a reliable history. Therefore, information from prehospital personnel and family members is essential to the diagnostic workup. In the clinical scenario, the family provided the necessary historical background and documented the history of diabetes and noncompliance with insulin therapy. Knowing this history narrows the differential to a metabolic etiology, specifically DKA.

Further symptoms consistent with DKA include a history of polyuria, polydipsia, fatigue, lethargy, and weakness, which are caused by hyperglycemia and subsequent osmotic diuresis. Accompanying complaints of anorexia, nausea, vomiting, and abdominal pain, which are caused by ketoacidosis and gastric stasis, are also common. The duration of symptoms can range from hours to days. In the clinical scenario, the etiology was likely twofold. The patient may have first developed an underlying viral syndrome. This was coupled with noncompliance of insulin therapy, leading to DKA. Incidentally, infection and lack of insulin therapy together contribute to more than 50% of cases of DKA. In the clinical scenario, the patient presented with lethargy and a change in mental status as the illness progressed. Up to 10% of patients present in coma, whereas more than 60% may be obtunded and lethargic.

Further history, if obtainable, should include a complete review of systems. Specific attention should be paid to possible causes of DKA including infection, abdominal pathological conditions, and cardiac disease. History of the patient's diabetes, any complications of the illness, and all medications should be noted.

Physical Examination

In the absence of a reliable history in a patient with a change in mental status, performing a thorough and accurate physical examination is imperative. Patients with DKA have variable physical findings depending on the severity of the illness. In general, they are young, lean individuals, who are insulin dependent and in a perpetual catabolic state. Vital signs are usually abnormal. As in the clinical scenario, the heart rate is usually elevated, consistent with dehydration. Orthostatic hypotension is not uncommon.

To compensate for the underlying metabolic acidosis, Kussmaul's respirations and tachypnea are present. Kussmaul's respirations are deep breaths causing hyperventilation and are the body's attempt to rid itself of excess carbon dioxide (CO_2), thereby inducing a respiratory alkalosis that compensates for the extreme metabolic acidosis. These patients appear air hungry. The serum acetone causes a musty, fruity odor of the breath, which is also characteristic of DKA. Further signs of dehydration include dry mucous membranes and poor skin turgor. The ketoacidosis causes gastric stasis with an abdomen that can be mildly tender and distended. For both DKA and HHNS, it is also important to look for signs of infection, that is, check the urine for urinary tract infection, the extremities for diabetic foot ulcers, and the lungs for pneumonia.

Diagnostic Evaluation

For a quick initial assessment in a diabetic patient with a change in the level of consciousness, a finger stick for rapid blood glucose measurement and a urine dip stick for glucose and ketones are recommended. If the blood glucose level is greater than 250 mg/dL and ketones are present in the urine, DKA is highly likely. The complete workup should include a CBC count with differential; electrolytes including calcium, magnesium, and phosphorus; serum ketones; ABG; UA; ECG; and in a febrile patient, two sets of blood cultures. Table 33.1 lists the

differences in the clinical evaluation of DKA versus HHNS.

Arterial Blood Gas Results

Patients in DKA have an arterial pH less than 7.30 with respective decreased partial pressure of CO_2 (pCO_2) and bicarbonate levels. The metabolic acidosis is secondary to the production of ketones. The pCO_2 is low because of the compensatory respiratory alkalosis. Recent literature suggests that a venous blood gas sample can substitute for ABG sample in the assessment of pH in the emergency department.

Electrolyte Levels

Knowing that a metabolic acidosis is present, the next step is to calculate the AG. The AG is a reflection of the presence of unmeasured anions. It is elevated in patients with DKA and represents the degree of ketoacidosis. It is calculated as follows:

$$AG \ (mEq/L) = Na^+ - [Cl^- + HCO^{-3}]$$

The AG is monitored closely as treatment is initiated, and it is expected to normalize as the body rids itself of ketoacids. The criteria for the differential diagnosis for an AG are given in Table 33.2. Because they are quite extensive, the mnemonic MUDPILES can be used.

The typical serum glucose value is greater than 350 mg/dL. In HHNS it is greater than 700 mg/dL.

Serum sodium (Na^+) is falsely low and is seen in the presence of dehydration, but

---

Table 33.1.

Diagnostic criteria for differentiating diabetic ketoacidosis from hyperglycemic hyperosmolar nonketotic syndrome

Diabetic Ketoacidosis
ph <7.30
Serum bicarbonate <15 mEq/L
Serum glucose >250 mg/dL
Presence of ketones: urine and serum

Hyperglycemic Hyperosmolar Nonketotic Syndrome
Absence of ketones
Serum glucose >400 mg/dL
Serum bicarbonate >15 mEq/L
Elevated plasma osmolality >315 mOsm

Table 33.2.

MUDPILES: differential of anion gap acidosis

Methanol
Uremia
Diabetic ketoacidosis
Paraldehyde
Isoniazid
Lactic acidosis
Ethylene glycol
Salicylates

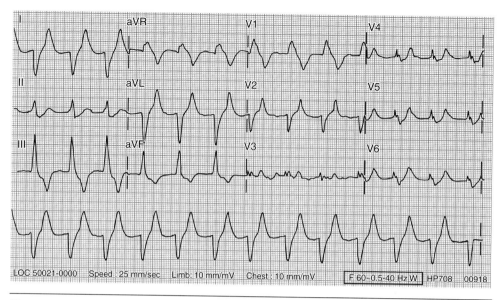

Figure 33.1
This electrocardiogram demonstrates the tall peaked T waves and markedly widened QRS of hyperkalemia. In addition there is loss of the normal sinus mechanism (no P waves). If untreated this patient, with a potassium of 9.2 mEq/L, will likely go into ventricular fibrillation.

hyperglycemia forces the movement of water from intracellular to the extracellular space, creating a dilutional hyponatremia. The serum Na^+ is corrected via the following equation:

$$Corrected\ Na^+ = 0.016(measured\ glucose - 100) + measured\ Na^+$$

This equation is also helpful in calculating the free water deficit.

Serum K^+ is often elevated (i.e., >5.2 mEq/L), even though there is total body K^+ depletion, because of acidosis, vomiting, osmotic diuresis, and the lack of insulin. The hydrogen ions are driven intracellularly, while the K^+ is driven extracellularly.

The serum phosphate and magnesium levels tend to be severely depressed and should be obtained on admission.

Electrocardiogram Findings

Hyperkalemia can be life threatening. It alters depolarization and repolarization of the cardiac membrane, producing ECG abnormalities. The evolutionary changes begin with tall, peaked T waves in the precordial leads, progressing to widening of the QRS interval, first- and second-degree atrioventricular (AV) block, and eventual ventricular fibrillation. The ECG shown in Figure 33.1 demonstrates the tall peaked T waves and markedly widened QRS of hyperkalemia.

Complete Blood Count Results

If there is no underlying infection, it is common to see leukocytosis without a left shift because of the stress-induced demargination of leukocytes.

Serum Ketone Levels

Serum ketone levels are a measure of acetoacetate. Serum ketones are present in DKA but not in HHNS.

Serum Osmolality Level

Serum osmolality is represented by the following equation:

$$Osmolality = 2(serum\ Na^+) + serum\ glucose/18 + serum\ blood\ urea\ nitrogen\ (BUN)/2.8$$

Alterations in mental status are directly related to the serum osmolality level. Alcohols (ethylene glycol, methanol, etc.) are low-molecular-weight solutes that increase the serum osmolality. A normal osmolality is 280 to 300 mOsm/kg. Once the patient's osmolality is calculated, it is subtracted from the expected osmolality. If there is a difference greater than approximately 10 mOsm, this is known as the osmolal gap. The gap can be used to determine whether an alcohol has been ingested by the patient, which would account for the change in mental status.

Differential Diagnosis

The differential diagnosis for metabolic disorders is illustrated in Table 33.3.

Treatment

The goal of therapy is repletion of the extracellular fluid losses, improved tissue perfusion, decreased serum glucose, reversal of the acidosis, and correction of electrolyte imbalances (Table 33.4).

Table 33.3.

Differential diagnosis for electrolyte-induced change in mental status

Hyperosmolar states
DKA
HHNS
Hypoglycemia
Not associated with respiratory distress
Presents with altered mentation, cool sweaty skin, focal neurological deficits, and seizure

Hyponatremia
Often caused by diuretics and volume overload particularly in the elderly.
Presents with lethargy, weakness, and confusion

Hyperkalemia
Laboratory error, acidosis, chronic renal failure, excessive potassium intake, medications, burns, and traumatic injuries
Presents with weakness, paralysis, and cardiac arrhythmias

Hypokalemia
Common causes include medications, alkalosis, magnesium deficiency, diarrhea, or Cushing's syndrome
Presents with muscle weakness, paralysis, and arrhythmias.

Hypercalcemia
Main etiologies: primary hyperparathyroidism and cancer
Presents with muscle weakness, fatigue, depression, and lethargy

Alcoholic Ketoacidosis
Malnourished alcoholic patients who have recently refrained from alcohol
Presents with abdominal pain, vomiting, and fruity odor on breath
Lactic acidosis: sepsis and emotional stress are common causes
Other alcohol ingestion: methanol, isopropyl alcohol, and ethylene glycol
Hepatic failure
Uremia
CVA

CVA, cerebrovascular accident; DKA, diabetic ketoacidosis; HHNS, hyperglycemic hyperosmolar nonketotic syndrome.

Table 33.4.

Treatment guidelines for diabetic ketoacidosis

Assessment of airway, breathing, and circulation

Two liters of oxygen via nasal cannula

IV access with at least an 18-gauge needle

Cardiac monitor and pulse oximetry

CBC count with differential, electrolytes, serum ketones, ABG, urinalysis, and ECG

Electrolyte levels every 4 hours

Hyperkalemia: calcium to stabilize the cardiac membrane; insulin and glucose, bicarbonate and inhaled bronchodilators to drive the K^+ intracellularly; Kayexalate, a K^+-binding resin, to remove K^+ from the body; hemodialysis only in extreme situations

IV regular insulin, may start continuous drip

Foley with strict measurement of ins and outs

Finger-stick glucose every hour

Treatment of any underlying infections

Flow sheet for accurate monitoring

Individualized therapy for every patient

ABG, arterial blood gas; CBC, complete blood count; ECG, electrocardiogram; IV, intravenous; K^+, potassium.

These goals are accomplished by the administration of IV fluids and insulin and by replenishment of K^+ losses.

Intravenous Fluid

The preferred IV fluid is normal saline. It is given initially as a bolus with 1 to 2 L in the first 2 hours, then normal saline (0.45% NaCl), at 250 to 500 mL/hour; dextrose is added when serum glucose is less than 250 mg/dL.

Insulin

Regular insulin is given initially as a bolus of 0.1 U/kg IV. If needed, an insulin drip is begun at 0.1 U/kg/hour and decreased to 0.05 U/kg/hour when the glucose level is between 250 and 300 mg/dL. Insulin is continued until the ketoacidosis resolves and the AG normalizes.

Potassium

There is an underlying total body K^+ depletion. Measure the K^+ level every 4 hours. If it is greater than 5.5 mEq/L, do not add K^+ to IV fluids. When the K^+ level is 3.3 to 5.5 mEq/L, add 20 to 30 mEq/L of IV fluids. If the K^+ level is less than 3.3 mEq/L, add 40 mEq to each liter of IV fluids.

Bicarbonate

Treatment of dehydration and lowering serum glucose is usually all that is needed for the acidosis. However, if the pH is less than 7.0, many authors advocate the use of bicarbonate.

Complications of Therapy

The treatment of DKA is not without risk and requires close supervision. A potentially fatal side effect is cerebral edema. Although more common in the pediatric population, it must be suspected if the patient develops a headache or undergoes any change in mental status once treatment is initiated. Additional complications include hypokalemia, hypophosphatemia, and hyperchloremic acidosis.

Disposition

All patients with DKA or HHNK must be admitted to the hospital. Different hospitals have differing policies on who belongs in the ICU and who can be safely treated on a general medical floor. Patients who are extremely acidotic, require frequent adjustments in insulin administration and electrolyte management (including Na^+ and K^+), or have an altered mental status should be admitted to the ICU. Some hospitals with adequate nurse-to-patient ratios on the medical floors, or sufficient house officer observation, will allow patients with mild DKA to be admitted to the general wards. When in doubt, it is better to err on the side of caution and to admit to the ICU.

Pathophysiology

The β-cells of the pancreas are responsible for insulin production. Patients who experience insulin resistance, or type 2 diabetes mellitus, may have some dysfunction in the production of insulin but also do not respond appropriately to insulin at the target organs.

This explains the very high serum glucose levels seen in patients with type 2 diabetes who present with HHNK states. These patients tend to be elderly; the slow decline with age of renal function sets the stage for the metabolic spiral downward, leading to the retention of glucose and hyperosmolar state and ensuing electrolyte imbalance and change in mental status. The high concentration of glucose acts like a diuretic (osmotic diuresis), further dehydrating the patient and causing electrolyte shifts, most often K^+ and Na^+. This is important to remember because the urine output may be significant, especially in HHNK states, but the patient may be severely volume depleted.

The lack of circulating insulin, insulin resistance, and subsequent elevation of counterregulatory hormones constitute the pathophysiological basis of DKA. These hormones work by opposing biochemical mechanisms to insulin and include catecholamines, cortisol, growth hormone, and glucagon. Ultimately, this counterregulatory process prevents peripheral glucose uptake in the muscle, while stimulating liver glucose production via gluconeogenesis and glycogenolysis pathways. This leads to profound hyperglycemia. In addition, free fatty acids (FFA) released as triglycerides are broken down from adipose tissue. The liver metabolizes these FFA and produces ketone bodies. The ketogenesis leads to ketoacidosis and a metabolic acidosis. These ketone bodies are the unmeasured anions, which produce the AG.

The hyperglycemia leads to the departure of water from cells, causing extracellular fluid expansion at the expense of the intracellular volume. An osmotic diuresis causes loss of urine, dehydration, volume depletion, and eventual retention of serum glucose. Patients with undiagnosed diabetes sometimes try to replete the severe dehydration by drinking fluids full of sugar; this only aggravates the hyperglycemia and hastens the decline in mental status.

Suggested Readings

Adrogue HJ, Madias NE. Hyponatremia. *N Engl J Med* 2000;342:1581–1588.

Bell DSH, Alele J. Diabetic ketoacidosis. *Postgrad Med* 1997;101(4):193–203.

Brandenburg MA, Dire DJ. Comparison of arterial and venous blood gas values in the initial emergency department evaluation of patients with diabetic ketoacidosis. *Ann Emerg Med* 1998; 31:459–465.

Bushinsky DA, Monk RD. Calcium. *Lancet* 1998; 352:306–311.

Chan FK, Koberle LM, Thys-Jacob S, et al. Differential diagnosis, causes, and management of hypercalcemia. *Curr Prob Surg* 1997;34:445–473.

Gonzalez-Campoy MJ, Robertson PR. Diabetic ketoacidosis and hyperosmolar nonketotic state. *Postgrad Med* 1996;99(6):143–152.

Kitabchi A, Wall BM. Management of diabetic ketoacidosis. *Am Fam Physician* 1999;60:455–464.

Lebovitz HE. Diabetic ketoacidosis. *Lancet* 1995; 345:767–772.

Matz R. Management of the hyperosmolar hyperglycemic syndrome. *Am Fam Physician* 1999; 60:1468–1476.

Miller J. Management of diabetic ketoacidosis. *J Emerg Nurs* 1999;25:514–519.

Rosen P. *Emergency medicine.* St. Louis: Mosby-Year Book, 1998:2463–2470.

Umpierrez GE, Khajari M, Kitabichi AE, et al. Review: diabetic ketoacidosis and hyperglycemic hyperosmolar nonketotic syndrome. *Am J Med Sci* 1996;311:225–233.

34

Seizure Disorders

Joel M. Wasserman, MD

Clinical Scenario

A 35-year-old man is brought to the emergency department (ED) by emergency medical services (EMS) after being found unresponsive by his wife on the floor of their bathroom. She heard him fall and found him foaming at the mouth and shaking violently. The event lasted about 1 to 2 minutes and then resolved. Afterward, he appeared to pass out. She tells you that he has a history of seizures for which he takes phenytoin (Dilantin). She is unsure how regularly he takes his medication. His cervical spine is immobilized, and he is transported to the ED. On arrival, he is confused and combative. Physical examination reveals only a hematoma of the occipital scalp and a laceration of the tongue. He is alert but confused.

He is placed on a monitor, oxygen at 2 L/minute is administered, and intravenous (IV) access is established. Glucose is checked by fingerstick and is 120 mg/dL. After 20 minutes of observation, his mental status has cleared. When a repeat physical examination reveals a nontender cervical spine, the cervical collar is removed. Repeat neurological examination is normal. A phenytoin level is obtained and found to be low. He is given supplemental IV Dilantin, and after several hours of observation is discharged home.

Clinical Evaluation

Introduction

Seizures are a common presenting complaint in the ED, accounting for 1% to 2% of visits.

Approximately 1.65 million individuals in the United States have a seizure disorder. This figure excludes those who experience secondary seizures as a manifestation of an underlying primary medical illness. With these cases included, it is estimated that 6% to 10% of the population will experience a seizure during their lifetime.

A seizure may be defined as a sudden excessive disorderly discharge of neurons in the brain. The discharge produces particular clinical manifestations observed by the practitioner or witness. Different types of seizures produce their own unique clinical manifestations. The term epilepsy is used to define seizures that occur spontaneously over a span of years.

History

With the exception of status epilepticus, which is defined as any seizure lasting longer than 30 minutes or three consecutive seizures without return of normal consciousness, most seizures last seconds to minutes. Commonly, the ED physician encounters a patient who has recovered or who is in the postictal phase. Direct observation of the seizure, unless it recurs in the ED, is often impossible. In addition, the patient is often amnestic for the event. Hence, the history may rely on accounts given by witnesses or EMS personnel (Table 34.1).

For patients presenting with their first seizure, the ED physician should elicit information to aid in classifying the seizure. Ask the patient or witness to describe what they saw, noting if all extremities were moving or only one. Did the patient remain awake? Was there any incontinence, tongue biting, loss of consciousness, or confusion?

Table 34.1.

Historical evaluation of seizure

Classification	*Patients with Epilepsy*
Type of activity	Comparison to previous seizures
Interruption of consciousness	Compliance with medication
Aura	Changes in medication dose
Postictal phase	New medications
Predisposing Conditions	*Secondary Injury Assessment*
Previous seizures	Musculoskeletal
Cerebrovascular disease	Neurological
Neoplastic disease	Facial
Metabolic disease (diabetes, renal)	Oral
HIV	
Recent trauma	
Neurological symptoms	
Fevers	
Medications and ingestions	
Alcohol or recreational drugs	

HIV, human immunodeficiency virus.

The patient should be questioned regarding medical conditions that predispose to seizures. History of neoplasm, cerebrovascular disease, human immunodeficiency virus (HIV) infection (which can predispose to intracranial lesions), and diabetes or renal disease (which cause metabolic abnormalities) should be sought. Ascertain whether trauma, headache, focal neurological changes, or fever has occurred recently. Is the patient taking anticoagulant medication that increases the risk of intracranial hemorrhage?

For patients with known seizure disorder, determine whether the current seizure activity is similar to previous seizures in type, frequency of occurrence, and duration. Review compliance with anticonvulsant medication, recent change in dose, or the addition of medications that interact with anticonvulsants. Exacerbating conditions such as intercurrent illness or fatigue should be sought.

For alcoholic patients, a history of alcohol related seizures and time of last drink may aid in determining the cause of the seizure. The diagnosis of alcohol-related seizure is based on history and physical findings, but other etiologies should be considered. Any history of falls should be elicited from the alcoholic patient who is at risk for occult head injury, such as chronic subdural hematoma.

All patients should be questioned regarding use of other drugs, particularly stimulants such as cocaine and other recreational drugs that may cause seizures. A history of depression or suicidal ideation should initiate a search for possible drug ingestions.

Finally, a comprehensive review of systems should be done to assess for injuries sustained during the seizure. Symptoms or signs of long bone, hip, facial, or jaw fracture; intracranial injury; cervical spine injury; and intraoral injury should be pursued.

Physical Examination

The general physical examination of the seizure patient is directed toward discovery of any illness that may have precipitated the seizure and any injuries resulting from the seizure. Review the vital signs. A patient with tachycardia, hypertension, and fever may have alcohol withdrawal, infection, or drug ingestion. Examine the pupils for size and reactivity. An intracranial lesion should be suspected in a patient with unequal pupils. Pinpoint pupils suggest narcotic overdose or pontine bleed. Large pupils may be found in certain drug overdoses. Assess the optic discs for papilledema, a sign of increased intracranial pressure. Examine the head for any signs of trauma, such as contusions, abrasions, hemotympanum, or battle's sign (bruising behind the ear, a sign of basilar skull fracture). The tongue and teeth should be examined for trauma, and the jaw should be evaluated for malocclusion. Examination of the neck must include evaluation for meningeal irritation, midline tenderness, and deformity. Auscultation of the lungs may reveal evidence of aspiration that occurred during the seizure. A careful extremity examination is required to rule out dislocation and fracture, because humeral fracture and shoulder dislocation are common complications. A careful neurological examination is mandatory and should include serial evaluations of the patient's level of consciousness to document resolution of the postictal phase, to rule out an ongoing neurological process, and to watch for additional seizures.

Diagnostic Evaluation

Other than initial determination of blood glucose, which should be obtained for all patients, the use of laboratory tests is guided by the history and examination (Table 34.2).

Table 34.2.

Laboratory tests in seizure

Recommended in all cases
Blood glucose
Anticonvulsant drug levels (if taking)

Considerations for First Seizure and Individual Cases
Electrolyte levels
Complete blood count
Toxicology assay
Lumbar puncture
Pregnancy test
Neurological imaging: CT scan and/or MRI scan
    if indicated

CT, computed tomography; MRI, magnetic resonance imaging.

For the known epileptic patient presenting after a typical seizure with no abnormal findings, all that may be required is an anticonvulsant drug level. However, the patient presenting with either a clear change in seizure history or a first seizure requires more extensive investigation. It has been reported that a significant number of patients will have an abnormal electrolyte level relevant to the etiology of the seizure and one third of patients with an unremarkable medical history and examination will have abnormal levels of electrolytes, glucose, blood urea nitrogen (BUN), or creatinine Hence, it is recommended that these studies be obtained. Whether other tests are obtained is guided by individual circumstances. Lumbar puncture after computed tomography (CT) scan of the brain is mandatory when meningitis is suspected and should always be considered in the immunocompromised patient. A pregnancy test is recommended for women of childbearing age. Toxicology assays are useful if drug use is suspected.

Laboratory values also may help confirm that a seizure has occurred. Patients with generalized convulsions will have lactic acidosis with anion gap for 30 to 60 minutes following the event. Prolactin levels may also be elevated in the hour following the seizure.

Magnetic resonance imaging (MRI) or CT scanning of the brain is a standard part of the workup for a patient with new-onset seizures. However, the indications for neuroimaging in the ED are few. For the epilepsy patient presenting with a typical seizure, imaging is unnecessary unless significant head trauma is suspected. Additional indications for brain imaging in known epilepsy patients include new focal deficits, persistently altered mental status, fever, recent trauma, persistent headache, history of cancer, anticoagulation, and known or suspected HIV disease. When indicated, a noncontrast CT scan is the imaging modality of choice in the ED to rule out hemorrhage, cerebral edema or intracranial mass, causing seizures. If a specific entity is suspected that requires contrast or MRI, these tests are occasionally performed during the ED visit. More frequently these tests are performed later on an outpatient basis.

Table 34.3.

Differential diagnosis in seizure

Epilepsy
CNS infection

Neonatal Conditions
Hypoxia
Ischemia
Hypoglycemia
Inborn errors of metabolism
Genetic abnormalities

Pediatric (6 months–5 years) Conditions
Febrile seizure

Adolescent Conditions
Recreational drug or overdose

Adult Conditions
Alcohol withdrawal
Head trauma
CNS tumor
CNS infection
Metabolic abnormalities
Recreational drug, therapeutic, or overdose
  of medication
Cerebrovascular disease: ischemia or hemorrhage

CNS, central nervous system.

Differential Diagnosis

The differential diagnosis for seizure disorder is illustrated in Table 34.3.

Treatment

Most seizures are short-lived and resolve spontaneously. Hence, the ED physician may encounter an actively seizing patient or a patient whose seizure resolved before arrival in the ED. In all cases, initial interventions include administration of oxygen, establishment of cardiac monitoring and IV access, initial blood glucose determination, and correction of hypoglycemia if present.

First Seizure

For the patient presenting with a first-time seizure, a decision must be made whether or not to start anticonvulsant treatment. The decision hinges on the physician's estimate of the risk of recurrence. If the seizure was a primary event, not resulting from secondary causes, the risk of recurrence is estimated at 36% to 77%. Risk factors for recurrence include known neurological injury or deficit, a sibling with epilepsy, focal neurological deficits in the postictal period (Todd's paralysis), or an abnormal electroencephalogram (EEG). These facts along with the risks of injury from seizures and the side effects of medications should be reviewed with the patient. The choice of anticonvulsant medication for long-term use is determined by the seizure characteristics. Decisions regarding initiating treatment and choice of medication are best made in consultation with a neurologist (Table 34.4).

Epilepsy

For the patient with known seizure disorder, subtherapeutic anticonvulsant levels should be corrected. If levels are therapeutic, any secondary causes should be evaluated and treated. If no etiology is found, discussion with the patient's primary care provider or neurologist is warranted to inform them of the breakthrough seizure, discuss possible medication change, and ensure proper follow-up.

If the patient is actively seizing, the initial approach is to protect the patient from secondary injury while waiting for the seizure to resolve. The patient should be placed in the lateral decubitus position to minimize aspiration risk. Gentle restraint to prevent trauma and control of movement to avoid falls is required.

Some authors recommend considering use of a short-acting anticonvulsant to terminate seizure activity lasting longer than 5 minutes. Benzodiazepines, most commonly diazepam and lorazepam, are often used as first-line therapeutic agents to terminate seizure activity. They rapidly enter the central nervous system (CNS) and exert anticonvulsant effects by inhibiting the spread of the seizure activity. Seizures that fail to abate after initial treatment, or last beyond the expected time frame, should be treated as status epilepticus (see later).

Alcohol Withdrawal

Alcohol withdrawal seizures have a demonstrated recurrence rate of 24% within 6

Table 34.4.

Medications used in seizure therapy

Drug	Seizure Type	Daily Dose	Therapeutic Level
Phenytoin	Partial, GCS	3–8 mg/kg	10–20 µg/mL
Carbamazepine	Partial, GCS	15–25 mg/kg	8–12 µg/mL
Phenobarbital	GCS, partial	2–6 mg/kg	15–40 µg/mL
Primidone	GCS, partial	10–20 mg/kg	5–15 µg/mL
Valproate	GCS, partial, absence	15–60 mg/kg	50–100 µg/mL
Ethosuximide	Absence	10–30 mg/kg	40–100 µg/mL
Gabapentin	Partial	≈4,800 mg/day	Not defined

GCS, . generalized convulsive seizure

hours. Administration of lorazepam (and presumably other rapidly acting benzodiazepines) significantly reduces the risk of recurrent seizures, and its use is appropriate in this setting.

Febrile Seizure

A significant number of children with febrile seizures require treatment for prolonged seizure activity, and febrile status epilepticus is a common first presentation. Diazepam is the first-line agent in these cases. Common routes of administration include IV and rectal. Recent studies have found midazolam administered via buccal and nasal routes to be efficacious. Cooling and antipyretics should be instituted.

Status Epilepticus

Status epilepticus occurs at some time in 5%–8% of patients with epilepsy. It is a potentially life-threatening condition that requires emergent management. Although the definition relies on lack of interictal recovery or a seizure lasting longer than 30 minutes, any patient who arrives with ongoing seizure activity or who is observed to seize for more than 10 minutes should be considered to be in status epilepticus.

The goal of treatment of status epilepti-

cus is control of seizures within 30 minutes (Table 34.5).

As with all seizures, initial measures include establishing airway, breathing, and circulation (ABCs); administering oxygen; monitoring cardiac status and blood pressure; establishing IV access, and determining serum glucose. If serum glucose cannot be determined, the adult patient should be treated empirically with thiamine and 50 g of 50% glucose solution. Children should receive 2 mg/kg of 25% glucose. Intubation may be necessary to protect the airway and to ensure adequate ventilation if anticonvulsants that cause respiratory depression are to be administered. Careful monitoring of vital signs is mandatory. Hyperthermia is common, and the patient should be cooled to normalize body temperature. Blood pressure may be labile, and pressors may be required to treat hypotension and maintain cerebral perfusion. Hydration should be done cautiously, because status epilepticus is associated with cerebral edema. A Foley catheter should be placed to monitor urine output.

Anticonvulsant therapy should be started immediately. The drug selected is determined by the clinical situation. For the actively seizing patient, benzodiazepines are the first line choice. If the seizures have resolved, therapy may be initiated with a long-acting medica-

Table 34.5.

Treatment protocol for status epilepticus

Therapeutic Measure	Time Frame
Establish and maintain airway IV, oxygen, monitor Dextrose 25–50 g IV, thiamine 100 mg IV lorazepam 2 mg/min IV up to 0.1 mg/kg or diazepam 5 mg IV q 5 minutes up to 20 mg	0–5 minutes
phenytoin 20 mg/kg IV or fosphenytoin 20 mg/kg IV Additional phenytoin 5–10 mg/kg IV or additional fosphenytoin 5–10 mg/kg IV phenobarbital up to 20 mg/kg IV	10–20 minutes

Additional phenobarbital 5–10 mg/kg IV
General anesthesia: midazolam 0.2 mg/kg IVP then
    0.75–10 µg/kg/min or propofol 1–2 mg/kg IV then
    1–15 mg/kg/h or phenobarbital 10–15 mg/kg IV
    then 0.5–1.0 mg/kg/h
	30 minutes

IV, intravenous; IVP, intravenous push.

tion. Diazepam and lorazepam are equally efficacious, although diazepam has a shorter duration of action. Side effects include hypotension and respiratory depression. If diazepam is used, it should be followed by a long-acting agent such as phenytoin.

Phenytoin is also effective in terminating seizure activity. Because it requires a loading dose and a slow infusion rate, it is less useful than benzodiazepines in active seizures. Phenytoin is the second-line drug given if seizures persist after administering benzodiazepines. Side effects include hypotension, bradycardia, and widening of the QT interval with possible subsequent arrhythmia. Sedation and rash are also common. Fosphenytoin is equally effective and may be infused faster. Hypotension and sedation are common side effects.

The patient who fails to respond to these measures is said to be in refractory status epilepticus. These patients require intubation if it was not done earlier. Treatment progresses to induction of an anesthetic coma to suppress seizure activity. They may be started on a midazolam, propofol, or pentobarbital. Continuous EEG monitoring is required to monitor progress toward reso-

lution of seizures and to define an endpoint for this type of treatment.

Disposition

For patients presenting with a first-time seizure, admission is recommended when any of the following are present: persistent altered mental status, CNS infection, new intracranial lesion, underlying correctable medical problem, acute head trauma, status epilepticus, or eclampsia. Neurological consultation should be obtained for all patients with new onset seizures, a focal neurological examination, persistent altered mental status, new intracranial lesion, change in seizure pattern, or poorly controlled seizures. Pregnant patients should also receive a neurology consultation.

The known epileptic patient with an uneventful postictal course may be discharged home after measurement and correction of anticonvulsant levels, evaluation for underlying illness or injury, and discussion with the patient's primary care provider. Patients with alcohol withdrawal seizures should be observed for 6 hours before discharge to a detoxification facility.

Pathophysiology

Although it is known that seizures result from the inappropriate discharge of cerebral neurons, why these groups of neurons behave abnormally is incompletely understood. The fact that seizure activity can be generated from neurons at the site of a structural lesion and also from neurons that appear to be completely normal implies that seizures are the end result of more than one process. Neurons in epileptic foci are thought to be hyperexcitable because of partial depolarization of their membranes. This can result from abnormalities of ion channels or neurotransmitter receptors or local scarring from injury and other factors. The neurons in epileptic foci are often spontaneously active. This stimulates inhibitory interneurons in the surrounding area, which act to contain and inhibit the abnormal activity. EEG recordings can detect the presence and location of the spontaneous activity in the seizure focus. During seizures, there is increasing amplitude and frequency of the abnormal firing of the neurons in the focus. Once the discharge reaches a given intensity, it overcomes the inhibitory influence of the surrounding neurons and spreads to adjacent regions along synaptic connections or simultaneously to wide areas of cortex via the thalamus. It is believed that any event that activates neurons within the focus or that inhibits those surrounding it will lead to the spread of the seizure activity.

Seizures are classified based on their clinical and electroencephalographic characteristics (Table 34.6).

Partial seizures are those with a localized onset in a limited area of the cortex. These are further classified as *simple partial,* in which no disturbance of consciousness oc-

---

Table 34.6.

Seizure classification

Type of Seizure	Clinical Features	Electroencephalographic Features
Simple partial	Signs and symptoms may be motor, sensory, autonomic, or psychic, depending on the location of seizure; consciousness is not impaired.	Focal slowing, sharp-wave activity, or both
Partial complex	Features similar to simple partial but consciousness is impaired and automatisms may be present. There may be a postictal period.	Focal slowing, sharp-wave activity, or both
Secondarily generalized	Seizure begins as in previous two cases but progresses to generalized tonic-clonic activity with loss of consciousness and postictal confusion. Accounts for aura phenomenon.	Focal slowing, sharp-wave activity, or both
Generalized nonconvulsive (absence, petit mal)	Seizure begins acutely with a brief period of unresponsiveness followed by rapid recovery.	Spike-wave pattern
Convulsive (grand mal)	Rapid onset of loss of consciousness followed by tonic clonic activity and postictal confusion.	Spike-wave pattern

Modified with permission from Brown TR, Holmes GL. Epilepsy. *N Engl J Med* 2001;344:1145–1151.

curs, or *partial complex*, in which there is a change in mental status. Partial complex seizures generally originate in the temporal or frontal lobe and can produce periods of altered thought and behavior. The seizure often has a motor component, which can take the form of stereotyped oral movements, such as lip smacking or other automatisms. Patients are usually amnestic for the events. A partial seizure may spread to involve the entire cortex of both hemispheres, a phenomenon termed *secondary generalization*. When a simple partial seizure occurs before generalizing, it can produce an aura that becomes known to the patient as a harbinger of the convulsion to come.

Generalized seizures are subclassified as convulsive (grand mal, tonic-clonic) or nonconvulsive (absence). The ED physician will encounter the convulsive form most commonly. The seizure begins with extension of the back and neck and then spreads to the limbs. As the thoracic musculature becomes involved, air may be expelled through the larynx, causing a cry. Breathing is erratic or absent, and the patient may become cyanotic. This tonic phase lasts approximately 10 to 20 seconds. Next comes the clonic phase, which is characterized by violent flexion of the muscles of the entire body. Facial grimacing and tongue biting are common. Tachycardia, hypertension, sweating, and emptying of bowel and/or bladder are typical. After 30 to 60 seconds, the convulsive activity stops and the postictal phase begins. Typically the patient is unconscious and still, except for breathing. Vital signs normalize. Generally, the patient can be aroused within about 5 minutes, but sleep may make the postictal period seem longer. The patient will have no recall of the seizure.

Febrile seizures are a common form of generalized convulsive seizure in infants and children. These are usually a brief, single event occurring as the fever rises or peaks. They have a good prognosis and are usually not associated with any underlying neurological abnormality. Alcohol withdrawal seizures are another common example of generalized seizure. These occur in patients with a history of chronic alcohol use who abruptly stop drinking. They occur 7 to 48 hours after the last drink in 90% of patients. These patients are generally neurologically normal unless they have sustained brain injury from some other cause.

Seizures may result from a variety of processes. The most common causes are idiopathic, posttraumatic, neoplastic, cerebrovascular, and metabolic. Head injuries account for 5% to 15% of secondary seizures. The seizures may begin anytime after the injury but generally occur within the first year. Tumors account for approximately 10% of cases of adult-onset seizures and are the most common cause of new-onset seizures in middle-aged adults. Metabolic abnormalities are common in certain populations. For example, diabetics and alcoholic patients may present with seizures secondary to hypoglycemia. Electrolyte abnormalities causing seizures are common in patents with renal failure. Many drugs, both prescribed and illicit, can produce seizures. Common offenders include hypoglycemic agents, antipsychotics, tricyclics, cocaine, alcohol, and certain antibiotics.

Specific causes of seizures tend to occur at different ages (Table 34.7). In the neonatal age range, most seizures result from antepartum or peripartum hypoxia and ischemia, or from genetic or metabolic abnormalities. Febrile seizures are the most common form in children age 6 months to 5 years. Idiopathic epilepsy tends to present after age 3 and most commonly in adolescence. Beyond age 20, common etiologies include head injury and tumor. In elderly pa-

Table 34.7.
Evaluation of seizure in children
Birth to 6 months
Hypoxia
Drugs
Infection
Trauma
Hypoglycemia
Intracranial hemorrhage
Metabolic abnormality
6 months to 3 years
Febrile seizures
Toxin related
Causes noted previously

tients, the most common etiologies are trauma, neoplasm, and cerebrovascular and neurodegenerative disease.

Suggested Readings

American College of Emergency Physicians (ACEP), Clinical Policies Committee Clinical Policies Subcommittee on Seizure. Clinical policy for the initial approach to patients presenting with a chief complaint of seizure who are not in status epilepticus. *Ann Emerg Med* 1997;29:706–724.

American College of Emergency Physicians (ACEP); American Academy of Neurology (AAN); American Association of Neurological Surgeons (AANS); American Society of Nephrology (ASN). Practice parameter. Neuroimaging in the emergency patient presenting with seizure. *Ann Emerg Med* 1996; 28:114–118.

Browne, TR Holmes GL. Epilepsy. *N Engl J Med* 2001;344:1145–1151.

Delanty N, Vaughan CJ, French JA. Medical causes of seizures. *Lancet* 1998;352:383–390.

D'Onofrio G, Rathlev NK, Ulrich AS, et al. Lorazepam for the prevention of recurrent seizures related to alcohol. *N Engl J Med* 1999;340:915–919.

Epilepsy and disorders of consciousness; Epilepsy and other seizure disorders. In: Adams RD, Victor M, Ropper AH eds. *Principles of neurology*, 7th ed. New York: McGraw-Hill, 2000: 329–404.

James JL. Epilepsy emergencies: the first seizure and status epilepticus. *Neurology* 1998;51: S34–S38.

Kelly KM, Valeriano JP, Solot JA. Seizures. In: Sgah SM, Kelly KM, eds. *Emergency neurology: principles and practice.* New York: Cambridge University Press, 1999:154–172.

Lowenstein DH, Alldredge BK. Current concepts: status epilepticus. *N Engl J Med* 1998; 338:970–976.

Pollack PV, Pollack PS. Seizures. In: Rosen P, Barkin R, Danzl DF, eds. *Emergency medicine: concepts and clinical practice*, 4th ed. St. Louis: Mosby, 1998:1221–1242.

Schierhout G, Roberts I. Anti-epileptic drugs for preventing seizures following acute traumatic brain injury. *Cochrane Database Systematic Rev.* In: Cochrane Library, Issue 3, 2004. Chichester, UK: John Wiley & Sons, Ltd.

Stephen LJ, Brodie MJ. Epilepsy in elderly people. *Lancet* 2000;355:1441–1446.

CHAPTER 35

Psychiatric Emergencies

Brendan G. Magauran, Jr., MD, MBA

Clinical Scenario

A 22-year-old man is brought to the emergency department (ED) by emergency medical services (EMS). The patient is acutely agitated and diaphoretic and is swearing loudly while EMS personnel physically restrain him on the stretcher. The emergency medical technician (EMT) states that the patient was uncooperative, refusing to answer medical questions or to allow vital signs to be taken. The EMT notes that the patient's mother had called the police initially because her son was acting strangely at home and the mother feared for her safety and the safety of younger children in the home. The mother stated that her son had no medical problems and took no medications. She did say that he smoked marijuana and occasionally drank alcohol.

At ambulance triage in the ED, the patient refuses to answer questions and verbally threatens the triage nurse and ambulance staff. The patient remains diaphoretic and restless and continues to attempt to leave the ED. Attempts to calm the patient and to reason with him are unsuccessful. The patient is brought back to the treatment area and is transferred to a hospital stretcher with security personnel present in an attempt to deescalate the situation. The patient becomes more agitated and fights being transferred while swearing and spitting at staff. The attending physician orders the patient to be restrained for the safety of the staff and patient and to enable an emergency evaluation to determine the etiology of this patient's altered mental status. The patient is placed in four-point restraints and administered a parenteral (intravenous [IV]) dose of haloperidol (Haldol). The patient is placed on cardiac monitoring and pulse oximetry. A trained observer (medical technician, security person, or hospital sitter) is assigned to the patient to monitor vital signs and response to treatment. Vital signs are obtained as soon as possible and rechecked every 15 minutes. IV access is obtained, blood is drawn for laboratory testing, and oxygen is administered via nasal cannula. Finger-stick blood sugar level is normal. Laboratory testing includes complete blood cell (CBC) count, electrolytes, blood urea nitrogen (BUN), creatinine, glucose, liver function tests, and alcohol (ethyl alcohol [ETOH]) and toxicological screen.

Physical examination shows a healthy-appearing young man with no obvious trauma. Vital signs are normal with the exception of a pulse of 110 beats/minute. His head, ear, eye, nose, and throat examination shows no evidence of trauma. Pupils are 4 mm and reactive to light. There is no hemotympanum (blood behind the tympanic membrane). The airway is patent.

The neck is atraumatic, and there is no lymphadenopathy, thyromegaly, mass, palpable bony deformity, or crepitus. Lungs are clear to auscultation bilaterally. Heart rate is regular with normal S_1 and S_2 and no murmur, rub, or gallop. There are normal bowel sounds. The abdomen is soft, nontender, and nondistended; no masses or hepatosplenomegaly are palpated. The back is nontraumatic, with no costovertebral angle (CVA) tenderness.

Genitourinary examination reveals a normal circumcised man. Rectal examination reveals normal prostate, and Hemoccult-negative stool. He moves all extremities, and there is no evidence of cyanosis, clubbing, or edema. Neurological examination is notable for not answering questions initially, and the patient is now sedated with haloperidol. Initially, it was noted that he did move all extremities with good motor strength. Completion of examination is deferred for now until the patient is more cooperative.

The patient gradually became more awake and less agitated over the next 3 hours in the ED. The laboratory analysis, including toxicological testing, was completely normal. Information was obtained by telephone from the patient's mother, who had not come to the ED because she had five younger children at home. The mother noted that her son had been increasingly more irritable at home over the past few weeks. He was barely sleeping more than a couple of hours per night, had stopped bathing, and ate relatively little. He had stopped watching TV and refused to allow anyone else to turn it on. Today, he had smashed the TV set with a hammer after his youngest sibling had turned on the TV. The patient had not harmed his mother or siblings, but his mother was afraid that he might after he attacked the TV. His mother had not noted drug use other than marijuana. She denied that her son had a psychiatric history or prior hospitalization for a psychiatric condition.

On reexamination of the patient, the neurological examination was normal. The patient was oriented times three. The patient admitted to destroying the TV because "it was telling me to kill myself or someone else." He had received these messages from the TV for the first time several weeks ago. He had not attempted to kill himself or anyone else, but he was worried about what would happen if he were to be near any TV.

Clinical Evaluation

Introduction

Psychiatric emergencies make up 10% of ED visits. The ED evaluation of psychiatric patients can be difficult and frustrating. Pa-

tients can be uncooperative, manipulative, and threatening. They may have a pure psychiatric condition; a psychiatric disorder exacerbated by drugs, alcohol, or medical conditions; or a medical condition masquerading as a psychiatric one. Common ED psychiatric complaints include anxiety; depression; mania; and, like the patient in the clinical scenario, psychosis. *Acute psychosis* is a descriptive term and does not specify cause. This chapter concentrates on the workup and evaluation of the psychotic patient.

Psychosis is defined as a condition whereby a patient is not in touch with reality and may respond to visual or auditory hallucinations. These patients may regard medical personnel as threatening and respond in a hostile and uncooperative manner. Therefore, the physician must first address the behavior and provide a safe environment for the workup of these patients.

History

Taking an extensive in-depth history may be the most important aspect of the appropriate diagnosis and disposition of the psychiatric patient. In addition, it may be helpful in ruling out or discovering active medical conditions that need attention. In some cases, the initial history must be deferred until the patient is calm and cooperative. When the patient is able, or when family is available, they should be thoroughly questioned on any medical complaints and the history of present illness. A complete review of systems should be done, with attention to systems that may present with psychiatric-like illnesses. Those include central nervous system (CNS) complaints such as headaches, cognitive impairment, visual changes, focal neurological weakness, or alterations in sensation. Endocrine disorders may present as a psychiatric condition, including hypothyroidism and hyperthyroidism. Pertinent questions would include weight gain or loss, cold or heat intolerance, hair loss, change in skin condition, and neck swelling or pain. Occult cancer or CNS metastasis should be considered in any patient with a remote or recent cancer history, unexplained weight loss, or other constitutional symptoms. Unfortunately, pure psychiatric conditions may present with many of these constitutional conditions, and each case must be carefully evaluated and screened. If a patient has a known psychiatric history, the ED physician must still rule out concurrent medical problems. The patient should be questioned for any new symptoms or complaints unrelated to their psychiatric condition.

Once it is felt the patient does not have a preexisting or new medical condition that needs attention, the psychiatric evaluation can be attended to. This requires a thorough historical evaluation, as follows.

Chief Complaint and History of Present Illness

Allow the patient to explain why they are in the ED today, focusing on the chief complaint ("Why now?"). Identify precipitants. If the patient is unable or unwilling to explain, then this information and the following information must be obtained from other sources, including police, EMS, family, friends, or bystanders who witnessed the events before the patient was brought to the ED.

Determine the onset, duration, and severity of symptoms and whether this has happened before.

- Psychosis: ascertain the presence of delusions or hallucinations, or behavioral observation of responding to internal stimuli.
- Depression: remember the mnemonic SIGECAPS (Sleep, Interest (motivation/pleasure), Guilt, Energy, Concentration, Appetite, Psychomotor agitation or retardation, Suicidality). Four or more symptoms for at least 2 weeks are diagnostic for major depressive episode.
- Suicidality and homicidality: ascertain current ideation, intent, plan, and previous attempts.
- Psychiatric history: a history of previous psychiatric hospitalization and outpatient treatment should be elicited directly.
- Substance abuse: current and former substance abuse with attention to change in use, dependency, and withdrawal.

Past Medical History and Medications

Determine current medical conditions and active problems and any medications being taken for those conditions.

- Pay attention to recent changes in medication dosages, new prescription medications, psychiatric medications, and nonprescription medications. Ask specifically how the medicines are being taken with attention to inadvertent or intentional overdose possibilities.
- Consider drug–drug interactions and duplicate medications, especially if there are multiple medical providers.
- Ask whether the patient is allergic to any medications
- If the patient had prior hospitalizations, ask about the diagnosis and outcome.
- Obtain the patient's past surgical history.
- Obtain the patient's obstetric history, with attention to recent delivery and postpartum state.

Family and Social History

- Family history: ask about major medical and psychiatric conditions.
- Social history: ascertain the patient's current functioning and best level of functioning, education, occupation, work history, living arrangements, marital status, and social support.

Physical Examination

Patients with psychiatric illness may be reluctant to be examined. They may be hostile, delusional, or paranoid. Your first concern must be the safety of the patient, staff, and physician. All threats should be taken seriously and appropriate steps initiated to ensure safety for all concerned. The physician should be positioned between the patient and the door. Help should be close by in case it is needed. Do not keep medical equipment visibly displayed. Even a stethoscope can be used as a weapon. Avoid wearing it around your neck when examining potentially violent patients.

Note the patient's vital signs, including pulse oximetry. Observe the patient's appearance, affect, and ability to cooperate with the examiner. Establish the patient's airway, breathing, and circulation (ABCs) and level of consciousness. Perform a complete physical examination, with focus on neurological examination and areas relevant to the current symptoms and chief complaint. Finally, note any signs of physical abuse, trauma, or exposure.

Mental Status Examination

The mental status examination includes level of consciousness, appearance and behavior, attention, mood and affect, language, thought form and content, memory, insight and judgment, and cognition.

Use the Folstein Mini-Mental Status to assess cognitive status. This brief, practical, and quantifiable examination focuses on the cognitive state of the patient. Points are assigned for each task completed correctly, with a total possible score of 30 points. Scores of 20 or lower suggest cognitive dysfunction resulting from dementia, delirium, or psychotic state such as schizophrenia.

- Orientation: ask, "What is date, day, month, year, and season?" (5 points).
- Location: ask the patient to name the hospital or department, location, town or city, county, and state (5 points).
- Registration: introduce this to the patient as a test of memory. State three unrelated objects that the patient must repeat back to the examiner. First repetition determines score (0 to 3 points). Allow up to six attempts to correctly state the three objects. Recall cannot be tested if the patient is unable to perform this task in six tries.
- Attention and calculation: serial 7 subtraction from 100 (100, 93, 86, 79, 72, 65). Stop after five subtractions (0 to 5 points). If the patient is unable or unwilling to perform this task, ask the patient to spell the word "world" backward (0 to 5 points).
- Recall: recall the three objects the patients was asked to remember earlier (0 to 3 points).

- Language:
  - Naming: wristwatch and pencil/pen (0 to 2 points).
  - Repetition: repeat "No ifs, ands, or buts" (0 to 1 point).
  - Three-stage command: "Take a piece of paper in your right hand, fold it in half, and place it on the floor" (0 to 3 points).
  - Reading: print, "Close your eyes" on a piece of paper and give it to the patient, instructing him or her to read the paper and follow the command (0 to 1 point).
  - Writing: ask the patient to write a sentence. The sentence must contain a subject and a verb and be sensible. Correct grammar and punctuation are unnecessary (0 to 1 point).
  - Copying: draw intersecting pentagons with 1-inch sides and ask the patient to copy the drawing exactly (0 to 1 point).

Compute the patient's score out of the possible total of 30 points

Diagnostic Evaluation

Radiology

Computed tomography (CT) scan of the head is indicated for patients with suspected intracranial bleed, mass, midline shift, or infection. History of immunocompromised state, malignancy, trauma, bleeding disorders, anticoagulation therapy, and/or focal neurological findings on examination; physical evidence of head trauma; or seizure activity should raise suspicion for an occult intracranial process.

Laboratory

Toxicological and metabolic screens for organic etiology must be considered. Decisions to order these tests are dependent on patient presentation, physical examination findings, institutional preference, and psychiatric receiving facility preferences. Screens for reversible causes of a change in mental status include CBC count, glucose, electrolytes, renal studies, liver function tests, thyroid profile, rapid plasmin reagin (RPR) test, ETOH, toxicological screen, and appropriate drug levels.

Lumbar Puncture

Any evidence of a possible CNS infection warrants a lumbar puncture.

Differential Diagnosis

The differential diagnosis for psychiatric emergencies is illustrated in Table 35.1.

Treatment

Medications for Agitated Patients

Two medications commonly administered to agitated patients are haloperidol (Haldol) and lorazepam (Ativan).

The initial dose of haloperidol is 5 mg intramuscular (IM), and may be repeated every 10 minutes until patient is calm. The maintenance dose for the next 12 hours is generally half of the dose initially required to calm the patient

The initial dose of lorazepam is 1 to 2 mg IM/IV and may be repeated in 20 minutes. Lorazepam is a benzodiazepine metabolized by glucuronidation with no active metabolites; therefore, it can be used in patients who have liver disease and patients who are elderly. Lorazepam can also be given to more mildly agitated patients in a dose range of 0.5 to 2.0 mg per dose (po) (Table 35.2).

Medications for Chronic Psychiatric Illness

There are dozens of medications prescribed for the many psychiatric diagnoses. The ED physician usually is not responsible for prescribing these medications, and it is beyond the scope of this book and chapter to discuss them. Generally, these medications should not be prescribed without psychiatric consultation. It should be remembered that many of these medications have side effects and toxicities, and their use should be carefully considered and monitored.

Disposition

The initial question that arises with psychiatric patients is disposition within the department (Table 35.2). All ED patients are

---

Table 35.1.

Differential diagnosis of psychiatric disorders

Common Medications That Cause Psychosis
Antianxiety agents
Isoniazid and rifampin
Anticonvulsants
Antidepressants
Antihistamines
Antineoplastic agents
Corticosteroids
cimetidine
Drugs of abuse
Cardiovascular drugs including captopril, digitalis, and propranolol

Psychiatric Disorders
Psychotic depression
Postpartum depression
Mania and bipolar disorder

Medical Disorders
Brain tumor
Cushing's syndrome
Alcoholic hallucinosis
Wernicke-Korsakoff syndrome
Delirium tremens
Thyroid disorders
Electrolyte disorders
Hypoglycemia
Hypoxia
Hypercarbia
Hepatic encephalopathy
Atypical migraine
Organic brain disease

Table 35.2.

Treatment summary of the agitated or psychotic patient

Ensure staff and patient safety
   Security personnel
   Sitter
   Physical restraints
   Pharmacological restraints: haloperidol (Haldol) 5 mg IV or IM, lorazepam (Ativan) 1–2 mg IV or IM
Medical evaluation
Psychiatric evaluation

IM, intramuscular; IV, intravenous.

triaged to a specific site of care in the ED and assigned a priority level indicating whether the presenting condition is emergent, urgent, or nonurgent. Most EDs have a specific room or set of rooms specifically dedicated for patients with psychiatric conditions. Generally, patients must be cooperative to be placed in these rooms. Uncooperative patients requiring physical and/or chemical restraints must be directly observed in an acute care area.

Once a patient is considered medically clear, disposition should be determined along with a psychiatric consultation. The major psychiatric conditions that require ED psychiatric evaluation and hospitalization include suicidal or homicidal ideation/gesture and psychosis. Inpatient admission depends on many factors, including whether the patient is a danger to himself or herself or to others, availability of social support systems, first psychotic episode, availability of beds including med-psychiatric and dual diagnosis, and availability of outpatient care.

Pathophysiology

The pathophysiology of the acutely confused patient depends on the etiology. Once the nonpsychiatric disorder has been ruled out, the pathophysiology becomes less known. Psychiatric illnesses are still relatively poorly understood. Schizophrenia, a thought disorder, and bipolar disorder, a mood disorder, both have a well-described genetic component. Studies of twins and families show that there is increased prevalence of psychiatric disease in families. Bipolar disorder is seven times more likely to occur in first-degree relatives of a person with the disease.

There is some evidence based on pharmacological and neuroimaging studies that schizophrenia is related to dysfunction in the prefrontal cortex and limbic system. The neurotransmitters dopamine, glutamate, and serotonin may be involved as well. Many pharmacological agents used to treat schizophrenia and other psychiatric disorders have neurotransmitter action. In general, the understanding of psychiatric disease pathophysiology has a long way to go and may yet provide better treatment along with understanding.

Suggested Readings

American Psychiatric Association. *Diagnostic and statistical manual of mental disorders*, 4th ed. Washington, DC: American Psychiatric Association, 1994.

Allen M, ed. *Emergency psychiatry*. Washington, DC: American Psychiatric Press, 2002. Available at http://www.appi.org/ (accessed 4/16/04).

Lamberg L. Psychiatric emergencies call for comprehensive assessment and treatment. *JAMA* 2002;288:686–687.

Massachusetts General Hospital handbook of general hospital psychiatry, 3rd ed. Stern TA, Fricchione GL, Cassem NH, et al., eds. St. Louis: Mosby 1992.

Merck manual of diagnosis and therapy, chapters 185–196. Beers MH, Berkow R, eds. Medical Services, USMEDSA, USHH. Available at http://www.merck.com/pubs/mmanual/section15/chapter194/194a.htm (accessed 4/16/2002).

Change in Mental Status
Questions and Answers

Questions

A patient with a known history of ethanol abuse presents to the emergency department (ED) with confusion, shaking, diaphoresis, and lethargy. Which of the following should be obtained in the initial management of this patient?

A. Blood alcohol level

B. Blood glucose concentration

C. Drugs of abuse toxicology screen

D. Hemoglobin and hematocrit concentration

2. A 38-year-old woman presents to the emergency department (ED) acutely confused. She has been hearing voices telling her to kill herself. She believes God is speaking to her through the telephone. She has no significant past medical history and denies using drugs or alcohol. She refuses a physical examination. Which of the following treatments is the most appropriate?

A. Restrain the patient and commit to a psychiatric unit.

B. Place the patient in a room and return when she is calm.

C. Order laboratory tests including a toxicological screen, thyroid-stimulating hormone (TSH), complete blood count (CBC) and electrolytes, and pregnancy test.

D. Place the patient in a quiet supervised setting. Order 1 mg of lorazepam. Return

when the patient is calm to continue the workup.

3. Which of the following statements best describes the symptoms associated with "the DTs"?

A. Piloerection, diarrhea, and decreased mental status

B. Nausea, vomiting, and "the shakes"

C. "The shakes," hallucinations, and agitation

D. Incontinence, tremors, and decreased mental status

4. A 35-year-old man with a past medical history of insulin-dependent diabetes presents to the emergency department (ED) dehydrated. Three days ago he ran out of insulin and ever since has been complaining of excessive urine output with the desire to drink large quantities of fluid. Which of the following laboratory tests is most consistent with a patient in diabetic ketoacidosis?

A. pH >7.4

B. Glucose <200 mg/dL

C. Anion gap >12

D. Excess total body potassium

E. High sodium

5. A 50-year-old man with a history of alcoholism is brought to the emergency department (ED) with a witnessed tonic-clonic seizure. He is initially postictal. After a short period of observation, his mental status improves. He has no evidence of trauma and denies any recent falls. He denies

taking any medications. He thinks he may have had a seizure in the past. He is tachycardic but stable. He is tremulous. He has no neck pain. His neurological and physical examination is otherwise unremarkable. Which of the following would be appropriate medical therapy in this patient?

A. Phenytoin 1,000 mg intravenously then discharge

B. Hospital admission

C. Two milligrams lorazepam IV observation then discharge

D. Observation for 6 hours then discharge

E. One liter normal saline then discharge if stable

6. A known alcoholic patient presents with generalized weakness and appears dehydrated and emaciated. Which of the following would be important to include in the management of this patient?

A. Potassium

B. Calcium

C. Magnesium

D. Thiamine

Directions: There are three sets of response options for the following scenario. You will be required to select one best answer from each question set.

7. A 35-year-old woman is brought to the emergency department (ED) after a witnessed tonic-clonic seizure. The patient is unable to provide any history. It is not known if this patient has any medical problems or prior seizures. Her physical examination reveals an unresponsive female. Pupils are 4 mm and equal. Her vital signs are significant for a blood pressure of 90/60 mm Hg, heart rate of 120 beats/minute, respiratory rate of 20 breaths/minute, temperature of 100°F, and 100% oxygenation. Lungs, cardiac, and abdominal examinations are normal. Extremities are normal. She responds to pain but is unable to follow commands. Her only medication is a tricyclic antidepressant.

7.1. Which of the following interventions should be done first?

A. Place an intravenous (IV) line

B. Place oxygen

C. Administer intramuscular (IM) lorazepam (Ativan)

D. Perform fingerstick for glucose

E. Administer IM naloxone (Narcan)

7.2. Which intervention listed is contraindicated in this patient?

A. Complete blood count (CBC), arterial blood gas (ABG), electrolytes, blood and urine cultures

B. Toxicological screen and electrocardiogram (ECG)

C. Antibiotics

D. Fluid resuscitation

E. Lumbar puncture (LP)

7.3. Further history from the family elicits a history of depression and prior suicide attempts. Which of the following is the next test or intervention that should be done?

A. Electrocardiogram (ECG)

B. Urine and blood toxicological screens

C. Placement of nasogastric (NG) tube and administration of charcoal

D. Intravenous (IV) sodium bicarbonate

E. IV naloxone (Narcan)

Answers and Explanations

1. B. A change in a patient's mental status can be the result of many etiologies. Consider all of them and investigate early the most common and most easily rectifiable. The symptoms presented here are more consistent with hypoglycemia than with acute ethanol intoxication. A bedside glucometer measurement, if low, is easily treated with intravenous (IV) solution containing dextrose. Glucose is metabolized differently in the alcoholic patient than in nondrinkers. Even in the context of malnutrition, the metabolism of alcohol increases the ratio of reduced nicotinamide adenine dinucleotide to oxidized nicotinamide adenine dinucleotide (NADH/NAD$^+$ ratio), inhibits gluconeogenesis, and increases the production of CO_2 and lactate. Therefore, hypoglycemia is a frequent consequence of acute or chronic alcohol use and is often the cause of altered mentation, particularly in an already malnourished and dehydrated alcohol-abusing patient. Blood alcohol levels may be elevated or zero in this patient and would not likely affect initial management. Toxicology screens and complete blood counts including hemoglobin and hematocrit will take considerably longer to obtain from the laboratory and will not generally change your *initial* management of this patient. Anemia does not cause a change in mental status.

2. D. The patient is suicidal and psychotic and cannot be placed in a nonsupervised setting. She appears stable and in no life-threatening condition, and time may be taken to calm her and do a good history, physical examination, and screening laboratory tests. In the event that the patient continues to be uncooperative, she will require restraints and forced evaluation; however; it is better to elicit the patient's cooperation when possible.

3. C. "DTs" are a potentially dangerous consequence of prolonged ethanol use. Given the morbidity and mortality rates associated with this syndrome, its recognition early in the patient's evaluation can be lifesaving. The "DTs" include altered mental status, marked confusion and disorientation, frightening hallucinations, tremors (known as "the shakes"), and severe agitation. The onset usually begins 48 hours to several days following the last drink and is generally accompanied by tachycardia, hyperthermia, tachypnea, and hypertension.

4. C. Although there are constellations of symptoms that are consistent with diabetic ketoacidosis (DKA), the diagnosis of DKA is based on laboratory findings. They include a serum glucose >300 mg/dL, serum bicarbonate <15 mEq/L, arterial pH <7.3, and ketosis. Patients will also have an anion gap >12 and total body potassium depletion. It is important to emphasize that patients will often present hyperkalemic with the potential for life-threatening cardiac arrhythmias; however, that is reflective of the extracellular serum potassium not the total body potassium that is depleted in DKA. Although the serum potassium is elevated on presentation, it can precipitously drop if not carefully replenished during the treatment period. The sodium is usually

artificially low on laboratory analysis because of the high glucose level.

5. C. This patient shows a classic example of alcohol withdrawal seizures. He does not take anticonvulsant medications despite having a prior history of seizures. He is tremulous, consistent with alcohol withdrawal. Patients presenting with alcohol withdrawal seizures are at high risk of recurrent seizure. The administration of lorazepam greatly reduces the risk of a second seizure. Alcohol withdrawal seizures are not amenable to treatment with anticonvulsant medications such as phenytoin. They do not indicate a primary seizure disorder and resolve with the resolution of the risk behavior. None of the other choices will help to diminish this patient's risk of a second seizure or his withdrawal symptoms. Hospital admission is only required if withdrawal symptoms do not respond to therapy, or he has symptoms of delirium tremens.

6. D. Chronic alcohol abusers are frequently malnourished as well. Therefore, the most common deficiency in this population is that of thiamine. Deficiency of thiamine in the alcoholic can precipitate a dangerous condition called Wernicke-Korsakoff encephalopathy. To avoid this complication, thiamine is commonly added with folate and multivitamins to the intravenous (IV) fluids in these patients. This combination renders the fluid a bright yellow, hence the popular name "banana bag." Deficiencies of magnesium, potassium, and calcium are less common but do occur. Deficiencies of magnesium and potassium tend to occur together in the alcoholic; you will encounter these deficiencies more frequently than that of calcium.

7.1. D. In the patient with altered mentation or seizure, hypoglycemia should always be ruled out immediately. The test is very fast and does not require time-delaying intravenous (IV) access. In addition, the treatment can completely cure the patient and stop a prolonged workup. In addition, the longer the brain goes without glucose, the more possibility exists for long-term consequences. Therefore, glucose should be administered as quickly as possible in the profoundly hypoglycemic patient. Oxygen and intravenous access are needed, but they should not delay the fingerstick. Lorazepam is not needed because the patient is no longer seizing and may further depress the mental status. Naloxone could be administered; however, the pupils are wide, decreasing the likelihood that this is a narcotic overdose.

7.2. E. In the patient with altered mentation and seizure, central nervous system causes should be strongly considered along with toxicological, infectious, and metabolic causes and epilepsy. A lumbar puncture (LP) should be considered in this patient only after a computed tomography (CT) scan of the head has been performed. In any patient with neurological abnormalities, a space-occupying lesion must be ruled out before LP. Antibiotics should be given before CT and LP in any patient where meningitis is suspected. The patient requires fluid resuscitation for the hypotension. Cultures of blood and urine are required because of her fever, and a toxicological screen may help determine the cause of the seizure.

7.3. A. Although many substances, when ingested, can cause seizure and altered mentation, a tricyclic overdose should be considered early because it is associated with high morbidity and mortality. In addition, treatment cannot wait for blood testing. The electrocardiogram (ECG) changes found in tricyclic use are quite specific and sensitive. Any suspected tricyclic overdose with a widened QRS (QRS >100 ms) should be treated with sodium bicarbonate until the QRS normalizes. Other ECG findings include tachycardia, rightward terminal 40-msec QRS axis deviation, and QT and PR prolongation. Toxicological screens should be sent; however, treatment often has to occur before return of results. Charcoal should be given as well, but in this patient, airway protection would require intubation before giving charcoal because of the risk and consequences of charcoal aspiration.

Weakness and Dizziness

To be weak is miserable.

Milton 1607

INTRODUCTION
Neils K. Rathlev, MD
Section Editor

Complaints of vague, generalized weakness or dizziness frequently lead to anxiety and frustration among emergency providers because of their nonspecific nature. The symptoms conjure up images of a futile maze of investigation with no "light at the end of the tunnel." However, a meticulous approach to the patient interview is frequently rewarded with a clear sense of direction in physical examination and further diagnostic evaluation. The terms *dizzy* and *weak* are poorly descriptive and imply different connotations for different individuals. Therefore, the patient initially should be asked to describe the symptoms in detail without using the words weak or dizzy. This is a time to allow the patient to speak without interruption. Open-ended questions should be posed that do not lead the interview in the direction of a preconceived bias. Accordingly, do not ask whether the room was "spinning" or whether the patient "lost consciousness" or developed an "unstable gait" because the interviewer is likely to obtain an affirmative but possibly misleading response to these questions. Pull up a chair, sit down, and listen as the patient explains the problem in his or her own words.

Dizziness can variably refer to syncope, presyncope, vertigo, ataxia, or ill-defined lightheadedness. Syncope and near-syncope imply the loss or near loss of consciousness as reported by bystanders or may be described subjectively as amnesia for a defined time period by the subject. The etiologies range from benign "fainting spells" or vasovagal episodes to life-threatening cardiac arrhythmias or blood loss. Vertigo involves the expressed sensation of movement of the surrounding environment, the individual, or both simultaneously. The sensation may involve a to-and-fro, retropulsive, or "sinking" movement without the more typical rotational component. Vertigo caused by central nervous system dysfunction or disease is virtually always accompanied by other abnormalities that are detectable by a detailed history and neurological examination. Ataxia can be distinguished from other categories of dizziness by the exacerbation of symptoms with ambulation. The balance impairment may resolve when lying down or sitting and may only manifest as a wide-based, unsteady gait. The astute clinician will distinguish a primary problem of proprioception versus cerebellar dysfunction by physical examination. Patients who cannot describe their symptoms with greater clarity than ill-defined "lightheadedness" typically have a very favorable long-term prognosis. These individuals often suffer from multiple sensory deficits such as senile hearing and visual loss, psychiatric disorders, or adverse effects from medications.

The symptom of weakness is similarly difficult to evaluate and is defined as the inability of muscles to exert a normal force. Difficulty in performing normal activities that previously required little effort is an important clue to the diagnosis. Weakness may be caused by loss of muscle, peripheral nerve, or upper motor neuron function. The most serious consequence of neuromuscular weakness is respiratory failure, which is essentially a form of restrictive lung disease. The patient must be carefully monitored for tachypnea and respiratory distress, and spirometry should be performed at the bedside in questionable clinical situations.

Primary muscle disease or myopathy commonly presents as proximal weakness of the hip girdle and shoulders and may manifest initially as difficulty in rising from a seated position, walking up stairs, or raising the arms above the head. Inflammatory disorders cause distinct muscle tenderness in the absence of preceding exertion. Disorders of the neuromuscular junction prevent muscle contraction by disturbing either the release or the postsynaptic binding of the neurotransmitting agent. Radiculopathy and peripheral neuropathy present with variable sensory dysfunction and hyporeflexia. Because of upper motor neuron involvement, anterior horn cell disorders result in hyperactive reflexes, fasciculations, and intact sensory function on physical examination. Hyperactive reflexes and extensor plantar responses (Babinski sign) are characteristic of spinal cord, brainstem, and cerebral hemispheric lesions. The latter frequently present with unilateral weakness, whereas myelopathy often produces bilateral symptoms.

Few presenting complaints test the skill and patience of the emergency provider to a greater extent than weak and dizzy. Outstanding clinicians will consider the patient a worthy diagnostic challenge that must be met with a rigorous approach to history-taking and physical examination, as opposed to a random series of laboratory and radiological tests. The following chapters provide a more detailed description of selected common causes of weakness and dizziness. Emphasis has been placed on a discussion of entities that may require emergency intervention, such as thrombolytic therapy in hemispheric stroke, brainstem infarction that presents as vertigo, antiarrhythmic therapy in cardiac syncope, and mechanical ventilation in neuromuscular disorders.

CHAPTER **36**

Cerebrovascular Accident

Ron Medzon, MD

Clinical Scenario

Emergency medical services (EMS) calls over the radio to inform the emergency department (ED) that they are bringing in a 74-year-old woman with a history of 90 minutes of slurred speech and right-sided weakness. Family members noted her to be in her usual state of health before dinner, approximately an hour and a half before EMS arrival. At the dinner table, she appeared ashen, was having difficulty using her right hand, and began to slur her words. Her symptoms have slowly worsened, and the family became concerned and called 911. EMS confirms that their physical examination is significant for aphasia and a right hemiparesis.

Past medical history includes hypertension, diabetes, high cholesterol, and a history of chronic stable angina. Social history reveals a 40-pack-year history of tobacco use. Medications include diltiazem, pravastatin (Pravachol), glyburide (Micronase), sublingual nitroglycerin as needed, and aspirin once a day.

Before the patient's arrival, the ED physician confirms with radiology that the computed tomography (CT) scanner is available for immediate head CT scan. On arrival, the patient is placed in a resuscitation room and initial evaluation is begun immediately. Two large-bore intravenous catheters are placed, an electrocardiogram (ECG) is obtained, blood samples are drawn and are sent for complete blood cell (CBC) count, electrolytes, international normalized ratio (INR), and partial thromboplastin time, and the patient is placed on 2 L/minute of oxygen via nasal cannula. Vitals signs are a temperature of 98.7°F, blood pressure (BP)

of 178/92 mm Hg, pulse of 98 beats/minute and regular, and a respiratory rate of 12 breaths/minute. The patient is ill appearing and is mumbling incoherently. There is a right facial droop, and she is unable to follow commands or move her right arm or leg. The right arm and leg are hyperreflexic, and she has an upgoing toe on the right. ECG reveals nonspecific ST-segment changes with no change from a prior tracing. The physician completes the physical examination, which is otherwise unremarkable, and the patient is rushed to a noncontrast CT scan of the head, which is negative for an intracranial bleed. The neurology service is contacted, and it is agreed to start thrombolysis with tissue plasminogen activator (t-PA) because the patient is having an acute left middle cerebral artery distribution stroke with an onset less than 3 hours before presentation. She is transferred to the intensive care unit, where she is stabilized. Three days later, at discharge to a rehabilitation facility, she has a marked improvement in symptoms, with the ability to converse and some residual weakness in her arm and leg.

Clinical Evaluation

Introduction

Strokes are defined as a sudden loss of brain function resulting from an interference with the blood supply to the brain. The National Institute of Neurological Disorder and Stroke (NINDS) limits this definition to acute vascular incidents, including ischemic and hemorrhagic lesions. Strokes are the third leading cause of death in the United States. They are the leading cause of disability, resulting in more than $51 billion in direct and indirect costs. The mortality rate is between 20% and 50%, and up to 70% of stroke patients do not return to gainful employment even 7 years after their strokes. The greatest advance in stroke treatment is the use of thrombolytic agents. For a select group of stroke patients, thrombolytics can potentially return the patient to normal function from the brink of a devastating illness.

History

The median age of onset of stroke is 65 years. Patients typically are older and present with a sudden onset of a focal neurological deficit, which is usually maximal at the time of onset of symptoms. Patients may complain of headaches (30%) and may present with a new-onset seizure, although this occurs less than 5% of the time. Patients with a history of a transient ischemic attack (TIA), atrial fibrillation, or prior stroke are at higher risk for stroke. Risk factors for stroke are similar to those of patients with coronary artery disease: (a) hypertension, (b) diabetes, (c) high cholesterol, and (d) tobacco use. It is essential to determine the time of onset of symptoms. Ask witnesses when the patient last appeared functionally normal. Patients who awaken with stroke symptoms are considered to have started their strokes at the time they went to sleep. Because the time window for delivering thrombolytic drugs is 3 hours from onset of symptoms, these questions are critically important.

Physical Examination

The physical examination for the suspected stroke patient obviously focuses on the neurological examination. Observe the patient carefully and compare the findings with that of the witnesses and EMS. Any signs of improvement point toward a TIA and do not warrant thrombolysis. The National Institutes of Health Stroke Severity Scale (NIHSSS) is a list of signs that stratifies patients according to risk and aids in the decision making regarding thrombolysis. It does not replace the detailed neurological examination. Keep in mind that a proximal aortic dissection involving the root of the carotid artery can mechanically occlude blood flow through the artery and cause symptoms mimicking a stroke. Check the blood pressure in both arms and examine peripheral pulses for symmetry.

An irregularly irregular pulse indicates atrial fibrillation, which is a risk factor for stroke. A patient presenting with sudden onset of severe headache, neck stiffness, and photophobia should raise suspicion of an acute intracranial bleed rather than an ischemic stroke. Palpate the carotids for diminished pulses, and then listen over the carotid arteries with the bell of the stethoscope for bruits, indicating carotid stenosis and the possible presence of plaque or thrombosis.

Neurological examination includes a mini mental status examination assessing for language and memory disturbances. An isolated seventh cranial nerve disturbance would present with a facial droop and inability to wrinkle the forehead on the affected side. This is the classic presentation of an isolated cranial nerve palsy (i.e., Bell's palsy) and is not a stroke. The seventh cranial nerve fibers crossover centrally to innervate the musculature of the forehead, thus a central nervous system lesion might spare the forehead, because the still functioning contralateral seventh nerve would innervate the affected forehead as well. This finding is not 100% reliable. Middle cerebral artery lesions typically cause a contralateral facial droop and paresis or weakness. Thus, the patient will have marked weakness or inability to move the arm and leg opposite the side of the brain lesion. Loss of central inhibitory innervation to the reflex synapses in the spinal cord results in hyperreflexia of the affected side, although the reflexes may initially be normal. Scratching the sole of the foot contralateral to the brain lesion will result in an upturning of the great toe (Babinski response), which is a more primitive reflex seen in infants before full neurological development. The normal response is for the toe to turn downward.

Visual field defects and changes in visual acuity occur in posterior cerebral artery circulation strokes. Personality disturbances may be noted in anterior cerebral artery circulation strokes because of the role of the frontal lobes in behavior, and motor and speech deficits may be seen. Basilar artery distribution strokes are almost universally fatal, because of the lack of compensatory blood flow from the circle of Willis. Patients may show signs of vertigo, nystagmus, dysarthria, and ataxia and may present with syncope. The neurological examination is incomplete until the patient stands up (if able) and is assessed for balance and gait.

In order for a patient to be eligible for thrombolysis, physical examination must demonstrate a significant neurological deficit. Isolated ataxia, isolated sensory findings, isolated dysarthria, or minimal weakness are not strong enough findings to warrant thrombolysis.

Diagnostic Evaluation

A noncontrast CT scan of the head is an emergent study in acute stroke of less than 3 hours' duration. The primary objective is to rule out intracerebral bleeding (which is an absolute contraindication for thrombolysis) and signs of a massive embolic stroke. The NINDS stroke consensus group recommends that a head CT scan be obtained no later than 25 minutes after the arrival of the patient in the ED and that the scan be read within 45 minutes, thereby allowing adequate time if the patient is a candidate and consents to thrombolysis.

Blood tests, which include CBC count, electrolyte levels, and coagulation studies, are useful in excluding candidates for thrombolysis and for determining other causes for a change in mental status, such as hypoglycemia. An ECG should be obtained to look for evidence of ischemia or infarction. Diffuse T-wave inversions sometimes occur in severe strokes (cerebral Ts) and should not be mistaken for ischemia. A chest x-ray film should be examined for widening of the aorta, which may be evidence of a dissection.

Differential Diagnosis

The differential diagnosis for cerebrovascular accident is illustrated in Table 36.1.

Table 36.1.

Differential diagnosis of stroke

Subdural hematoma
Epidural hematoma
Subarachnoid bleed
Intracranial tumor
Intracranial abscess
Seizure/postictal state (Todd's paralysis)
Meningitis and encephalitis
Multiple sclerosis
Hypoglycemia
Complicated migraine
Hypertensive encephalopathy
Cranial nerve palsy (Bell's palsy)
Hypertensive encephalopathy
Aortic dissection with carotid involvement
Carotid dissection
Ménière's disease/labyrinthitis (posterior circulation)

Treatment

The primary objective in treating the stroke patient is to determine their eligibility for thrombolysis. Treatment guidelines are listed in Table 36.2. Any patient older than 18 years who has an ischemic stroke with a measurable deficit on the NIHSSS with a clearly defined time of onset less than 3 hours to treatment is eligible. The absolute contraindications are evidence of intracranial bleed on CT scan of the head or a clinical presentation consistent with intracranial hemorrhage despite normal CT, uncontrolled hypertension, known arteriovenous malformation, prior intracranial bleed, head trauma or neurosurgery within the last 3 months, pregnancy, active internal bleeding, or post myocardial infarction pericarditis. Warning signs that should cause you to reevaluate the need for thrombolysis include clinical improvement signifying a possible TIA, recent very high or very low blood glucose (<50 or >400 mg/dL), recent lumbar puncture, or gastrointestinal or genitourinary bleed.

There is still some controversy surrounding the decision of the American Heart Association (AHA) and National Institutes of Health (NIH) guidelines considering thrombolysis in eligible stroke patients as standard

---

Table 36.2.

Treatment guideline for acute stroke

EMS call notifies ED of potential stroke patient
Physician evaluates patient in first 10 minutes
CT scan of head obtained within 25 minutes of arrival
CT scan interpreted within 45 minutes of arrival
Confirmed stroke <3 hours of symptoms and no absolute contraindications for thrombolysis

   Administer intravenous rt-PA

   Admit to ICU for minimum of 24 hours

ASA 325 mg po within 48 hours (hold 24 hours if t-PA given)
Hypertension: treat BP >220/115 mm Hg with labetalol 20 mg IV, may double each
   subsequent dose, add sodium nitroprusside if refractory to labetalol
Hypertension and t-PA: keep BP <185/110 mm Hg using previously listed medications
Seizure: phenytoin 17 mg/kg IV load
Fever: treat aggressively with acetaminophen or ibuprofen; identify source of fever
Hyperglycemia: treat aggressively with insulin

ASA, acetylsalicylic acid (aspirin); BP, blood pressure; CT, computed tomography; ED, emergency
department; EMS, emergency medical services; ICU, intensive care unit; IV, intravenous; po, by mouth;
rt-PA, recombinant tissue plasminogen activator; t-PA, tissue plasminogen activator.

---

of care. The discussion is beyond the scope of this text; however, the studies to date demonstrate the following: (a) there is an 11% to 13% greater chance of return to normal function in stroke victims who receive thrombolytics compared with age-matched controls who do not receive thrombolytics and (b) the rate of symptomatic intracranial hemorrhage is 10 times greater in the thrombolytic treatment group (6.4% vs. 0.6%) versus patients who do not receive thrombolytics, with no change in overall mortality. The clinician must discuss these issues carefully with the patient if possible and with the family or health care proxy if the patient cannot understand the complex issues of treatment. Recombinant tissue plasminogen activator (rt-PA) is the current medication of choice. Specialized centers with interventional neuroradiologists on call have started to use intraarterial thrombolysis with prourokinase for stroke patients who fall within the 3- to 6-hour time window from onset of symptoms. The initial results are promising.

Aspirin has been proven effective and safe in strokes if given within 48 hours of onset of stroke and continued for at least 2 weeks. It decreases the rate of recurrent strokes and decreases the mortality rate from strokes. Aspirin should be withheld from patients receiving t-PA for the first 24 hours, although the NINDS group did not find a difference in complications or mortality of patients who were on aspirin and were given thrombolysis. Other antiplatelet agents (ticlopidine, clopidogrel) are slightly better than aspirin with respect to aiding stroke victims and reducing side effects. Detailed cost-benefit analyses demonstrate that aspirin is by far the most cost-effective drug and that alternative agents should be used for those patients who cannot take aspirin.

Heparin given within 48 hours of ischemic stroke reduces the rate of deep venous thrombosis and pulmonary embolism and also decreases the rate of recurrent ischemic stroke; however, it does this at the expense of a higher rate of intracranial hemorrhage, without significantly affecting mortality or disability at 6 months. Its use is currently controversial.

Hypertension should not be treated in acute stroke. It generally resolves untreated in 2 to 4 days. The exceptions include some patients with intracranial hemorrhage and thrombolysis candidates with blood pressures in excess of 185/110 mm Hg. The AHA and National Stroke Association (NSA) both recommend treating blood pressures greater than 220/115 mm Hg. The initial drug of choice is labetalol, followed by sodium nitroprusside, if necessary. Hyperglycemia should be treated aggressively, because stroke patients do worse if their blood sugars are poorly controlled irrespective of a prior history of diabetes. The patient's volume status should be assessed, and a euvolemic state should be maintained. Dehydrated patients require volume to maintain lower blood viscosity. Fever is dangerous in stroke and should be treated with antipyretics such as acetaminophen. The cause for the fever should be sought as well. Seizures are treated with phenytoin; however, there is no benefit to seizure prophylaxis in stroke. Oxygen is given only to patients who are hypoxic because there is no added benefit to supplemental oxygen as a standard measure.

Disposition

Stroke patients who are stable can be admitted to a general medical floor or neurology floor. Patients who are unstable or receive thrombolysis require at least one night's stay in a neurological intensive care unit (ICU), or a medical ICU with neurology expertise available on call. Patients with TIA require prompt testing, possibly including magnetic resonance brain imaging (MRI) and magnetic resonance angiogram (MRA), carotid Doppler ultrasound scan, and cardiac ultrasound scan to look for a source of embolic stroke. Discretion can be exercised whether to admit the patient to the hospital for this testing or whether to place the patient on an appropriate antiplatelet agent and discharge with follow-up testing scheduled.

Pathophysiology

The brain does not store its own energy. It requires a constant supply of glucose and oxygen. Normal cerebral blood flow is 50 mL/100 g tissue/minute, from which the brain extracts approximately 50% of the oxygen and 30% of the glucose. To accommodate for the loss of oxygen and glucose

that occurs when a blood vessel in the brain occludes, the extraction fraction increases as determined by the size of the clot and the number of collateral vessels available. The remaining vessels vasodilate and the collaterals open. Once cerebral blood flow drops below 50% expected, the synapses stop transmission to conserve energy. As cerebral blood flow decreases further, the ion pumps do not receive the energy supply they need to continue functioning. The sodium/potassium ATPase pumps fail, and the normal ion gradients and membrane potentials are lost. There is an uncontrolled release of excitatory amino acids, namely aspartate and glutamate. Aspartate causes the opening of calcium channels, and calcium, sodium, and chloride influx into the cells. Intracellular potassium in turn leaks out. The calcium stimulates proteases, endonucleases, phospholipase, and nitric oxide synthetase, which are all destructive to the cells. The acidic pH increases free radical formation and also activates pH-dependent endonucleases, causing further cellular damage. Mediators such as cytokines, interleukins, tumor necrosis factor, and platelet-activating factor initiate chemotaxis. Polymorphonuclear cells, macrophages, and platelets are drawn to the site of injury, causing microvascular occlusion.

The *penumbra* describes the area of brain tissue surrounding the necrotic neurons that still has marginal blood flow. It is known that an ischemic cellular membrane can maintain its integrity for 6 to 8 hours provided the area receives at least 25% to 50% of expected blood flow. Thus, any treatment within the first 6 hours of a stroke that can lead to return of normal flow to the penumbra would greatly improve the patient's functional outcome. It is precisely this concept that led to the present use of thrombolytics in stroke.

Suggested Readings

American Heart Association. *2000 Heart and stroke statistical update.* Dallas, TX: American Heart Association, 1999:13–14.

Chinese Acute Stroke Trial (CAST) Collaborative Group. CAST: randomized placebo-controlled trial of early aspirin use in 20,000 patients with acute ischemic stroke. *Lancet* 1997;349: 1641–1649.

Clark WM, Wissman S, Albers GW, et al. Recombinant tissue plasminogen activator (alteplase) for ischemic stroke 3 to 5 hours after symptom onset, the ATLANTIS study: a randomized controlled trial. *JAMA* 1995;274:2019–2026.

Hacke W, Kaste M, Fieschi C, et al. Intravenous thrombolysis with recombinant tissue plasminogen activator for acute stroke study (ECASS). *JAMA* 1995;274:1017–1025.

National Institute of Neurologic Disorders in Stroke: rt-PA Stroke Study Group. Tissue plasminogen activator for acute ischemic stroke. *N Engl J Med* 1995;333:1581–1587.

CHAPTER 37

Vertigo

Frank Michael Carrano, MD

Clinical Scenario

A 68-year-old woman is transported by ambulance to the emergency department (ED) complaining of dizziness, nausea, and three episodes of vomiting, which began after waking from sleep. She states that apart from a recent "head cold" from which she has now recovered, she felt well until this morning. On rolling over and attempting to rise from her bed, she suddenly felt extremely dizzy and nauseated, to the point that she was forced to lie back in her bed and remain still. There was no loss of consciousness. She further explains that lying motionless seems to alleviate the dizziness within a few minutes, although she has continued to feel mildly nauseated; she vomited during another attempt at rising and also when being moved onto a stretcher by prehospital personnel. There was no blood noted in the emesis. Further questioning reveals that her dizziness is the sensation that the room is moving around her although she is not actually moving. She does not feel light-headed or as though she might faint. The patient denies any prior history of these symptoms. She denies double or blurred vision, difficulty swallowing, change in her speech, or hearing loss.

She has a history of mild hypertension, controlled with diet and exercise, and osteoarthritis but no history of head trauma, diabetes, anemia, thyroid disease, or stroke. She takes only an aspirin and a multivitamin daily. She has no drug allergies.

Physical examination reveals a pale-appearing female clutching an emesis basin. She is afebrile. Her supine blood pressure is 142/85 mm Hg, with a pulse of 88 beats/minute while seated at the edge of the bed (which exacerbates her symptoms). Her standing blood pressure is 140/82 mm Hg with a pulse of 94 beats/minute. Her temperature is 98.7°F with a respiratory rate of 12 breaths/minute and a room air oxygen saturation of 97%. The skin turgor is normal. Her pupils are equally reactive at 4 mm and her conjunctivae are pink; her tympanic membranes are pearly gray with a sharp light reflex and no effusion or bulging. Her mucous membranes are moist. Lung sounds are clear, and cardiac examination yields a regular rate and rhythm without evidence of murmur. No bruits are heard on auscultation of her carotid arteries. Her abdomen is soft and nontender; a rectal examination reveals brown stool without blood. On neurological examination, the patient is uncomfortable but alert and oriented times three. Her cranial nerve examination is normal, as is her strength and sensory examination; the reflexes are brisk and equal bilaterally. Examination of her extraocular movements causes her symptoms to return, and lateral gaze of her eyes in either direction generates binocular horizontal nystagmus. A Dix-Hallpike maneuver is performed, which generates a sensation of vertigo and horizontal nystagmus. She is unwilling to allow gait testing as attempted ambulation precipitates severe symptoms.

An intravenous (IV) line is placed and a complete blood cell (CBC) count and basic electrolyte panel are drawn. A bedside glucose test reveals a serum glucose level of 116 mg/dL. The patient feels she is too nauseated to swallow oral medications, so she is given diphenhydramine 50 mg IV. Within 20 minutes, the patient reports great improvement in her symptoms, and she is able to sit up in bed and walk to the bathroom without return of her symptoms. After a period of observation, she is discharged home with an oral antihistamine, an antiemetic suppository, and a diagnosis of benign paroxysmal positional vertigo.

Clinical Evaluation

Introduction

The patient in the clinical scenario presents a classic example of benign positional vertigo. Vertigo is the sensation of movement when none actually takes place, and patients may feel that either they or their surroundings are in motion. They may describe a sensation of leaning to one side, staggering, sinking, or that the "ground is rushing up toward them." When true vertigo is present, the initial priority is to determine whether the origin is central (associated with deep brain structures such as the cerebellum and brainstem) or peripheral (associated with the eighth cranial nerve and vestibular apparatus). This is an important distinction, because central vertigo is often associated with serious dysfunction and consequences. This chapter addresses the approach to diagnosing these entities.

History

Peripheral Vertigo

Classically, peripheral vertigo is sudden in onset and worsened by change in body or head position, with episodes lasting seconds to minutes. Patients frequently complain of nausea, vomiting, and diaphoresis and may also describe tinnitus or hearing loss. You should ask about current symptoms of headache, a history of migraine headaches, a recent history of head trauma, and active medication use, all of which could be associated with vertiginous symptoms.

Other causes of peripheral vertigo include Ménière's disease, a degenerative disease, which leads to excess endolymph in the cochlea and labyrinth of the inner ear. The pathophysiology is not well understood; however, the disease can present almost identically to benign paroxysmal positional vertigo. The vertigo of Ménière's disease tends to be sudden and is associated with nausea and vomiting. Vertiginous symptoms usually last 5 to 40 seconds in benign paroxysmal positional vertigo, whereas they typically last between 2 and 8 hours in Ménière's disease. Attacks occur anywhere from two to three times per week to once a month. Ménière's disease is also accompanied by hearing abnormalities and frequent tinnitus.

Vestibular neuronitis is a peripheral cause of vertigo that is thought to be of viral origin. Inflammation of the eighth cranial nerve is suspected to be the pathological lesion. Although the symptoms of vestibular neuronitis are similar in intensity and onset to other forms of peripheral vertigo, they last only a few days and do not recur. Patients may present with an upper respiratory infection, and although the disease typically abates in dramatic fashion, older patients may be left with a persistent, residual gait disturbance.

Labyrinthitis is another form of peripheral vertigo, which is similar to vestibular neuronitis because a viral infection of the labyrinth of the middle ear is the suspected cause. Patients present with hearing loss, intense sudden-onset vertigo, and evidence of middle ear infection.

Peripheral vertigo can be caused by an extensive list of medications and drugs; aminoglycoside antibiotics accumulate in the endolymph and can destroy cochlear and vestibular hair cells, leading to ataxia and oscillopsia (the inability to fixate on a stationary object while in motion). Quinine-derived drugs and loop diuretics are among medications that can cause irreversible ototoxicity. Vertigo is less common than ataxia or oscillopsia as a presenting complaint in patients with drug-induced toxicity, because both inner ears are damaged equally. Erythromycin, minocycline, and some fluoroquinolones can cause reversible ototoxicity, and drugs such as phenytoin and phencyclidine can cause central vestibular symptoms.

Lastly, lesions such as meningiomas and acoustic schwannomas, which involve the eighth nerve or the cerebellopontine angle, can precipitate peripheral vertigo. Symptoms caused by tumors involving the eighth nerve tend to be very gradual in onset. Vertigo is preceded by hearing loss. Tumors involving the cerebellopontine angle may also cause loss of the corneal reflex, ipsilateral facial weakness, and cerebellar dysfunction.

Central Vertigo

Central vertigo tends to be gradual in onset and unrelated to position change; it presents over a longer period. It is likely to be associated with other neurological findings including cranial nerve abnormalities such as diplopia, dysphagia and dysarthria, and ataxia. Central vertigo can be caused by a variety of disorders, including cerebellar hemorrhage or infarction, which tend to produce less severe vertigo accompanied by an abnormal Romberg test and gait and truncal ataxia (loss of balance of the trunk).

Central vertigo may be caused by vertebrobasilar insufficiency. In this instance, positional changes precipitate symptoms, unlike other causes of central vertigo. For example, a patient with stenosis of the vertebral artery on the left may transiently occlude the vessel on turning his or her head to the right. The resulting loss of blood flow to the brain and brainstem can cause vertebrobasilar insufficiency. Previously established risk factors for atherosclerotic vascular disease predispose patients to this disorder. Multiple sclerosis may create focal areas of demyelination in the brainstem and can cause vertiginous symptoms (see Chapter 39). In multiple sclerosis, symptoms can last from hours to weeks but tend to be less severe than in cases of peripheral vertigo. Nystagmus is also associated with vertigo caused by this disorder.

Lastly, any neoplasm that involves or compresses the brainstem can cause vertigo. A history of chronic headaches, worse in the morning and abating as the day progresses, may be a symptom of a brain tumor (see Chapter 31).

Physical Examination

The physical examination of the dizzy patient should initially focus on vital signs, including orthostatic blood pressure measurements (a systolic decrease of more than 20 mm Hg when the patient is moved from a supine to a seated or standing position suggests postural hypotension). A careful cardiac examination must be performed to search for signs of arrhythmia or valvular disease. The carotid arteries should be auscultated for bruits because occlusion can precipitate dizziness, near-syncope, and syncope. Neurological, vestibular, and ear examinations are essential for the patient with true vertigo.

The tympanic membranes should be evaluated for erythema, bulging, or other abnormalities suggestive of otitis media. Hearing loss can be uncovered while whispering in one ear and covering the other. If the patient has hearing loss, Rinne and Weber tests are indicated to help identify sensorineural or conductive hearing losses. The neurological examination includes testing of cranial nerves, deep tendon reflexes, and sensation including proprioception. Rapid alternating movements of the hands test cerebellar function, and both the Romberg test and tandem gait evaluate the function of the cerebellum and vestibulospinal system.

If central vertigo is suspected, the clinician should look for the absence of the corneal reflex, motor or sensory deficits of the face, loss or depression of the gag reflex, and difficulty swallowing (Table 37.1).

The most important means of diagnosing benign paroxysmal positional vertigo is the history and physical examination. The Dix-Hallpike maneuver is a simple positional test that can assist in establishing the diagnosis, and it is performed according to the following procedural steps. The patient is initially positioned on the examining table, seated upright. The examiner then brings the patient's head down over the edge of the table and turns the head to one side. If the patient has benign paroxysmal positional vertigo, after a few seconds, the examiner will witness characteristic, rhythmic movements of the eyes, called nystagmus. The ear that is pointing toward the floor has disrupted otoconia if nystagmus is seen, and the patient becomes dizzy. The examiner repeats the test, this time turning the head to the opposite side while testing the other ear. The nystagmus and perception of vertigo will fatigue (i.e., slow down) and

Table 37.1.

Signs and symptoms of peripheral versus central vertigo

	Peripheral	Central
Symptoms		
Onset	Sudden	Gradual
Related to position of head and body	Yes	No
Duration	Brief	Chronic
Associated symptoms	Nausea, vomiting, earache, tinnitus, hearing loss	Symptoms of CNS disease (e.g., headache)
Habituation (decreased response) with repeated provocative maneuvers	Yes	No
Intensity	Severe	Mild
Signs		
Cranial nerve deficits	No	Common (e.g., diplopia, dysphagia, dysarthria and facial numbness)
Ataxia	No	Possible, unilateral
Motor/sensory deficits	No	Possible
Nystagmus on provocative maneuvers	Yes	Variable or no response
Direction	Horizontal, rotatory, unidirectional	Possibly vertical, convergent multidirectional
Fatigability	Yes	No
Latency (delay in onset)	2–20 sec	No
Suppression with gaze fixation	Usually	No

CNS, central nervous system.

cease after 15 to 20 seconds. If the head is not moved, further symptoms will not develop. If the process is repeated, vertigo will recur, but will last a shorter period. This phenomenon is known as "habituation."

Diagnostic Evaluation

Routine laboratory studies and imaging studies are not necessary in the patient with benign paroxysmal positional vertigo; however, in the course of a general evaluation of nonspecific dizziness, a CBC count should be checked to rule out anemia or a bacterial cause of labyrinthitis. The serum glucose level should be measured to exclude hypoglycemia.

Dizziness, syncope, and vertigo associated with head trauma or focal neurological deficits are indications for a computed tomography (CT) scan or a magnetic resonance imaging (MRI) study of the brain to rule out an intracranial lesion or bleed. Imaging studies of the brain are mandatory for patients with a strong suspicion of central vertigo. Possible cerebellar infarction or hemorrhage is an indication for an immediate CT scan of the brain because definitive treatment may involve emergent surgical decompression. An urgent CT scan or MRI may not be necessary if a tumor is suspected and the patient does not manifest signs of increased intracranial pressure. An electrocardiogram (ECG) should be obtained and cardiac monitoring should be instituted if vertebrobasilar insufficiency is a concern; ultrasound examination of the carotid arteries and MRI or magnetic resonance angiography should be considered.

Differential Diagnosis

The differential diagnosis for vertigo is illustrated in Table 37.2.

Treatment

A variety of medications are currently in use for suppression of peripheral vertigo and concomitant nausea and vomiting (Table 37.3). The most common class of medications used is the antihistamines (specifically the histamine-1 [H_1] antihistamines), such as diphenhydramine (Benadryl), dimenhydrinate, and meclizine (Antivert). Their mechanism of action is not fully understood. Other medications used to treat vertigo include anticholinergic medications such as scopolamine and the medium-duration benzodiazepines such as diazepam. The benzodiazepines are thought to suppress the function of vestibular pathways. For nausea and vomiting, antiemetic medications such as promethazine and hydroxyzine may be helpful; however, single-agent therapy with an antihistamine may be all that is required as successful treatment of vertigo and often reduces or eliminates nausea and vomiting as well.

In addition, a nonpharmacological treatment known as the canalith repositioning or Epley maneuver is effective for benign

Table 37.2.

Differential diagnosis of vertigo

Vestibular Disorders
Benign peripheral vertigo/benign paroxysmal positional vertigo
Trauma/post-head injury
Infection: labyrinthitis, vestibular neuronitis, Ramsay-Hunt syndrome

Syndromes
Ménière's syndrome
Neoplasia
Vascular disease
Paget's disease
Drug-induced (aminoglycoside antibiotics)

Neurological Disorders
Vertebrobasilar insufficiency
Cerebellopontine angle tumor
Basal ganglia disease
Multiple sclerosis
Infection: tuberculosis, neurosyphilis
Epilepsy
Migraine headache
Cerebrovascular disease/accident

General
Hematological disease: anemia, polycythemia
Alcohol intoxication
Chronic renal failure
Metabolic disorder: hypoglycemia, thyroid disease

paroxysmal positional vertigo. The Epley maneuver involves rotating the patient's head in a predetermined succession of four movements. These are designed to force any free-floating particles in the posterior semicircular canal of the inner ear to move into the utricle, where they are less likely to cause vertigo. The success rate of abolishing symptoms of vertigo with this technique is approximately 80%. Unfortunately, benign paroxysmal positional vertigo often recurs. Repeated episodes occur in approximately one third of patients in the first year and in 50% within 5 years after treatment. Surgical intervention, which is reserved for refractory cases, is associated with a cure rate that approaches 100%.

Ménière's disease is treated symptomatically, because no method for halting the

Table 37.3.

Table 37.3.

Treatment guidelines for vertigo

Peripheral/benign positional

Oral H$_1$-blocker (e.g., diphenhydramine 50 mg, meclizine 12.5–25 mg)

Anticholinergic (e.g., scopolamine)

Benzodiazepine (e.g., diazepam [Valium] 5 mg po)

Antiemetic (e.g., promethazine)

Antibiotics for bacterial labyrinthitis

Repositioning maneuver (optional)

If vomiting, medications may be administered IV

Ménière's disease

All of the previously listed medications are options but in addition a low salt diet and diuretic (hydrochlorothiazide, triamterene) may be used

Central Vertigo

Vertebrobasilar Insufficiency/CVA

Treatment in conjunction with neurologist and/or neurosurgeon

Antiplatelet agents include aspirin, ticlopidine, or clopidogrel

Carotid stenosis may require surgery

Neoplasm

Treatment in conjunction with neurologist and neurosurgeon

Radiation therapy

Neurosurgery

Migraine

Treatment discussed in Chapter 29

Multiple Sclerosis

Treatment guided by neurologist

Immunomodulators (e.g., interferon)

CVA, cerebrovascular accident; H$_1$, histamine-1; IV, intravenous; po, by mouth.

degenerative process exists at present. Anticholinergic and antihistaminic medications have been shown to reduce symptoms in the acute phase. The combination of two diuretics, triamterene and hydrochlorothiazide, has been shown to improve symptoms, as has a low-salt diet.

Vestibular neuronitis and labyrinthitis are also treated symptomatically, with antinausea medications, anticholinergics, and antihistamines. Bacterial labyrinthitis is uncommon but may require antibiotics and evaluation by an otolaryngologist for surgical drainage. The treatment of causes of central vertigo depends on the etiology.

Neoplasms are managed either surgically or with cytotoxic agents. Multiple sclerosis is treated with a number of immunomodulating agents. Interventions for vertebrobasilar insufficiency are aimed at treating and preventing progression of atherosclerotic disease of the vertebral and basilar arteries.

Disposition

Patients with peripheral vertigo are usually discharged home from the ED to follow-up with their primary care physician or an otolaryngologist. Patients who are treated with the Epley maneuver should seek specialty follow-up. If the origin of the symptoms cannot be reasonably determined, neurological consultation is warranted. Suspected bacterial labyrinthitis or persistent vomiting that cannot be controlled is an indication for admission to the hospital. Patients with suspected or confirmed central vertigo are usually admitted to the hospital for further evaluation. The service that they are admitted to depends on the diagnosis, but often they are admitted to the neurology service.

Pathophysiology

The vestibular labyrinth is responsible for detecting both linear and angular head movements (Figure 37.1). Each labyrinth is composed of three semicircular canals and two otolithic organs called the saccule and the utricle. The semicircular canals (lateral, superior, and posterior) are oriented at right angles to each other and detect rotational movement. The utricle and saccule detect linear acceleration. Stereocilia function as mechanical transducers of these stimuli and are termed hair cells. In the semicircular canals, the hair cells are organized under a gelatin film called the cupula. Angular acceleration causes deflection of the cupula and the hair cells and subsequent hyperdepolarization or depolarization, depending on the

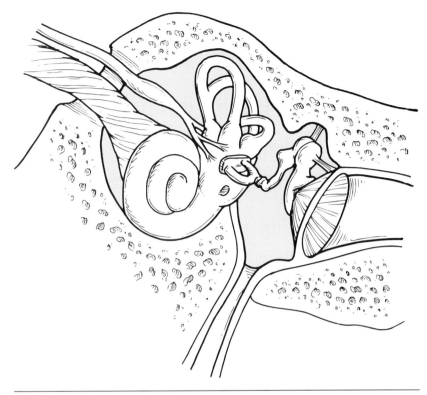

Figure 37.1
The vestibular labyrinth is located in the petrous portion of the temporal bone. The three semicircular canals are attached to the globule-shaped utricle. The superior, lateral, and posterior canals contain the endolymph. The saccule is attached to the cochlea.

direction of movement. In the otolithic organs, the hair cells are attached to a layer of crystalline particles known as the otoconia. The otoconia remain stationary relative to the head with linear acceleration, which causes deflection and stimulation of the underlying hair cells.

In addition to an appropriately functioning vestibular system, normal balance requires input from the visual (vestibulo-ocular) and proprioceptive (vestibulo-spinal) systems. Vestibular input is compared and balanced with this input. Any insult that disrupts the calibration or balance between the peripheral vestibular systems or between the vestibular system and visual and proprioceptive input leads to the sensation of vertigo or loss of balance. If the process is acute, vertigo usually results. In a more chronic situation, dysequilibrium may be the primary symptom. Therefore, the goal of treatment is to restore balance between the various input systems. In addition, intimate linkage of the brainstem pathways serves to process vestibular and visceral inputs. These systems converge in the nucleus of the solitary tract, the parabrachial nucleus, and the rostral ventrolateral medullary reticular formation. The connection between parabrachial nucleus and brainstem sympathetic output pathways, neuroendocrine regions of the hypothalamus, and limbic regions of the forebrain provides a potential neurological basis for the affective, autonomic, and neuroendocrine manifestations of vestibular dysfunction.

Benign paroxysmal positional vertigo was previously explained as cupulolithiasis (i.e., calcific deposits embedded in the cupula, rendering the semicircular canal dependent on gravity). Substantial evidence now indicates that the disorder results from canalolithiasis, which is calcific debris (presumably displaced otoconia) in the semicircular canal that is not adherent to the cupula. Head movements, particularly looking up, lying down, or rolling onto the side of the affected ear, result in displacement of this canal "sludge" and movement of endolymph away from the cupula. This results in a "plunger-like" effect with distraction of the cupula.

Suggested Readings

Froehling DA, Bowen JM, Mohr DN, et al. The canalith repositioning procedure for the treatment of benign paroxysmal positional vertigo: a randomized controlled trial. *Mayo Clin Proc* 2000;75:695–700.

Froehling DA, Silverstein MD, Mohr DN, et al. Benign positional vertigo: incidence and prognosis in a population-based study in Olmsted County, Minnesota. *Mayo Clin Proc* 1991;66:596–601.

Furman JM, Cass SP. Benign paroxysmal positional vertigo. *N Engl J Med* 1999;314:1590–1596.

Healy GB. Hearing loss and vertigo secondary to head injury. *N Engl J Med* 1982;306:1029–1031.

Herr RD, Zun L, Mathews JJ. A directed approach to the dizzy patient. *Ann Emerg Med* 1989;18:664–672.

Hotson JR, Baloh RW. Acute vestibular syndrome. *N Engl J Med* 1998;339:680–685.

Koelliker P, Summers RL, Hawkins B. Benign paroxysmal positional vertigo: diagnosis and treatment in the emergency department—a review of the literature and discussion of canalith-repositioning maneuvers. *Ann Emerg Med* 2001;37:392–398.

Marill KA, Walsh MJ, Nelson BK. Intravenous lorazepam versus dimenhydrinate for treatment of vertigo in the emergency department: a randomized clinical trial. *Ann Emerg Med* 2000;36:310–319.

CHAPTER **38**

Syncope

Tara D. Director, MD

Clinical Scenario

The patient is a 48-year-old woman who presents to the emergency department (ED) with a complaint of "fainting." The patient states that she was eating dinner with friends when she began to feel dizzy and nauseated for several minutes. She also states that her vision narrowed to the point at which "everything went black." She denies chest pain, palpitations, or shortness of breath. She next recalls awaking on the floor surrounded by her friends and the paramedics. She reports vomiting once after waking. She did not feel groggy, confused, or tired after the event. According to a friend, the patient had stated, "I don't feel well" before the event. Her eyes then rolled upward and she became unresponsive for 30 to 60 seconds. The friend did not note tonic-clonic activity or incontinence. The patient now feels completely well. She recalls fainting on one prior occasion 3 years ago, but she did not seek medical attention at that time. She has no cardiac history or history of seizures. She has no family history of sudden death. The patient's past medical history is noncontributory. She takes no medications and has no drug allergies.

Physical examination reveals a thin, well-appearing African-American woman in no distress. Her temperature is 97.5°F, blood pressure is 109/74 mm Hg, heart rate is 88 beats/minute and regular, respiratory rate is 12 breaths/minute, and oxygen saturation is 99% on room air. The patient's blood pressure and pulse do not change when she moves from a sitting to standing position. The patient has a normal physical examination

including clear lungs, a regular heart beat without murmur, a nontender abdomen, and a nonfocal neurological examination (i.e., intact cranial nerves, motor, and sensory function, symmetrical reflexes, and downgoing toes on plantar reflex examination). Her stool is Hemoccult negative. Her electrocardiogram (ECG) reveals a normal sinus rhythm at 70 beats/minute with normal intervals and axis; there is no evidence of ischemia or arrhythmia. After review of her history, examination, and ECG, the patient is diagnosed with vasovagal syncope. She is reassured and educated about her diagnosis; she is warned about a possible recurrence of syncope and is discharged home with instructions to follow up with her primary care doctor.

Clinical Evaluation

Introduction

Syncope is the transient and sudden loss of consciousness associated with the loss of postural tone and is caused by cerebral hypoperfusion. Episodes are typically brief and recovery is rapid, complete, and spontaneous. Presyncope is the prodromal symptom to fainting or the feeling that syncope is imminent before complete loss of consciousness occurs. Patients experiencing presyncope may complain of dizziness, nausea, sweating, or visual changes as common premonitory symptoms. Both presyncope and syncope are symptoms and differ only in their severity. The diagnostic evaluation is the same for both complaints. Syncope is a common presenting problem in health care settings; it accounts for 3% to 5% of ED visits and 1% to 3% of hospital admissions.

These figures undoubtedly underestimate the true incidence of syncope because many individuals do not seek medical evaluation.

History

Initial history taking should focus on the following questions about the circumstances before the attack: (a) Was the patient sitting or in a standing position? (b) Was the patient resting, exercising, coughing, urinating, eating, shaving, or turning his or her head? (c) Was the patient afraid, in pain, in a warm room, or standing for a long time? and (d) Did he or she feel chest pain or palpitations? The presence of prodromal symptoms such as nausea, sweating, cold, blurred vision, or an aura at the onset of the attack should be noted. Witnesses should be questioned as follows about the episode: (a) How did the patient fall? (b) Was the patient pale, moving abnormally (tonic-clonic movements, myoclonus, automatisms), or incontinent? and (c) How long was the patient unresponsive? Details of the recovery from the episode are also important, including the presence of nausea, vomiting, confusion, muscle aches, or injury. The patient's past medical and family history must also be investigated. Ask whether the patient has any of the following: (a) a cardiac history or family history of sudden death, (b) a neurological history such as generalized tonic-clonic seizures or Parkinson's disease, (c) a psychiatric illness, (d) a prescribed regimen of medications such as antihypertensives or antidepressants, or (e) a history of similar previous events.

Cardiac Syncope

The presence of heart disease is an important factor that should lead to careful consideration of a cardiac cause of syncope. A recent study concluded that the absence of heart disease excluded a cardiac cause in 97% of patients with syncope. Palpitations, syncope during exertion or in the supine position, brief intervals between syncopal episodes (less than 4 years between first and last episodes), and a family history of sudden death suggest a cardiac cause.

Centrally Mediated Syncope

Neurally mediated syncope is a transient malfunction of the blood pressure regulatory centers in the brain (medulla and pons) leading to a slowing of the heart rate and a drop in blood pressure enough to cause loss of consciousness. It is suggested by an interval of 4 years or longer between syncopal episodes, abdominal discomfort before loss of consciousness, and nausea and sweating in the recovery phase.

Vasovagal Syncope

Vasovagal syncope commonly occurs with prolonged standing; in warm or crowded places; or while experiencing unpleasant sensations such as pain, distress, or fear. This type of syncope is often associated with nausea, vomiting, and blurred vision.

Situational Syncope

Situational syncope is likely if syncope occurs during or after activities such as urination, defecation, coughing, or swallowing. These physiological functions may trigger a strong vagal stimulus that creates hypotension and bradycardia without a compensatory response.

Carotid Sinus Sensitivity Syncope

Carotid sinus sensitivity syncope occurs on triggering the carotid sinus reflex, which also slows the heart rate and reduces the blood pressure. This should be suspected when syncope occurs in an older patient or in association with head turning, shaving, tight collars, or the like.

Orthostatic Syncope

Orthostatic hypotension or syncope occurring shortly after standing from a sitting position suggests orthostatic syncope; medications such as antihypertensives and antidepressants can predispose patients to orthostatic syncope. A history suggestive of blood loss or dehydration should be sought including recent vomiting, diarrhea, black stools or poor po intake. Other symptoms of hypoperfusion include dizziness, sweating, or nausea.

Seizure

Symptoms such as an identifiable aura, disorientation after the event, or a slow return to baseline consciousness, oral trauma, and rhythmic movements suggest seizure activity rather than syncope. However, cerebral hypoxia can cause myoclonic movements, which an inexperienced, untrained witness may confuse with tonic-clonic movements.

Physical Examination

The physical examination should focus on signs of cardiac disease and other serious causes of syncope. The patient's vital signs should be evaluated carefully for abnormalities of the heart rate. Tachycardia or bradycardia suggests arrhythmia and cardiac syncope. Tachycardia and hypotension suggests orthostatic syncope resulting from either dehydration or blood loss. Blood pressure and pulse should be obtained in the supine and standing positions to check for orthostatic hypotension. The respiratory rate and oxygen saturation must be assessed, because a rapid respiratory rate or low oxygen saturation with tachycardia suggests a pulmonary embolism. It is imperative that a careful cardiac examination be performed looking for signs of cardiac syncope, which include the following: (a) an irregular heart rhythm, (b) evidence of aortic stenosis (a systolic ejection murmur with radiation to the neck, delayed carotid upstroke, a single S_2 and an S_4), (c) signs of hypertrophic obstructive cardiomyopathy (a systolic ejection murmur that increases with Valsalva and a "spike and dome" carotid upstroke), and (d) findings consistent with congestive heart failure (elevated jugular venous pressure [JVP], crackles on lung examination, and peripheral edema). Significant blood pressure differences between the patient's arms suggest subclavian steal or acute aortic dissection. Neurological examination is important to evaluate for signs of transient ischemic attack, stroke, or seizure. Skin should be assessed for hydration status. Evidence of ane-mia may be noted by very pale conjunctiva or sallow skin. Abdomen may reveal tenderness, which along with Hemoccult-positive stool, indicates gastrointestinal bleeding. In pregnant patients, a pelvic examination should be considered for the evaluation of ruptured ectopic pregnancy.

Diagnostic Evaluation

Initial assessment of the patient, including a comprehensive history and physical examination, may lead to the diagnosis without additional laboratory evaluation. However, the ECG is important in identifying the cause of syncope and is recommended in all patients who present to the ED; 45% of all patients have a diagnosis established following these initial steps. ECG tracings are often normal when obtained for patients with syncope; however, a "normal" interpretation may be falsely reassuring because of the transient nature of many arrhythmias. A pathologically abnormal ECG that is diagnostic of arrhythmia or cardiac ischemia is highly suggestive of cardiac syncope. Arrhythmias that are considered diagnostic of syncope include the following: (a) sinus bradycardia less than 40 beats/minute, (b) sinus pauses longer than 3 seconds, (c) repetitive sinoatrial blocks, (d) Mobitz II second-degree or third-degree atrioventricular (AV) block, (e) rapid supraventricular tachycardia, (f) ventricular tachycardia, (g) alternating right and left bundle branch block, and (h) pacemaker malfunction with sinus pauses. A long QT on ECG is suggestive of torsades de pointes or the long QT syndrome (Fig. 38.1). The ECG may also indicate myocardial infarction, pulmonary hypertension, left ventricular hypertrophy, and Wolff-Parkinson-White syndrome.

Basic laboratory tests such as a complete blood cell (CBC) count, electrolytes, blood glucose, blood urea nitrogen (BUN), and creatinine are indicated only if syncope resulting from anemia, hypovolemia, or metabolic causes such as hypoglycemia is suspected. These tests rarely yield helpful information and are not routinely recommended. Further evaluation should be guided by the history

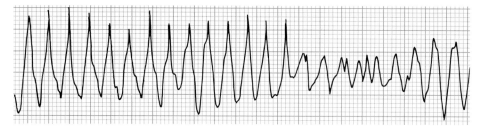

Figure 38.1
Electrocardiogram (ECG) rhythm strip of a 47-year-old woman with long QT syndrome. The rapid ventricular rhythm reveals an undulating "twisting about a point" morphology. The peaks of the QRS (spindle) appear to shift from one side to the other of the isoelectric base (node).

and physical examination; specific testing is recommended only to confirm a suspected diagnosis. All women of childbearing age should have a pregnancy test.

The next step in the evaluation is directed toward differentiating cardiac from noncardiac causes of syncope. Patients with known or suspected heart disease, abnormal ECG, suspected arrhythmia, or palpitations associated with the event should undergo echocardiography and prolonged ECG monitoring. The echocardiogram is useful to evaluate for valvular disease, cardiomyopathy, wall motion abnormalities suggestive of infarction, cardiac tumors, and infiltrative diseases such as amyloidosis. The yield from echocardiography is low in the absence of clinical, physical, or ECG evidence suggestive of a cardiac abnormality.

The purpose of continuous ECG monitoring is to diagnose intermittent arrhythmias. Continuous monitoring is useful for patients with a high pretest likelihood of arrhythmia. ECG monitoring is diagnostic only if a direct correlation is found between syncope and a significant ECG abnormality. Several options exist for continuous monitoring including Holter, event, and implantable monitors. Holter monitors are external cassette recorders worn for 24 hours; they record beat to beat for the entire time. Symptoms in conjunction with arrhythmia occur in 4% of those tested (a diagnostic result), symptoms without arrhythmia in 17%, and no symptoms accompanied by insignificant or no arrhythmia in 79%. However, symptom recurrence may

not develop during the testing period, which may not provide the opportunity to correlate symptoms with arrhythmias. Event monitors are worn for up to several weeks. They are also external recorders, which record only on demand. Event monitors have a retrospective or "looping" ability that can be activated after the patient regains consciousness to record the heart rhythm experienced during the syncopal event; the monitor records the previous 2 to 5 minutes and subsequent 60 seconds of rhythm. Arrhythmias during syncope are found in 8% to 20% of patients with this modality. Implantable ECG monitors have recently become available and are similar to event monitors. They also retrospectively record ECG patterns after an episode but have the advantages of a longer battery life (18 to 24 months) and greater convenience for patients. It is likely that the implantable monitors will become the future standard of evaluation when arrhythmic syncope is suspected.

Electrophysiological (EP) studies are recommended if the initial previously described tests suggest, but do not prove, cardiac arrhythmia as the cause of syncope. EP studies use electrical stimulation and monitoring to uncover conduction abnormalities that predispose patients to arrhythmia; the testing is both invasive and expensive. An EP study is considered diagnostic if the test reveals sinus bradycardia, bifascicular block, ventricular tachycardia, and rapid supraventricular arrhythmia with hypotension. Positive results occur predominantly in the setting of organic heart disease and are rare when patients present with a negative cardiac history and a normal ECG. However, the sensitivity of EP for bradyarrhythmias is low, and patients with a negative EP study may benefit from event or loop monitoring.

Signal-averaged ECG may be an aid to using EP studies. This type of ECG detects ventricular late potentials that can promote ventricular arrhythmias and may help identify patients with recurrent syncope resulting from ventricular tachycardia (Fig. 38.2). Patients with chest pain suggestive of myocardial ischemia or infarction should have stress testing in addition to echocardiography and ECG monitoring. Cardiac enzyme testing should be performed and interventional studies such as cardiac catheterization may be indicated. Exercise stress testing may also benefit patients who experience exertional

syncope after echocardiographic evaluation has excluded an obstructive cardiac lesion or hypertrophic obstructive cardiomyopathy.

Patients with a suspected noncardiac etiology of syncope may benefit from carotid massage and tilt-table testing. Carotid sinus massage is used to evaluate elderly patients with syncope of unknown cause and a history suggestive of atherosclerotic carotid disease. This test is performed by placing pressure on the carotid artery with concurrent monitoring of blood pressure and ECG. Investigators look for hypotension or sinus pauses. The test is performed in both the supine and upright position; it is considered positive if symptoms are reproduced in the presence of asystole longer than 3 seconds or a drop in systolic pressure greater than 50 mm Hg. Carotid testing should not be performed on patients with a carotid bruit,

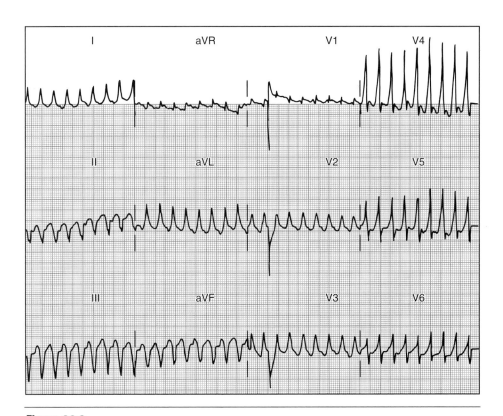

Figure 38.2
Electrocardiogram (ECG) of 55-year-old man with syncope and a history of congestive heart failure. Atrioventricular dissociation is noted in leads I, II, and III. Nonconducting P waves are noted to be marching through at a rate of 75 beats/minute independently of the QRS complexes. This is diagnostic of ventricular tachycardia.

recent myocardial infarction, transient ischemic attack, or stroke, or a history of ventricular tachycardia.

Tilt testing is another modality used to evaluate patients with recurrent syncopal episodes in the absence of clinically evident cardiac disease or for patients with unexplained syncope after cardiac causes have been excluded. It is a method of evaluating the body's ability to adjust to changes in blood volume caused by changes in body positioning. Tilt testing evaluates the appropriateness of the compensatory response; an abnormal test consists of hypotension and/or bradycardia. Patients are placed in a supine position for 20 to 45 minutes and then tilted upright; blood pressure and heart rate are monitored. Drug provocation with isoproterenol or nitroglycerin is added if the initial evaluation is negative. The test is considered positive if syncope occurs.

Adenosine triphosphate (ATP) testing is an additional way to evaluate patients with unexplained syncope. ATP administration provokes a short cardioinhibitory response resulting from vagal stimulation at the AV node. Patients are given a bolus of ATP, and a cardiac pause of longer than 10 seconds is considered positive. Testing is positive in 28% to 41% of patients with an unknown etiology for syncope. ATP testing may be useful in the older population suspected of vasovagal syncope, but further investigation is needed to evaluate its diagnostic value.

Elderly patients are a difficult population to evaluate. Syncope in this group is often multifactorial, including cardiac disease, co-existing illnesses, and medications. A search for a single cause should be pursued as previously outlined before multiple abnormalities are treated. Neurological testing, including electroencephalogram (EEG) and computed tomography (CT) scan and/or magnetic resonance imaging (MRI) of the head, are rarely helpful in the evaluation of syncope. A detailed history and physical examination should guide the physician toward a diagnosis of neurological origin such as seizure, vascular headache, or stroke. Some patients with recurrent, unexplained syncopal episodes with negative tilt-table testing may benefit from

Table 38.1.

Differential diagnosis of syncope

Cardiac Disorders
Ventricular arrhythmias
Supraventricular arrhythmias
Tachybrady syndrome

Orthostatic Disorders
Ectopic pregnancy
Aortic dissection
GI Bleeding
Dehydration

Neurological Disorders
Transient ischemic attack
Migraine
Seizure

Other Disorders
Pulmonary embolus
Hyperventilation
Hypoglycemia
Subclavian steal
Drop attack

Psychiatric Disorders
Anxiety
Depression
Panic attack
Hysteria

GI, gastrointestinal.

psychiatric evaluation for anxiety, depression, and panic disorder.

Differential Diagnosis

The differential diagnosis for syncope is illustrated in Table 38.1.

Treatment

The treatment of syncope depends entirely on its etiology (Table 38.2). Initial treatment of neurally mediated syncope is reassurance and education.

Vasovagal Syncope

Patients with vasovagal syncope should be taught to recognize preceding symptoms and to avoid triggers such as volume depletion, prolonged standing, and so forth. β-Blockers

Table 38.2.

Treatment of syncope

All Patients—Initial Approach[a]
IV
Oxygen
Continuous cardiac monitor
ECG
Finger-stick blood sample monitored for glucose
Hematocrit

Cardiac Syncope
Bradycardia

   Transcutaneous pacer pads for any
   bradycardia, type 2, second- or third-degree
   heart block, or tachy-brady syndrome

   Atropine 0.5–1 mg for bradycardia, may repeat

Tachycardia: unstable patients with tachycardia
   may require cardioversion
Ventricular tachycardia: amiodarone 150 mg IV
   or lidocaine 0.5–0.75 mg/kg bolus IV
Supraventricular tachycardia: adenosine 6 mg IV
   push
Atrial fibrillation: β-blocker, calcium channel
   blocker, or amiodarone

Orthostatic Syncope
IV saline bolus
Type and crossmatch for suspected anemia
Type-specific or uncrossmatched blood products
   for profound hemodynamic instability from
   suspected blood loss

ECG, electrocardiogram; IV, intravenous.
[a]All patients must be treated for the individual etiology
of their syncope. Treatment will vary by other factors
including age, persistence of symptoms, and general
health.

are currently used for treatment; however, their mechanism of action is poorly defined and the current literature is equivocal in terms of their efficacy. Serotonin uptake inhibitors like sertraline, paroxetine, and fluoxetine are being investigated as possible beneficial treatments.

Carotid Sinus Sensitivity

The treatment of choice for carotid sinus syncope is cardiac pacing and avoidance of precipitating factors.

Situational Syncope

Treatment of situational syncope relies on avoiding the trigger event. When the scenario cannot be avoided, patients are counseled about protective postures, maintenance of intravascular volume, slow positional changes, and so forth.

Orthostatic Syncope

A thorough review of the patient's medications is vital; drug-induced autonomic failure is a very frequent cause of hypotension, especially in the elderly population. If possible, treatment of orthostatic syncope should consist of eliminating potential offending medications (commonly antihypertensives and antidepressants). Volume expansion is the next step in treatment. Options to expand volume include higher salt intake, high fluid intake, or volume expanders such as fludrocortisone or midodrine. Older patients tolerate volume-expanding medications poorly and should be monitored for edema. Decreasing vascular pooling by using support stockings can also help. Leg crossing may reduce venous pooling while standing. Orthostatic syncope resulting from dehydration can be treated with intravenous volume replacement in the ED. Syncope resulting from blood loss should be treated according to the etiology and may require volume replacement with blood products in the ED. Fluid resuscitation should be initiated aggressively in these patients.

Arrhythmia

The choice of treatment for arrhythmia depends on the underlying rhythm abnormality. As an initial step, the patient's medication list should be reviewed to eliminate any contributing drugs (e.g., β-blockers, calcium channel blockers, and cardiac glycosides, which can cause sinus node dysfunction); antiarrhythmic drugs and psychoactive agents can promote arrhythmias such as torsades de pointes. Bradyarrhythmias and AV nodal disease require cardiac pacing, and supraventricular tachycardias may be treated with ablation. Ventricular tachycardias may be managed with antiarrhythmic medications or with implantable cardioverter-defibrillators.

Structural Heart Disease

The most common structural heart disease causing syncope is myocardial infarction. This can be treated medically or with revascularizing interventions such as angioplasty or coronary artery bypass surgery. Other structural abnormalities such as valvular disease or cardiac tumors require surgical correction.

Disposition

Admission to the hospital allows for observation and prevention of serious consequences. It should be considered for patients with a high risk of cardiac syncope or for treatment of the underlying cause. In general, an abnormal ECG, symptoms suggestive of arrhythmia, a history of cardiac disease, chest pain, and a family history of sudden death are important markers for cardiac syncope and warrant admission. One recent study attempted to stratify the risk for patients with syncope presenting to the ED. The study found four factors useful to evaluate the risk of mortality and sudden death: age older than 45, history of ventricular arrhythmia, history of congestive heart failure, and an abnormal ECG. A recent study evaluated patients with syncope with the purpose of developing criteria for predicting possible serious outcomes including death, myocardial infarction, arrhythmia, pulmonary embolus, stroke, and subarachnoid hemorrhage. The investigators found the following predictors of poor outcome: (a) age older than 75 years, (b) an abnormal ECG, (c) hematocrit less than 30 mL/dL, (d) respiratory rate greater than 24 breaths/minute, (e) shortness of breath, and (f) a history of congestive heart failure. Patients with isolated or rare syncope, no evidence of structural heart disease, and a normal ECG have a low risk of cardiac syncope and may be evaluated as outpatients.

Pathophysiology

Syncope is a symptom of cerebral hypoperfusion. Loss of consciousness has been shown to result from cessation of blood flow for a period as brief as 6 to 8 seconds. Cerebral perfusion pressure depends mainly on systemic arterial pressure; a decrease in systolic pressure to 60 mm Hg is associated with syncope. Systemic arterial pressure is a factor of cardiac output and peripheral vascular resistance. Cardiac output, a product of stroke volume and heart rate, therefore depends on (a) venous filling, which can be altered by excessive pooling in the lower extremities, decreased blood volume, and valvular disorders and (b) arrhythmias such as bradyarrhythmias and tachyarrhythmias. Peripheral vascular resistance is determined by the current state of peripheral vasodilation or vasoconstriction.

Syncope is categorized by pathophysiological mechanism. The most important task is to distinguish being between cardiac and noncardiac syncope. Noncardiac syncope includes neurally mediated syncope, which occurs because of an inappropriate reflex vasodilatation, bradycardia, or both. Examples include vasovagal syncope and carotid sinus sensitivity syncope in addition to situational syncope, which occurs during cough, micturition, and defecation. Orthostatic syncope is another form of neurally mediated syncope, which results from hypotension when the autonomic nervous system fails to trigger vasoconstriction during positional change. Cardiac syncope includes syncope resulting from bradyarrhythmia and tachyarrhythmia or structural heart disease such as coronary artery disease (e.g., acute myocardial infarction), valvular disease (e.g., severe aortic stenosis), cardiomyopathies (e.g., hypertrophic obstructive cardiomyopathy), congenital heart disease, and pulmonary embolus.

Vasovagal syncope is the most common etiology, followed by cardiac syncope. The prognosis for the patient is related to the underlying cause. The 1-year mortality for cardiac syncope is higher (18% to 33%) than for noncardiac causes (0% to 12%), as is the risk for sudden death (24% vs. 3% to 4%). Structural heart disease, such as hypertrophic obstructive cardiomyopathy, valvular disease, and congestive heart failure, is a major risk factor for sudden death in patients presenting with syncope, but individuals with malignant ventricular arrhythmias are also at very high risk. Patients with ventricular dysfunction have the worst prognosis, whereas patients with noncardiac syncope typically have a very good prognosis.

Suggested Readings

Alboni P, Brignole M, Menozzi C, et al. Diagnostic value of history in patients with syncope with or without heart disease. *J Am Coll Cardiol* 2001;37:1921–1928.

Brignole M, Alboni P, Benditt D, et al. Guidelines on management (diagnosis and treatment) of syncope. *Eur Heart J* 2001;22:1256–1306.

Heaven D, Sutton R. Syncope. *Crit Care Med* 2000;28:116–120.

Kapoor W. Primary care: syncope. *N Engl J Med* 2000;343:1856–1862.

Linzer M, Yang E, Estes N, et al. Clinical guideline: diagnosing syncope: Part 1: value of history, physical examination, and electrocardiography. *Ann Intern Med* 1997;126:989–996.

Linzer M, Yang E, Estes N, et al. Clinical guideline: diagnosing syncope: Part 2: unexplained syncope. *Ann Intern Med* 1997;127:76–86.

Martin T, Hanusa B, Kapoor W. Risk stratification of patients with syncope. *Ann Intern Med* 1997;29:459–466.

Quinn J, Stiell I, McDermott, DA, et al. The San Francisco Syncope Rule to predict patients with short-term serious outcomes. *Ann Emerg Med* 2004;Feb;43(2)233–237.

Neuromuscular Weakness

Kerry K. McCabe, MD

Clinical Scenario

A 55-year-old man presents to the emergency department (ED) with generalized weakness that started 2 to 3 days prior. He had been feeling ill the previous week, with a runny nose, nasal congestion, transient sore throat, and cough. His cold symptoms have resolved, but over the past few days he has noticed "heaviness" in his arms and legs. He notes that he has been stumbling today and that he must look at his feet to be sure "where they are." He denies fever, chills, back pain, chest pain, numbness, tingling, incontinence, and visual changes. He admits that he feels more short of breath than usual when walking up stairs.

Past medical history includes hypertension and hernia repair. He takes diltiazem (Cardizem) and an aspirin a day. He has no known drug allergies. He does not smoke or use recreational drugs but drinks alcohol occasionally. There is no significant family medical history.

His blood pressure is 146/ 75 mm Hg, heart rate is 82 beats/minute, temperature is 98.8°F, respiratory rate is 24 breaths/ minute, and his oxygen saturation is 99% on room air. His head is normocephalic and atraumatic, and the oropharynx is without erythema, edema, or exudates. The tympanic membranes are clear. The neck is supple and nontender and exhibits full range of motion. His chest is clear to auscultation bilaterally. Examination of his heart reveals a regular rate and rhythm; no murmurs, rubs, or gallops; and no jugular venous distension. The abdomen is soft, nontender, and nondistended, and the bowel sounds are normoac-

tive. There is no clubbing, cyanosis, or edema of the extremities. He demonstrates full passive and active range of motion of all extremities.

Pupils are equal, round, and reactive to light. Extraocular movements are intact. There is no facial asymmetry. Motor examination is notable for 4+/5 strength in both upper extremities but only 3+/5 strength in the lower extremities bilaterally. The patient has a normal sensory examination of the arms, but decreased light touch and proprioception is noted in both feet. Finger-to-nose examination and rapid alternating movements are intact. He is ambulatory with a slightly widened gait and has a mildly positive Romberg with his eyes closed. Examination of the reflexes reveals a 1+ biceps and triceps, absent patellar and Achilles responses, and an equivocal Babinski sign on plantar reflex testing. An electrocardiogram (ECG) shows no change from previous tracings, his chest x-ray film is clear, and there are no abnormalities on blood testing, including toxic screen, Monospot, Lyme titer, and heavy metals screen. Computed tomography (CT) examination of the head is negative. A lumbar puncture is performed and cerebrospinal fluid (CSF) shows a mildly elevated protein level, normal glucose, and no white or red blood cells.

The patient is admitted to the hospital, and serial pulmonary function tests show progressive deterioration over the course of several days. Arterial blood gas results reveal an increasing PCO_2. The patient is transferred to the intensive care unit and he is electively intubated. His neurological examination deteriorates to the point of total flaccid paralysis with absent reflexes on hospital day 12. He receives plasma exchange therapy during this time. Over the next 20 days, his neurological examination gradually improves and he is extubated on hospital day 32. He is able to move his upper extremities, although fine motor control is abnormal, and with time he is increasingly able to move his lower extremities. He is discharged to a rehabilitation facility on hospital day 36. After several weeks of rehabilitation, he is ambulatory with a walker. One year later, the patient is fully engaged in his normal daily activities, although he is not able to participate in his customary weekly basketball game.

Clinical Evaluation

Introduction

Generalized weakness is a nonspecific and often frustrating symptom to sort out in an ED setting. The variety of causes includes toxic, infectious, nutritional deficiency, and autoimmune etiologies. Historical clues to the etiology of a specific case of weakness are provided by the duration and location of symptoms, speed of progression, whether symptoms come and go, past medical history, and social history. Physical examination findings are also very important when diagnosing complaints of weakness.

In the clinical scenario, the patient was diagnosed with Guillain-Barré syndrome (GBS). The main characteristics are ascending flaccid paralysis and absent or decreased reflexes. The disease has a bimodal distribution pattern and typically affects young adults (ages 15 to 35) and older adults (50 to 75). The male-to-female ratio is 1.5:1. It seems temporally related to a variety of medical conditions, including low-grade infectious symptoms (e.g., upper respiratory infection, diarrhea) or immunizations. It is thought to be autoimmune in nature and results from demyelination of peripheral nerves. Some people with GBS have relatively low-grade symptoms that resolve entirely in a matter of weeks without any specific treatment. A small subgroup can go on to have permanent disability from the disease. Most patients have a range of residual long-term neurological findings that do not impair their usual activities. Early diagnosis of the disease requires a high index of suspicion, because physical examination findings may be subtle. However, it is important to identify these patients because the muscular and respiratory sequelae of the syndrome can be rapidly progressive and life threatening.

History

Patients with GBS typically present with complaints of weakness, loss of coordination, and possibly sensory changes. On questioning, the complaints are typically symmetrical, gradually progressive, and often predated by some other illness. The weakness starts in the distal lower extremities and progresses cephalad, thus giving the syndrome one of its other names, Landry's ascending paralysis.

Atypical cases of GBS occur, with either a descending motor paralysis or cranial nerve paralysis as the initial presentation (Miller-Fisher variant). Some patients complain of pain in the back, buttocks, shoulders, or thighs, which can be confused with intervertebral disc disease. Occasionally, patients with GBS can present with asymmetrical complaints. If the asymmetry of the complaints persists, other diagnoses, including stroke, must be ruled out.

Taking a careful history will help to rule out other causes of generalized weakness. Recent history of sore throat may lead to consideration of diphtheria; fevers and headache should prompt suspicion of meningitis or encephalitis. A recent history of camping should remind the provider to consider Lyme disease or tick paralysis; eating canned foods makes botulism more likely; industrial exposures can lead to heavy metal poisoning. Symptoms that worsen as the day goes on or with exertion may indicate myasthenia gravis; symptoms that wax and wane over weeks to months suggest multiple sclerosis, whereas symptoms that gradually progress over several months may be due to nutritional deficiencies or alcoholic or diabetic neuropathy.

Physical Examination

The physical examination of patients with GBS is frequently normal with the exception of the neurological examination. It is important to note the vital signs, because the disease can affect the autonomic nervous system. Blood pressure, heart rate, and temperature can fluctuate widely. Urinary hesitancy and lack of sweating may be present and patients should be observed for signs of ileus.

Neurological examination findings can range from the very subtle, which require careful assessment and a high index of suspicion, to obvious paralysis. The hallmarks of GBS are symmetrical deficits and absent reflexes. The major exceptions to this are the cranial nerves, which often are asymmetrically affected. If all reflexes are preserved in a patient with motor paralysis, other diagnoses must be considered. Examination of the distal lower extremities typically reveals the most obvious neurological deficits, which gradually become less prominent as one moves toward the head. The upper extremity reflexes can be preserved after the lower extremity reflexes have been lost. Sensory examination abnormalities may be found but are not as common as motor findings.

It is very important to examine the fundi of patients with GBS, because they can develop papilledema caused by pseudotumor cerebri. Case reports of descending paralysis have been described. In these cases, the presentation usually starts with cranial nerve symptoms such as drooling or difficulty speaking or swallowing.

Physical examination findings can be helpful in detecting other causes of generalized weakness. A rash or tick found on the body can indicate Lyme disease or tick paralysis. Descending symmetric paralysis with a prodrome of gastrointestinal symptoms and intact reflexes is suggestive of botulism. Cranial nerves and bulbar muscles are often affected first, and patients may initially present with diplopia, dysarthria, and dysphagia, followed later by generalized weakness. Focal or patchy neurological findings raise the likelihood of multiple sclerosis. A classic sign of multiple sclerosis is intranuclear ophthalmoplegia. The sign consists of a unilateral malfunction of the medial rectus muscle innervated by cranial nerve III. When a patient is asked to look to the right, for example, the right eye would move laterally, while the left eye might stop at center gaze. The patient would complain at that moment of double vision. This is a result of a sclerotic lesion in the medial longitudinal fasciculus that controls coordinated lateral gaze patterns in the brain.

Asymmetric neurological findings may indicate a stroke, whereas a neurological deficit below a defined sensory level is indicative of a spinal cord injury or transverse myelitis. A fever must immediately raise the suspicion of meningitis or encephalitis, and empiric treatment should be started concurrently with further diagnostic evaluation. Patients who fatigue when asked to do repetitive motor tasks may suffer from myasthenia gravis. Often the first subtle sign is lagging of the eyelids during rapid blinking.

Diagnostic Evaluation

There is no single test that confirms an initial suspicion of GBS. The diagnosis is primarily based on the presence of a defined clinical syndrome. It is wise to rule out other treatable diagnoses that can be life threatening. Early diagnosis of stroke or spinal cord injury significantly affects the treatment plan and can improve patient outcome. Neuroimaging is important in differentiating these entities. Stroke victims may have focal cerebral edema sufficient to produce a regional hypodensity on CT scan of the head, if the symptoms of ischemic stroke have been present for more than 6 to 12 hours. Spinal cord magnetic resonance imaging (MRI) is the study of choice for defining a focal spinal cord injury or lesion. In addition, spinal cord MRI reveals enhancement of the cauda equina nerve roots in 95% of people with GBS. Decisions regarding diagnostic imaging on an emergent basis are guided by the acuity and severity of the patient's illness and whether rapid diagnosis and treatment will improve outcome.

Major electrolyte abnormalities can be an indicator of the syndrome of inappropriate antidiuretic hormone secretion (SIADH), which is sometimes associated with GBS. This diagnosis can be confirmed by measurement of urine and serum osmolarity. Patients with GBS may also have mildly elevated liver function tests. Patients presenting with weakness may have electrolyte changes such as low or high potassium. Elevated creatinine kinase (CK) indicates muscle breakdown and is frequently found in patients with myopathies and some neuropathies. Serum and urine toxin screens should be sent and an assessment for heavy metals toxicity should be specifically requested. A B_{12} level and hematocrit should be checked to rule out pernicious anemia with neurological complications. The ECG may be normal in patients with GBS but may also show signs of delayed conduction, ST depression, or arrhythmias. A pregnancy test should be performed in women of childbearing age, because pregnancy can trigger the onset of the syndrome.

CSF evaluation is crucial when meningitis or encephalitis feature prominently in the differential diagnosis. In patients with GBS, the CSF reveals a normal cell count and glucose levels, thus ruling out meningitis. The CSF may have an elevated protein level, especially if symptoms have been present for several days. However, a normal protein level does not rule out the diagnosis because the protein spike may be delayed by 1 to 2 weeks. Antibody testing of the CSF may be helpful, because many patients have antibodies to central and peripheral nerves. Patients with multiple sclerosis frequently have a larger proportion of mononuclear cells, normal glucose and possible elevated protein, and elevated IgG. Patients with myasthenia gravis have elevated CSF protein.

Pulmonary function should be assessed, because one fourth of patients with GBS develop respiratory muscle paralysis. Although other neuromuscular disorders can affect pulmonary function (e.g., muscular dystrophies), patients with these diseases will not present acutely to the ED without a known diagnosis, because these diseases are not characterized by rapid deterioration. Peak flow measurements and incentive spirometry are available in the ED. A pulmonary consultation should be requested from the ED when abnormalities are uncovered on screening testing, because the results may affect the disposition of the patient. Formal pulmonary function testing should always be performed early during the hospital course. Nerve conduction studies should also be done because the presence of characteristic changes will support the diagnosis. Absence of these classic abnormalities must trigger consideration of other pathological entities.

Diagnostic testing is important to rule out diseases that are a potential threat to life or that can cause significant morbidity. It is also crucial to identify individuals with treatable diseases, regardless of whether they require admission to the hospital. In addition to GBS, botulism, tick paralysis, paralytic shellfish, and heavy metal poisoning can all be fatal because of suppression of respiratory drive. Lyme disease, diphtheria, and meningitis can result in serious sequelae, including communicability and even death. Fortunately, they can all be treated effectively if recognized early. Indolent diseases that still may improve with treatment include myasthenia gravis, Eaton-Lambert syndrome, nutritional deficiencies, alcoholic and diabetic neuropathies, and multiple sclerosis. It is important to create a differential diagnosis for each patient presenting with generalized weakness to stratify the risk of his or her illness and develop an appropriate disposition and treatment.

Differential Diagnosis

The differential diagnosis for neuromuscular weakness is illustrated in Table 39.1.

Treatment

There is unfortunately no curative treatment available for GBS. The initial goals are to maintain a high index of suspicion for the diagnosis, institute supportive care, and initiate appropriate testing. Adequate support of the patient may require intensive care in a monitored setting. All patients in whom this

Table 39.1.

Comparison of clinical findings in neuromuscular diseases

Spinal Cord	Peripheral Neuropathy	Myoneural Junction	Muscle Disease
Limbs weak	Limbs weak	Cranial nerves weak initially	Proximal weakness
Absent DTRs	Decreased/absent DTRs	DTRs intact	DTRs intact
Sharp sensory level	Stocking/glove sensory loss	No sensory loss	No sensory loss
Bowel/bladder incontinence	Bowel/bladder function normal	Bowel/bladder function normal	Bowel/bladder function normal
Examples			
Transverse myelitis	Polio	Eaton-Lambert syndrome	Periodic paralysis
Disc herniation	Guillain Barré syndrome	Myasthenia gravis	Polymyositis
Tumor	Acute intermittent porphyria	Botulism	Alcohol myopathy
Hemorrhage	Tick paralysis	Organophosphate	Electrolyte abnormality
Abscess	Arsenic toxicity	Toxicity	
Infarction	Paralytic shellfish poisoning	Aminoglycosides	
	B_{12} and folate deficiency		
	HIV		
	Diphtheria		
	Lyme disease		

DTR, deep tendon reflex; HIV, human immunodeficiency virus.

diagnosis is suspected should have an intravenous line placed and should receive supplemental oxygen. Cardiac monitoring should be initiated. A patient with significant respiratory compromise requires intubation and mechanical ventilation. Symptomatic bradycardia can be treated successfully with atropine, whereas tachycardia is not usually treated. Pacing may be required if heart block develops. Short-acting intravenous medications can be used if widely fluctuating blood pressures are noted; however, hypotension frequently responds to fluid boluses. Deep venous thrombosis prophylaxis should be considered, and all patients with urinary complaints or paralysis should have a urinary catheter placed.

Patients with severe disease may receive plasma exchange or intravenous immune globulin. Both have been proven to shorten the course of the disease and are approximately equal in cost. Patients with mild disease usually improve spontaneously over time with supportive therapy and are not typically offered these interventions because of the cost and risks involved. Steroids have not been found beneficial in the management of this disease.

Treatment of other causes of neuromuscular weakness spans a wide range of modalities and is determined by the specific diagnosis. Supportive care, antimicrobials, steroids, pain control, and chelating agents are examples of the diversity of treatment options. The treatment strategies frequently evolve as new medications are found and as the pathophysiology is clarified.

Disposition

All patients with GBS should be admitted to the hospital. It is not initially possible to accurately predict the progression of symptoms. Telemetry monitoring is appropriate until possible cardiac involvement has been fully evaluated and excluded. Any patient with a forced vital capacity (FVC) of less than 20 mL/kg, problems with handling secretions, or cardiac abnormalities should be admitted to the intensive care unit.

For patients with weakness of other etiologies, disposition depends on the patient's condition, access to appropriate follow-up, and suspected etiology. Many patients require hospital admission to facilitate a diagnostic workup and to monitor progression of symptoms. For those patients who have a complete workup in the ED, are hemodynamically stable, and have a condition that is chronic or slowly progressive, discharge with appropriate follow-up may be considered.

Pathophysiology

GBS is an autoimmune disease that can result from a variety of triggers. Two thirds of patients with the syndrome report having had either an upper respiratory illness or a gastrointestinal illness preceding the onset of symptoms by 1 to 4 weeks. *Campylobacter jejuni* appears to be a frequent inciting pathogen. The other one third of patients may have had one of a long list of possible preceding conditions, including recent vaccinations. Some individuals do not recall preceding symptoms of any kind.

Because of the inciting event, the body's immune system "erroneously" attacks peripheral nerves, nerve roots, and cranial nerves, causing demyelination. This process causes disruption of the electrical signal traveling down the nerve, leading to the sensory and motor problems typical of the disease. Rarely, the disease attacks the axon of the nerve.

It is not understood how or why this process is initiated, and it is not known what specific inciting features are common to predisposing conditions. Once initiated, the reaction can be indolent or rapidly progressing. Increased morbidity and mortality is associated with rapidly progressive symptoms, advanced age, autonomic instability, cardiac involvement, and prolonged intubation and hospitalization. The mortality rate is on the order of 5% to 10%.

Suggested Readings

Drachman DB. Myasthenia gravis. *N Engl J Med* 1994;330:1797–1810.

Furukawa T, Peter JB. The muscular dystrophies and related disorders. *JAMA* 1978;239:1537–1542, 1654–1659.

Lasky T, Terracciano GT, Magder L, et al. The Guillain-Barré syndrome and the 1992–1993 and 1993–1994 influenza vaccines. *N Engl J Med* 1998;339:1797–1802.

Noseworthy JH, Lucchinetti C, Rodriguez M, Weinshenker BG. Multiple sclerosis. *N Engl J Med* 2000;343:938–952.

Ropper AH. The Guillain-Barré syndrome. *N Engl J Med* 1992;326:1130–1136.

Schmidt RD, Markovchick V. Nontraumatic spinal cord compression. *J Emerg Med* 1991;10:189–199.

Van der Meche FGA, Schmitz PIM, and the Dutch Guillain-Barré Study Group. A randomized trial comparing intravenous immune globulin and plasma exchange transfusion in Guillain-Barré syndrome. *N Engl J Med* 1992;326:1123–1129.

Williams DB, Windebank AJ. Motor neuron disease. *Mayo Clin Proc* 1991;66:54–82.

Weakness and Dizziness
Questions and Answers

Questions

1. Which of the following conditions suggest the central cause of vertigo?

  I. Absent response to the Dix-Hallpike maneuver

  II. Recent viral illness

  III. Deficits of cranial nerve or cerebellar function

  IV. Tinnitus or hearing loss

  V. Nystagmus that fatigues after 15 seconds

   A. I, II, and III

   B. I and III

   C. II and IV

   D. V only

   E. All of the above

2. Which of the following factors suggest cardiac syncope?

   A. Electrocardiogram (ECG) tracing diagnostic for sinus bradycardia less than 40 beats/minute or acute cardiac ischemia

   B. Family history of sudden death

   C. Syncope during exertion

   D. Preceding palpitations

   E. All of the above

3. A 78-year-old man is brought to the emergency department with new onset of left-sided weakness in both arms and legs and a left facial droop. Nursing home attendants stated to emergency medical services (EMS) that he was walking

with a cane and had no weakness 1 hour before contacting EMS. Past medical history includes myocardial infarction, hypertension, transient ischemic attack (TIA) with no residual deficit, and diabetes. He was discharged 2 months ago for an upper gastrointestinal (GI) bleed. On arrival, the patient has a left hemiparesis and right facial droop. Abdomen is benign, and rectal examination is negative for trace blood in his stool. Vital signs are blood pressure of 167/98 mmHg, pulse of 89 beats/minute, temperature of 98.6°F, and respiratory rate of 12 breaths/minute. Which of the following treatments is most appropriate?

   A. Thrombolysis following recent GI bleed, head computed tomography (CT) scan, aspirin, and hospital admission.

   B. Head CT; if no bleed is evident, aspirin and thrombolysis if all tests are completed less than 3 hours from symptom onset.

   C. Head CT; if no bleed is evident, labetalol to control hypertension, and thrombolysis if all tests are completed less than 3 hours from symptom onset.

   D. Head CT; if no bleed is evident, thrombolysis, if all tests are completed less than 3 hours from symptom onset.

Directions: There are three sets of response options for the following scenario. You will be required to select one best answer from each question set:.

4. A 45-year-old man presents to the emergency department (ED) complaining of weakness and dizziness. He states that for the past several weeks he has had progressively worsening weakness in his right leg and right arm. On further questioning, he admits to several months of intermittent numbness of the right arm and leg and describes bouts of "dizziness," which make him feel as if he might pass out; he has fainted once in the past month. Physical examination reveals normal vital signs. Cranial nerves are normal, but there is noted weakness of the right deltoid, biceps, and handgrip. The right leg seems mildly weaker than the left, and on walking, the patient has a mild limp.

4.1. Which of the following diagnoses is correct?

A. A cerebrovascular accident (CVA) is the likely diagnosis considering the findings of unilateral weakness.

B. Guillain-Barré syndrome is a probable diagnosis because of the gradual nature of the weakness and because it is unilateral.

C. The patient may have a lower motor neuron spinal cord lesion on the left.

D. A cerebellar stroke could produce vertigo, aphasia, and unilateral weakness.

E. Multiple sclerosis can present with intermittent sensory symptoms and develop motor signs.

4.2. What is the most appropriate diagnostic step?

A. Complete blood count (CBC), chest x-ray examination, and admission to the hospital

B. CBC, electrolytes, chest x-ray film, and admission to the hospital

C. Computed tomography (CT) scan of the head to rule out subdural/subarachnoid hemorrhage

D. Magnetic resonance imaging (MRI) study of the brain to rule out chronic subdural hemorrhage and to look for multiple sclerosis lesions, and admission to the hospital

E. MRI study of the brain and spinal cord, laboratory tests, and admission to the hospital

4.3. The patient's electrocardiogram (ECG) shows a normal sinus rhythm without ST abnormalities. Which of the following statements about his syncopal episode is true?

A. An arrhythmia is the most likely cause.

B. Despite the normal ECG, an ischemic arrhythmia at the time of syncope is possible.

C. The presence of dizziness and weakness in the limbs rules out cardiac syncope.

D. The patient did not experience true syncope but was suffering from weakness and collapsed.

E. The syncopal episode was not a seizure because there is no history of urinary incontinence or tongue biting.

Answers and Explanations

1. B. Benign paroxysmal positional vertigo usually responds to the Dix-Hallpike maneuver, which provokes lateral nystagmus, and can be used as a diagnostic test in selecting patients suitable for positional therapy. Any patient with focal findings on neurological examination should undergo workup for central causes of vertigo. Recent viral illnesses often precede labyrinthitis, a peripheral cause of vertigo. Tinnitus, or ringing in the ears, is a hallmark of Ménière's disease, although it can be caused by some central processes. Hearing loss, on the other hand, is usually a problem of the ear or the peripheral nerves leading to it. Nystagmus occurs in patients with peripheral vertigo and in patients with central vertigo. If the central nervous system is unaffected, then as the patient is asked to hold his or her gaze in either lateral direction, the brain will be able to suppress the nystagmus after a number of beats.

2. E. Many arrhythmias can induce syncope. Bradycardia causes syncope when the cardiac output drops the pressure gradient sufficiently that the brain is temporarily not perfused. A number of familial arrhythmia syndromes can cause syncope; thus, all patients with a syncopal event and a family history should be investigated for a cardiac source. When a patient describes exertional syncope, especially a younger patient, you should consider the possibility of hypertrophic cardiomyopathy. Hypertrophic cardiomyopathy is an entity in which the interventricular septum is enlarged and actually interferes with aortic outflow during exertion, so much so that in some instances the person has syncope. Palpitations obviously are a symptom originating from the heart, and although not all palpitations are serious, a patient with syncope and palpitations has a high likelihood of a cardiac source.

3. D. The patient possesses risk factors for stroke including diabetes, hypertension, and prior transient ischemic attack (TIA). If thrombolysis is to be given, it must be within the first 3 hours of presentation. The patient must have a computed tomography (CT) scan of the head to rule out a bleed. The National Stroke Association recommends treating blood pressure greater than 185/110 mm Hg if thrombolysis is considered or 220/115 mm Hg if no thrombolysis is indicated; thus, labetalol is not required in this patient. Aspirin should be held for 24 hours if thrombolysis is to be given, although there is no increase in mortality or complications if the patient is currently on aspirin. A history of gastrointestinal (GI) bleeding is a warning sign for thrombolysis not an absolute contraindication. The GI bleed in this patient was 2 months prior, and there is no evidence at this time of active bleeding. If the symptoms are severe enough to warrant thrombolysis, then it may be administered.

4.1. E. Multiple sclerosis is a disease characterized by sclerotic deposits in the brain and spinal cord. Symptoms stutter and progress over time, sometimes years may pass without symptoms before another exacerbation. A cerebrovascular accident (CVA) is an acute event that stops blood flow to an area of brain and produces clinical symptoms and signs. This history is very atypical for a stroke, because the symptoms were not acute but gradual. Guillain Barré syndrome is a progressive demyelinating process that classically presents with symmetric ascending paralysis that is not unilateral. Lower motor neurons innervate the ipsilateral side of the spinal cord. Thus, left-sided fibers would cause left-sided weakness. A viral syndrome is a classic prodrome, which was not elicited in the history for this patient. A cerebellar stroke would produce ataxia and possibly unilateral or bilateral weakness, but the cerebellum has no role in speech production; thus, aphasia would not occur.

4.2. E. A magnetic resonance imaging (MRI) of the brain and spinal cord is necessary to evaluate this patient. His intermittent symptoms and weakness in the extremities may be from a spinal cord lesion and would be missed if only the brain was imaged. MRI study of the head is better to pick up chronic bleeds. A spinal cord lesion, quite possibly related to multiple sclerosis, may cause the weakness. The brain MRI would also rule out central nervous system (CNS) masses. A complete blood count (CBC) is helpful to look at the hematocrit for anemia, because the patient reported a syncopal episode. The electrolyte, calcium, and magnesium levels would be helpful to rule out metabolic causes of weakness, although those are rarely unilateral. Although a computed tomography (CT) scan of the head is the test of choice to rule out an acute intracranial bleed, this patient's symptoms have persisted for weeks. He has had no headache or trauma, and bleeding is an unlikely diagnosis.

4.3. B. An otherwise healthy man in his forties is not at high risk for coronary artery disease. He gave no history of angina-like symptoms, nor did he complain of palpitations at the time of the event. In fact, very little history is given surrounding the event. A normal electrocardiogram without evidence of ischemia or prior myocardial infarction (MI) cannot rule out ischemic heart disease, because the patient is not experiencing the symptoms at the time that he is being evaluated. There is not enough history to rule out the fact that no true syncope occurred. Tongue biting and incontinence are hallmarks of seizures if present, but their absence does not confirm the absence of a seizure. Arrhythmia may cause global feelings of weakness but not focal weakness. There is insufficient history to determine whether the patient truly had syncope or collapsed, because it was unwitnessed.

Fever

Fever in the morning
Fever all through the night

Blackwell and Cooley

INTRODUCTION
Brian J. Hession, MD

Fever is a common symptom and presenting complaint to the emergency department. It is a systemic response to an enormous range of clinical entities and therefore presents a challenging diagnostic puzzle for the clinician to solve.

The "normal" human core body temperature has long been cited to be 37°C (98.6°F). Several factors should be considered when evaluating a recorded temperature. A rectal temperature most closely reflects the true core body temperature and usually varies by approximately +0.7°C from a simultaneous accurate oral temperature. Oral temperatures are affected by many factors that can influence the accuracy of the reading. These factors include probe position within the oral cavity, mouth breathing, ingestion of hot or cold food or liquid immediately before temperature measurement, use of supplemental oxygen, and heart rate. Tympanic temperatures may also be falsely low from poor positioning, cold exposure, and cerumen impaction. In addition, there is a circadian temperature variation of 0.5°C to 1.0°C throughout the day. In addition, premenopausal women experience a slight variation in their normal temperature according to their menstrual cycle.

Why do we develop fever? One hypothesis suggests that fever is largely a protective feature for the human host. Neutrophil and lymphocyte activity is greater at temperatures higher than 37°C. Furthermore, fever can inhibit the survival of several bacteria and viruses, either by direct effect or by starvation. Circulating levels of iron and zinc are lowered during the febrile response, depriving invading microbes of these growth factors. This section reviews some of the many causes of fever seen in the emergency department.

40

Traveler's Fever

Nannette M. Lugo-Amador, MD, MPH

Clinical Scenario

A 32-year-old man presented to the emergency department (ED) with a complaint of fever, chills, and body aches. He returned from a safari trip to the Congo region in central Africa 2 weeks ago. He began feeling sick 4 days ago, with headaches, high fever, anorexia, and malaise. He also complains of diffuse abdominal pain and low back pain.

He has no past medical history, is on no medications, and has no allergies to medications. He denies use of intravenous (IV) drugs, tobacco, or alcohol. He is sexually active, has one female partner, and uses condoms. Travel history is significant for his recent safari trip where he stayed in tents. Only the Congo region was visited, and his vaccines are up to date. He was started on chloroquine chemoprophylaxis by his primary physician before his trip and finished the therapy 1 week after his return.

On physical examination, his vital signs are as follows: oral temperature of 40°C (104°F), heart rate of 125 beats/minute, blood pressure of 110/60 mm Hg, respiratory rate of 20 breaths/minute, and room air pulse oximeter of 95%. He is a diaphoretic man who appears acutely ill. His skin is warm and flushed with no rashes. His sclerae are icteric (yellow/jaundiced), and there is no photophobia. His mucous membranes and lips are dry. His neck is supple without rigidity. Lung examination reveals crackles (rales) at the bases but otherwise clear. His abdomen is soft and is tender to palpation in the right upper quadrant without guarding or rebound. His spleen is palpable, slightly enlarged, and tender. The rest of the

examination, including a neurological examination, is unremarkable.

An IV line is established, blood is drawn for laboratory testing, including blood cultures, a complete blood cell (CBC) count with differential, thick and thin blood smears, electrolyte levels, and liver function tests, and a normal saline infusion is started. The patient is given 1 g of acetaminophen orally.

The laboratory calls to report a positive blood smear for red blood cell (RBC) rings suggestive of malaria, with further identification pending. The patient is admitted with a diagnosis of falciparum malaria presumably caused by multiple-drug resistant *Plasmodium falciparum*. He fully recovers after appropriate antibiotics are administered.

Clinical Evaluation

Introduction

Traveler's illness is common. In one study of approximately 10,000 travelers, 15% of them reported health problems. The most common infectious symptoms and diseases reported by travelers to developing countries, in decreasing order of frequency, are severe diarrhea, acute respiratory tract infection with fever, giardiasis, viral hepatitis, amebiasis, gonorrhea, malaria and other tropical diseases, salmonellosis, helminths, syphilis, and shigellosis. The diseases that have dire treatment and epidemiological consequences if missed are discussed in more detail in the section on selected tropical diseases. Because of the speed of today's transportation, many of these infected patients return to their country of origin before manifesting any symptoms. When these patients develop symptoms, medical care is provided in EDs and primary care settings, posing a diagnostic challenge to clinicians.

History

The most important historical information for these patients is a history of travel to an area that is endemic for one or more of these diseases. Once a history of travel is obtained and an etiology is suspected, the clinical history may help to narrow down the individual pathogen. The area of travel, combined with clinical features and laboratory testing, usually allows the clinician to make an accurate diagnosis. You are unlikely to encounter most of the tropical diseases described in the following paragraphs, the exception being is if you work in areas populated by immigrants from endemic areas. Nevertheless, it is useful to be aware of these diseases and keep a higher index of suspicion in anyone who has traveled to endemic areas.

Selected Tropical Diseases

Malaria

Malaria is a disease with different presentations. However, most commonly, it presents with paroxysms of fever, chills, anemia, and splenomegaly.

Malaria has an incubation period of approximately 6 to 16 days. A prodrome consisting of fevers, headaches, myalgias, malaise, and anorexia lasts for 2 to 3 days. Fever paroxysms are the classic presentation and can be synchronous or asynchronous. Synchronous paroxysms refer to the occurrence of fever in a regular time pattern, usually every 48 to 72 hours. The patient feels much better between paroxysms. Asynchronous paroxysms refer to the occurrence of fever episodes in an irregular time pattern. The use of chemoprophylaxis may affect the presentation of the fever paroxysms. A fever paroxysm typically starts with a sensation of coldness, chills, and teeth chattering followed by high fever, sweats, and malaise. Nausea, vomiting, diarrhea, abdominal pain,

dyspnea, and cough can also be part of the paroxysms. Severe hemolysis may occur, which causes hemoglobin to be passed through the urine, turning it dark ("blackwater" fever). Hemolysis is a potential cause of renal failure.

Viral Hemorrhagic Fevers

The viral hemorrhagic fevers are a group of infections caused by different viruses. These infections are characterized by early fever presentation and, in severe cases, subsequent shock and disseminated bleeding. The most common of these infections are dengue fever and yellow fever. Other viral hemorrhagic fevers are Marburg disease, Lassa fever, Ebola virus disease, and Hanta virus.

Dengue Fever

Classic dengue fever is also known as "breakbone fever" because its febrile spasms can be so severe that the patients actually fracture their bones. The incubation period is approximately 1 to 7 days and is followed by the abrupt onset of fever, chills, headache, eye pain, joint pain, lumbosacral pain, and transient erythematous rash for the first 24 to 48 hours. Patients can also have gastrointestinal symptoms, such as nausea and vomiting. The symptoms last from 3 to 5 days, after which the fever resolves.

Dengue hemorrhagic fever has a similar presentation to classic dengue fever; however, it is further complicated by abnormalities in capillary permeability, coagulation, and hemostasis. Ninety percent of the time dengue hemorrhagic fever and dengue shock syndrome occurs in second-time infections; therefore, it does not represent a major health risk for occasional travelers.

Dengue shock syndrome is the most severe form of the spectrum of dengue infection. It is characterized by hypotension and circulatory shock that can occur during the second to fifth day of illness. Patients can have disseminated intravascular coagulation and decreased levels of clotting factors; less commonly, patients exhibit encephalitis, renal failure, and fulminant hepatitis.

Yellow Fever

The incubation period of yellow fever is from 3 to 6 days. Most cases are self-limited with flu-like symptoms, fever, and myalgias. Twenty-five percent to 50% of the yellow fever cases are fatal and have the full syndrome. Yellow fever has three clinical stages: infection, remission, and intoxication. The period of infection consists of the initial abrupt onset of fever, headache, and myalgias. Patients either fully recover after the initial infection period or have a temporary remission followed by recurrence of fever and symptoms. Following remission, the intoxication stage begins with high fever, lumbosacral back pain, abdominal pain, nausea, vomiting, and changes in mental status. The patient is lethargic and often dehydrated from vomiting. The patient manifests bleeding abnormalities such as epistaxis, oral mucosal bleeding, hematemesis, and petechial or purpuric hemorrhages. Clinical deterioration continues, including the development of hepatitis, renal failure, hypotension, and bleeding. Encephalopathy and coma are a common consequence of the metabolic abnormalities and cerebral edema. Death occurs 7 to 10 days after onset of symptoms.

Physical Examination

Although the physical examination may provide clues to infectious etiologies, it is almost never diagnostic in traveler's diseases. It is primarily the history of travel combined with a high index of suspicion on the clinician's part that leads to the appropriate care of the patient.

As in the clinical scenario, the presence of episodic fevers, a tender liver edge, enlarged spleen, and jaundice after a recent African trip prompted the physician to send blood for a thick smear, which ultimately confirmed the diagnosis of malaria. Cerebral malaria can cause neurological symptoms such as nystagmus, focal and generalized seizures, and coma.

Physical examination should always be used to look for signs of meningitis in febrile patients who appear toxic.

The diagnosis of dengue fever can be made based on the history and physical examination in a patient who visited a dengue-endemic area. Patients with hemorrhagic fever are jaundiced and have clinical manifestations of bleeding, rashes, and palpable lymphadenopathy. A morbilliform rash develops in the trunk area and spreads centripetally to the face and extremities with a possible brief fever recrudescence. Hemorrhagic phenomena, such as petechial hemorrhage and epistaxis, may present during the illness.

Yellow fever is a disease of variable severity characterized by a triad of hepatitis, hemorrhagic diathesis, and proteinuria. Apart from the rash, yellow fever shares many physical findings of dengue fever on physical examination.

Diagnostic Evaluation

Malaria

The gold standard for the diagnosis of malaria is the thick and thin blood smears from the acutely ill patient. Most patients' initial blood smears are positive for malaria. Newer techniques for detecting malaria include polymerase chain reaction (PCR), the antigen detection technique, fluorescent staining of the parasite nuclei, and the malaria antibody test.

Dengue Fever

Minimal diagnostic criteria for dengue hemorrhagic fever are a positive tourniquet test, leukopenia, thrombocytopenia with a platelet count of less than 100,000/mm^3, and plasma leakage reflected by an increase in the hematocrit by 20% from its baseline, ascites, and pleural effusions. (A positive tourniquet test is the appearance of hemorrhagic phenomena, such as petechiae, in the skin when a tourniquet is placed on an extremity.)

The diagnosis can also be confirmed with virus isolation from the serum of an infected patient during the febrile illness. Different virus identification techniques are available: cell cultures, live mosquito inoculation, immunotest for serotype, and reverse PCR.

Serology tests can also help in the identification of a dengue infection. There is an increase in IgM against dengue antibody 1 to 3 months after infection. Other tests are complement fixation, neutralizing antibody titers, and heme-agglutination inhibition tests.

Yellow Fever

Diagnostic tests include viral isolation and serological tests. Virus isolation is possible during the first 12 days of illness and can be done by cell cultures or inoculation of mosquitoes. Serological tests include detection of IgM by enzyme-linked immunosorbent assay (ELISA) and the neutralization test.

Differential Diagnosis

The differential diagnosis for traveler's fever is illustrated in Table 40.1.

Treatment

Malaria

Patients presenting with malaria acutely should be treated for falciparum malaria until laboratory confirmation of the *Plasmodium* species. Drug resistance should be assumed if there is any history of travel to a drug-resistant region. Acute uncomplicated malaria caused by all species of *Plasmodium* except chloroquine-resistant species should be treated with oral chloroquine.

Table 40.1.
Differential diagnosis of the traveler's fever
Abdominal abscess
Amebic hepatic abscesses
Brucellosis
Dengue fever
Ebola virus
Hepatitis, viral
Influenza
Leishmaniasis
Malaria
Toxoplasmosis
Tuberculosis
Tularemia
Typhus

The recommended treatment for chloroquine-resistant uncomplicated falciparum malaria is a regimen consisting of oral quinine sulfate and pyrimethamine sulfadoxine. Uncomplicated falciparum malaria resistant to pyrimethamine and sulfa should be treated with oral quinine sulfate and a tetracycline or clindamycin. An alternative treatment for chloroquine-resistant or pyrimethamine sulfa-resistant falciparum malaria is mefloquine. For severe falciparum malaria, IV treatment with quinidine gluconate should be used. Vivax and ovale malaria should be treated with primaquine, in addition to the chloroquine, to prevent relapses. The recommended drugs and dosages of antimalarial drugs are summarized in Table 40.2. Chemoprophylaxis is the prevention of a disease by the use of chemicals or drugs. For all *Plasmodium* species except chloroquine-resistant falciparum, the recommended chemoprophylaxis agent is chloroquine phosphate 300 mg orally once a week 2 weeks before visiting a malaria-endemic area and continued for 4 weeks after returning. Persons visiting areas known to have chloroquine-resistant falciparum malaria can use mefloquine or doxycycline as chemoprophylaxis.

Dengue Fever

Treatment of dengue fever is supportive. Sicker patients who require hospital admission need to have their platelets and hematocrit monitored and blood products replaced as needed.

Yellow Fever

The treatment of yellow fever is totally supportive. There are no specific therapies for this infection. Treatment of dehydration and correction of electrolyte abnormalities are important. Immunoprophylaxis for yellow fever is available. There is a live attenuated vaccine, which offers protective immunity to 95% of its recipients 10 days after vaccination.

Prevention

Reducing insect bites reduces the transmission of diseases. Using protective clothing,

Table 40.2.

Recommended antimalarial drugs and dosages

Drug	Adult Dosage	Pediatric Dosage
Chloroquine phosphate, chloroquine sulfate, or hydroxychloroquine sulfate	600 mg base (1 g) po, then 300 mg base (0.5 g) 6 hours after first dose, then 300 mg base qd for 2 days	10 mg/kg of base po, then 5 mg/kg of base at 6, 24, and 48 hours
Chloroquine dihydrochloride	200 mg of base IM every 6 hours for a maximum of 3 days	5 mg/kg of base IM every 12 hours for a maximum of 3 days
Pyrimethamine sulfadoxine	3 tablets po × 1, each tablet contains 25 mg of pyrimethamine and 500 mg of sulfadoxine	0.5–4 yr = ½–1 tablet po × 1 5–8 yr = 1 tablet po × 1 9–14 yr = 2 tablets po × 1
Mefloquine	750–1,250 mg po × 1, or 500 mg po every 6 hours × 3 doses; repeat in 7 days	15 mg/kg po × 1
Doxycycline	100 mg po bid × 7 days	2 mg/kg po bid × 7 days
Quinidine sulfate	650 mg of base po tid × 3–7 days	10 mg/kg po tid × 3–7 days
Quinidine gluconate	10–15 mg/kg (IV) (salt) loading dose in 500 mL of isotonic saline with glucose over 1–2 hours, then 1–1.5 mg/kg/hr constant (IV) infusion for a maximum of 72 hours. Patient should be on cardiac monitoring.	Same as adults
Primaquine	15 mg of base po qd × 14 days	0.25 mg/kg of base po qd × 14 days
Tetracycline	250–500 mg po qid × 7 days	10 mg/kg po qid × 7 days
Clindamycin	900 mg po tid × 3 days	20–40 mg/kg/day po in 3 divided doses × 3 days

bid, two times a day; IM, intramuscular; po, by mouth; qd, daily; qid, four times a day; tid, three times a day.

mosquito nets, and insect repellent and avoiding exposure during mosquito feeding times (at dawn and dusk) will protect against mosquito bites.

Disposition

The disposition of a patient presenting with any traveler illness depends on the severity of the condition. Mild presentations can be treated with oral hydration, antipyretics, and rest as outpatients. Sicker and dehydrated patients can be admitted to the hospital for IV fluids and closer monitoring. Hospital admission should be considered for pregnant patients and immunocompromised patients. Patients with severe presentations, such as cerebral malaria, respiratory distress syndrome, dengue shock syndrome, and severe yellow fever, should be admitted to an intensive care unit for more aggressive supportive care and monitoring.

Pathophysiology

Malaria

Malaria is caused by a protozoan of the genus *Plasmodium*. Four species of *Plasmodium* are capable of infecting humans: *P. falciparum, Plasmodium vivax, Plasmodium malariae,* and *Plasmodium ovale. P. falciparum* is associated with more severe disease and complications. *Plasmodium* is transmitted to humans by female *Anopheles* mosquitoes. The malaria-endemic areas are Central and South America, sub-Sahara Africa, India, South East Asia, the Middle East, and some areas of the Caribbean.

Transmission of malaria usually occurs with the bite of an infected female *Anopheles* mosquito. Malaria can also be transmitted (although less commonly) through a blood transfusion and infected needles. When an infected female *Anopheles* mosquito bites a person, it injects saliva that contains *Plasmodium* life forms, which invade the liver cells and replicate. Infected liver cells eventually rupture, liberating more life forms to the circulation, which in turn infect more RBCs. The paroxysms of fever and chills occur during this acute rupture. *P. vivax* and *P. ovale* can remain dormant; however, infected liver cells eventually rupture after weeks, months, and even years.

Malaria affects multiple organ systems. RBC destruction (hemolysis) occurs as part of the life cycle of *Plasmodium* and causes anemia. Hemolysis causes hemoglobin to be released to the circulation; the hemoglobin, in turn, is excreted by the kidneys. Large amounts of hemoglobin excretion can cause renal failure, one of the complications of severe malaria.

RBCs infected with *P. falciparum* adhere to the blood vessel inner surface and, in sufficient amounts, can obstruct blood flow. Microcirculation obstruction in the organ tissues can cause multiorgan failure. In acutely ill malaria patients, respiratory distress syndrome causes hypoxemia; these patients require assisted mechanical ventilation. In patients with severe cases of falciparum malaria, the brain tissue is highly parasitized. Obstruction to the cerebral blood flow causes central nervous system dysfunction, presenting with focal or generalized neurological deficits.

Dengue Fever

Dengue is caused by four different types of dengue virus, which belong to the genus *Flavivirus*. Dengue fever is transmitted by the mosquito *Aedes aegypti* and is common in tropical and subtropical areas of the Americas, Asia, Africa, Australia, and the Caribbean. There are approximately 100 million reported cases of dengue fever every year. The severity and the course of dengue fever infection differentiates three different entities: classic dengue fever, dengue hemorrhagic fever, and dengue shock syndrome.

After an infected mosquito bites a person, viral replication occurs in regional lymph nodes. The virus is disseminated to other tissues through blood and lymph, and it further replicates in the reticuloendothelial system and in the skin. The hemorrhagic complications that are seen in dengue hemorrhagic fever and in dengue shock syndrome are secondary to coagulation, capillary permeability, and hemostasis abnormalities.

Yellow Fever

Yellow fever is endemic in the tropical forests of South America and Africa. The disease is caused by an arbovirus of the genus *Flavivirus* transmitted to humans by the mosquito *Aedes aegypti*. Viral replication occurs in regional lymph nodes, and the virus is spread via blood and lymph to other tissues. The virus replicates in the liver, spleen, and bone marrow. The hemorrhagic manifestations of this infection are a consequence of the depletion of hepatic clotting factors, platelet dysfunction, and intravascular coagulation. Shock occurs, possibly caused by vasoactive cytokines and parenchymal damage to the kidneys, myocardium, and other organs.

Suggested Readings

Doezema D, Hauswald M. Infection in the traveler and immigrant. In: Brillman JC, Quenzer RW, eds. *Infectious disease in emergency medicine*, 2nd ed. Philadelphia: Lippincott-Raven, 1998:401–436.

Magill AJ. Travel medicine, fever in the returned traveler. *Infect Dis Clin North Am* 1998;12: 445–469.

Magill AJ, Strickland GT. Fever in travelers. In: Strickland GT, ed. *Hunter's tropical medicine and emerging infectious diseases*, 8th ed. Philadelphia: WB Saunders, 2000:1049–1057.

Steffen R, Rickenbach M, Wilhelm U, et al. Health problems after travel to developing countries. *J Infect Dis* 1987;156:84–91.

Suh KN, Kozarsky PE, Keystone JS. Travel medicine, evaluation of the fever in the traveler. *Med Clin North Am* 1999;83:997–1017.

Taylor TE, Strickland GT. Malaria. In: Strickland GT, ed. *Hunter's tropical medicine and emerging infectious diseases*, 8th ed. Philadelphia: WB Saunders, 2000:614–643.

Tsai T. Yellow fever. In: Strickland GT, ed. *Hunter's tropical medicine and emerging infectious diseases*, 8th ed. Philadelphia: WB Saunders, 2000:272–275.

Vaughn DW, Green S. Dengue and dengue hemorrhagic fever. In: Strickland GT, ed. *Hunter's tropical medicine and emerging infectious diseases*, 8th ed. Philadelphia: WB Saunders, 2000:240–245.

Wyler DJ. Plasmodium and Babesia. In: Gorbach SL, Barlett JG, Blacklow NR, eds. *Infectious diseases*, 2nd ed. Philadelphia: WB Saunders, 1998:2407–2416.

41

HIV and Fever

Thea James, MD

Clinical Scenario

A 24-year-old woman who is a graduate student presents to the emergency department (ED) complaining of a low-grade fever and fatigue for 2 weeks. She also complains of a productive cough, shortness of breath worsening over the past 3 days, and loss of appetite. She states that she has not felt like her usual self for almost 2 weeks. She feels disinclined to carry out her usual activities. She states that she does not want to go to the museum and have lunch with her friends because she has difficulty breathing just walking around in her apartment. Her closest friend has convinced her to come to the ED and has accompanied her there. Her friend says that the patient had a 10-day flulike illness 1 year ago. At that time, the patient had a low-grade fever, muscle aches, a sore throat, and loss of appetite. She attributed it to a viral illness and to heavy involvement in aerobics. The patient says she has never been ill, and her only time spent in a hospital was when she made daily visits to see her ex-boyfriend when he developed pneumonia 1 year ago. He has since moved back to his hometown to live closer to his family.

The patient denies chest pain, abdominal pain, neck pain, or back pain. She denies nausea, vomiting, diarrhea, or dysuria. She has no neurological complaints, except a mild headache that occurs when she is coughing. Her last menstrual period was 14 days ago, and she does not always use a condom when engaging in sexual intercourse.

The patient has no past medical illnesses and takes no medications, except oral contraceptive pills. She has no allergies.

Physical examination reveals a tachyp-neic young woman, who appears weak and pale. Her blood pressure is 99/50 mm Hg, heart rate 120 beats/minute, respiratory rate 30 breaths/minute, temperature 103°F, and room air oxygen saturation 88%. Her skin is warm and dry. Examination of her head, ears, eyes, nose, and throat (HEENT) is unremarkable, and her neck is supple and nontender. Her heart examination reveals a regular tachycardia without murmurs. Her lungs are clear on the left, and the base of her right lung is notable for a marked decrease in breath sounds. Her abdominal and extremity examinations are unremarkable. She has mild generalized adenopathy.

An intravenous (IV) line is placed and blood is obtained for cultures, complete blood cell (CBC) count, and electrolyte levels. An arterial blood gas (ABG) sample is obtained and the patient is placed on 2 L/minute of oxygen via nasal cannula Her pulse oximetry improved to 95% and she was sent for a posteroanterior (PA) and lateral chest x-ray examination. The x-ray film showed a right lower lobe patch infiltrate. The patient was begun on antibiotics and admitted. The white blood cell count returned low at 1,800/mm^3. An HIV test was done and returned positive. After improving she is dischrged to follow up in an infectious disease clinic.

Clinical Evaluation

Introduction

Fever or flulike illness is the most common presenting complaint in patients on initial presentation of HIV but is often missed because of its benign appearance to the clinician. Fever is also a common presenting complaint in the patient with known HIV disease. Fever in the HIV-infected patient should always be taken seriously. Fever may be acute, with focal or systemic symptoms; later in HIV disease, the patient may have intermittent spiking temperatures or low-grade fevers. Any acute fever, or unexplained fever of longer than 2 weeks' duration, should be thoroughly evaluated. Fever in any patient with a CD4 count of less than 200/ml may herald an opportunistic infection and should be carefully evaluated.

Infection is the number one cause of death in HIV patients. Infectious etiologies include fungal, bacterial, parasitic, and viral. Noninfectious causes of fever in patients with HIV disease include drug reactions and neoplasm. This chapter focuses on the workup of the HIV-positive patient who presents with fever.

History

The emergency medicine physician should begin the evaluation by taking a thorough history from the patient presenting with fever. It is important to ask about the duration, severity, and pattern of the fever: how long the patient has had the fever, whether it is constant or intermittent, and its numerical measurement in degrees. A thorough social and medical history should be obtained. Patients should be asked about the following: associated symptoms in addition to the fever, any prior medical illnesses, any medications being taken currently or recently, travel to areas endemic for mycoses or tuberculosis (TB), active IV drug use, medication use, and whether the patient has adhered to prophylactic medication use. The social history should include a sexual practice history including safe-sex practices, such as the use of condoms currently and historically.

Any patient who presents with a fever of unknown origin and who is at risk for HIV (i.e., less than 100% condom use, IV drug use, recipient of blood transfusion in the past 20 years, intimate exposure to anyone at risk for HIV, and prior or current residence in an HIV-endemic area), should have HIV in the differential diagnosis until proven otherwise. As an emergency physician, it is important to maintain a high index of suspicion in anyone at risk for HIV.

In the patient with known HIV disease and fever, it is important to ascertain information about his or her HIV status. Does the patient know his or her CD4 count and viral load? Is he or she taking any medications for HIV disease? Has he or she had any prior infections or HIV-related illnesses? The CD4 count can be very helpful in predicting a differential. Those patients with a high CD4 count are not at increased risk for opportunistic infections; however, they are at increased risk for common community infections, such as community-acquired pneumonia and sinusitis. A CD4 count less than 200/ml increases the risk of opportunistic infection; in fact, there is an inverse relationship between CD4 count and risk of opportunistic infections.

In the HIV-infected patient, certain illnesses should be suspected with certain complaints. For those with complaints of fever and cough or dyspnea, consider community-acquired pneumonia, *Pneumocystis carinii* pneumonia (PCP), TB, or bacterial pneumonia. Systemic symptoms present more often than respiratory symptoms in the early course of PCP; therefore, it should always be suspected and included in the differential diagnosis, particularly in patients with a CD4 count less than 200. For complaints of fever and headache, neck pain, or altered mental status and behavior, the differential diagnosis should include toxoplasmosis, sinusitis, cryptococcal meningitis, herpes encephalitis, and central nervous system (CNS) lymphoma. Patients who complain of fever with abdominal pain and hepatosplenomegaly should have an expanded differential diagnosis to include disseminated *Mycobacterium avium* complex (MAC), histoplasmosis, lymphoma, and bacillary peliosis. Asymmetric or unilateral lymphadenopathy should raise suspicion for TB, non-Hodgkin's lymphoma, and bacillary angiomatosis.

Physical Examination

When a patient with known or suspected HIV infection presents to the ED with fever, the physical examination must be complete with focus on any area notable on review of systems or chief complaint. Particular attention should be paid to the skin, sinuses, IV catheter sites, lungs, retina, lymph nodes, heart, abdomen, and CNS, all areas that can harbor unsuspected infection or disease.

Patients with fever and nonspecific viral symptoms, especially at-risk patients (multiple sexual partners, unprotected sexual activity, IV drug use) should have a careful examination for diffuse lymphadenopathy, which may be the only physical finding pointing to underlying HIV infection.

Mild neck stiffness or midline back pain when flexing the neck could be the only finding for a CNS infection. Patients with acquired immunodeficiency syndrome (AIDS), defined by HIV disease with a CD4 count below 200/ml and the appearance of opportunistic infection, may harbor more indolent CNS pathogens, such as cryptococcus, or CNS toxoplasmosis for example. IV drug users are at risk for epidural abscess; thus, midline back pain and fever, especially in HIV positive individuals, should make you highly suspicious for this diagnosis. Listen carefully for cardiac murmurs as well in the IV drug using population, because they are at risk for endocarditis, an infection of the valves.

Diagnostic Evaluation

In the early stages of HIV disease, routine laboratory studies should be done, and specific tests should be added according to local signs and symptoms. Routine laboratory tests include a CBC count with differential, urinalysis, two sets of blood cultures, and a chest x-ray film. For more focal complaints such as abdominal pain, vomiting, headache, neck pain, or difficulty breathing, other tests should be obtained, such as computed tomography (CT) scan, electrolyte panel, liver function tests, lumbar puncture, or ABG levels. Fever evaluations in patients with CD4 counts less than 100 cells/ml will often not render an etiology for fever through routine testing. For these patients, further testing might be required, for example, mycobacterial blood cultures, fungal blood cultures, and serum cryptococcal antigen. For sustained fever in patients with advanced HIV disease, bone marrow aspiration and tissue biopsy might be necessary to obtain an etiology for fever; these tests have a very high yield.

Differential Diagnosis

The differential diagnosis for HIV disease and fever is illustrated in Table 41.1.

Bacterial Infections

Bacterial infections often occur early in symptomatic HIV disease. Community-acquired pneumonias are common pulmonary manifestations of HIV disease. Pathogens such as *Streptococcus pneumonia*, *Staphylococcus aureus*, *Haemophilus influenzae*, *Mycobacterium tuberculosis*, *Chlamydia pneumonia*, and *Legionella* and *Klebsiella* species are often the cause of pneumonia in HIV-positive patients. Another cause of pulmonary infection in HIV disease is *Pseudomonas aeruginosa*. PCP is a severe and commonly diagnosed AIDS-related infection in the United States. It generally occurs gradually but on occasion can occur abruptly. Patients usually present with fever, dyspnea, malaise, nonproductive cough, chills, and chest pain. Some patients can have a productive cough.

Mycobacterial Infections

Mycobacterial infections are common in HIV-infected patients, and HIV disease has contributed to the rise in TB in the United States since the middle 1980s. TB can disseminate (extrapulmonary TB); however, the most common presentation is pulmonary TB. Patients present with cough, fever, weight loss, and night sweats. A patient's degree of immunodeficiency generally dictates the severity of signs and symptoms. Chest x-ray films can help in the diagnosis of pulmonary TB; however, up to 10% are normal. Some nontuberculous mycobacterial pathogens are MAC and *Mycobacterium kansasii*. Both of these diseases occur in advanced stages of AIDS. Both can also disseminate.

Viral Infections

A viral cause of fever in HIV disease is cytomegalovirus (CMV) infection. CMV can disseminate and can manifest as encephalitis, esophagitis, hepatitis, colitis, pneumonitis, adrenalitis, and chorioretinitis. Herpes virus infections (herpes simplex, varicella and zoster) can cause pneumonitis or pneumonia in HIV-infected patients.

Table 41.1.

Differential diagnosis and the relationship between type of infection and T-cell levels[a]

300–499 T Cells	<200 T Cells	<100 T Cells
Bacterial and Viral respiratory infections	PCP	All of infections seen in patients with <200 T cells
Sinusitis	Fungal diseases	CMV
Otitis	Encephalitis	MAC
Cellulitis	Cryptococcus	Disseminated KS
Pyelonephritis	Toxoplasmosis	Coccidioidomycosis
PID	Histoplasmosis	Salmonella sepsis
Herpes zoster	Lymphoma	Cryptosporidiosis
Condyloma acuminata	Cervical or anal dysplasia	
Molluscum contagiosum		
Bacillary angiomatosis		
HIV acute syndrome		
Candidiasis		

CMV, cytomegalovirus; HIV, human immunodeficiency virus; KS, Kaposi's sarcoma; MAC, *Mycobacterium avium complex*; PCP, *Pneumocystis carinii* pneumonia; PID, pelvic inflammatory disease.
[a]Some opportunistic infections that typically occur in advanced stages of HIV, (lower T-cell counts) have occurred atypically in patients with higher T-cell counts.

Fungal Infections

Fungal presentations of HIV disease are cryptococcus, histoplasmosis, coccidioidomycosis, candidiasis, and pulmonary aspergillosis. Most of these pathogens can disseminate and can have a range of presentations, including pulmonary and neurological (meningitis). Candidiasis also has a mucocutaneous presentation.

Parasitic Infections

Examples of parasitic infections in HIV disease are toxoplasmosis and cryptosporidiosis. Patients with toxoplasmosis usually present with necrotizing encephalitis. It appears as ring-enhancing lesions on CT scans or magnetic resonance imaging (MRI).

Neoplasms

Patients with HIV infection are at risk for particular neoplasms. Two of the most common are Kaposi's sarcoma (KS) and non-Hodgkin's lymphoma. In general, fever is only present in KS when it has disseminated to viscera. Fever can often accompany clinical presentations of lymphoma.

Other Causes of Fever

Women with HIV infection may present with certain gynecological complaints. They typically present with vulvovaginal candidiasis, cervical dysplasia, and human papillomavirus. Cervical dysplasia is often an omen for the presence of HIV infection.

Other causes of fever in HIV-infected patients are drugs (prescribed and illicit) and self-injected bacteria by IV drug users. Patients with HIV have increased sensitivity to several medications, including antibiotics. They are often prescribed multiple drugs to prevent and treat HIV-associated clinical problems.

Treatment

Treatment should be based on a suspected etiology and also depends on the patient's CD4 count and stage of HIV disease. It is beyond the scope of this book to discuss the treatment of the many HIV-related illnesses.

The treatment of HIV-related infections would not be complete without a mention of new treatments for HIV disease and the use of potent antiretroviral drugs as a method of suppressing the HIV virus. There are four major classes of antiretroviral drugs: nucleoside reverse transcriptase inhibitors, nonnucleoside reverse transcriptase inhibitors, protease inhibitors, and fusion inhibitors. They have become widely used and available since 1996. The term HAART is a common acronym seen under the list for medications of HIV-infected individuals. It represents highly active anti-retroviral treatment and consists of the use of three or more antiretroviral agents in various combinations. There are presently 20 approved antiretroviral medications at time of publication, and fusion inhibitors are reserved for patients who show resistance to other medications. These drugs have changed the classic clinical presentations of HIV infections. Many clinicians have noticed marked decreases in the occurrence of AIDS-related opportunistic infections and unusual presentations and manifestations of previously common infections.

Disposition

Patients who are at risk for HIV infection, and who present with complaints of fever lasting longer than 10 days and complaints consistent with the acute or seroconversion stage of HIV, should have a conversation with the emergency physician about possible HIV infection. The physician should compassionately and thoroughly explain reasons for concern and the importance of further evaluation (testing for the HIV virus). It should be stressed that a diagnosis of HIV has not been found and is not certain and only must be ruled out. If the patient has a primary care physician, he or she should be advised to follow-up with the physician immediately. If the patient does not have a primary care physician, the patient should be provided with resources for seeking a primary care physician or a clinic that performs HIV testing. The emergency physician's discharge plan depends on the social situation of the patient. Patients with questionable social situations often require more directed discharge planning.

Patients who are known to have HIV infection and who have CD4 counts greater than 200 with local signs or symptoms should be evaluated, and the specific signs and symptoms treated accordingly. The decision to either discharge the patient to home or admit to the hospital depends on the severity of the symptoms. For example, patients who have respiratory compromise with difficulty breathing and decreased oxygen saturation (<95%), patients who are vomiting and unable to tolerate drinking fluids, or patients who are severely volume depleted and compromised by severe weakness should be admitted to the hospital. In the hospital, they can be treated more aggressively with the use of IV fluids, IV antibiotics, or continuous oxygen. Patients who are not compromised physically can generally be discharged to home with a prescription for the appropriate antibiotic, instructions appropriate for their diagnosis, and primary care follow-up.

Patients with known HIV disease and CD4 counts less than 200/ml generally require a more thorough inpatient evaluation. Fever in these patients often portends an opportunistic infection.

Pathophysiology

An understanding of the natural history and progression of HIV infection is key to diagnosing and appropriately evaluating febrile illnesses associated with HIV disease. As the immune system becomes more compromised, the differential diagnosis evolves. The disease and its sequelae changes from early-stage HIV to advanced-stage HIV; specific processes present in each stage. Therefore, the most important factor in evaluating a patient who has HIV infection and a fever is understanding the natural progression of HIV and understanding the patient's presenting clinical complaints as it relates to his or her stage of HIV.

The manifestation of HIV infection maintains a broad spectrum, depending on the stage. It is helpful to approach fever in the setting of possible HIV infection by categorizing the infection into three stages: acute stage, or seroconversion (initial HIV presentation); asymptomatic stage; and symptomatic stage.

In the acute stage (seroconversion), HIV disseminates throughout the body, to lymph nodes and other organs. The first clinical manifestation of HIV infection is often a self-limited febrile illness. It usually presents as a viral-like or mononucleosis-like syndrome occurring from 8 to 12 weeks after the initial exposure to HIV. Patients may present with malaise, fatigue, pharyngitis, headache, diffuse adenopathy, diarrhea, or rash. The seroconversion stage can also be associated with peripheral neuropathy or symptoms of aseptic meningitis. There have been reports of vaginal, rectal, oral, penile, and esophageal ulcers. Some patients may be asymptomatic. This illness can last from 1 to 5 weeks.

The progression of HIV disease after the seroconversion stage can vary. Although patients with HIV infection usually remain asymptomatic after the seroconversion phase, active viral replication occurs with damage to the immune system and progressive depletion of the CD4 lymphocyte count. When an HIV-positive patient's CD4 count decreases to a level of 200/ml, he or she is at great risk for opportunistic infections. At this level of immunodeficiency, patients are also reclassified as having AIDS (in addition to being HIV positive). These opportunistic infections are also referred to as AIDS-defining diagnoses.

High-grade viremia heralds the onset of symptomatic HIV disease. Bacterial infections can be early symptomatic manifestations of HIV. Some patients who are HIV positive present with recurrent bacterial infections, such as sinusitis and pneumonia. Patients give a history of cough, cold, or sinusitis symptoms that last for an extended period or continue to recur. Other manifestations of symptomatic HIV disease are intermittent fever, diarrhea, weight loss, and lymphadenopathy. As the disease progresses and the virus ravages the immune system, symptomatic disease is characterized by opportunistic infections, neoplasms, and HIV-related dysfunction of organs.

Suggested Readings

Fauci AS, Bartlett JG, Kaplan JE, et al. Guidelines for the use of antiretroviral agents in HIV-1-infected adults and adolescents. Panel on Clinical Practices for Treatment of HIV Infection convened by the Department of Health and Human Services, March 23, 2004. Full text available online at http://aidsinfo.nih.gov (last accessed 9/23/04).

Jacobson MA, French M. Altered natural history of AIDS-related opportunistic infections in the era of potent combination antiretroviral therapy. *AIDS* 1998(12 Suppl A):S157–163.

Kilby JM, Goepfert PA, Miller AP, et al. Recurrence of the acute HIV syndrome after interruption of antiretroviral therapy in a patient with chronic HIV infection: a case report. *Ann Intern Med* 2000;133:435–438.

Mandell GL, Douglas RG, Bennett JE, eds. Human immunodeficiency virus-associated fever of unknown origin. In: *Principles and practice of infectious diseases*, 5th ed. New York: Churchill Livingstone, 2000.

Mandell GL, Douglas RG, Bennett JE, eds. Classic fever of unknown origin. In: *Principles and practice of infectious diseases*, 5th ed. New York: Churchill Livingstone, 2000.

Perlmutter BL, Glaser JB, Oyugi SO. How to recognize and treat acute HIV syndrome. *Am Fam Physician* 1999;60:535–542, 545–546.

Skiest DJ, Kaplan P, Machala T, et al. Clinical manifestations of influenza in HIV-infected individuals. *Int J STD AIDS* 2001;12: 646–650.

Walker AR. HIV in children. *Emerg Med Clin North Am* 1995;13:147–162.

Wormser GP. *AIDS and other manifestations of HIV infection*, 3rd ed. Philadelphia: Lippincott Williams and Wilkins, 1998.

Bacterial Source of Fever

Michael Snyder, MD

Clinical Scenario

A 72-year-old woman is brought to the emergency department (ED) by emergency medical services (EMS) from a local nursing home. She has been febrile to 102°F for about 2 days and has become pale and mildly lethargic over the last 6 hours. Her urine was reported to be foul smelling and cloudy over the past few days. She has taken very little to eat or drink recently, and the nursing staff reports her systolic blood pressure to be 80 mm Hg.

The patient's past medical history is significant for a prior ischemic stroke with residual left-sided weakness, noninsulin-dependent diabetes, and hypertension. Her social history is significant for a remote smoking history. She has been living in a nursing home since the stroke 5 years ago. Her medications include coumadin, aspirin, lisinopril, Glucotrol, Colace, and Dulcolax suppositories. She has no known drug allergies.

Her physical examination is notable for an oral temperature of 102°F, a blood pressure of 80/45 mm Hg, a pulse of 120 beats/minute, a respiratory rate of 22 breaths/minute, and an oxygen saturation of 97% on room air. When you first observe her, she is diaphoretic and lethargic; is taking somewhat rapid, shallow breaths; and has mottled skin. She is thin, pale, and drowsy, but arousable. Her head shows no evidence of trauma. Her eyes, ears, nose, and mouth are notable only for dry mucous membranes. Her neck is supple. On auscultation, her heart is tachycardic with normal heart sounds, and her lungs are clear. Her abdomen is soft and is not tender or distended.

Her skin shows poor turgor and is mottled, with no rashes, ulcers, or edema. Neurological examination is significant for a left hemiparesis. Stool obtained by digital rectal examination is negative for occult blood.

Oxygen is administered by nasal cannula, and intravenous (IV) access is obtained and a normal saline infusion is started. Continuous pulse oxymetry and cardiac monitoring are established. Electrocardiogram and chest x-ray film are obtained. Blood is drawn and is sent for culture, complete blood cell (CBC) count, electrolyte levels, blood urea nitrogen (BUN) and creatinine (Cr) levels, and coagulation studies. A Foley catheter is inserted and urine is sent for urinalysis (UA) and culture. Antibiotics are started.

The chest x-ray film is clear. The UA is positive for large leukocytes and nitrites, 3+ bacteria, and 100 white blood cells (WBCs)/high-powered field (HPF). The serum WBC count is 18,000 cells/mm^3 with a left shift (increased neutrophils). BUN and Cr levels are mildly elevated. Her blood pressure improves with IV fluids and she is admitted to the floor. Antibiotics are begun in the ED for treatment of urosepsis.

Clinical Evaluation

Introduction

Although the diagnosis in this particular clinical scenario is urosepsis, many different bacterial causes of fever are possible. In this patient, certain key features, including the chronic indwelling Foley catheter; increased WBCs in the urine; and lethargy likely resulting from hypoperfusion, fever, and hypotension, point to sepsis from a urological source as the most likely etiology. Antibiotics, antipyretics, and IV fluids for volume and blood pressure support are the main treatment modalities. Vasopressors are often required for cardiovascular support, especially in a patient with cardiac disease who cannot tolerate a large volume of IV fluid. It is very important to treat both the infection and the clinical manifestations, specifically the fever and the cardiovascular compromise.

History

Many factors in the history are indicative of sepsis from a bacterial infection. The patient's temperature, of course, is an important finding in infection, but you must be aware that elderly patients can often present afebrile even when they have a serious infection (they may not always mount a WBC response, either). It is important to look at all aspects of the history and presentation and the past medical history. In the clinical scenario, cloudy urine, fever, indwelling Foley catheter, and altered mentation guide the clinician toward a urinary tract infection as the most likely culprit. For any patient with fever and signs of bacterial sepsis, a complete review of systems should be obtained. It may be simplest to start from the head and work down, so that nothing is missed. The patient should be asked about headache, earache, sore throat, and sinus pain. Neck pain may indicate meningitis or epidural abscess. Pulmonary symptoms include cough, shortness of breath, and chest pain. Back pain may be unilateral as in pyelonephritis. Abdominal pain and pelvic pain, including genitourinary symptoms, should be elucidated. Any history of skin rashes, open wounds, or painful extremities and joints should be obtained. It is also important to find out a history of alcohol abuse; IV drug use; human immunodeficiency virus (HIV) infection risks; and social history, such as where the patient lives (or whether they are homeless), and family support systems.

Physical Examination

The physical examination for a patient presenting with the chief complaint of a fever must be broad and very thorough, not focused. Vital signs are important both for the temperature and for the cardiovascular status. Tachycardia may accompany the fever, volume depletion, or hypoxia. Hypotension can signal volume depletion, vasodilation, or cardiac compromise, guiding the clinician toward certain types of bacteria, such as gram negatives, and a more serious infection. The head, ears, eyes, nose, and throat (HEENT) examination may yield signs of ear infection or erythema, exudate, and edema of the oropharynx, which could indicate systemic infection, local infection, or a deep space infection of the pharynx with possible airway compromise. The neck examination may demonstrate lymphadenopathy, nuchal rigidity, or thyroid edema or tenderness, suggesting thyroiditis, a noninfectious cause of fever. The heart examination may elicit murmurs, rubs, tachycardia, or muffling, leading to a diagnosis of endocarditis, pericarditis, or pericardial effusion. The pulmonary examination may demonstrate areas of infiltrate or consolidation. It is important to listen for signs of alveolar fluid (rales) and consolidation (egophony, inspiratory to expiratory ratio [I:E] changes). On abdominal examination you should look for focal areas of tenderness over specific organs or peritoneal signs. Tenderness in the right lower quadrant is suspicious for appendicitis; in the right upper quadrant, cholecystitis; and in the left lower quadrant, diverticulitis. In addition, tenderness in the suprapubic region may be found in urinary tract infections and uterine infections. All sexually active women with abdominal pain and fever should have a pelvic examination looking for cervical motion tenderness, purulent discharge, or adnexal pain, to rule out pelvic inflammatory disease or tubo-ovarian abscess. In men, lower abdominal or groin pain should prompt a genitourinary examination to rule out epididymitis and orchitis. The genitourinary examination may yield discharge, sores, abscesses, testicular edema, or tenderness. Examination of the back should search for pain with palpation over the kidneys (pyelonephritis) or midline spinal tenderness (epidural abscess). The extremity examination may yield ulcers, wounds, or vascular abnormalities. The skin examination should focus on any erythema, rashes, ulcers, fluctuance, wounds, or mottling. The neurological examination may demonstrate mental status changes or meningeal signs, as discussed later. The rectal examination should look for guaiac status, masses, abscesses, fistulas, or prostate tenderness.

The characteristics of specific infectious etiologies are summarized in Table 42.1.

Diagnostic Evaluation

The diagnostic evaluation should be guided by clinical presentation, history, and physical examination. When the presentation does

---

Table 42.1.

Characteristics of specific infectious etiologies

Disease	Characteristics
Abscess	Fever, erythema, fluctuant mass
Appendicitis	Fever, anorexia, pain that starts periumbilically and moves to RLQ at McBurney's point
Biliary tract infection	Right upper quadrant tenderness, jaundice, Murphy's sign (in which tenderness is elicited when the patient inhales bringing the gallbladder up against the examiner's hand, which is palpating the right upper quadrant), possibly with fever. If the triad of fever, jaundice, and right upper quadrant tenderness is present, this is known as Charcot's triad, indicative of ascending cholangitis.
Cellulitis	Erythema, fever, possible edema, tenderness, blanching
Endocarditis	Fever, murmur or rub, possible rash, Osler's nodes (painful nodules at the finger tips), splinter hemorrhages (red or brown longitudinal lines in the nail), petechiae (small red or purple skin lesions suggestive of vascular emboli to the skin)
Gastroenteritis	Abdominal pain, fever, diarrhea, vomiting
Meningitis	Fever, rash, change in mental status, stiff neck, positive Kernig's (involuntary resistance to knee extension when the hip is flexed) or Brudzinski's (flexion at the hips and knees when the neck is flexed) signs
Otitis	Erythematous and bulging eardrum, fever
Pharyngitis	Erythematous pharynx, exudates, pain, fever
Pelvic inflammatory disease	Fever, pain, discharge through the cervical os, cervical motion tenderness, ovarian mass or tenderness
Pneumonia	Fever, focal crackles on lung exam, egophony (patient says "ee" and it is heard as "ay" on auscultation), decreased or asymmetric fremitus (vibrations noted on palpation of the chest wall while the patient speaks), decreased breath sounds
Septic arthritis	Fever; erythematous, painful, inflamed joint
Sepsis	Fever, rigors, hypotension
Sinusitis	Sinus tenderness, nasal discharge, fever
Urinary tract infection	Fever, possible abdominal pain, CVA tenderness if pyelonephritis
Wound infection	Fever, erythema, pus

CVA, costovertebral angle; RLQ, right lower quadrant.

not point in an obvious direction, a broad workup must be initiated.

Radiological Studies

The chest x-ray film is done primarily to look for airspace disease suggesting an infiltrate in the lungs; however, an enlarged heart, vascular congestion, effusions, tumor, or a wide mediastinum may also be observed as other sources of pulmonary and cardiovascular abnormalities.

A computed tomography (CT) scan of the abdomen may be done to look for a source of infection such as appendicitis, diverticulitis, a pancreatic pseudocyst or necrosis, signs of cholecystitis or cholangitis, an abscess, or a fistula.

An ultrasound scan may illustrate a uterine, fallopian tube, or ovarian source of infection or cholecystitis and may be diagnostic in testicular pathological conditions.

Laboratory Tests

Laboratory tests should be ordered based on the suspected source of infection. A WBC count with differential should always be ordered to look for signs of infection and an increase in neutrophils, indicating a bacterial etiology. The cerebrospinal fluid should be sent for cell count, culture, and other pertinent studies in the case of a potential central nervous system (CNS) infection. Sputum should be sent for a Gram stain and culture if any pulmonary symptoms are present. Blood cultures should always be sent for assessment when septicemia is suspected. They are not necessary if the source of the fever is obvious and easily treated, as in pharyngitis or otitis, for example. The electrolytes may be altered with significant dehydration, diarrhea, or vomiting. The BUN and Cr levels may increase with dehydration or disease of the kidney. Liver enzyme results may indicate intrinsic liver disease or obstructive disease of the gallbladder. Coagulation studies should be done, along with blood typing, if there is any need for procedures or surgery. A UA is done to look for a urological or renal source of infection.

Diagnostic Procedures

Diagnostic procedures include lumbar puncture for a suspected CNS infection, a paracentesis for suspected spontaneous bacterial peritonitis, a thoracentesis for a parapneumonic effusion of the lung, a biopsy or débridement of an abscess, an arthrocentesis of a possible joint infection, or other major surgical procedures. Be cautious of introducing a needle into a potential sterile space or cavity if the overlying skin looks infected. Doing an arthrocentesis of a joint in a cellulitic knee may turn a sterile knee into a septic knee.

An electrocardiogram should be done to look for any cardiac etiology of hypotension, signs of pericarditis, ischemia in response to vascular deficiency, or changes indicative of a valvular lesion as a source of infection.

Differential Diagnosis

The differential diagnosis for bacterial infection is illustrated in Table 42.2.

Treatment

As discussed previously, treatment includes antibiotics, treatment of symptoms, and

Table 42.2.

Differential diagnosis of bacterial infection

Abscess
Appendicitis
Biliary tract infection (cholecystitis, cholangitis)
Cellulitis
Diverticulitis
Endocarditis
Gastroenteritis
Meningitis
Necrotizing fasciitis
Otitis
Pharyngitis
Pelvic inflammatory disease
Pneumonia
Septic arthritis
Sepsis
Sinusitis
Pyelonephritis
Wound infection

Table 42.3.

Treatment guidelines for febrile diseases of bacterial origin

Stable Vital Signs

Antipyretic: acetaminophen 1,000 mg, ibuprofen 400–600 mg orally

Consideration focused laboratory testing: complete blood cell (CBC) count, possible need for blood cultures (e.g., suspected endocarditis), urinalysis and culture

Chest x-ray film for pulmonary source

Other studies: directed by history and physical examination (e.g., ultrasound scan for suspected cholecystitis)

Procedures: Diagnostic and/or therapeutic

 Incision and drainage of abscess

 Operating room for operative treatment

 Arthrocentesis for suspected septic joint

 Lumbar puncture for suspected meningitis

Oral antibiotics for outpatient treatment

IV antibiotics for inpatient treatment

Unstable Vital Signs/Sepsis: Hypotension, Tachycardia, and Tachypnea

Antipyretic: acetaminophen 1,000 mg orally or per rectum, ibuprofen 400–600 mg orally

IV access: administration of normal saline fluid bolus (1–2 L)

Vasopressors IV (If persistent hypotension despite fluids)

 Dopamine IV

 Dobutamine if CHF present

 Norepinephrine

Oxygen for hypoxia: consider of intubation for persistent hypotension and hypoxia, despite fluids, oxygen, and IV pressors

Laboratory testing: CBC count, blood chemistries levels, two sets of blood cultures, liver function tests for suspected biliary source, amylase and lipase for pancreatitis

Foley catheter placement, urinalysis and urine culture

Chest x-ray film for pulmonary source

ECG for secondary cardiac ischemia

Other studies directed toward suspected diagnosis (e.g., ultrasound scan for cholecystitis, CT scan of abdomen for suspected appendicitis or diverticulitis, and so forth)

IV antibiotics (Directed to specific source)

 If unknown source and septic patient, use broad-spectrum antibiotic coverage that can be narrowed once source is known:

 Imipenem or meropenem

 Aminoglycoside plus antipseudomonal penicillin or third-generation cephalosporin plus clindamycin or metronidazole (e.g. ampicillin, gentamicin, and metronidazole)

 Third- or fourth-generation cephalosporin plus clindamycin or metronidazole

 Vancomycin 1 g IV for methicillin resistant *Staphylococcus aureus*

CHF, congestive heart failure; CT, computed tomography; ECG, electrocardiogram; IV intravenous.

cardiovascular support (Table 42.3). Current research supports the length of time until antibiotics are administered as being very significant in improving outcomes.

Antibiotics must be chosen based on the etiology of the infection. If the source is not readily identified and the patient is exhibiting signs of sepsis, broad-spectrum antibiotics must be initiated before identifying the source based on the cultures and other studies. Prior history of significant infection and antibiotic use should be examined to avoid potential resistant organisms. For sepsis in a nonimmunocompromised adult, *The Sanford Guide to Antimicrobial Therapy 2003* recommends antipseudomonal penicillin, imipenem or meropenem; an aminoglycoside plus anti-pseudomonal penicillin or a third-generation cephalosporin plus clindamycin or metronidazole; or either a third- or fourth-generation cephalosporin or a fluoroquinalone plus clindamycin or Flagyl. Vancomycin should be added whenever methicillin-resistant *Staphylococcus aureus* (MRSA) is suspected. All the antibiotic therapies mentioned should be in IV form regardless of absorption rates, because of the potential inability to swallow oral medications, possible gastrointestinal (GI) tract hypoperfusion, and other potential GI abnormalities.

Sometimes it is possible to remove the source of infection, for example, by surgically opening an abscess, performing an appendectomy, or débriding or amputating infected tissue. Oxygen should be administered to support the patient with hypoxemia. Care should be taken whenever using supplemental oxygen to avoid causing carbon dioxide retention in certain patients with chronic obstructive pulmonary disease (COPD).

Cardiovascular support initially is in the form of IV fluids, usually an isotonic solution such as normal saline, or blood products if indicated. High volumes are often necessary to overcome the very low systemic vascular resistance common in septic shock. You must be aware of the possibility of potential fluid overload after the patient recovers, if the cardiovascular and renal system are unable to excrete the excess (usually in a patient with preexisting renal failure or congestive heart failure). Vasopressors and inotropic agents are often needed in addition to fluids. Dopamine is usually the first-line drug, because it has both inotropic β-effect and vasopressor α-effect. The second-line drug is either dobutamine for more inotropic support, which is especially helpful in patients with a history of poor myocardial ejection fraction or congestive heart failure, or norepinephrine for more vasopressor effect. The addition of epinephrine when all else fails is usually the last line of support, correlating with a very poor outcome because of the severity of disease. Pulmonary support and airway protection with intubation may be required in the hypoperfused patient because of the severely depressed mental status and inability to protect the airway. In addition, patients who are severely hypoxic from either pneumonia or pulmonary edema may need intubation. Caring for the septic patient who is designated "do not resuscitate/do not intubate" (DNR/DNI) should proceed without compromise as in any other patient. The exception is the patient who has taken care to specify that he or she does not wish to receive pressors. Otherwise, the "R" in DNR refers to the resuscitation of the "newly dead," that is, it refers to the treatment reserved for the advanced cardiac life support (ACLS) protocols in a patient who has lost all vital signs. If there is time, and the patient is unable to communicate, it is helpful to contact the patient's health care proxy for guidance should intubation be necessary.

Disposition

The disposition of the patient with a fever related to infection of bacterial origin is dependent on the patient's comorbidities and the extent of the infection. Young healthy patients with single-lobe pneumonia, small areas of cellulitis, or abscesses that have been drained, for example, can often be treated on an outpatient basis if no other significant comorbidities or vital sign abnormalities exist. Similar presentations in an older, diabetic patient may require a brief hospital observation admission. Patients with more significant infection requiring IV antibiotics, continuous oxygen saturation monitoring, and aggressive pulmonary treatments or requiring frequent wound assessment and treatment may require longer hospital admissions. Patients requiring aggressive fluid resuscitation and possible vasopressor and inotropic support require an intensive care unit admission. The individual patient must also be assessed for the home support system, homelessness, alcohol or drug addiction, or nursing home support system, guiding one either toward or against admission in borderline cases. Care should also be taken not to discharge that patient who at present appears stable but may decline rapidly. This is a skill acquired with experience.

Pathophysiology

Sepsis is largely the result of the body's response to infection, not simply the direct result of the presence of bacteria. Septic shock occurs when sepsis leads to a decrease in tissue perfusion with or without hypotension. Although hypoperfusion may be related to fluid losses (e.g., diarrhea or vomiting), it is more commonly the result of the systemic response to the infection.

In patients with septic shock, there is an initial decrease in systemic vascular resistance along with a state of high cardiac output. However, the cardiac function is eventually depressed. Capillary leak often leads to shunting, which can contribute to hypoxia. These changes all lead to a drop in blood pressure, which may be refractory to administration of fluid, inotropic agents, and vasopressors. Tachypnea and hyperventilation are often present because of the hypoxemia that is related to shunting. Severe shock can lead to multisystem organ failure and death resulting from severe end-organ hypoperfusion.

The host immune system reacts in response to an endotoxin, in the case of gram-negative bacteria, or an exotoxin, in the case of gram-positive bacteria. Endotoxemia may correlate with illness severity.

The endotoxin can induce arterial dilation and venous constriction, causing pooling of the blood in the capillary beds. Gram-positive bacterial components can mimic the activity of the gram-negative endotoxin. Either the toxin or the antibody-antigen complexes can also activate the complement system, which in turn can result in vasodilation, capillary leak, activation of phagocytes, and direct attack of the bacteria. The mechanism of the vasodilatation is unclear, but an increase in nitric oxide production and a deficiency in the hormone vasopressin are thought to play roles. Vascular leaking can occur in both the pulmonary and systemic vasculature, contributing to a decrease in the circulating intravascular volume.

Macrophages release specific cytokines, including tumor necrosis factor (TNF)-α, interleukin (IL)-1, and IL-6, which further enhance the inflammatory responses. TNF-α potentially increases the effect of tissue factor on endothelial cells, stimulates extrinsic coagulation, and decreases protein C and S activity, leading to hypercoagulation and eventually decreasing the activity of the fibrinolytic system. Microthrombi can form in the skin and end organs, prothrombin time (PT) and partial thromboplastin time (PTT) may increase, and disseminated intravascular coagulation (DIC) may occur, characterized by uncontrollable bleeding. TNF-α and IL-1 have a potentially synergistic effect; they also increase the effects of other cytokines. Cytokines play a role in endothelial cell injury, leading to vascular leak and decreased vascular tone and increasing nitric oxide production and therefore vasodilation. Cytokines can also alter cardiac function, further affecting the circulatory system. IL-6 increases acute phase responses and is one of the cytokines that has been shown to correlate with outcome.

Suggested Readings

Barriere SL, Lowry SF. An overview of mortality risk prediction in sepsis. *Crit Care Med* 1995; 23:376–393.

Bates B. *A guide to physical examination and history taking*, 5th ed. Philadelphia: JB Lippincott, 1991.

Berkow R, ed, Fletcher MB, asst. ed. *The Merck manual of diagnosis and therapy*, 16th ed. Rahway, NJ: Merck Research Laboratories, 1992.

Editors of Market House Books Ltd. *The Bantam medical dictionary*, rev. ed. New York: Bantam Books, 1990.

Gilbert DN, Moellering RC, Sande MA, eds. *The Sanford guide to antimicrobial therapy 2000*, 30th ed. Hyde Park, VT: Antimicrobial Therapy, Inc, 2000.

Levinson WE, Jawetz E. *Medical microbiology and immunology*, 3rd ed. Norwalk, CT: Appleton & Lange, 1994.

Opal SM, Cohen J. Clinical gram-positive sepsis: does it fundamentally differ from gram-negative bacterial sepsis? *Crit Care Med* 1999;27: 1608–1616.

Rosen P, ed, Barkin R, sr. ed. *Emergency medicine concepts and clinical practice*, 4th ed. St. Louis: Mosby, 1998.

Wiessner WH, Casey LC, Zbilut P. Treatment of sepsis and septic shock: a review. *Heart Lung* 1995;24:380–393.

CHAPTER 43

Fever of Uncertain Etiology

Brian J. Hession, MD

Clinical Scenario

A 78-year-old woman with a past medical history significant for adult-onset diabetes mellitus and hypertension presented to the emergency department (ED) complaining of a 3-week history of subjective fever and intermittent chills. On review of systems, she denied headache, neck stiffness, photophobia, cough, shortness of breath, chest pain, abdominal pain, nausea, dysuria, or frequency. On presentation, her vital signs demonstrated a tympanic temperature of 101.4°F, a blood pressure of 113/61 mm Hg, a regular heart rate of 114 beats/minute, and a respiratory rate of 15 breaths/minute, with a room air pulse oximetry reading of 96%. Her fingerstick glucose level was 142 mg/dL.

On physical examination, she demonstrated a normal head, ears, eyes, nose, and throat (HEENT) examination. Her neck was nontender and supple. Examination of her lungs showed full and equal breath sounds. Auscultation of the heart revealed a regular rate with a grade II/VI systolic murmur at the upper sternal border radiating toward the carotids. Her abdomen was soft and nontender with normal bowel sounds. Her extremities were unremarkable. Pulses were full and equal. No rashes or lesions were evident on her skin. She was oriented to person, place, and date and the remainder of her neurological examination was nonfocal. This patient was given a 1-g dose of acetaminophen. Intravenous (IV) access was established, and blood was drawn for laboratory analysis, including blood cultures and a complete blood cell (CBC) count. A urinalysis was obtained, and findings were normal.

A chest x-ray film was also obtained and was interpreted as normal. A second blood culture was ordered, and the patient was admitted to the general medical service for further workup and observation.

Clinical Evaluation

Introduction

Fever is a relatively common reason for patients to present to the ED, accounting for 6% of adult and 20% of pediatric visits. Fever is not a diagnosis but rather suggests an underlying disease. The entity of "fever of unknown (or uncertain) origin," also known as FUO, is a challenging condition. The definition of FUO is at least 3 weeks of fever with temperature elevations of 101°F (38.3°C) and 1 week of investigation in the hospital. This challenges the physician to use clues from the patient's history and physical examination findings and results of diagnostic testing to arrive at a diagnosis explaining the presentation of fever. For the purposes of this chapter, we concentrate on any patient who presents with fever without obvious source, instead of the narrowly defined condition of FUO.

Special consideration is needed for a few groups of patients presenting to the ED with fever. The extremes of age, both old and young, often have atypical presentations of common illnesses. Immunocompromised patients not only have atypical presentations of typical illnesses but also present with infections that would not be considered in the immunocompetent host. In addition to a thorough physical examination, history, and review of systems, these patients must be approached with a broad differential diagnosis.

This section discusses the ED approach to the patient presenting with fever without an obvious source.

History

Historical information should begin with the fever. This includes how long the fever has been present, whether the patient has documented fever at home, any antipyretics used and when last taken, and any cyclical nature of the fever. Past medical conditions may help direct the workup and should be elicited, along with any recent travel, past infections, or surgeries. In addition, all medications and allergies should be noted.

The most common source of fever is infectious and is often readily discovered by history, review of systems, and physical examination. The initial history should focus on infectious causes of fever (see Chapter 42). If an infectious source is not obvious or has been ruled out, further history should include a broader differential.

A history of intravenous drug use (IVDU) is important to elicit. Back pain (epidural abscess), skin infections, endocarditis, and human immunodeficiency virus (HIV) infection are all associated with IVDU and may require more extensive workup. In addition, a recent history of IV drug injection, with the drug drawn up through a piece of cotton, may suggest "cotton fever." An entity unique to IVDU, cotton fever is thought to be due to a reaction to foreign material drawn up from the cotton and injected. It is usually a diagnosis of exclusion, with a history as noted previously. The fever is self-limited but the patient's temperature may be very high.

Occult Infections

Infectious causes of fever are discussed in earlier chapters; however, a review of the signs and symptoms of occult infections with serious morbidity and mortality is worth repeating. They include endocarditis, central nervous system (CNS) infections, and septic arthritis. The severity of signs and

symptoms in patients presenting with infective endocarditis often depends on the virulence of the offending organism and whether the pathological condition is acute or subacute. Fever is a defining and often the most obvious feature of infective endocarditis. Other symptoms may include chills, rigors, dyspnea, chest pain, fatigue, malaise, and/or arthralgias.

CNS infections carry such significant morbidity that they should be included in the differential diagnosis of every patient presenting with fever of unproved etiology. Bacterial meningitis classically presents with fever, headache, nuchal rigidity, altered mental status, and photophobia. In many cases of CNS infection, some of these symptoms may be absent; therefore, the presence of one or more of these symptoms in the setting of fever warrants consideration of meningitis and initiation of the appropriate confirmatory workup (see Chapter 30).

Septic arthritis is another emergency that may present with fever. However, patients with septic arthritis typically present to the ED because of acute joint pain rather than because of fever. Any patient presenting with a complaint of arthralgia or joint effusion (with or without fever) should be carefully assessed for any evidence of a septic joint.

Fever is often the most common presenting sign of intraabdominal infections and abscesses. Spontaneous bacterial peritonitis is an infection that typically occurs in the presence of ascites. Ascites is often a result of hepatic cirrhosis. Offending organisms are typically enteric gram-negative bacilli. The patient typically reports a history of ascites that predates the complaint of fever or abdominal pain.

Intraabdominal abscesses are also a source of fever that may not be obvious. Liver, splenic, renal, and perinephric abscesses are the most common intraabdominal abscesses. In addition to fever, these patients may present with a leukocytosis and abdominal pain referable to the anatomic site of infection.

Patients with sinusitis typically complain of pain in an anatomic distribution that correlates to an underlying sinus space, which is inflamed. Fever, chills, or rigors in this setting may be attributable to the sinusitis or may suggest a more concerning extension of this infection. Such patients are typically more toxic and may present with orbital cellulitis, periorbital cellulitis, facial cellulitis, or facial abscess.

Noninfectious Causes of Fever

A history of toxic ingestions or illicit drug use should be discussed. Many drugs cause fever. In addition, common medications can cause drug fever at any point in their use.

Fever may be present in approximately half of patients with pulmonary embolus. Although fever would not be the only finding expected in such a patient, it may be the patient's main complaint. Additional history might include chest pain and shortness of breath (see Chapter 5).

Malignancies can cause fever; however, a more common scenario is the cancer patient who presents with fever referable to an infectious process in the setting of chemotherapy- or radiation-induced immunosuppression. Occult malignancy should be considered in the differential diagnosis of a patient presenting with fever without any obvious etiology. A history of chronic pain, night sweats, unexplained weight loss, or neurological symptoms (in the patient with a CNS tumor) may lead you to investigate possible cancers.

Factitious fever may be considered when the patient's history of present illness sounds suspicious or implausible or when the magnitude of fever appears disproportionate to vital signs and physical findings. The term *factitious fever* is used to indicate cases in which the mechanism of measuring body temperature has been manipulated to indicate a false elevation of body temperature.

Physical Examination

As in any patient with fever, infectious sources must be sought. The physical examination must include a thorough examination of the oropharynx, ears, neck, and teeth. Lungs may reveal decreased breath sounds and rales or rhonchi associated with pneumonia. A new heart murmur in a patient with a fever may be the first evidence of endocarditis. Abdominal tenderness may indicate specific infections in organ systems or intraabdominal abscess. The skin may reveal abscesses or rashes consistent with cellulitis.

Endocarditis

A thorough physical examination may elicit physical manifestations of endocarditis. Heart murmurs are typically identified in the course of the disease. Any new murmur or change in a preexisting murmur is suggestive of endocarditis until proven otherwise. Less common manifestations of endocarditis include splinter hemorrhages, Janeway lesions, Osler nodes, and Roth spots. Splinter hemorrhages are subungual linear streaking hemorrhages. Janeway lesions are small nodular hemorrhagic lesions found on the palms or soles of the feet. Osler nodes are small painful nodules typically found on the fingertip or toe pads. Roth spots are oval retinal hemorrhages with a pale center seen in a small percentage of endocarditis cases.

Septic Arthritis

On physical examination, the involved joint typically is exquisitely tender; may have a palpable effusion, erythema, and warmth (or "hot"); and demonstrates a limited range of motion. Patients who provide a history of IVDU, are immunocompromised, have prior joint infection, and have any underlying joint abnormality are of particular interest. These patients are at increased risk for infective arthritis. Patients can have both septic and crystalline arthritides simultaneously.

Pulmonary Embolism

Patients presenting with a pulmonary embolism often have lowered oxygen saturation, tachypnea, and tachycardia. Findings such as rales, gallop, fever, and phlebitis may also be observed. The classic presentation and findings cannot be relied on.

Drug Fever

Drug fever has no specific findings on physical examination, although it may be associated with a diffuse erythematous maculopapular rash. There may be a history of starting a new medication recently; otherwise, only the suspicion of drug fever can lead you to its eventual diagnosis.

Neuroleptic Malignant Syndrome

Neuroleptic medications are used primarily as antipsychotics. Neuroleptic malignant syndrome (NMS) usually manifests within the first week of therapy initiation. Muscular rigidity is due to extrapyramidal effects of the central dopaminergic blockade, and thus may also present with involuntary muscular movements and/or dysarthria. Autonomic instability manifests as tachycardia, labile blood pressure, and cardiac rhythm disturbances.

Toxic Ingestions

Toxic ingestions may be diagnosed during physical examination by observing constellations of signs and symptoms known as toxidromes (see Chapter 52).

Diagnostic Evaluation

Laboratory Studies

Evidence has demonstrated that the white blood cell (WBC) total count is neither sensitive nor specific for identifying persons with a serious bacterial infection; thus, caution must be used not to rule out a serious infection if the WBC count is normal. Several noninfectious entities can elevate the WBC count, including burns, corticosteroid use, Cushing's syndrome, diabetic ketoacidosis, epinephrine administration, and fractures. The differential may be helpful. A high percentage of bands suggest bacterial etiologies. High eosinophilia count may suggest drug reaction or parasite infection. A high lymphocyte count or atypical lymphocytes may suggest viral etiologies such as infectious mononucleosis.

Blood cultures should be considered on any patient with fever of unknown source. Typically, two sets are sent to the laboratory before administration of antibiotics, if any are to be given.

One may consider obtaining an erythrocyte sedimentation rate (ESR) on a patient with fever of uncertain etiology. The ESR is a nonspecific test with poor sensitivity, which may reflect a variety of inflammatory states including infection. The Westergren ESR is the most commonly used test. This is performed by diluting a sample of anticoagulated blood, allowing it to settle in a standardized 200-mm glass tube for a time period of 1 hour, and then measuring the "rate of sedimentation" in units of millimeters per hour (mm/hour). Generally, red blood cells (erythrocytes) aggregate and settle slowly (0 to 20 mm/hour). However, in the presence of acute-phase products, the aggregation and sedimentation of erythrocytes is much more rapid (>30 mm/hour). The ESR is elevated not only in infection but also in collagen vascular disorders, neoplasms, thyroid disorders, rheumatic illness, temporal arteritis, and rheumatoid arthritis. Other processes, namely hemoglobinopathies, predictably lead to decreased ESR results. Even in the setting of proven infection, the ESR value can be difficult to interpret because it may not rise immediately and may remain elevated even after the infection resolves. However, the ESR is another laboratory tool at your disposal in the evaluation of fever. Like the ESR, the C-reactive protein (CRP) is another laboratory test with some utility in confirming an infectious process. CRP is an acute-phase reactant and is elevated in many inflammatory conditions including infectious arthritis. Like the ESR, it is very nonspecific and can be elevated in a broad array of inflammatory and infectious diseases.

A urinalysis must be obtained on all patients with fever of unknown source. The populations most likely to harbor an occult urinary tract infection include those in the pediatric or elderly groups and immunocompromised patients.

Toxicology screens should be obtained to search for drugs that produce fever such as tricyclic antidepressants (TCAs), amphetamines, and cocaine.

Determining arterial blood gas levels may be helpful to estimate severity of illness (acidosis) or hypoxia in particular cases.

Radiographic Studies

The haphazard ordering of radiological studies is not supported in the absence of any history or physical examination findings pointing toward a specific diagnosis. However, using a chest radiograph as a screening tool in the appropriate population may be supported, given the frequency of pulmonary sources of fever. Any patient with unclear etiology of fever should have posteroanterior (PA) and lateral chest x-ray films to rule out pneumonia, atelectasis, elevated hemidiaphragm, pleural effusion, or undiagnosed cancers.

A focused computed tomography (CT) scan may help diagnose a neoplasm, pulmonary embolus, intraabdominal infection, or an abscess when indicated by history or physical examination.

Diagnostic Evaluation of Select Etiologies

When endocarditis is suspected, the patient should have three sets of blood cultures, each taken from a different site. In addition, the patient should have an echocardiogram or transesophageal echocardiogram (TEE) to look for vegetations on the leaflets of the heart valves.

When septic arthritis is suspected, plain radiographs of the acute infected joint are typically normal and nondiagnostic. Arthrocentesis is the diagnostic test of choice. Synovial fluid culture does not always yield the offending organism but is estimated to do so in approximately half of cases. The usual infectious agents include *Staphylococcus* and *Streptococcus* species, *Haemophilus influenzae*, and *Gonococcus* or *Meningococcus* species. Antibiotic therapy is warranted to prevent destruction of the joint with significant functional loss. Wide-spectrum antibiotic therapy with a penicillinase-resistant penicillin with or without an aminoglycoside is the recommended therapy. Orthopedic consultation is required, and surgical intervention may be necessary as well.

The diagnosis of spontaneous bacterial peritonitis is confirmed by the isolation of a pathogen from a sample of ascites fluid obtained by paracentesis. Because results of cultures and Gram stain may be negative for organisms, the finding of 300 polymorphonuclear neutrophils (PMNs) per microliter of fluid is also considered a positive paracentesis. Broad-spectrum antibiotic therapy with penicillinase-resistant penicillin, an aminoglycoside, and metronidazole is recommended to cover for the usual enteric pathogens.

If an occult intraabdominal abscess is suspected, an imaging study such as ultrasonography or CT scan is indicated. Morbidity and mortality of these infections is high; thus, hospital admission for IV antibiotics is warranted.

If a complicated sinusitis is suspected, a CT scan of the head is an appropriate diagnostic modality. IV antibiotics and hospital admission are also indicated.

Differential Diagnosis

Table 43.1 lists a broad differential diagnosis. Many of these conditions have been discussed in earlier chapters. In addition to the table, some of the noninfectious causes of fever are discussed in this section.

Drug Fever

Drug fever is a diagnosis of exclusion without any confirmatory diagnostic test. Any medication is capable of producing a febrile response. Drug fever is produced through a variety of mechanisms, but the most common is a hypersensitivity reaction in which the end result is production of endogenous pyrogen. The initial host immune response may be directed toward the active ingredient of the medication, an impurity, or an inert component. Antibiotics are perhaps the most common medications that elicit drug fever. Penicillins, cephalosporins, and sulfonamides have been implicated as more common precipitants of drug fever. Cessation of therapy with the offending agent will eliminate the fever.

Toxic ingestions include use of illicit drugs and intentional and unintentional overdoses of prescription medicines. Stimulants like cocaine, amphetamine, and other sympa-

Table 43.1.

Differential diagnosis of fever of unknown etiology

Infectious Diseases (not just bacterial infection)
Tuberculosis
Bacterial endocarditis
Intraabdominal infections (liver, subphrenic, renal, splenic, or perinephric abscess)
Others: subacute cholangitis, chronic prostatitis, hepatitis, infectious mononucleosis, fungal
    infections (histoplasmosis, cryptococcosis), malaria, brucellosis, babesiosis, Lyme disease,
    AIDS, Q fever, Rocky Mountain spotted fever, psittacosis, LGV, ehrlichiosis, amebiasis,
    toxoplasmosis, osteomyelitis, leishmaniasis

Collagen-Vascular Diseases
Vasculitis, hypersensitivity vasculitis
Polymyalgia rheumatica, giant cell arteritis
SLE
RA, adult Still's disease
Others: polyarteritis nodosa, juvenile RA, Wegener's granulomatosis, polymyositis

Drugs
Barbiturates
Antibiotics (sulfonamides, penicillins, nitrofurantoin, amphotericin B, isoniazid [INH],
    cephalosporins, rifampin, paraaminosalicylic acid, vancomycin, tetracyclines)
Antihypertensives (methyldopa, diuretics, nifedipine, hydralazine)
Antiarrhythmics (procainamide, quinidine)
Drugs of abuse (amphetamines, cocaine, anticholinergics, PCP)
Phenytoin
Others: antihistamines, salicylates, cimetidine, bleomycin, allopurinol, heparin, meperidine,
    propylthiouracil

Oncological Conditions
Tumor lysis
Occult malignancy

Miscellaneous
Factitious fever
Cotton fever
Pulmonary emboli
Hyperthermia
Malignant hyperthermia
Periodic fever, central fever (rare)
IBD
Others: subacute thyroiditis, FMF, retroperitoneal hematoma, alcoholic hepatitis,
    granulomatous hepatitis, aortic-enteric fistula, thyrotoxicosis, Kawasaki disease, sarcoidosis,
    hyperimmunoglobulinemia D syndrome

AIDS, acquired immunodeficiency disease syndrome; FMF, familial Mediterranean fever; IBD,
inflammatory bowel disease; LGV, lymphogranuloma venereum; PCP, phencyclidine; RA, rheumatoid
arthritis; SLE, systemic lupus erythematosus.

thomimetics cause patients to present with agitation, tachycardia, and sometimes fever. Neuroleptics, salicylates, anticholinergics, and lithium all may cause fever as part of their respective toxidromes.

Neuroleptic Malignant Syndrome

NMS is most often attributable to the use of the phenothiazine antipsychotic medication haloperidol, but it can be seen with use of many neuroleptic medications. NMS may be mediated by central dopaminergic blockade. There is no confirmatory diagnostic test; the diagnosis is made on a clinical basis and by exclusion of other causes of fever or hyperthermia. The cornerstone of NMS treatment is the cessation of neuroleptic therapy, followed by provision of symptomatic treatment. Hypotension should be addressed with fluid resuscitation and α-agonists, if necessary. Hypertension secondary to vasoconstriction may be responsive to nitroprusside therapy. Cardiac abnormalities, if present, may mimic TCA overdose and should be treated with bicarbonate if appropriate. The profound hyperthermia requires cooling with measures such as a cooling blanket, fans, ice, and antipyretics. Muscular rigidity may be treated with dantrolene. Patients with NMS warrant admission to the hospital in an intensive care setting.

Neoplasm and Fever

Several malignancies are capable of generating fever in the host. Lymphoma (Hodgkin's and non-Hodgkin's), leukemia, renal cell tumors, hepatoma, and CNS tumors are the most common tumors implicated as the source of neoplastic fever. These neoplasms typically elicit fever either by directly producing and liberating endogenous pyrogen or by initiating a host immune response with the subsequent elaboration of endogenous pyrogen. Tumor fever is another diagnosis of exclusion without any specific confirmatory diagnostic test.

Heat Stroke

Heat stroke is a disorder in which the body's capability to dissipate heat is overwhelmed by a dysfunction of thermoregulation. Exertional heat stroke typically affects younger patients who engage in strenuous physical activity during periods of high ambient temperature and humidity. These individuals are commonly healthy athletes or military personnel. Heat stroke is a clinical diagnosis and a diagnosis of exclusion. Laboratory work should be performed to assess for potential end-organ damage. An electrocardiogram (ECG) and chest radiograph should be performed. A head CT scan or lumbar puncture may be needed to evaluate altered mental status. Continuous cardiac monitoring is warranted. When suspected, heat stroke should be immediately treated with cooling techniques.

Factitious Fever

Although factitious fever should not be high on your list of differential diagnosis, it should be noted here that there are psychiatric causes for "fever." Direct observation, use of an electronic tympanic thermometer, comparison of two temperatures from two different anatomic sites, and measurement of fresh voided urine temperature are all measures that can help determine if a fever is factitious.

Treatment

Treatment is entirely dependent on cause. When an infectious etiology is known, appropriate therapy should be initiated. Antibiotics should be chosen to target the responsible agent or location of infection. When indicated, surgical intervention may be required. The difficulty in treatment comes when the etiology of fever is not certain. In some patients, a diagnosis may be suspected. It is the individual clinician's decision whether to treat the patient to cover a broad range of possibilities while awaiting laboratory test results, or to wait and watch with close follow-up. In any patient who appears ill, has underlying medical conditions, or is at the extremes of age, it may be prudent to treat with antibiotics while awaiting results of final cultures and any other tests (Table 43.2).

Disposition

Disposition depends on the patient's general state of health, and the suspected diagnosis.

Table 43.2.

General treatment summary

All patients: Place on IV, and begin hydration if indicated. Obtain blood tests as indicated.

- For most patients this step includes CBC count with differential, electrolyte levels, and two sets of blood cultures.
- When indicated include liver function tests, ESR, CRP, coagulation studies, and a third blood culture.
- Specialized laboratory testing when indicated, such as HIV test, collagen vascular disease testing, and thyroid studies. For the purposes of the ED visit, these are not usually indicated but are sent as inpatient studies.

All patients: Obtain urinalysis and chest radiograph.

Attempts at cooling the patient should be made as follows:

- For all patients with no evidence of liver failure, 1 g of acetaminophen. Alternatively ibuprofen 600–800 mg can be given or ketorolac 15–30 mg IV or IM can be given.
- For patients with suspected cocaine or amphetamine fever, malignant hyperthermia, or hyperthermia, external cooling techniques should be undertaken.
- For patients suspected of malignant hyperthermia: dantrolene 2.5 mg/kg IV should be given.

For patients with suspected joint infection: arthrocentesis.

For patients with suspected CNS infection: lumbar puncture after CT scan (if indicated)

For patients with suspected intraabdominal pathology: abdominal imaging as indicated (abdominal ultrasound or CT scan).

Patients with suspected bacterial infection should receive etiology driven antibiotics.

Patients who are ill appearing, have comorbidity, or immunocompromised status should be admitted.

CBC, complete blood cell; CNS, central nervous system; CRP, C-reactive protein; CT, computed tomography; ESR, erythrocyte sedimentation rate; HIV, human immunodeficiency virus; IM, intramuscular; IV, intravenous.

For any patient who appears ill, may be immunocompromised, or is chronically ill, admission is suggested. Patients who may not require admission, but in whom the diagnosis is not known, should have close follow-up. Patients who are septic or have depressed mental status may require intensive care admission. Patients with fever of a toxicological etiology that resolves after a period of observation may be safely discharged.

Pathophysiology

The human thermoregulatory center lies in the preoptic region of the anterior hypothalamus. The hypothalamus tightly controls body temperature by sensing local blood temperature and coordinating this information with the input of neurons from more peripheral temperature receptors. Fever is an elevation of body temperature above this hypothalamic set point, caused by an imbalance between heat production by the body tissues and heat dissipation. It is believed that upregulation of prostaglandin (PG) E_2 synthesis by vascular endothelial cells surrounding the hypothalamus causes elevations in body temperature. The diffusion of PGE_2 into the hypothalamus triggers a cyclic-adenosine monophosphate (cAMP) second messenger that ultimately resets the hypothalamic thermostat to a higher temperature. Fever is then produced when the central message is sent out to increase heat production in the muscles and liver and to increase heat conservation via peripheral vasoconstriction, which inhibits heat dissipation.

Substances that cause fever are referred to as pyrogens. Endogenous pyrogens are fever-causing substances that are produced by the host, typically in response to infection or inflammation. Exogenous pyrogens are generated outside the host and initiate a fever when incorporated into the internal milieu.

There are several endogenously derived polypeptides known as cytokines that are capable of producing fever. The cytokines most commonly implicated are the interleukins. The interleukins play an important role in mediating the local host immune response by promoting activation and chemotaxis of neutrophils, phagocytes, and lymphocytes. These cytokines also initiate the acute-phase response, inducing the hepatic synthesis of factors such as CRP, fibrinogen, ferritin, haptoglobin, and complement components. Lastly, these cytokines cause an increased hypothalamic prostaglandin synthesis that mediates an elevation of the hypothalamic temperature set point via cAMP.

Exogenous pyrogens arise outside of the human host but have the capacity to induce fever when incorporated within that host. These substances include microorganisms, their toxins, or their products and are best characterized by the gram-negative bacteria. All gram-negative bacteria contain a lipopolysaccharide (LPS) as a component of their cell outer membrane. LPS has been shown to produce fever when introduced into the systemic circulation in very small amounts. It is believed that the mechanism of fever production is via a direct effect on brain endothelial cell prostaglandin synthesis. Gram-positive bacteria are also capable of causing fever attributable to cell wall constituents.

Suggested Readings

Barkin RM, Rosen P. Fever in children. In: Barkin RM, Rosen P., eds. *Emergency pediatrics: a guide to ambulatory care*, 5th ed. St Louis: Mosby, 1999.

Berkowitz CD. Fever. In: Tintinalli JE, Kelen GD, Stapczynski JS, et al, eds. *Emergency medicine a comprehensive study guide*, 4th ed. New York: McGraw-Hill, 1996:749–753.

Blum FC. Fever. In: Marx J, Hockberger R, Walls R, eds. *Rosen's emergency medicine concepts and clinical practice*, 5th ed. St. Louis: Mosby, 2002.

Dinarello CA, Wolff SA. Fever of unknown origin. In: Mandell GL, Douglas RG, Bennett JE, et al, eds. *Principles and practice of infectious diseases*, 3rd ed. New York: Wiley, 1990.

Gallagher EJ, Brooks F, Gennis P. Identification of serious illness in febrile adults. *Am J Emerg Med* 1994;12:129–133.

Gelfand JA, Dinarello CA, Wolff SA. Fever, including fever of unknown origin. In: Isselbacher KJ, Martin JB, Braunwald E, et al, eds. *Harrison's principles of internal medicine*, 13th ed. New York: McGraw-Hill, 1994:125–133.

Leinicke T, Navitsky R, Cameron SA, et al. Fever in the elderly. *Emerg Med Pract* 1999;1(5): 1–15.

Yarbrough B, Vicario S. Heat illness. In: Marx J, Hockberger R, Walls R, et al, eds. *Rosen's emergency medicine concepts and clinical practice*, 5th ed. St. Louis: Mosby, 2002.

Fever
Questions and Answers

Questions

1. Which test is considered the "gold standard" to diagnose malaria in a patient presenting to the emergency department (ED) with high fevers after a recent trip to Central Africa?

A. Chest x-ray film

B. Blood culture

C. Blood smear

D. Urinalysis

E. Stool culture

2. A patient with known human immunodeficiency virus (HIV) disease and a CD4 count of 250 presents to the emergency department (ED) complaining of fever, cough, shortness of breath, and generalized malaise. The most likely diagnosis in this patient is:

A. *Pneumocystis carinii* pneumonia (PCP)

B. Community-acquired pneumonia

C. Mycobacterial pneumonia

D. Toxoplasmosis

E. Upper respiratory infection

3. Which of the following is not a viral hemorrhagic fever?

A. Yellow fever

B. Dengue hemorrhagic fever

C. Malaria

D. Ebola

4. A 45-year-old man is sent to the emergency department (ED) from a detox facility for evaluation of fever. The patient complains of fever, chronic cough with green sputum, and weakness. He denies headache. He has a history of alcoholism. He denies intravenous drug use (IVDU). He is a smoker. His vital signs include a temperature of 102°F, pulse of 120 beats/minute, blood pressure of 160/90 mm Hg, and oxygen saturation of 93% on room air. He is moderately ill appearing. Head, ears, eyes, nose, and throat (HEENT) examination is unremarkable, neck is supple, and lungs show coarse breath sounds with rales in the right upper lobe area. He is mildly tremulous. The rest of his examination is unremarkable. Which is the best choice for his workup?

A. Chest x-ray film, intravenous (IV) line, O$_2$, blood samples for complete blood count (CBC) and culture

B. IV with blood for culture and CBC, chest x-ray film, and admission to hospital

C. IV; O$_2$; CBC and culture; chest x-ray film; consideration of benzodiazepines, antibiotics, and hospital admission

D. IV, O$_2$, CBC and blood culture, urine culture, chest x-ray film, head computed tomography (CT) scan, lumbar puncture (LP), antibiotics, and admission

5. A patient presents to the emergency department (ED) with complaint of fever. The patient is a 33-year-old woman with a long history of intravenous drug use (IVDU). She has myalgias, arthralgias, headache, generalized fatigue, and a 3-day history of fevers to 103°F. On physical examination, she is noted to have no obvious source of infection. The most appropriate workup and disposition of this patient is:

A. Discharge to home with good instructions and follow-up.

B. Check a complete blood count (CBC). If the patient has elevated white blood cell (WBC) levels, admit to the hospital.

C. Obtain a urine specimen, chest x-ray film, CBC, and blood culture. If all are normal, send her home.

D. Obtain at least two blood cultures, CBC, and urinalysis; obtain chest x-ray film; and admit the patient to the hospital.

E. Obtain blood cultures, CBC, urinalysis, chest x-ray film, sedimentation rate, and lumbar puncture. Send the patient home if all are negative.

Directions: There are three sets of response options for the following scenario. You will be required to select one best answer from each question set.

6. A 70-year-old woman is sent to the emergency department (ED) for decreased appetite, loss of interest in activities, and weakness. Her past medical history includes hypertension, mild dementia, and arthritis. She lives alone with family close by. She takes atenolol and Celebrex. On arrival in the ED, she is a frail-appearing woman. Her vital signs are blood pressure of 100/50 mm Hg, pulse of 60 beats/minute, respiratory rate of 20 breaths/minute, oral temperature of 101°F, and oxygen saturation of 95%. Her physical examination is remarkable for dry mucous membranes, decreased breath sounds, normal cardiovascular examination, tenderness in the lower abdomen with a soft belly, heme-negative stool, and a nonfocal neurological examination.

6.1. The patient is given intravenous (IV) hydration, acetaminophen, and oxygen by nasal cannula. What is the most appropriate next step?

A. IV ampicillin, gentamicin, and Flagyl. Coverage can be narrowed once pathogen is discovered.

B. Chest x-ray film

C. IV Lasix

D. Ceftriaxone 1 g IV

6.2. An intravenous (IV) is established and blood samples are sent for complete blood count (CBC), electrolytes, and culture. A chest x-ray film is obtained, which is clear. What diagnostic test should be done next?

A. Head computed tomography (CT) scan and lumbar puncture

B. Abdominal CT scan

C. Renal ultrasound scan

D. Gallbladder ultrasound scan

E. Foley catheter for urinalysis

6.3. The patient improves with intravenous (IV) fluids and her temperature has decreased. She wants to go home. Her current vital signs are blood pressure of 90/60 mm Hg, pulse of 60 beats/ minute, respiratory rate of 22 breaths/ minute, oral temperature of 99°F, and oxygen saturation of 98%. She is found to have a urinary tract infection. Of the following choices, which would be the best disposition?

A. Admit to the hospital for IV fluids, observation, and antibiotics.

B. Discharge to a skilled nursing facility with antibiotics.

C. Discharge to home in the care of family with oral antibiotics.

Answers and Explanations

1. C. The blood smear can be performed as a thick or thin smear. The thick smear has the advantage of capturing many more red blood cells, making the likelihood of finding an intracellular *Plasmodium* higher. Patients with malaria may have high bilirubin content in the urine, creating dark urine (blackwater fever). Patients may present with pneumonia; however, the chest x-ray film is not diagnostic for a malaria infection. Neither stool cultures nor blood cultures are helpful in diagnosing malaria.

2-B. Community-acquired pneumonia. In this patient, the CD4 count is greater than 200, which virtually rules out opportunistic infections and eliminate answers A, C, and D. However, patients with human immunodeficiency virus (HIV) disease are at an increased risk of developing community-acquired pneumonia, so although an upper respiratory infection might be correct, community-acquired pneumonia would be more likely with this presentation.

3. C. Malaria is the only disease listed that is a parasitic infection caused by the *Plasmodium* species. All the others are caused by viral pathogens.

4. C. This patient is at high risk for pneumonia by history and physical findings. He is in a detox center and is likely to be withdrawing, as evidenced by his vital signs and tremulousness. He should be treated for both withdrawal and infection. He should be admitted because of his co-morbidities. Answer A is incorrect because he should not get the chest x-ray film before initiation of fluid resuscitation and oxygen, because he is both hypoxic and tachycardic. Answer B is wrong because it does not address his withdrawal symptoms or antibiotics. Finally, answer D is incorrect because this patient has no indication for computed tomography (CT) scan, lumbar puncture (LP), or even urine culture if his chest x-ray film is positive for pneumonia.

5. D. This patient is at high risk for occult infection, in particular endocarditis. Any patient with a history of recent intravenous drug use (IVDU) and fever should be admitted and cultured to rule out endocarditis. A complete blood count (CBC) will be elevated in many febrile illnesses and is a useful test, but it cannot be used to diagnose an illness and it is not sufficient workup to send a patient home if it is normal. Although a lumbar puncture may be indicated in a patient with a history of IVDU and high fever, it is still prudent to admit and observe the patient; thus, this response (C) is incorrect.

6.1. B. This patient is a classic elderly nursing home patient with a fever and failure to thrive (FTT). At this point, there is no obvious source of infection. She is hypoxic, has abnormal lung sounds, and should get a chest x-ray film to look for pneumonia. If she had a history of congestive heart failure, had elevated neck veins, peripheral edema, and crackles on lung examination, then her hypoxia might be due to failure and Lasix would be appropriate. Nonetheless, she is stable and should have a chest x-ray film to help diagnose whether there is heart failure. Antibiotics will likely be needed; however, they should not be given until the patient has blood and urine cultures obtained. If the patient is not septic

appearing, she should undergo diagnostic evaluation to focus antibiotics on the likely source. In the event that the patient is too ill or the source is not identified, the patient should receive wide-spectrum antibiotics.

6.2. E. A urinary source of infection is very common in elderly women. This etiology should be ruled out before subjecting the patient to testing in the radiology suite. In addition, this patient had mild lower abdominal pain, which can be caused by urinary retention or infection. A Foley catheter should be used to ensure a sterile and accurate urinalysis and to monitor fluid status. If the urine is clean, further workup may include visualization of the abdomen to rule out appendicitis, diverticulitis, and cholecystitis. The need for computed tomography (CT) head scan and lumbar puncture (LP) would depend on the patient's response to fluids, mental status, neck examination, and other findings. In any patient with markedly compromised mental status, and no other source, an LP should be performed. Although an ultrasound examination is the test of choice to diagnose cholecystitis, the patient is not jaundiced and has no tenderness over her gallbladder in the right upper quadrant. If none of the other testing turns up a diagnosis and the liver function tests are elevated, including alkaline phosphatase, then a right upper quadrant ultrasound examination is indicated. A renal ultrasound examination can look for hydronephrosis, but it will not give any significant information that would acutely change the patient's management. If she were to have urolithiasis and infection, the stone would appear on abdominal CT, as would the hydronephrosis in most instances.

6.3. A. Although the patient feels better, her vital signs are concerning. She still has a low blood pressure and a rapid respiratory rate. Her pulse is normal; however, she takes a β-blocker, which slows her heart rate. These vital signs may herald early sepsis; therefore, she should be admitted to the hospital for observation. Most nursing homes do not have the skilled nursing to monitor vital signs and deliver intravenous (IV) fluids and medications with sufficient attention to an individual patient to safely discharge her to a nursing home. Similarly, she requires more aggressive hydration and blood pressure monitoring and could not receive this at home.

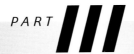
Topics in Emergency Medicine

Prehospital

44

Prehospital Emergency Medical Services Systems

Alexander P. Isakov, MD, MPH

Historical Perspective

Prehospital emergency medical services (EMS) serve the community by responding to calls for medical assistance, evaluating the medical needs of the individuals, rendering medical care in the austere environment of the prehospital setting, and transporting the sick and injured to an appropriate medical facility.

Although the earliest ambulance service dates back to 1865, it is in the last 35 years that development of a hospital-based prehospital system has seen its greatest growth. As late as the 1960s, ambulances were generally a means of transport only, operated by drivers with no standardized training or equipment, and often run by funeral services simply because their vehicles could accommodate a patient lying flat. The federal government took an interest in prehospital medical care after the development of the nation's interstate highway system and the realization that no system was in place to respond reliably to the victims of tragic automobile accidents. In 1966, the National Academy of Sciences–National Research Council report titled "Accidental Death and Disability: The Neglected Disease of Modern Society," identified the inadequate delivery of emergency care and the lack of an emergency services infrastructure. From this

document came recommendations for a funded prehospital medical delivery system and the birth of EMS systems as we have come to recognize them today.

Emergency Medical Services Education

The federal interest in EMS development in the 1960s spawned national standard educational curricula for the training of ambulance attendants or emergency medical technicians (EMTs). The first national standard curriculum developed by the National Highway Traffic and Safety Administration (NHTSA) was promulgated in 1971 (EMT-A) and was the minimum initial training expected of ambulance attendants. As more sophisticated medical evaluation and treatment options became available to street providers, more advanced training curricula emerged. There are currently four national standard training curricula promulgated by NHTSA. They are (a) the First Responder, (b) EMT-B (basic), (c) EMT-I (intermediate), and (d) EMT-P (paramedic). The first responder curriculum trains providers to perform basic patient assessment, manage airway obstruction, control external hemorrhage, administer cardiopulmonary resuscitation (CPR), and apply an automatic external defibrillator (AED) device. The length of training is approximately 20 hours. The next level of training, EMT-B (basic), has become nationally recognized as the minimum level of training required for ambulance transport. It is also required training for a provider to advance to the intermediate or paramedic level. The provider is trained in ambulance operation, communications, documentation, scene assessment, initial patient assessment, triage, patient immobilization, basic airway maneuvers, and more. The ability to deliver medications is very limited. The curriculum requires approximately 110 hours of education. The EMT-I (intermediate) level adds approximately additional 300 hours of training, increasing the provider's basic pathophysiology knowledge base, increasing assessment skills, and training the provider in venous cannulation and the establishment of a secure airway. The EMT-P (paramedic) has the most rigorous and extensive prehospital training curriculum. It consists of approximately 1100 hours of training beyond the EMT-B level and includes advanced training in pathophysiology, intravenous access, definitive airway control, pharmacology, and the administration of a wide variety of pharmaceuticals. The paramedics are also trained in rhythm recognition, manual defibrillation, and synchronous cardioversion.

Although national standards exist, the training requirements for prehospital providers are regulated by the states, which have variably adopted them in whole or in part, establishing scopes of practice presumably suited to each state's needs. Therefore, although the tiered system of training is ubiquitous, in which the paramedic (EMT-P) is the most highly trained prehospital provider, the length of education and the scopes of practice of these providers vary from state to state. There exist approximately 40 different levels of EMT provides nationwide.

In addition to the initial training required to become a certified prehospital provider, continuing education is very important. Continuing education is often mandated and regulated by the state office of EMS to maintain one's certification.

Communication

Communication is essential to the proper delivery of prehospital emergency services. Communication must exist for the community to access EMS and for the service to properly dispatch and manage its resources.

One of the great initiatives for public access to emergency medical services was the introduction of the 911 system. Before the universal three-digit emergency number, dialing a seven-digit number was required to access EMS. These seven-digit numbers varied from region to region. With standardized 911 access, the public increased its likelihood of correctly contacting the EMS agency in the event of an emergency. The United States has 911 access for more than 95% of the population. An additional aid is the introduction of enhanced 911 (911E), which provides the 911 call-taker with the phone number and address of the caller. These 911 calls are routed with the assistance of the local phone company to a designated public safety answering point (PSAP). This is an emergency communications center, which is often managed by municipal government. The call is identified as a medical emergency and forwarded to a call-taker. It is the call-taker's job to determine the nature of the emergency, determine the urgency of the emergency so it can be prioritized for dispatch, forward the call to a dispatcher who can send an ambulance to respond, and also provide prearrival instructions to the caller if appropriate. Modern EMS systems use written or computer-assisted call-taking protocols to ensure a standardized approach, thus ensuring consistent and appropriate triage of calls. These protocols also reduce the amount of time spent questioning a patient before dispatch. For example if a man, older than 50 years, calls complaining of nontraumatic chest pain, no further information is required to determine that the call is high priority (of possible cardiac etiology). Further questioning to make a presumptive diagnosis before dispatch could be time consuming, possibly detrimental, and not relevant to the dispatch decision.

Once the call-taker has determined the priority of the call, it is forwarded to the EMS dispatcher. This individual must determine the closest ambulance available to respond to the call in a timely manner. In a small system with one or two ambulances, this would not be particularly challenging. However, as the number of ambulances serving the system increases, it becomes increasingly difficult to recognize which ambulances are available to respond to a call, which ambulances are already busy responding, and the location of all these ambulances in the community. To assist the dispatcher, computer programs are available that electronically chart the activities of all the ambulances in the service. The program indicates which ambulances are available and which are engaged and, with the help of a global positioning system (GPS), can locate the ambulances in the municipality and even recommend which in-service unit is closest to the call. The efficiency of the system is further increased by deploying ambulances to locations in the coverage area that historically have had the highest volume of calls and redeploying assets to these areas when the covering units are occupied. Furthermore, peak load staffing is employed, which puts a greater number of ambulances on the street during times of the day when, historically, the call volumes are the greatest.

The dispatcher communicates with the ambulances by radio. Depending on the community, they may use very-high-frequency (VHF), ultra-high-frequency (UHF), or 800-MHz radio systems. The advantage of VHF is its extremely long range; however, VHF is limited by its inability to penetrate solid structures, such as buildings in an urban environment. UHF and 800-MHz systems have shorter range but superior penetration. These radios are used for dispatch, ambulance-to-hospital communication, ambulance-to-ambulance communication, and so on. The U.S. Federal Communications Commission (FCC) has designated 10 medical control channels or frequencies in the UHF range for EMS use. These "Med Channels" 1 to 10 are nationally recognized and are often regionally controlled by a central medical communications center (C-MED).

System Structure

How responders are dispatched to a call is very much determined by the structure of the system, and this varies regionally. As discussed previously, prehospital providers

acquire varying levels of training, for example, first responders, basic, and advanced paramedics. Each EMS system determines which type of providers will be employed in their service depending on medical necessity and the resources available to the community. Some EMS systems operate an "all advanced life support (ALS)" system in which every ambulance has at least one paramedic and has the capability to deliver the most advanced prehospital care. Some EMS systems operate a "two-tiered" system, with ALS-staffed and equipped ambulances and basic life support (BLS)-staffed and equipped ambulances. In a two-tiered system, the nature of the call determines who gets dispatched, BLS, ALS, or both. The assumed advantage to this system is that with appropriate triage, the caller will receive the level of care required, and ALS units will not be occupied responding to BLS-level calls. In addition to ambulance transport services, some systems also have a first responder tier. First responders have fewer medical capabilities but often arrive more quickly; they are trained to initially manage life-threatening hemorrhage, airway obstruction, or full cardiac arrest with oxygen, CPR, and an AED. The structure of the EMS system is often determined by the responsibility to provide timely and appropriate medical assistance within the constraints of the community's fiscal realities.

The agencies involved in the delivery of prehospital care also have great regional variation. EMS may be fire department based, may exist as a separate municipal agency or "third service," may involve the police department, may be operated as a hospital-based service, or may be contracted out to a private enterprise. Some systems combine the various resources, for example, with the fire department serving as first responders and a hospital-based EMS service providing advanced care and transport. In some regions, EMS providers are paid professionals; in other regions, mostly rural areas, they are staffed by dedicated volunteers. Each system has its own strengths and weaknesses, some medically relevant and others economically relevant. There is much debate on the pros and cons of each system design. The lead EMS agency, however it is designed, should clearly have patient care as its top priority, ensure the skill of its prehospital medical providers, and have strong medical oversight.

Medical Oversight

Prehospital emergency medical services, by definition, perform medical assessments and deliver medical care in the out-of-hospital environment. Because EMS is essentially a health care delivery system, physician and emergency department involvement and oversight is essential for a quality system. Physicians provide guidance in the treatment of patients, are involved in the education of the prehospital providers, are essential to the quality improvement process in EMS, and can even directly become involved in the care of patients in the prehospital setting.

To standardize the care of patients, the medical director will develop patient care protocols to guide prehospital providers in the management of routinely encountered ailments. These protocols assume the EMT is skilled in the initial assessment of the patient and then present standing orders for the EMT to perform a procedure or deliver a medication depending on the condition of the patient. These protocols are often presented in an algorithm format, much as the American Heart Association presents its Advanced Cardiac Life Support (ACLS) protocols. Because the care of some patients can be complex and not every presentation straightforward, not every option in the patient care protocols is a standing order, but some require consultation with a medical control physician who is available by radio or telephone. The medical director ensures that a mechanism exists for EMTs to contact a physician when necessary. Some systems use one base hospital's emergency department to manage all such consultations in what is known as centralized medical control; others consult physicians in the emergency department to which the patient will be transported in what is called decentralized

medical control. Whatever system is used, it is important that the physicians providing consultation on the radio or phone are well versed in the medical director's prehospital protocols and understand the capabilities of the field prehospital providers and what resources are available to them.

The office of the medical director also ensures quality in the system by overseeing a quality assurance and quality improvement program. This may include timely review of patient care reports (PCRs) generated by the field personnel. The medical director will evaluate PCRs for appropriateness of the medical care rendered and compliance with the promulgated protocols. Other measures of quality, such as time to arrival on high-priority calls, or length of time providing care on the scene, can also be reviewed. Once issues are identified for correction or improvement, either individual remediation or perhaps system-wide training can be implemented.

To further ensure consistency and quality in the EMS system and to close the feedback loop in the quality improvement process, the medical director is very involved in the continuing education of field personnel. This can include overseeing the training of personnel, lecturing directly to the field providers, or negotiating with a hospital to provide clinical venues for skills retention, such as endotracheal intubation. Most states have continuing education requirements for their prehospital providers, as does the National Registry for EMTs. The medical oversight staff can be instrumental in providing the necessary training to meet these continuing medical education (CME) requirements and to improve quality in the system by dedicating time and energy to training.

Prehospital research is also an important aspect of physician involvement in prehospital systems. Much of the practice of prehospital medicine has originated from the emergency department and other parts of the hospital, although the prehospital environment is quite different. Many interventions have entered prehospital practice without rigorous prehospital study. Callaham reported that of the 5,842 scientific studies on

EMS in MEDLINE since 1985, only 54 were randomized controlled trials, only 1 examined a major outcome such as survival, and only 1 other compared the studied intervention with a placebo. There are many compelling reasons to aggressively pursue research in the prehospital arena. Interpretation of the culled data could improve patient care in the future, interventions with documented positive outcomes will likely weather fiscal scrutiny, and the science of prehospital medicine can expand as any science is obligated to do. The scientific basis for medical interventions in the field can only come from physician academicians dedicated to the study of prehospital care.

Historically, any interested physician, despite a lack of formal training, provided medical oversight. Now, emergency medicine residents receive some introduction to EMS and EMS systems in their residency core curriculum. However, this EMS experience varies greatly from one program to another. Postgraduate EMS fellowship training is now also available in 1- and 2-year formats. The fellowship programs train emergency medicine physicians in EMS operations, communications, legislation, education, research, finance, ground and air transport, and other skills that will be of benefit to provide competent medical oversight to a prehospital EMS system. Most 2-year programs offer a master's degree in public health, hospital administration, business, or other disciplines. Guidelines for a standard fellowship curriculum have been endorsed by the Society for Academic Emergency Medicine and the National Association of EMS Physicians.

EMS is interdisciplinary. The system responds to 911 emergency medical calls and scheduled and unscheduled medical transports with ground and air ambulances. Beyond the daily oversight of prehospital patient care and transport, many EMS physicians are also involved in planning for mitigation of mass casualty incidents, more widespread community disasters of natural or industrial origin, or the medical consequences of weapons of mass destruction. Furthermore, the interface of the EMS system with the community provides many opportunities for physicians to implement public health and injury prevention initiatives.

Emergency medicine physicians, by virtue of their training and their practice environment, are uniquely qualified to provide leadership in this science and improve the delivery of health care in the prehospital environment.

Suggested Readings

Callaham M. Quantifying the scanty science of prehospital emergency care. *Ann Emerg Med* 1997;30:785–790.

Emergency Medical Services agenda for the future. Washington, DC: NHTSA and the Health Resources and Services Administration, 1996.

Krohmer JR, Swor RA, Benson NM, et al. Prototype core content for a fellowship in emergency medical services. *Ann Emerg Med* 1994;23:109–114.

National Academy of Sciences–National Research Council. *Accidental death and disability: the neglected disease of modern society.* Washington, DC, 1966.

Verdile VP, Krohmer JR, Swor RA, et al. Model curriculum in emergency medical services for emergency medicine residency programs. *Acad Emerg Med* 1996;3: 716–722.

45

Disaster Management

Kathyrn Brinsfield, MD, MPH, FACEP

Disasters vary from natural disasters, such as floods and hurricanes, to human-made disasters, such as industrial accidents and terrorism. Disasters may be different in their length, breadth, life lost, and property damage. However, all disasters share the following basic elements: the phases of the event, the types of injuries and public health issues, and the basic tenets of disaster response. This chapter explores the different types of disasters, their similarities and differences, and the universal response to any disaster.

Basic Principles

A disaster is usually defined as a multiple or mass casualty incident (MCI) that overwhelms the local emergency response. In this light, a 10-car accident with 20 serious injuries may be considered a disaster in a rural area, whereas an explosion with 100 casualties may not overwhelm a city's response system. Another way to look at the issue is experience: a 2-foot snowstorm may cause a disaster with loss of life in a southern city, whereas a flood in an area experienced with flooding may hardly interrupt normal routines.

All disasters share four basic elements: warning, event, response, and recovery.

Different disasters may exhibit different patterns; for example, a hurricane may have a prolonged warning and event cycle, whereas a terrorist event may have little to no warning, and an event phase that is over in minutes. Recovery, although an important aspect of returning an area to the predisaster normalcy, may take hours to months and is often overlooked in medical planning.

Most disasters share a prevalence of certain types of injuries. These include crush injuries, soft tissue injuries, and orthopedic injuries. For instance, the type of crush injury that results from a building collapse is the same whether an earthquake or an engineering failure caused the collapse. Soft tissue injuries caused by flying glass are similar whether they are the result of high winds from a hurricane or concussion from an explosive device. The exception to this rule is the potential for nuclear, biological, or chemical terrorism, which may require a new type of medical proficiency.

Certain issues recur despite historical lessons:

- Unfamiliarity with paper plans: This results when a plan exists that satisfies planners and administrators but is never read or tested by the personnel who must carry out the plan.

- Difficulty in coordinating the response of multiple agencies: Because many disasters bring about overlapping responses from local, state, and federal agencies, the Incident Command System (ICS) was developed to help structure the coordination of agencies at a disaster site.

- Difficulty with communication at disaster sites: For example, at the MGM

Grand Hotel fire in Las Vegas, difficulty with radio communication from the front to the back of the building required disaster responders to use runners. In New York City on September 11, 2001, the local hospitals were overwhelmed by victims, many of whom needed transfer, but were without internal and external phone systems because of the collapse of the twin towers of the World Trade Center.

- Flooding of the closest medical facility with casualties while hospitals within a reasonable distance remain unaffected. There are many modern examples of this, including Oklahoma City after the 1995 bombing of the Murrah Federal Building, in which most patients were taken or self-triaged to the nearest hospital, leaving hospitals a short distance away virtually untouched.

- Difficulties of coordinating volunteer response and donations at a disaster site: during the 1989 San Francisco earthquake, and the collapse of the San Francisco-Oakland Bay Bridge, volunteers from the surrounding neighborhoods completed most of the rescues, while several tons of concrete hung perilously above.

- A lack of appreciation for logistical issues and planning: Predisaster medical care at a disaster site is only as good as the materials for making it happen. On September 11, 2001, many doctors and nurses arrived at Ground Zero in an effort to help, with limited medical supplies and a lack of protective equipment.

Natural Disasters

Natural disasters are often weather related, such as floods, hurricanes, tsunamis, tornadoes, and mudslides. They may also be geology based, such as earthquakes and volcanoes.

Although most natural disasters are high on property and infrastructure damage, and low on loss of life, recent and historical examples exhibit the potential for profound physical injury. Most recently, the earthquake in Bam, Iran saw life losses of more than 40,000 individuals. An 1871 forest fire in Peshtigo, Wisconsin resulted in 1,182 deaths, and the hurricane that hit Galveston, Texas in 1900 resulted in about 5,000 deaths. Improvement in emergency warning systems and weather predictions have certainly helped to limit the loss of life, but some of these improvements may have been offset by increased population density in at-risk areas.

Not all injuries and loss of life occur immediately after the event in a natural disaster. Loss of hospital facilities, difficulty in response and travel, loss of food and contamination of water supply, extremes of climate, and injuries that result from cleanup and recovery activities may result in greater injury and loss of life after the event.

Human-made Disasters

Industrial Accidents

Human-made disasters can be industrial accidents or acts of terrorism. Although acts of terrorism grab much of the current headlines, industrial accidents have resulted in massive loss of life in recent years. The Hyatt Hotel-Kansas City Skyway collapse resulted in the death of 111 people. During a regular Friday evening dance event, patrons lined the suspended balconies that hung in the four-story-tall atrium. As they swayed to the music, the top balcony failed, crashing down onto the other three balconies and the dance floor below. In another example, the Union Carbide plant in Bhopal, India had an accidental release of a chemical because of a mechanical failure. This resulted in a cloud of methyl isocyanate dispersing over the sleeping city, killing up to 3,800 people.

Acts of Terrorism

Terrorist disasters are still primarily conventional weapons, meaning that most injuries are from explosive devices. Bombs depend on pressure waves and direct trauma to cause injury. The pressure waves can result in lung, ear, and hollow organ damage. Direct trauma can be caused from objects packed around the bomb (e.g., the metal objects in the Olympic Park bombing in Atlanta); from victims being thrown against solid objects; from flying glass; or from building collapse, such as the Nairobi embassy bombing, which resulted in 4,000 deaths. The severity of the overpressure injury depends markedly on the surroundings of the victim: Open-air areas result in fewer deaths, whereas enclosed spaces, such as the bus bombings in Israel, can result in more severe injuries.

Weapons of mass destruction (WMD) include nuclear, biological, and chemical terrorism. These events have been relatively rare, despite the growing concern in the press. Chemical terrorism is hard to distinguish from an industrial chemical accident, except for the place and persons exposed. For instance, the Sarin gas release in the Tokyo subway system affected thousands of commuters, but killed only a few persons. Chemical terrorist agents are usually divided into four categories:

- Nerve agents: These behave much like insecticides, causing a relative excess of acetylcholine, resulting in bronchorrhea, rhinorrhea, and gastric distress.
- Blood agents: Cyanide blocks cellular respiration.
- Vesicants: Blister-causing agents such as sulfur mustard and lewisite. They can cause DNA damage and skin and lung injury.
- Riot control agents: Include a variety of chemical mixtures commonly labeled as tear gas. Although more annoying than deadly, these agents disable individuals from functioning normally by irritating their eyes, mouths, noses, and lungs. In crowds, this can cause widespread panic and be very disruptive to any efforts to control the crowd.
- Biological terrorism would include the release of virus or bacteria into a population. Biological events could present insidiously, with initial victims presenting first with flulike symptoms and eventually differentiating to be victims of agents such as anthrax or smallpox.
  - Anthrax: Although it is not transmissible from human-to-human, anthrax

bacteria can form spores that remain infectious for up to 70 years. Mortality of the respiratory form can be as high as 95%.
  - Smallpox: A virus that is easily transmitted from human-to-human, smallpox has 30% to 40% mortality in the immune population.
- Nuclear terrorism involves the release of radioactive material into the population. This could present insidiously, if a source is left in a populous place, or with explosives. Two types of explosives have been a recent concern: the "dirty" bomb and the "suitcase" bomb.
  - Dirty bomb: Any type of explosive ordinance contaminated with nuclear material, such that the explosion causes blast damage and spreads the nuclear material.
  - Suitcase bomb: Theoretically, nuclear devices small enough to be hand carried (as in a suitcase); these would cause a large explosion and spread many types of radioactive isotopes.

Disaster Planning

Planning for the medical consequences of either natural or human-made events involves similar issues. First, will medical personnel best serve by augmenting the hospital staff or by responding to the disaster scene? Medical personnel who respond to active incidents must have safety training, protective equipment, portable medical equipment, and training in and an agreement with the local incident command. Second, the hospitals must plan and prepare for potential disasters. This planning includes setting up a hospital incident command system; stockpiling food, water, and medical supplies; establishing policies and procedures for recalling personnel and using volunteers; and planning for responding safely to potential contaminated patients.

Every disaster increases interest in disaster planning and disaster medicine, but the challenge is keeping continued interest in disaster planning when there is no immediate threat. Every disaster plan needs to be read, understood, periodically revised, and practiced to be a useful part of decision making in those first few chaotic minutes of a disaster.

Summary

Disasters do happen, and the timing and type of disaster are not always predictable. However, the principles of response are similar for the different types of disasters. Medical personnel should develop generic emergency plans, which encompass recovery and response and deal with the universal injuries and issues in disasters. This includes planning for logistical needs, communication, and personnel. All disaster plans must be simple enough to be read and understood by the people who will carry them out, and they should be regularly practiced with all agencies involved and action reports after the event.

Suggested Readings

Atomic suitcase bombs. Available at http://www .pbs.org/wgbh/pages/frontline/shows/russia/ suitcase/(last accessed 9/25/04).

Fact sheet on dirty bombs. Available at http://www .nrc.gov/reading-rm/doc-collections/fact-sheets/ dirty-bombs.html (last accessed 9/23/04).

Mitchell JK. *The long road to recovery: community responses to industrial disaster.* Tokyo/NY/ Paris: United Nations University Press, 1996.

Talking to each other in crisis. *Joint Commission Perspectives*, Vol 21(12) 2001 Dec:16.

Woodward S, Pessek RJ. The Hyatt horror: 111 dead, 188 hurt and a city in shock. *The Kansas City Star* 1981 July 19.

Hazardous Materials

K. Sophia Dyer, MD, FACEP

Chapter Outline

Hazardous Materials
Chemical Identification
Decontamination
Protective Gear

Chemicals surround us on a daily basis. At home, at work, and on the roadways, chemicals exist in their final form or as precursors to products that we depend on in both industrial and nonindustrial societies. In addition, the continuous creation of new chemicals stresses our ability to respond when things go wrong. Despite the continued thirst for new products, our society remains largely unaware or unwilling to accept the consequences of releasing chemical hazards into communities and the environment. Most hospitals and the medical profession in general are ill equipped to deal with patients exposed to a hazardous materials release, even from known hazards. Thankfully, most hazardous material releases involve only minor or no exposure and/or injury. Reminders of the human consequences of hazardous material exposures occur, both internationally (the Union Carbide pesticide plant leak in Bhopal, India) and nationally (the 26-ton release of hydrofluoric acid from a Texas plant in 1987). In the Bhopal incident, an estimated 3,800 people died either immediately or in the days after the release.

The emergency physician may become involved in a sudden hazardous materials release, such as a bioterrorist attack or an industrial accident. In addition, the physician may become aware of a less obvious release, such as chronic exposure in a workplace or contamination of a community water supply.

Hazardous Materials

What are hazardous materials? In addition to chemicals, biological agents and radioactive material also fall under the heading of hazardous materials (often abbreviated as HAZMAT). Most hazardous materials releases are unpredictable accidents. Thus, any emergency physician may be called on to assist in such an incident. In general, most accidental releases occur during weekdays and are from fixed facilities. Releases from transportation vehicles present a special threat, because of the chemical hazard and the trauma from the accident that caused the spill. Terrorists may use fixed or mobile hazardous materials as weapons, by placement of a detonation device in proximity to the container. In addition, terrorists could contaminate a bomb with radioactive or nonradioactive chemicals. Some believe that the planners of the first World Trade Center bombing that occurred in New York City on February 26, 1993 entertained a plan to add cyanide to the bomb.

Chemical Identification

The emergency physician is not completely at the mercy of chance happenings or terrorist acts. Although hospitals should prepare for the likelihood of patients contaminated with an unidentified chemical, many chemicals are identifiable at the time of the incident or shortly afterward. Various systems exist for the quick identification of chemicals; however, most of these are unfamiliar to the emergency physician. In most communities, the fire chief, or someone in an equivalent role, has knowledge about the various chemicals stored in the community. In 1986, the U.S. Environmental Protection Agency (EPA) required the development of local, state, and national emergency-response plans. Regional planning committees are required to have representatives of all parties that would be called on to respond to a hazardous materials spill. This was codified in the Superfund Amendments and Reauthorization Act (SARA) of 1986. A section of SARA (Title III) deals with community hazardous materials response; this section is also referred to as the Emergency Preparedness and Community Right-to-Know Act. The U.S. Occupational Safety and Health Administration (OSHA) uses similar occupational right-to-know rules that cover workers.

The U.S. Department of Transportation also carries regulations about the visible identification of chemicals on the roadways. These regulations dictate that carriers of certain amounts of chemical must identify the type of chemical on the outside of the container and vehicle. This identification is commonly referred to as a placard. Placards are diamond-shaped signs with a classification of the hazard (explosive, flammable solid, and so on) as indicated by a number; in addition, some containers may be marked with a United Nations (UN) number. The four-digit UN number is used in Canada, the United States, and Europe to identify the type of chemical. One can look up this number by using a manual titled the *North American Emergency Response Guidebook* and determine the general type of chemical and brief emergency response guidelines. Specific regulations dictate what amount and type of chemical need placarding, which is beyond the scope of this brief overview. The National Fire Protection Association (NFPA) 704M is another identification system that is used. The NFPA placard is divided into four separate diamonds, each color-coded with the type of hazard: health risk (blue), flammability (red), reactivity (yellow), and the bottom diamond (white) for information such as water reactivity. In each of the color-coded diamonds, a number lists the degree of the hazard, ranging from 0 (no risk) to 4 (greatest risk). The NFPA system can be used on containers of chemicals and on doors to rooms containing chemical hazards. The NFPA system and the UN system are two of the major hazardous materials identification mechanisms. Commercial trucks, planes, ships, and railcars also frequently have shipping papers describing the cargo carried.

Another helpful book for the emergency physician or EMS provider on scene is the *NIOSH Pocket Guide to Chemical Hazards* published by the National Institute for Occupational Safety and Health (NIOSH). This publication contains information about chemical properties and basic first aid and is a good source of information about personal protective equipment. The local poison control center has human health information available on particular chemicals and provides access to a medical or clinical toxicologist for assistance. Other phone resources are the Chemical Manufacturers Association's information service for transportation accidents (1-800-424-9300 in the United States). The Canadian government runs a similar service. A U.S. governmental agency that can assist with the medical care of victims of a hazardous materials exposure is the Agency for Toxic Substances and Disease Registry ([ATSDR], 1-404-488-4100; 404-498-0110; fax: 404-498-0093; toll-free phone: 1-888-422-8737). Most governmental agencies such as the Centers for Disease Control and Prevention (CDC) and the EPA also have Web sites with specific information on a large number of chemicals.

Decontamination

Decontamination of the exposed patient, regardless of whether the exposure is chemical, biological, or nuclear, is an issue that has catapulted to attention since the World Trade Center attacks of September 11, 2001 and the subsequent anthrax exposures. Many emergency departments are unprepared for decontamination procedures. Unfortunately, the nature of hazardous materials releases is that they are unplanned.

Prehospital decontamination may occur, but as many mass casualty events have demonstrated, patients tend to present to the hospital on their own. Even one contaminated patient could tax an emergency department's resources and potentially contaminate the department. Hospital-based decontamination does not have to be an insurmountable task. Every hospital should work out a plan for how one or multiple contaminated patients are dealt with and how to prepare and accommodate a mass casualty or terrorist attack.

Most simple decontamination can be accomplished by instructing a conscious patient to disrobe and brush off powder contaminants before entering the department. Early attempts at substance identification are imperative. Most substances are not water reactive, and the patient then can be instructed to wash. A simple outdoor shower or garden hose can accomplish this goal. Weather conditions and privacy should be considered. Some emergency departments have installed hot and cold water in an outdoor shower system with surrounding curtains for privacy. The patient who is too ill to self-decontaminate poses a special challenge to the emergency department. Most emergency departments have little to no capabilities to decontaminate an ill patient. The local fire department or EMS providers may be expected to complete this task. Much of the concern regarding decontamination of an ill patient centers on the potential harm to the caregivers from the contamination. Little hard data exist regarding the potential of asymptomatic contamination or potential harm to medical providers who have tended to a contaminated patient. In the Sarin (an organophosphate nerve agent) attack on the Tokyo subway, medical providers in the St. Luke's Hospital reported symptoms of miosis, eye pain, and nausea. None of the hospital staff was seriously harmed.

Protective Gear

One way to protect the hospital staff is to educate them on the methods of identifying hazardous chemicals and on the use of chemical protective gear. Such a project can be a significant expense to an emergency department budget, especially for a resource that may be used infrequently. Following is a review of the types of chemical protective gear for a general understanding. The choice of chemical protective gear can be complex. Many different materials exist for suits, gloves, and boots, and various levels of protection are available. Anyone making decisions about materials for specific conditions should consult available reference tables and/or a professional with experience in hazardous materials, such as an industrial hygienist. For example, some materials will not hold up to a potent acid exposure.

Level A is the highest level of chemical protection. This includes a fully encapsulating suit, inner and outer gloves, boots, and a self-contained breathing apparatus. A self-contained breathing apparatus is used in both Level A and Level B protection. Chemical protective gear use the same type of breathing apparatus that is used by firefighters. Air is supplied through a hose to a faceplate that extends from the hairline to the chin. Because there are many different shapes and sizes of people, each person must be individually fit tested. To use the equipment properly, a training course must be completed. The additional work of breathing and the weight of a steel or fiberglass tank on the worker's back make the use of Level A and Level B chemical protective gear a strenuous activity. Even in a temperate environment, the worker can quickly become overheated. Thus, prework and postwork hydration is essential. Some workplaces and emergency departments have supplied air on a wall connection, to which a hose can be attached, allowing the worker an extended period of air supply without changing bottles. Air bottles or tanks, in contrast, typically provide 30 or 60 minutes of air supply. Moreover, this amount can vary by the worker's minute ventilation. During strenuous operations, such as rescue or emergency containment work, the worker may quickly use most of the tank's content. On the other hand, air supplied via a hose connection permits the worker to reach only a limited area.

Level A chemical protective gear is indicated as the highest level of protection for any situation when the hazard is either unknown or known to be very hazardous. The science officer in a plant or the fire chief decides what level of protection is to be used. Level B chemical protective gear includes self-contained breathing apparatus, hooded suit (without the full encapsulation of a combined faceplate), inner and outer gloves, and boots. Level C chemical protective gear is the same as Level B, with the exception of the respiratory protection. With Level C, the respiratory protection uses the same faceplate as a self-contained breathing apparatus; however, instead of supplied air, level C uses a canister filter. Level C can be used only when the oxygen in the environment is sufficient and the contaminant is known. Level C can also contain a high-efficiency particulate air (HEPA) purifier; such an addition may be helpful when the contaminant is a biological agent.

Now that you are familiar with the various methods of chemical identification, decontamination, and personal protective gear and a general approach to hazardous materials, you may be interested in learning more about this topic. Many good texts, training programs, and Web-based resources exist. Although not a daily occurrence, a basic understanding of general topics in hazardous materials can benefit the patient and the entire hospital community.

Suggested Readings

Anonymous. *Managing hazardous materials incidents. Vol. 1 Emergency Medical Services.* Atlanta, U.S. Department of Health and Human Services, 2001.

Anonymous. *NFPA HazMat quick guide.* Quincy, MA: National Fire Protection Association, 1997.

Borak J, Callan M, Abbott W, eds. *Hazardous materials exposure.* Englewood Cliffs, NJ: Brady, 1991.

Cox RD. Decontamination and management of hazardous materials exposure victims in the emergency department. *Ann Emerg Med* 1994; 24:761–770.

National Institute for Occupational Safety and Health. *NIOSH pocket guide to chemical hazards* (NIOSH Publication No. 97-140 third printing), January 2003. A condensed version of a CD-ROM for this title is available online at http://www.cdc.gov/niosh/npg/npg.html (accessed 9/25/04). http://hazmat.dot.gov/guidebook.htm (accessed 9/25/04).

Sidell FR, Borak J. Chemical warfare agents: II. nerve agents. *Ann Emerg Med* 1992;21:865–871.

Sullivan JB, Krieger GR, eds. *Clinical environmental health and toxic exposures,* 2nd ed. Philadelphia: Lippincott, Williams & Wilkins, 2001.

Trauma

General Approach to Trauma

Simon Roy, MD

Millions of people are victims of trauma each year in the United States. Victims of violent crime alone measure in the several thousand victims per hundred thousand citizens in the United States. It is difficult to extract precise statistics, because each state and urban center has its own particular profile. Urban emergency departments (EDs) frequently see victims of penetrating trauma by gunshots or stabbing resulting from petty crimes, interpersonal violence including gangs, or domestic violence and disputes. Motor vehicle crashes, work-related injuries, and sports and recreation-related injuries all contribute to a major health problem that imposes a physical and financial burden on the victim and society. The only way to reduce trauma is to promote prevention. Many organizations exist to promote prevention, including government-led initiatives by the Centers for Disease Control and Prevention (CDC) to promote awareness of issues ranging from seatbelt and helmet use to prevention of falls to avoid hip fractures in the elderly.

It is impossible in an introductory text to cover the field of trauma in extensive detail. Several texts devoted solely to trauma fill multiple hardcover volumes. In this chapter, the general approach to the trauma patient is covered, with particular attention to the important general principles. The algorithms presented contain most of the significant "rules" to treat the trauma victim.

The preparation for treatment of the trauma victim begins even before the patient reaches the hospital (Fig. 47.1). Obtain as much information as possible from the emergency medical services (EMS) report while the patient is still in the field. Using this information wisely and having a trauma team with specific predetermined roles are the key to an organized, calm, and controlled approach to a clinical situation that can be stressful and chaotic. A report of hypotension in the field suggests that the patient is in shock. Such a report should trigger the standard approach from the Advanced Trauma Life Support (ATLS) course (offered by the American College of Surgeons) of ordering un-crossmatched blood to the trauma room. Moreover, it should also trigger a call to the trauma surgeon so that there will be no delay should the patient require surgery. If an acute hemothorax is suspected, preparation for placing a chest tube and setting up the autotransfuser from the chest tube output can also be started. Early preparation even before the patient arrives is essential for the rapid evaluation and treatment of the patient.

Major Blunt Trauma General Protocol

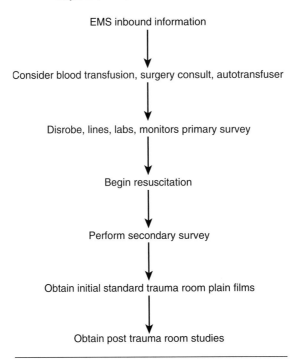

EMS inbound information

Consider blood transfusion, surgery consult, autotransfuser

Disrobe, lines, labs, monitors primary survey

Begin resuscitation

Perform secondary survey

Obtain initial standard trauma room plain films

Obtain post trauma room studies

Figure 47.1
General approach to major blunt trauma. EMS, emergency medical services.

Primary Survey

On arrival, the patient is completely disrobed and is placed on a blood pressure monitor, cardiac monitor, and pulse oximeter. Two large-bore (minimum 18-gauge) intravenous (IV) lines are started. If access is not instantaneously achieved and the patient is unstable, a large-bore central line often referred to as a trauma line is placed usually in the femoral vein using sterile technique. (see femoral line, Chapter 68). If central access fails, another location may be used, such as the subclavian or internal jugular vein central access. If access is still not achieved, a venous cutdown of the saphenous vein may be performed. When all else fails, particularly in children, an interosseous line should be obtained.

Next is the primary survey, which includes assessment of airway and breathing. (The general approach to resuscitation is discussed in detail in Chapter 2.) This involves checking the mouth for blood and secretions and removing these by suctioning if

they are present. Any signs of airway compromise or shock in the trauma patient requires immediate intubation. Look for tracheal deviation from the midline and jugular venous distension, which are found in patients who have a tension pneumothorax. Auscultation of the lung fields also provides initial clues to possible hemothorax or pneumothorax (decreased breath sounds). If the clinical signs strongly suggest that a tension pneumothorax is present, needle decompression should be performed and a chest tube inserted immediately, without waiting for a confirmatory chest x-ray film.

The primary survey continues with the assessment of the circulation by checking the pulse and blood pressure. Resuscitation must occur concurrently with the primary survey and may include endotracheal intubation for any signs of pulmonary insufficiency, needle decompression and chest tube placement for suspected hemothorax or pneumothorax, and volume and blood infusion for signs of

Table 47.1.

Classification system for hemorrhagic shock by percent of total blood loss and physical signs

Class	Percent Blood Loss	Clinical Signs
I	≤15	Mild increase in heart rate, 90–100 bpm Focal swelling, bleeding
II	15–25	Increased heart rate Prolonged capillary refill Increased diastolic blood pressure
III	25–50	Any of previous signs in addition to hypotension, confusion, acidosis, decreased urine output
IV	>50	Hypotension unresponsive to resuscitation Acidosis unresponsive to resuscitation

circulatory insufficiency. Any obvious ongoing bleeding must be controlled by direct pressure at this time. There is a simple classification for hemorrhagic shock that allows you to quickly assess how much blood the patient has been losing (Table 47.1).

Secondary Survey

The secondary survey includes a detailed head-to-toe examination of the patient and is the main determinant of what studies (e.g., computed tomography [CT] scans, arteriograms, ultrasound scans, detailed plain x-ray films of spine and extremities) will be undertaken after obtaining the initial standard plain x-ray films of the lateral cervical-spine, supine chest, and pelvis. The patient is assessed for neurological signs (D, disability). The mnemonic AVPU is often used for a quick reference. Is the patient Alert (A), Verbal (V), responding only to a Painful stimulus (P), or completely Unresponsive (U).

The patient is completely disrobed (E, exposure) (See Chapter 2). If the patient is on a backboard and has a cervical collar on, the clothing is cut off the patient to minimize any neck movement. Exposure may reveal other significant findings including extremity deformities, contusions, lacerations, and penetrating trauma. In some cases, action such as hemorrhage control may be re-

quired during the exposure. You can quickly see that the construct of the primary and secondary survey is an organizational one so that no injury is missed. In reality, much of the evaluation and treatment of the sick trauma patient occurs simultaneously.

If the patient is awake and conversant, obtain a brief history. Using the mnemonic AMPLE covers the most basic questions that need to be asked. Ask the patient if he or she has any drug Allergies (A), is on any Medications (M), has any Past medical history (P) or may be Pregnant (P), when the Last meal was eaten (L), and about the Events leading to the trauma (E). Ask about the last tetanus vaccination as well.

The Three-Compartment Approach to Trauma

The simplest way to approach the patient with blunt trauma and multiple-system injuries is to consider the problem broken down into three compartments: the central nervous system (CNS), the abdomen, and the chest (Fig. 47.2). You can see that the algorithms are designed to prioritize and manage the life-threatening issues first, then take care of other important but less emergent injuries. Extremity injuries are considered separately and are mentioned later under vascular injuries.

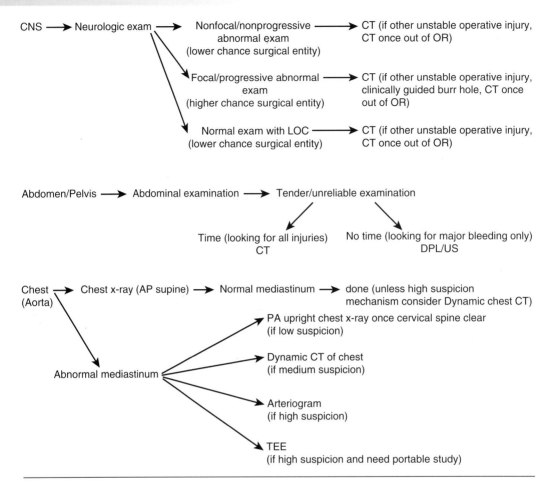

Figure 47.2
Three-compartment approach to blunt trauma. AP, anteroposterior; CNS, central nervous system; CT, computed tomography; DPL, diagnostic peritoneal lavage; LOC, loss of consciousness; OR, operating room; PA, posteroanterior; TEE, transesophageal echocardiography; US, ultrasound.

Central Nervous System

The CNS evaluation begins with a detailed neurological examination. If the patient has an abnormal neurological examination, but it is nonfocal and nonprogressive, the patient needs a CT scan of the head. An example would be a patient who is alert, talking, and able to move extremities to command but is repeatedly asking the same questions or is disoriented. If another issue in either of the other two compartments requires an immediate operation, then the head CT scan can be performed postoperatively, because the chances of the patient having a neurosurgical entity are low.

If the patient has an abnormal neurological examination *and* focal or progressive findings, a head CT scan is again indicated. Examples of concerning findings include single dilated pupils or decerebrate or decorticate posturing, suggesting that herniation is occurring in the brain. In these cases, however, if another issue in either of the other two compartments requires immediate surgery, the neurosurgeon can perform a clinically guided burr hole in the operating room (OR) while the trauma surgeons are operating on the chest or the abdomen at the same time. This temporizes the most dangerous but treatable CNS surgical entity, the epidural hematoma. A head CT scan can then be obtained postoperatively. This approach has become controversial with the advent of high-speed spiral CT scans. Many neurosurgeons insist on a positive head CT scan before placing a burr hole.

The patient with a normal neurological examination but transient loss of consciousness should be dealt with similarly to the patient in the first situation, because it is unlikely that an operative condition exists. Recent studies indicate that the patient with minor head injury with a normal neurological examination irrespective of loss of consciousness does not need a CT scan. The prospective validation of these findings is ongoing.

Abdomen

The patient with a tender or unreliable abdominal examination (resulting from intoxication or head injury) will need a diagnostic study. Ideally, this is a CT scan, which will delineate almost all injuries. There is no need to delay the study to administer oral contrast. If the patient is hemodynamically unstable, do not send the patient to radiology for a CT scan. An ultrasound or diagnostic peritoneal lavage (DPL) is an acceptable option, with the goal being to rapidly identify blood in the peritoneal cavity (hemoperitoneum) and expedite laparotomy. The focused abdominal sonogram in trauma (FAST examination) has been the subject of many studies and remains controversial when the examination is negative. When the ultrasound scan demonstrates fluid in the abdominal cavity by creating an anechoic stripe in Morrison's pouch, there is generally more than 250 mL of free fluid, presumably blood, and many centers use this result to take an unstable patient directly to the OR for exploration of the abdomen. Some sonographers believe that as little as 30 mL of blood can be detected by ultrasound.

Chest

The life-threatening injuries that involve the chest compartment include tension pneumothorax, active bleeding into the chest cavity (hemothorax or hemopneumothorax if accompanied by a pneumothorax) from a vascular injury, cardiac tamponade, and traumatic aortic dissection. If the patient has a suspected aortic arch tear seen on chest x-ray film, the chest compartment takes the lowest priority, because patients either die instantaneously or are inherently stable over a few hours, allowing time to evaluate all of the compartments as needed.

There are multiple approaches to this compartment, all beginning with a supine chest x-ray film. Pneumothorax, hemothorax, and pulmonary contusions are all seen on this study if they are significant. If there is a normal mediastinum on x-ray film, an aortic tear is extremely unlikely, unless there is a massive deceleration mechanism, in which case a dynamic CT scan should be performed even if the chest x-ray film is normal. Abnormal chest x-ray findings consistent with aortic tears include mediastinal widening, blunted aortic knob, apical pleural capping, tracheal deviation, depression of the left mainstem bronchus, esophageal deviation, and loss of the paratracheal stripe. If any of these abnormal findings are present, the diagnostic options include the following:

1. Clearing the axial spine of injury by performing cervical spine x-ray films with or without thoracic spine x-ray films, depending on bony tenderness or mechanism (see Chapter 48 for cervical spine injury and indications for x-ray). Once the spine is clear, the patient can be seated upright for an upright chest x-ray film. This is done because a supine film can create the appearance of a widened mediastinum by magnifying the chest contents, when in fact the mediastinum is normal. If the upright chest x-ray examination is normal, the chest is considered clear.

2. Performing a dynamic chest CT.

3. Proceeding to aortography.

4. Performing transesophageal echocardiography (TEE).

Which approach is used depends on the degree of suspicion for an aortic tear based on the initial chest x-ray film and is a somewhat subjective issue. However, you should keep in mind that a positive dynamic CT scan usually means simply that the patient has nonspecific mediastinal blood (venous or arterial); this is further investigated with aortography to confirm the arterial injury. TEE is used in the patient with a high suspicion for an aortic tear but who is too unstable to travel to the aortography suite.

Unstable Blunt Trauma

Assessing a patient for stability is a continuous process (Fig. 47.3). You must constantly recheck the blood pressure, pulse, respiratory rate, and oxygenation of the patient. Instability can be manifested in several ways. Most often, a low blood pressure or sudden drop in blood pressure in an otherwise healthy individual occurs with blood loss. The patient may appear to become confused when he or she was initially oriented. The patient's respiratory rate may be high and oxygen saturation low because of low circulation of oxygenating red blood cells, pneumothorax, pulmonary contusions, or poor respiratory effort because of exhaustion.

The unstable patient receives the standard bolus of 1 to 2 L of normal saline or Ringer's lactate solution intravenously or blood in class 3 shock (decreased blood pressure). This may be repeated if needed. If the patient does not stabilize, the most likely possibility is ongoing blood loss and a rapid assessment of the limited sources of hemorrhage is undertaken. This includes skin inspection for lacerations, persistent tachycardia, and hypotension. If the patient is brought in wearing a cervical collar, take down the collar while an assistant holds the head in midline traction. Look for hidden scalp lacerations that may still be bleeding. The long bones and pelvis are examined for fractures. The thigh alone can hold several units of blood from a femur fracture. Major vascular injuries may occur with a significant pelvic fracture, resulting in severe blood loss that can lead to irreversible shock. A chest x-ray film is performed for hemothorax and either DPL or ultrasound of the abdomen is done to search for hemoperitoneum. If these are negative, nonhemorrhagic traumatic causes of shock must be considered. Physical examination for tension pneumothorax must be undertaken, and a chest x-ray film is reviewed if not already done. Echocardiography for cardiac contusion and tamponade should be performed. Spinal evaluation for fracture and spinal shock must be considered, although this entity must always be the diagnosis of exclusion.

After all traumatic issues have been addressed, nontraumatic etiologies (e.g., myocardial infarction, toxicological issues) should be investigated with an electrocardiogram (ECG) and toxicological screens. This standard approach to the relatively limited causes of shock in the trauma patient allows rapid assessment and resuscitation of

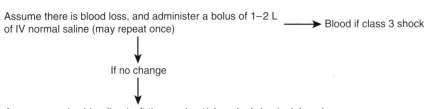

Assume there is blood loss, and administer a bolus of 1–2 L of IV normal saline (may repeat once) ⟶ Blood if class 3 shock

↓

If no change

↓

Assume ongoing bleeding (soft tissue, chest/pleural, abdominal, bony)

Nonbleeding traumatic cause (tension pneumothorax, cardiac tamponade, cardiac contusion, uncommonly neurogenic)

Nontraumatic (MI, toxicologic issues, etc.)

Always consider diversion to OR

Figure 47.3
General approach to the unstable trauma patient. MI, myocardial infarction; OR, operating room.

the unstable situation. As a final point, always consider transport to the OR for further evaluation and treatment in the persistently unstable patient.

Penetrating Trauma

Chest

Chest wounds can be broken down into stable and unstable, with each group being further subdivided into lateral (to the nipple line) and central. All gunshot wounds should be considered central. All other penetrating wounds should be classified as possibly central unless the point of entry is lateral to the nipple and is known to be from a short knife. Figure 47.4 describes the approach to the patient with penetrating chest trauma.

The Stable Patient

The initial step in evaluating the stable patient is to perform a chest x-ray examination. Obvious hemothorax and pneumothorax are treated with a chest tube. If the stab wounds are lateral and well above the diaphragm and below the clavicles (well away from the abdomen and root of the neck) and the initial chest x-ray film is normal, the patients can be managed by observation and a repeat chest x-ray examination in 6 hours. The patient can potentially be discharged if the repeat film is normal. After chest x-ray examination, central wounds in stable patients can be managed by observation or selective studies including echocardiography, angiography, esophageal studies, and occasionally bronchoscopy. The studies performed are those chosen by an experienced clinician using wound location, direction, and depth of

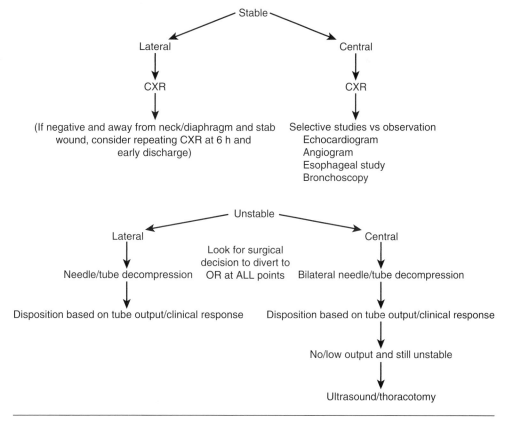

Figure 47.4
General approach to penetrating chest injuries. CXR, chest x-ray; OR, operating room.

penetration as determinants. With a low overall suspicion of deep structure violation, simple observation is also an option.

The Unstable Patient

Hemodynamically unstable patients with penetrating trauma require immediate surgical consultation, because there is a high likelihood of needing a thoracotomy. In the absence of a surgeon, empirical needle decompression followed by chest tube placement should be performed, unilaterally for lateral wounds and bilaterally for central wounds. Needle decompression uses a long, large-bore IV catheter (e.g., 14 gauge, 2.5 inches), which is inserted into the second intercostal space in the midclavicular line to the hub of the catheter. If no air is heard escaping from the catheter, there is a chance that the catheter is too short and has not entered the pleural space. Placing a chest tube on the same side must follow needle decompression. This eliminates a tension pneumothorax and provides vital information via chest tube output as to which side of the chest is bleeding and how much. Chest tube output that requires surgery is generally in the range of greater than 1,200 mL initially or greater than 200 mL/hour for 4 hours. If the patient loses vital signs in the department, the ED physician should perform an open thoracotomy. This procedure is only useful if there is immediate surgical backup available to take the patient to the OR.

In central wounds, if no obvious tension pneumothorax is found, and chest tube drainage is minimal, cardiac tamponade should be considered. An echocardiogram can be performed to confirm this, and thoracotomy in the ED (or preferably OR if time permits) must follow to repair the cardiac wound. You should keep in mind that all penetrating chest trauma in conjunction with hemodynamic instability, in the appropriate setting with a qualified surgeon, may be best served by rapid disposition to the OR for thoracotomy.

Abdomen

The initial evaluation of the patient who has sustained a penetrating injury to the abdomen is focused on identifying the usual indications for mandatory laparotomy (Fig. 47.5). These include hemodynamic instability, radiographic free air, evisceration, and peritonitis; most authors would also

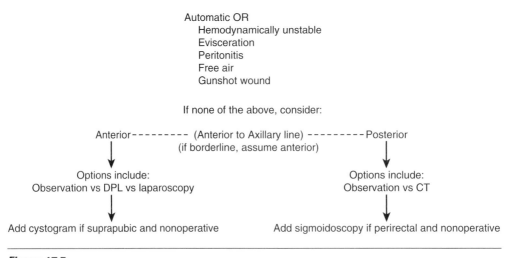

Automatic OR
Hemodynamically unstable
Evisceration
Peritonitis
Free air
Gunshot wound

If none of the above, consider:

Anterior - - - - - - - - (Anterior to Axillary line) - - - - - - - - Posterior
(if borderline, assume anterior)

Options include:
Observation vs DPL vs laparoscopy

Options include:
Observation vs CT

Add cystogram if suprapubic and nonoperative

Add sigmoidoscopy if perirectal and nonoperative

Figure 47.5
General approach to penetrating abdominal injuries. CT, computed tomography; DPL, diagnostic peritoneal lavage; OR, operating room.

include gunshot wounds. Assuming there is no immediate operative indication, the wounds are then classified as either anterior or posterior, using the mid axillary line as the dividing point.

Options for the evaluation of anterior wounds include either observation or DPL. There are no data to show that DPL is any more effective than observation in this situation, because DPL is relatively insensitive in detecting colonic wounds where early diagnosis can improve the patient's outcome. If a stab wound is thought to be relatively superficial, the wound opening may be extended and the wound explored to determine whether it has penetrated the peritoneal cavity. Another method for evaluating stab wounds is to do a laparoscopy to determine whether there is a violation of the peritoneum using direct visualization from the inside of the peritoneal cavity.

Options for evaluation of posterior wounds include either in-hospital observation or a "triple contrast" (IV, oral, and rectal) CT scan. There are no data to show that CT is any more effective than observation alone. This is predominantly because there are so few positive CT scans in the published literature that it is not possible to

develop a clear definition of what constitutes a positive scan, and as a result one cannot establish a course of action from that point onward (further studies, operation, angiography, and so forth). If a patient is deemed nonoperative, one should consider cystography for suprapubic wounds (to detect bladder wounds) and sigmoidoscopy (to detect rectal wounds) for perirectal wounds. Obviously, these are unnecessary if the patient is undergoing laparotomy, because direct inspection of the bladder and rectum can be performed in the OR.

Neck

Penetrating neck injuries are divided into three anatomic zones. Zone 1 extends from the clavicle to the cricoid cartilage. Zone 2 extends from the cricoid cartilage to the angle of the mandible. Zone 3 is from the mandibular angle to the skull base. Figure 47.6 describes the approach to the patient with penetrating neck trauma.

A wound is classified as penetrating if the platysma muscle is violated. Any wound with an expanding hematoma or hemodynamic instability is managed operatively, regardless of the zone of involvement. Wounds

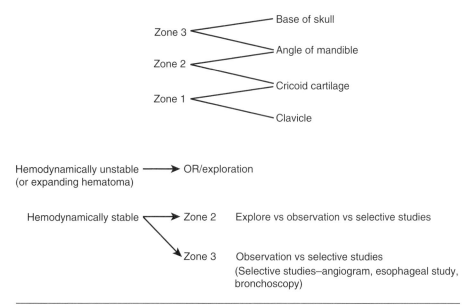

Figure 47.6
General approach to penetrating neck injuries. OR, operating room.

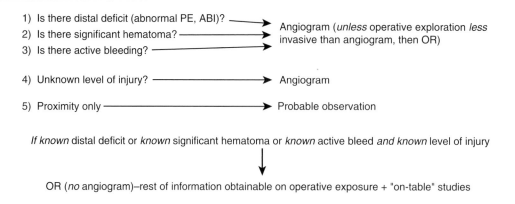

1) Is there distal deficit (abnormal PE, ABI)? ⟶

2) Is there significant hematoma? ⟶   Angiogram (*unless* operative exploration *less* invasive than angiogram, then OR)

3) Is there active bleeding? ⟶

4) Unknown level of injury? ⟶ Angiogram

5) Proximity only ⟶ Probable observation

If known distal deficit or *known* significant hematoma or *known* active bleed *and known* level of injury

↓

OR (*no* angiogram)–rest of information obtainable on operative exposure + "on-table" studies

Figure 47.7
General approach to peripheral vascular trauma. ABI, ankle-brachial index–leg systolic blood pressure divided by radial systolic blood pressure (normal = 1.1 to 0.8); OR, operating room; PE, physical examination.

in stable patients can be managed by observation or selective studies like angiography, esophagram or endoscopy, and occasionally bronchoscopy. The studies performed are those chosen by an experienced clinician using wound location and direction and depth of penetration as determinants. With a low overall suspicion of deep structure violation, simple observation is also an option. For zone 2 wounds, operative exploration may also be undertaken in stable patients, because the surgical exposure of the structures in this area is relatively easy compared with zones 1 and 3.

Peripheral Vascular Injuries

The initial question with peripheral vascular injuries is whether the patient needs an operation without any further diagnostic studies (Fig. 47.7). Assessment for serious vascular injuries can be remembered by the 5 Ps. A Pale, Painful, Poikilothermic (cold), Pulseless extremity with Paresthesias is a limb that is in danger of irreversible damage. Lower extremities can be assessed using the ankle-brachial index (ABI). This is simply a ratio of the systolic pressure auscultated at the ankle versus that of the brachial pulse using the same cuff. A normal ABI is usually greater than 0.8; however, in patients with a history of arterial insufficiency, it is only useful if prior evaluations demonstrated significantly different ABIs.

If there is an obvious vascular deficit (loss of pulse or low ABI) or obvious major bleeding and the level of injury is known (e.g., local fracture, penetrating wound), then operative exploration and repair is indicated without preoperative arteriographic studies. On-table studies in the OR may be performed if needed. When you are examining a wound and cannot decide whether there is a definite deficit or major bleeding or cannot determine the level of injury (possibly two or more levels of injury), then a diagnostic arteriogram is indicated. If the only issue with respect to a wound is its proximity to a major vessel, simple observation is warranted.

Suggested Readings

Beitsch PD, Flynn E, Easley S, et al. The role of physical exam and arteriography in patients with penetrating zone 2 neck wounds. *Arch Surg* 1994;129:577.

Demetriades, et al. The management of penetrating wounds of the back. *Ann Surg* 1988;207:72.

Feliciano, et al. 500 open taps or lavages in patients with abdominal stab wounds. *Am J Surg* 1984;148:772.

Gavant ML, Menke PG, Fabian T, et al. Blunt traumatic aortic rupture, detection with helical CT of the chest. *Cardiovasc Radiol* 1995;Oct, 197(1)125–133.

Gomez, et al. Suspected vascular trauma of the extremities: the role of arteriography in proximity injuries. *J Trauma* 1986;26:1005.

Kerr TM, Sood R, Buckman RF, et al: Prospective trial of the six-hour rule in stab wounds of the chest. *SGO* 1989;169(3)223–225.

McKenney MG, Martin L, Levitz K, et al. 1000 consecutive ultrasounds for blunt abdominal trauma. *J Trauma* 1996;40(6)607–612.

Phillips, et al. Use of the contrast enhanced CT enema in the management of penetrating trauma to the flank and back. *J Trauma* 1986;26:593.

Saletta S, Lederman E, Fein S, et al. Trans-esophageal echocardiography for the initial evaluation of the widened mediastinum in trauma patients. *J Trauma* 1995 July;39(1): 137–141.

Scalafani, et al. The role of angiography in penetrating neck trauma. *J Trauma* 1991;31: 557.

Smith MD, Cassidy JM, Sonther S, et al. Trans-esophageal echocardiography in the diagnosis of traumatic rupture of the aorta. *N Engl J Med* 1995;332(6)356–362.

Stiell IG, et al. The Canadian CT head rule for patients with minor head injury. *Lancet* 2001; 358:1013–1034.

Wood, et al. Penetrating neck injuries: Recommendations for selective management. *J Trauma* 1989;29:602.

Musculoskeletal Trauma

Elizabeth L. Mitchell, MD

Musculoskeletal trauma is one of the most common presenting complaints to the emergency department (ED).

Although these injuries are rarely life threatening, they may be limb threatening. In addition, the proper identification and treatment of these injuries may speed a good recovery and limit long-term morbidity and functional impairment. A careful focused history with an emphasis on mecha-

nism of injury may allow the physician to predict quite accurately the type of injury that a patient has sustained. As the physician most often first to see and diagnose musculoskeletal injury in the acute setting, the emergency physician must be able to accurately diagnose, initiate treatment, and determine the need for consultation. In addition, the emergency physician should be able to definitively treat a large number of orthopedic injuries. For those injuries requiring orthopedic consultation or follow-up, the emergency physician must know how to describe the injury in the precise terminology used by the orthopedic surgeon. This chapter attempts to familiarize the student with the general principles used in the evaluation and management of orthopedic trauma and the terminology used to describe those injuries.

Clinical Evaluation: General Principles

History

Mechanism of Injury

In evaluating an isolated orthopedic injury, the emergency physician should take an in-depth focused history. The history of the patient with an orthopedic injury is often underused, instead the physician depends entirely on x-ray films for diagnosis. In soft tissue injuries, in which x-ray films are rarely helpful, the history of injury is a primary diagnostic tool. Because much of orthopedics can be understood by the principles of physics, a firm understanding of the forces placed on a particular part of the skeleton may lead one to postulate not only the primary injury but associated injuries as well. For example, a patient has fallen 10 feet from a ladder. He complains of heel pain in one foot consistent with a calcaneous injury. From our knowledge of the force of this mechanism, we know that he has a 50% chance of having another injury. He has a good chance of having either a lumbar fracture or a fracture of the calcaneus of the other foot. He may not notice the pain of the secondary injury because of the distracting pain of the primary injury. He also may be intoxicated, which will lessen his ability to feel pain. The mechanism of injury always points you in the direction of the appropriate and complete diagnosis.

Time of Injury

Time of injury can be an important factor in diagnosis, treatment, and prognosis. As time from the injury increases, the ability to accurately diagnose may be confounded by local swelling and inflammation. For example, in an ankle sprain, early evaluation may elicit tenderness over one or more involved ligaments, but as time goes on generalized swelling expands the tissues and decreases the specificity of the examination. Time to swelling can add important information as well. A knee that swells immediately may indicate a ligament tear; one that swells after many hours may indicate a less severe soft tissue injury. Time may also hamper your treatment. The longer a joint is dislocated, the more spasm occurs in the surrounding muscles. This often makes the joint more difficult to reduce. In addition, time can worsen the prognosis of certain injuries, for example, leading to increased risks of infection in open fractures or avascular necrosis in hip dislocations.

Symptoms

Asking a patient about specific symptoms helps to focus the diagnosis and treatment. It is important to ask about swelling, muscle strength, range of motion, and sensory loss. What exacerbates or improves the injury? In addition, certain conditions have specific associated symptoms; for example, patients

Table 48.1.

History of musculoskeletal injury

Mechanism of injury
Time since injury
Symptoms
Age
Sex
Past medical history
Medications
Allergies
Type of work, activity level
Prior orthopedic injuries
Last food, drugs, or alcohol
Last tetanus shot

with meniscal tears often complain of the knee locking or giving out.

These are the important focused points of the orthopedic history. Additional information that is important to the patient's history includes age, sex, general level of activity and type of work, past medical history, medications and allergies, prior orthopedic injuries or treatment, drug or alcohol use, last meal, and last tetanus immunization (Table 48.1).

Physical Examination

The physical examination of the injured extremity should be performed before any manipulation. It is especially important to ascertain vascular and neurological deficits, because even simple movement can result in neurovascular damage.

Inspection

Before the laying on of one's hands, it is wise to inspect the involved area for any deformities, swelling, bruising, lacerations, or redness. Always compare sides, as this shows subtle changes more easily.

Palpation

Examination of soft tissue and bone injury can be very uncomfortable for the patient. One should begin with light touch to feel for warmth, crepitus, subcutaneous air, the tenseness of the soft tissues, and underlying hematomas. Areas of maximal tenderness should be found by gentle palpation. In a patient with obvious deformity, range of motion and palpation should be delayed until after radiographs and pain control. Neurovascular assessment should not be delayed.

Vascular Assessment

The vascular integrity of a limb should be assessed. Distal to the injury, the skin should be examined for warmth, color, and capillary refill. Pulses should be palpated. If pulses cannot be felt, a Doppler should be used to locate a pulse. Compare pulses on the uninjured side to detect differences in strength. If there is no pulse present, one must assume a vascular injury and take appropriate action to salvage the limb.

Neurological Assessment

Orthopedic injuries are often associated with specific nerve injuries. It is necessary to know the distribution of specific nerves and to know which injuries have a high association of neurological injuries. For example, ankle sprains may be associated with sural nerve injury. The sural nerve wraps around the lateral malleolus and may stretch or contuse in an inversion mechanism. Nerves can be contused, stretched, crushed, or severed. The type of injury determines the prognosis. Sensation distal to the injury should always be evaluated. Light touch, pinprick, and two-point discrimination in the fingers are usually adequate. Two-point discrimination measures the patient's ability to discriminate between two simultaneously placed points in a vertical direction, at the volar aspect of the distal finger. Normal discrimination is 4 to 5 mm. The uninjured side can be used as a comparison.

Motor Strength

Strength testing is done using a rating scale. In some instances, motor testing may be delayed for pain control, radiographs, or limb stabilization. Following is the rating scale commonly used:

0 = no contractility

1 = slight contractility but no motion

2 = complete motion without gravity

3 = complete motion against gravity, but none against resistance

4 = moves against resistance, decreased strength

5 = full resistance

Range of Motion

When possible, passive and active range of motion should be tested. All the motions of a particular joint should be tested in a passive manner by the examiner. When indicated, the patient should then be encouraged to actively range the joint.

Injury-Specific Testing

Many orthopedic injuries have examination techniques and tests specific to them. For example, the knee has specific tests to evaluate the integrity of the ligaments and the menisci (Table 48.2).

Diagnostic Evaluation

Plain radiographs are the mainstays of fracture diagnosis. Depending on the area being filmed, routine x-ray films include an anterior-posterior (AP) view and a lateral. In addition, some areas, such as the foot and fingers, require an oblique view. In most cases, the area above and below the injury should be included in x-ray films. Special views may be needed for particular injuries. For example, a suspected patellar view requires a "sunrise" x-ray film, taken with the knee bent 45 degrees and the x-ray beam originating from in front of the patient through the patella. When a certain diagnosis is suspected or discovered, x-ray films looking for associated injuries must be obtained. Other modes of diagnosis may be required in certain conditions. Injuries such as calcaneus fractures or hip fractures may require computed tomography (CT) scan.

Table 48.2.

Musculoskeletal physical examination

Inspection
Capillary refill
Skin temperature

Swelling
Color
Deformity
Skin integrity

Motor Functions
Strength
Range of motion

Palpation
Warmth
Crepitus
Hematoma
Tenderness

Neurovascular Assessment
Pulses
Sensation
Two-point discrimination

Special Tests

Although not typically performed in the ED, bone scan or magnetic resonance imaging (MRI) may be useful when occult fracture is suspected with normal x-ray films. Plain x-ray films are also useful to rule out foreign bodies in penetrating injury.

Prehospital Evaluation

The primary survey, evaluation of airway, breathing, and circulation (the ABCs) guides the initial prehospital approach to the orthopedic trauma patient. The primary survey is the evaluation of the ABCs. Once the prehospital provider has determined that there is no life-threatening injury, attention is turned to the injured area. Attention to neurovascular status is critical before any manipulation. The injured extremity should be splinted to provide stability in transport. If possible, the limb should also be elevated. In cases of bleeding from an extremity injury, direct pressure is the desired method of

hemorrhage control. This is usually effective. Tourniquets are highly undesirable and should only be used in the rare instance when direct pressure is ineffective and the patient is at risk of exsanguinating. When a tourniquet is used, the time of application should be noted. If the transport time to the hospital is unusually long, as in a rural area, the tourniquet should be let down periodically to allow distal perfusion.

In amputations, the amputated part should be transported to the ED. Any gross contamination should be washed off with sterile saline and the amputated part should be wrapped in saline-moistened gauze, placed in a plastic bag or container, and packed in ice.

Fractures

The topic of fractures is enormous. Multiple-volume textbooks have been written on this subject alone. There are numerous fractures possible in a given bone, multiplied by hundreds of bones. For the purposes of this book, the topic of fractures is too large to discuss diagnosis and treatment of individual injuries. However, there are general terms, goals of treatment, and special circumstances that can guide the initial evaluation of any patient with a potential fracture.

The terminology can be overwhelming. It is crucial for the emergency physician to understand and use the standard language of orthopedics. This avoids confusion and allows the emergency physician to accurately describe injuries. When the orthopedist and the emergency physician are able to communicate in precise language, the emergency physician can often treat the patient acutely with appropriate orthopedic follow-up. When the orthopedist is unclear about an injury, an unnecessary ED consultation may be required, or worse, a serious injury misdiagnosed. Select orthopedic terminology is illustrated in Fig. 48.1. Table 48.3 lists some of the common orthopedic definitions.

Treatment

Treatment depends on the nature of the injury. With the exception of some foot, clavicle, and humerus fractures, most fractures require immobilization to heal. Immobilization may take the form of splints, casts, pins, plates, or screws. Depending on the fracture, manipulation may be required to return the bones to anatomic position. This may be done under local anesthesia, regional blocks, conscious sedation, or operative reduction. Stable fractures that are nondisplaced (in anatomic position) and not intraarticular can usually be splinted in the ED and released with orthopedic follow-up. Splints or casts placed in the ED must cross the joint above and below a fracture, to keep the fragments from moving. Splinting is the immobilization of choice in the ED. (See Chapter 75.) It allows for the acute phase of swelling to occur and can be converted to a cast at a later time. In general, all fractures that are open, involve the joint, are unstable, or require reduction should have orthopedic consultation in the ED. There are other factors to consider as well. Patients who are elderly or have comorbid conditions such as diabetes require special attention and follow-up. Some patients may require admission if they live alone or are incapable of caring for themselves. In general, the treatment and disposition of each case must be considered on an individual basis.

Complications

Many complications are associated with fractures. Some of these are life threatening and some limb threatening. They include hemorrhage, vascular and nerve injuries, compartment syndrome, and avascular necrosis. Hemorrhage occurs to some extent in any fracture. The skeleton is highly vascular and bleeds extensively when injured. In a confined space, such as the wrist, hemorrhage is limited. However, in certain areas (pelvis, thigh), a large amount of blood can be lost, putting the patient at risk for shock. Isolated vascular injury can occur as well. Arterial injury may result from laceration by a bone fragment, significant force, or excessive swelling. If the patient exhibits signs of arterial insufficiency, arteriography or explo-

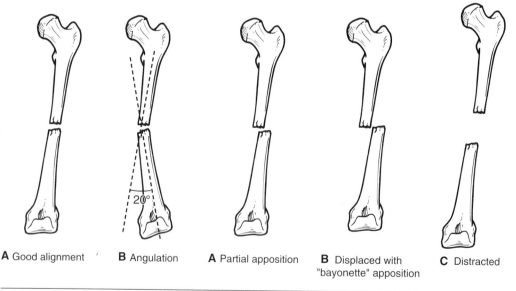

A Good alignment   **B** Angulation   **A** Partial apposition   **B** Displaced with "bayonette" apposition   **C** Distracted

Figure 48.1
Select orthopedic terminology.

Table 48.3.

Limited orthopedic glossary

Angulated: fracture whose two ends are no longer in a straight plane but are at an angle (described in degrees)

Avulsion: small fracture (chip) near a joint that usually has ligament or tendon attached

Closed: (simple) fracture that has no open wound to the skin

Comminuted: fracture with multiple fragments

Dislocation: disruption in the continuity of a joint whereby the bone ends are no longer in contact

Displaced: fracture whose ends are separated (usually described as percentage or in millimeters)

Distracted: fracture whose ends are separated in the vertical plane

Fracture: a break in the continuity of a bone

Impacted: fracture whose ends are driven into each other

Intraarticular: fracture that involves the joint surface of a bone

Ligaments: stabilizing structures that connect bone to bone, usually around a joint

Occult: fracture is clinically suspected but not radiographically evident

Open: (compound) fracture in which there is a communicating open wound of the skin and soft tissue

Pathologic: fracture resulting from an underlying illness, usually malignancy

Spiral: fracture results from a rotational force and presents as a spiral in a long bone

Sprain: injury to the supporting ligaments or capsule of a joint

Strain: overstretching of a muscle or tendon

Subluxation: incomplete dislocation

Tendons: pulley mechanisms that connect bone to muscle

Transverse: fracture occurs at a right angle to the long axis of a bone

---

ration may be required. Other complications occur after the initial presentation. Avascular necrosis occurs in bones with a tenuous blood supply and may lead to bone loss. Problems with healing can lead to malunion or nonunion, in which the two fracture fragments heal incorrectly or not at all. Chronic pain syndromes such as reflex sympathetic dystrophy (RSD), also known as complex regional pain syndrome (CRPS), may develop after traumatic injury. The syndrome is believed to be of nerve origin, which leads to pain, muscular atrophy, and skin changes, and can be permanently debilitating. In addition, immobilization has numerous risks, including pulmonary embolus, deep venous thrombosis, pneumonia, and muscle atrophy.

Open Fractures

In addition to all the information stated earlier, open fractures deserve a brief description of their own. An open fracture is any fracture that communicates with the skin. This can be as dramatic as a fragment of bone protruding out the skin or as subtle as a small puncture wound. Whenever there is disruption of the skin's integrity near a fracture, it is incumbent on the ED physician to determine whether or not it communicates with the bone. Similarly, any wound in close proximity to a joint must be evaluated for possible communication with the joint. This can be accomplished in several ways:

Inspection: There is obvious communication and bone is visible beneath a wound.

Exploration: Using a sterile technique, the wound is gently probed to determine the path of the opening and any communication with fracture below.

Fat droplets: If fat droplets are evident in the blood from a wound, it is fairly good evidence of communication with a fracture.

Saline arthrogram: To rule out joint involvement of a wound, saline is injected into the joint space, at a site distant from the wound. The wound is then inspected for any sign of saline leakage.

Open fractures are at high risk for infection and osteomyelitis. All open fractures and wounds communicating with a joint require intravenous antibiotics and copious irrigation, usually in the operating room. All patients should have orthopedic consultation in the ED as well.

Pediatric Fractures

Fractures in the pediatric population present unique problems. Children's bones are in a state of growth throughout childhood. They have a growth plate at or near the ends of the long bones, known as the epiphyses. The growth plate is cartilaginous and is not visible on plain x-ray film. This makes the diagnosis of fractures in the area of a growth plate very difficult. It also requires its own classification system to describe growth plate injuries. This is known as the Salter-Harris Classification, detailed in Table 48.4 and illustrated in Fig. 48.2. Epiphyseal injuries are common because of the weakness of the cartilaginous growth zone. They should be suspected in any child with pain in the epiphyseal aspect of a long bone. It is often helpful to get comparison views of the unaffected side. Types I and II have a good prognosis. Types III and IV require anatomic reduction and may still have growth disturbances. Type V causes growth arrest.

Pediatric patients have other unique qualities. The bones are generally softer than adults and may sustain incomplete fractures such as a "greenstick" or "torus" fracture. A greenstick fracture is an angulated long bone fracture that looks, aptly, like a green stick that has been bent. A torus fracture appears like a wrinkle and is a buckling injury. Finally, in pediatric fracture patients, one has to consider the possibility of nonaccidental trauma (NAT). Patients who present with a suspicious history or multiple episodes of fractures, and particularly infants with fractures, should be considered possible victims of abuse. If any question of NAT exists, social services and the appropriate state agency must be notified.

Compartment Syndrome

Complications of fractures include vascular injury, nerve injury, nonunion, osteomyelitis, avascular necrosis, skin breakdown, and long-term disability. In addition, there are several entities that can have life-threatening and limb-threatening complications. Pelvic fractures, femur fractures, and open fractures are at risk for major hemorrhage. The pelvis and the thigh can hide large volumes of blood loss. The pelvis in particular can cause a patient to exsanguinate with little outward evidence. The clinician must anticipate this complication and be ready with blood products as needed until bleeding can be controlled.

In addition, fractures and crush injuries are at risk for compartment syndrome. This can cause tissue ischemia and loss of limb. Compartment syndrome can be caused by

Table 48.4.
Salter-Harris classification of pediatric fractures

Type I: fracture through the growth plate, appears as widening on plain x-rays
Type II: fracture through growth plate, extends up into metaphysis
Type III: fracture through growth plate, extends into epiphysis
Type IV: fracture through growth plate, epiphysis, and metaphysis
Type V: crush injury of the epiphyseal plate

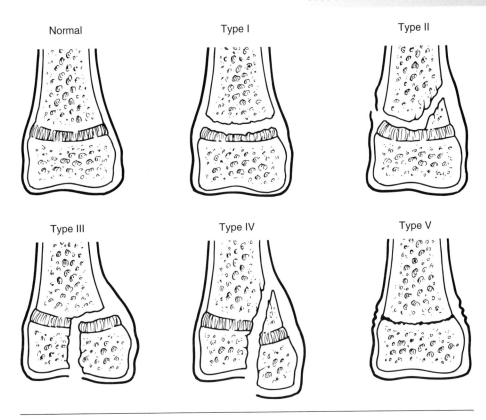

Figure 48.2
Salter-Harris classification of pediatric growth plate injuries.

several different entities. The injury is ultimately the same, whatever the cause: swelling within a muscular compartment (enclosed by fascial planes) that leads to obstruction of blood flow. When left untreated, this leads to muscle hypoxia and necrosis. When multiple compartments are involved, myonecrosis can lead to myoglobinuria, rhabdomyolysis, renal failure, and even death. The causes of compartment syndrome are many. Fractures, vascular injuries, prolonged use of a tourniquet, and high-voltage electrical injury are some examples.

Diagnosis of compartment syndrome requires clinical suspicion, because early treatment has the best prognosis. There are six classic signs, known as the six Ps of ischemia: pain with passive stretch, pallor, paralysis, pulselessness, paresthesias, and poikilothermia (cold extremity). Ideally, diagnosis is made early. One of the earliest and most sensitive physical examination findings is pain with passive stretch. Pulses are lost late in the course, and ideally, diagnosis should be made well before that. Measuring the compartment pressure can make the diagnosis. This can be done in several ways; one way is to introduce a needle into the involved compartment and measure tissue pressure. Normal pressures are between 12 and 20 cm H_2O. When intracompartmental pressure exceeds 30 torr (cm H_2O), decompression is indicated. Compartment syndrome is a surgical emergency and treatment is aimed at releasing compartment pressures with fasciotomy.

Dislocations

The primary treatment goal of all dislocations is successful reduction of the joint. Every joint is capable of dislocation. Some joints, such as the shoulder, interphalangeals, and temporomandibular, are more commonly dislocated. The shoulder is by far the most commonly dislocated joint, mainly because of its enormous range of motion and lack of constraining elements. Other joints dislocate less frequently but may have catastrophic results when they do. The knee, for example, if dislocated, may result in severe neurovascular damage. For a more complete discussion of dislocations, see Chapter 74.

Sprains

A sprain is defined as a stretching injury to a ligament supporting a joint. The most common sprain and one of the most common ED complaints is the ankle sprain. The role of ligaments is to provide support to joint motion. That means that a ligament works with other stabilizing structures, such as muscle, to restrain the movement of the bones in a joint complex. When the forces on a particular joint motion are greater than the tensile strength of a ligament, it is injured. For example, in the knee, the anterior cruciate ligament (ACL) restrains forward motion of the femur on the tibia. When a person runs or skis and is suddenly stopped or cut off, the femur continues to accelerate over the motionless lower leg, and the force often tears the ACL. There are three basic grades of sprain:

Grade I: microscopic tear, tenderness to palpation, stable

Grade II: macroscopic but incomplete tear, tender to palpation, moderately unstable

Grade III: complete rupture of the ligament, unstable joint

Diagnosis

Physical examination is the hallmark of diagnosis. Tenderness over a ligament, swelling, and joint instability are all signs of ligament injury. Radiographs should be obtained when a fracture cannot be confidently ruled out. In the case of ankle, foot, and knee pain, a set of rules—the Ottawa rules—have been developed and tested to guide the use of x-ray examination. The Ottawa rules were developed in Ottawa, Canada, using a series of studies that accurately predicted when radiographs were unnecessary. The initial studies were done on ankle pain and later developed for the knee and cervical spine. X-ray films should be ordered in the situations described in Table 48.5.

Treatment

Treatment depends on the specific area injured and extent of injury. General treatment is based on the mnemonic RICE (rest, ice, compression, and elevation). Usually a patient can be advised on range of motion and strengthening exercises. Physical therapy

---

Table 48.5.

The Ottawa rules for the ankle, foot, and knee describe the findings that indicate a need for x-ray examination

Ankle Pain
Bone tenderness posterior edge, distal 6 cm, or tip of either malleolus
Inability to bear weight for four steps immediately after injury and at evaluation

Foot Pain
Bone tenderness at the navicular or base of the fifth metatarsal
Inability to bear weight for four steps immediately after injury and at evaluation

Knee Pain
Age 55 years or older
Tenderness at the head of the fibula or patella
Inability to bear weight for four steps immediately after injury and at evaluation

may be helpful. For certain ligamentous injuries, orthopedic referral is advised. Some of the more common injuries that should be referred include the cruciate and collateral ligaments of the knee, grade two or three ankle sprains, and the collateral ligaments of the thumb (ski-pole or gamekeeper's thumb).

Complications

The complications of a ligament injury depend on the joint involved and degree of sprain. Pain and joint instability are the most common complications of any sprain. In addition, nerve injury—primarily stretch or contusion—may also occur. Some sprains may require surgical interventions. Long-term complications may include degenerative arthritis or repeat injury to the same joint.

Spine Injury

This chapter would be incomplete without mention of the enormous topic of injuries to the cervical, lumbar, and thoracic spine. These injuries range from minor muscle strain to life-threatening cervical spine injuries. In most cases of trauma, cervical spine protection is required until an injury can be ruled out. Injuries to the spine can result in death, quadriplegia, paraplegia, and chronic disability. Half of these injuries occur from motor vehicle and motorcycle accidents and the other half occur from falls, sporting activities, and intentional trauma. The elderly and those with malignancy or osteoporosis are at risk of injury from even minor falls. The cost to society, for the care of severely disabled spinal cord patients, is in the billions of dollars. In addition, the psychological and emotional impact to families is unfathomable.

By far the most devastating and most common injuries occur to the cervical spine. The cervical spine x-ray film is the most frequently ordered skeletal film in the ED. In this era of cost containment and overcrowding, decreasing x-ray ordering has significant implications. Several large studies have been undertaken to try to decrease the number of cervical spine x-ray examinations. They include the NEXUS Trial and the Ottawa group (the same group who developed the Ottawa ankle and knee rules). Each trial has devised a set of criteria for clearing the cervical spine. The Ottawa cervical spine rules can be seen in Table 48.6.

Table 48.6.

Ottawa cervical spine rules for radiography

---

1. Any high-risk factor that mandates radiography?
- Age greater than or equal to 65
- Dangerous mechanism
- Paresthesias in extremities

If Yes, radiography; if No, then go to part 2

2. Any low-risk factor that allows safe assessment of range of motion?
- Simple rear-end MVC
- Sitting position in ED
- Ambulatory at any time
- Delayed onset of neck pain
- Absence of midline cervical-spine tenderness

If No, then radiography

If Yes, then

3. Able to actively rotate neck 45-degrees right and left?

If able, no radiography

If unable, radiography

ED, emergency department; MVC, motor vehicle crash.

Suggested Readings

Hoffman, JR. Validity of a set of clinical criteria to rule out injury to the cervical spine in patients with blunt trauma. *N Engl J Med* 2000;343:94–99.

Marx JA, Hockberger R, Walls R, et al, eds. *Rosen's emergency medicine concepts and clinical practice*, 5th ed. St. Louis: Mosby, 2002.

Ruiz E, Cicero JJ. *Emergency management of skeletal injuries.* St. Louis: Mosby, 1995.

Stiell IG, McKnight RD, Greenberg GH, et al. Implementation of the Ottawa ankle rules. *JAMA* 1994;271:827–832.

Stiell IG, Wells GA, Vandemheem KL, et al. The Canadian C-spine rule for radiography in alert and stable trauma patients. *JAMA* 2001;286: 1841–1848.

49

Trauma During Pregnancy

Robert P. Collins, MD

All emergency physicians must be prepared to evaluate and treat pregnant patients who are victims of trauma. Trauma during pregnancy is not an uncommon occurrence; in fact, some type of trauma complicates 6% to 7% of all pregnancies. Furthermore, trauma is the leading cause of nonobstetric death in women of childbearing age. Injuries during pregnancy range from minor to catastrophic, including instances in which the life of the fetus is lost, and extreme cases in which the viable fetus is delivered but the mother does not survive.

Regardless of the severity of injury, all health care providers experience high levels of anxiety when caring for an expectant mother involved in the tragedy of a trauma. The pregnant trauma patient presents the emergency physician with a complicated and often vague clinical situation. Two patients are present at one time, both interrelated. Therapies directed at the expectant mother also have direct effects on the unborn child.

As the specialist most likely to care for pregnant trauma patients, the emergency physician must have a comprehensive understanding of trauma care. This must be combined with a thorough knowledge of the physiological and anatomic changes that take place during pregnancy. Attention should also be paid to details in the history and physical examination that may suggest physical abuse or domestic violence. This chapter familiarizes the student with the evaluation and management of the unique situation that exists when treating pregnant patients involved in trauma.

Evaluation of the Patient

Any female trauma patient of childbearing age presenting to the emergency department (ED) must be checked for pregnancy. Questions regarding menstrual history are often omitted by clinicians, and answers to these questions are often misleading and unreliable. Therefore, all female trauma patients of reproductive age should be screened with urine pregnancy tests. Until a negative result is obtained, it is prudent to assume that the patient may be pregnant.

Obtain a detailed history of the traumatic event when possible. This is true in any trauma patient but is especially pertinent in pregnancy. Whether the history is obtained from the patient, the family, or the paramedics, this information often provides valuable information to the emergency medicine team. As with any trauma patient, questions regarding the mechanism of injury, prehospital vital signs, and general questions about pain and discomfort are all appropriate. Ask about past medical history, any medications the patient is taking, or whether she has any drug allergies. Pay special attention to any complaints of abdominal pain or cramping, low back pain, or vaginal bleeding. These complaints have unique significance in pregnant trauma patients. Often these symptoms are associated with intraabdominal injuries or fetal complications.

Management

As with all injured patients, assessment of airway, breathing, and circulation (the ABCs of trauma management) should be rapidly and efficiently accomplished. The patient's airway is of primary importance in any trauma case. It should be quickly assessed and maintained. If the airway is compromised, it should be immediately managed with endotracheal intubation. Breathing should always be supported with supplemental 100% oxygen by facemask if the patient is not intubated. Because it is not known what level of hypoxemia is associated with fetal demise, maintaining a high level of maternal oxygen saturation is critical during the workup and resuscitation of the mother. A high level of maternal oxygen saturation directly increases fetal oxygen saturation. High fetal oxygen levels result in improved tolerance by the fetus of the stress of trauma. Regardless of the apparent stability of the mother, always maintain continuous oxygen saturation monitoring with pulse oximetry.

It is important to recall that fetal hemoglobin differs from maternal hemoglobin. The oxygen dissociation curve is shifted to the left so that fetal hemoglobin can effectively extract oxygen from the mother. Small increases in maternal oxygen content result in proportionately larger changes in fetal oxygen content. Maintenance of high levels of fetal oxygenation is the first and most crucial step in effective fetal resuscitation.

After all issues pertaining to the airway and breathing have been addressed, the emergency physician should turn his or her attention to ensuring that adequate maternal circulation is present. Two large-bore intravenous (IV) catheters should be inserted and infusion of normal saline or lactated Ringer's should be started. As maternal blood loss progresses, the mother shunts blood away from the uterus to maintain perfusion to her vital organs. Even relatively mild maternal blood loss can result in fetal distress and shock. Keep in mind that a well-appearing mother may be compensating at the expense of the fetus.

Management of the injured pregnant patient beyond the first trimester should be accomplished with her in the left lateral decubitus position. Supine hypotension occurs when the pregnant uterus lies on top of the mother's inferior vena cava, directly compressing it. This significantly reduces venous blood return to the right side of the heart. It can lead to rapid and, at times, large decreases in the maternal blood pressure. The simple maneuver of shifting the mother onto her left side, either with rolled towels under the backboard or by manually distracting the uterus to the left, can mean the difference between hemodynamic stability and hypotensive shock in the mother.

When performing a physical examination and assessment of a pregnant trauma patient, it is essential to remember that the signs and symptoms of shock may be delayed when compared with nonpregnant patients. There is a physiological increase in maternal blood volume that leads to the tolerance of significant blood loss by the mother before her vital signs deteriorate. The fetus, however, often shows signs of distress before the mother because uterine blood flow is decreased. Maternal vital signs often remain near normal until there has been a large volume of blood loss. Deterioration of the maternal vital signs is often followed by rapid hemodynamic failure and shock.

Care of the pregnant trauma patient is often an emotional and stressful situation for all providers. It is important to avoid the temptation to focus efforts on the unborn child and the pregnancy. A delay in either treatment or needed diagnostic tests because of concern for the fetus can lead to poor outcomes for both the mother and child. Pregnancy should never alter or delay resuscitation and treatment of the mother. The best and most effective care for the fetus is timely and aggressive resuscitation of the mother.

During the initial assessment, the ABCs of trauma care, severe or ongoing blood loss, and all major and life-threatening injuries are addressed. Only when this is accomplished is it suitable for the examining physician to move on to a secondary survey of the patient. At this point in the evaluation, examination of the mother from head to toe in an organized and detailed fashion is appropriate. During the secondary survey of the mother, the clinician should perform a first assessment of the fetus.

The gestational age can be estimated during the physical examination of the abdomen. It is important to recognize if the fetus is potentially viable. If viability is possible and signs of fetal distress persist despite treatment, emergent cesarean section by an obstetrician may be necessary to save the baby. Currently, a gestational age of 23 weeks is considered the lower limit of fetal viability. A measurement from the pubic symphysis to the top of the uterine fundus in centimeters roughly approximates the gestational age in weeks (Fig. 49.1). For example, 24 cm equals 24 weeks. A less accurate but faster and generally acceptable approach is to palpate three fingerbreadths above the umbilicus. If the uterine fundus is palpated at this level, fetal viability is possible. If the fetus is found to be previable (i.e., less than 23 weeks), an assessment of the fetal pulse is usually the extent of the fetal evaluation. If the pregnancy is determined to be greater than 23 weeks, continuous fetal heart rate monitoring and continuous monitoring of maternal uterine contractions are warranted. This external monitoring is known as cardiotocodynamometry (CTD). You must be aware of early signs of fetal distress in a fetus that has reached viability. Signs of distress in a viable fetus may

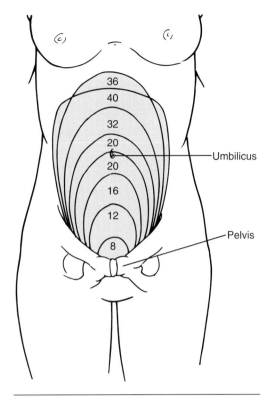

Figure 49.1
The size of the uterus relative to number of weeks' gestation.

necessitate immediate cesarean delivery by an obstetrician.

Anatomic and Physiological Changes During Pregnancy

For physicians who do not care for pregnant patients on a regular basis, recollection of the large number of anatomic and physiological changes that occur during a normal pregnancy is difficult at best. A thorough knowledge of these clinically important changes is critical to effective care and resuscitation of pregnant trauma patients. Significant physiological changes occur in the cardiovascular, respiratory, hematological, and gastrointestinal systems among others. Clinically significant anatomic changes occur in the abdomen, pelvis, and thoracic area. An understanding of these changes facilitates accurate and timely decisions that can make the difference between a good and bad out-come for both the mother and child.

Maternal Blood Volume

Maternal blood volume increases by 50% by the twenty-eighth week. Plasma volume increases proportionally more than the red blood cells. This results in a normal physiological anemia during the middle and late stages of pregnancy because of the dilutional effects on the red blood cell mass. Hematocrit levels tend to decrease. During late pregnancy a hematocrit of 32 to 36 ml/dl is normal. White blood cell counts also change and tend to be slightly higher in pregnancy, ranging from 5000 to 16,000/mm^3.

Hemodynamic Changes

Hemodynamic changes that occur in pregnancy include an increase in the resting heart rate and a decrease in blood pressure. The pulse is increased by an average of ten beats per minute. The systolic blood pressure decreases by an average of 2 to 4 mm Hg by the third trimester. These changes are minimal; therefore, any clinically significant drop in blood pressure or rise in pulse should be attributed to hemodynamic shock and not to normal variations that occur in pregnancy.

Significant Anatomic Changes

Significant anatomic changes occur within the abdomen and pelvis as pregnancy progresses. In nonpregnant women, the uterus is located within the pelvis, protected somewhat from injury by the pelvic bones. Uterine injuries in the nonpregnant woman are very rare in blunt and penetrating trauma. By the second trimester, the uterus transitions from the pelvis to the abdomen. This change in anatomic location leads to an increased susceptibility to injury during both blunt and penetrating trauma. There is a substantial increase in blood flow to the uterus during pregnancy. Uterine injuries may result in severe maternal hemorrhage. The enlargement of the uterus during pregnancy also alters the anatomic location of some abdominal organs. Bowel is pushed

away from the peritoneum. Pain fibers within the peritoneum are stretched and their density is decreased. This leads to blunting of abdominal pain and decreased sensitivity to free blood in the peritoneum. The abdominal examination is therefore misleading to the clinician and physical findings are often delayed or even absent.

Bowel is displaced into the upper abdomen as pregnancy progresses. During penetrating abdominal trauma, multiple bowel loops may be injured. The liver and spleen remain in the same position as in the nonpregnant state. Therefore the incidence and severity of injuries to the liver and spleen is not changed. The bladder, particularly when full, is more susceptible to injury because it is displaced from a pelvic to an abdominal organ after the twelfth week of pregnancy.

Gastric emptying time is increased and pressure is exerted on the stomach from the enlarged uterus and crowded bowel. The pressure is especially great when the patient is on her back, as in a trauma situation. This may lead to increased risk of vomiting and subsequent aspiration of stomach contents into the lungs. Early and frequent use of a nasogastric tube to decompress the stomach is prudent.

Assessment of the Fetus

Fetal Monitoring

In the previable fetus, documentation of fetal heart tones should be obtained in the secondary survey. If absent or unobtainable, no further action is required at this time.

The situation is different in the case of a potentially viable fetus. When it is determined that the fetus may have reached a gestational age of 23 weeks or more, CTD is required to monitor the fetus. CTD is an external monitor placed on the mother's abdomen. This monitor simultaneously records uterine contractions and fetal heart rate, and can alert the clinician to early signs of fetal distress. Subtle changes can occur over a short time; therefore, all emergency physicians should be familiar with interpretation of fetal monitor tracings before an obstetrician is available. CTD is the closest thing the clinician has to observe the fetus inside the maternal uterus. Continuous CTD is the most reliable indicator of how the fetus is tolerating the stress of trauma. A decrease in the beat-to-beat variability or a deceleration of the fetal heart rate indicates fetal distress.

Fetal Distress

When signs of fetal distress are detected, quick action must be taken. Optimization of maternal oxygenation and aggressive volume resuscitation should occur. As mentioned before, repositioning the mother onto her left side or manually pushing the pregnant uterus off the inferior vena cava may help. When these measures have failed, the consulting obstetrician should be notified immediately because emergency cesarean section may be indicated.

Fetomaternal Hemorrhage

Fetomaternal hemorrhage (FMH) is a unique problem specific to pregnancy. FMH often occurs during trauma when the normally separate fetal and maternal circulations are mixed across the placenta. When an Rh-negative (Rh⁻) mother is exposed to Rh-positive (Rh⁺) blood from the fetus, the mother can be sensitized. The mother then produces Rh antibodies to the Rh⁺ fetal red cells. Future pregnancies can be complicated by this sensitization. It is important to realize that the frequency of FMH and the volume of hemorrhage are not related to the severity of the trauma. All Rh⁻ mothers who present to the ED with a history of any abdominal trauma should receive prophylactic Rh immune globulin (RhoGAM) to prevent sensitization.

Blunt Trauma

Head Injury

The major cause of significant maternal trauma is motor vehicle accidents. The second most frequent cause is direct assaults on the abdomen, often from domestic violence. Falls also occur with increased frequency as pregnancy progresses. As the pregnancy

progresses, the mother's center of gravity is displaced and balance becomes more difficult.

As with nonpregnant trauma victims, head injuries are the primary cause of maternal morbidity and mortality. There is no evidence that isolated, severe head injuries are associated with fetal loss. All mothers with severe head injury and evidence of a live fetus should be aggressively supported. Delivery of a healthy baby is still possible even in the case of maternal brain death, and instances have occurred when the mother has been supported until fetal viability is reached. Decisions regarding withdrawal of support or maintenance of life support in severe head injuries should be made in accordance with the patient's and the family's wishes.

Abdominal Injury

In blunt abdominal trauma, placental abruption is often the cause of fetal demise and maternal blood loss. In placental abruption, the relatively stiff placenta separates from the inner wall of the flexible uterus. Significant bleeding usually occurs. Separation of 50% or more is frequently associated with fetal death. Signs of placental abruption may include vaginal bleeding, uterine tenderness, uterine contractions, and evidence of fetal distress on external fetal monitoring. Absence of vaginal bleeding should not lead you to rule out abruption. The uterus can sequester a large volume of blood with no external bleeding.

Uterine rupture is possible in blunt abdominal trauma. Although uncommon, it is associated with rapid maternal deterioration. Fetal survival is very unlikely when the uterus ruptures.

The fetus may also sustain direct injury during blunt abdominal trauma. Fetal head injuries are of special concern, especially when the mother suffers a pelvic fracture.

Penetrating Trauma

Penetrating abdominal trauma consists of stab wounds and bullet wounds. As with nonpregnant patients, stab wounds tend to have a better prognosis than gunshot wounds. The enlarging uterus does provide a protective shielding effect for the mother and often the penetrating object lodges within the uterine cavity or the fetus. As with nonpregnant patients, a trauma surgeon in the operating room should surgically explore all bullet wounds to the abdomen. Stab wounds are often managed with a diagnostic peritoneal lavage, ultrasound, or expectant management with frequent abdominal examinations. Surgical exploration of the abdomen is well tolerated by the pregnant patient and the fetus. A laparotomy does not necessarily require a simultaneous cesarean section.

Minor Trauma

A far more common situation encountered by the emergency physician is the pregnant patient involved in minor trauma. Whether from a minor fall, blow to the abdomen, or isolated extremity injury, even seemingly insignificant trauma requires a meticulous workup. Although minor maternal injury usually does not result in harmful effects to the fetus, any degree of maternal injury can be associated with fetal loss. This fetal demise is usually from placental abruption. For both medical and legal reasons, it is imperative that the emergency physician be familiar with current practice guidelines for care of the pregnant patient involved in minor trauma with a viable fetus. The first step involves managing the mother exactly as a nonpregnant patient. After the specific complaints and injuries have been addressed, all pregnant patients greater than 23 weeks' gestational age involved in trauma of any type should be monitored with external fetal monitoring for 4 hours. This monitoring should be done under the supervision of an obstetrician whenever possible. Symptoms of placental abruption can include abdominal pain or cramping, vaginal bleeding, uterine contractions, or signs of fetal distress detected by an external fetal monitor. Immediate obstetrical consultation is warranted should any of these occur. If no signs of placental abruption have occurred within 4 hours, it is safe to discharge the patient home with obstetrical follow-up and detailed instructions to return should pain, cramping, or bleeding occur.

Medications and Radiological Studies

As with every aspect of managing pregnant trauma patients, the first and foremost goal is to care for the mother. An indicated radiological study or medication should never be withheld or delayed because of concerns for the fetus. However, it is prudent to weigh the benefits of any medication or radiographic study against the risks to mother and child.

Most medications that are commonly administered in trauma patients are acceptable in pregnancy. Narcotics such as morphine and anesthetic agents are generally safe. Paralytic agents that are given for rapid-sequence intubations have not been well studied in pregnancy, but if indicated should not be withheld. These agents do cross the placenta, so their effects may be seen in the newborn if delivery occurs soon after their administration. Penicillin and cephalosporin antibiotics are safe. Aminoglycoside and tetracycline antibiotics should be avoided in pregnancy. The dose of fetal radiation exposure from x-rays performed during a trauma is well below the minimum threshold thought to cause fetal side effects. Most detrimental effects occur in the earliest few weeks of pregnancy during the period when fetal organs are formed. Common sense dictates that only necessary radiological studies should be performed at any stage of the pregnancy. Unnecessary views should not be performed, and appropriate pelvic shielding techniques should always be used. Computed tomography (CT) scanning of the mother's head and chest expose the fetus to very low levels of radiation and are generally not of concern. Direct CT scanning of the abdomen and pelvis do expose the fetus to a potentially significant dose of radiation, approaching the 5-rad dose felt to be the minimum at which fetal risk increases. CT scanning of the abdomen and pelvis should always be done when indicated, but other modalities, such as ultrasound, diagnostic peritoneal lavage, and magnetic resonance imaging (MRI) scanning should also be considered as an alternative if available. These modalities are safe and do not expose the fetus to the direct radiation of a CT scan. The underlying principle of "what is best for the mother is best for the unborn child" must always be remembered, and needed x-ray examinations and medications cannot be withheld or delayed.

Maternal Cardiac Arrest

Fortunately, the emergency physician is rarely confronted with a near-death or post-mortem pregnant patient. However, when this rare clinical situation does present, it requires immediate, decisive action to potentially salvage the unborn child. The decision to perform a perimortem cesarean section must be made swiftly and often with limited and incomplete information.

When presented with the critical pregnant trauma patient, initial airway measures and aggressive fluid resuscitation need to be accomplished rapidly. If there is no response, and maternal death is imminent or cardiac arrest has occurred, the immediate performance of a perimortem cesarean section must be considered. The prerequisites for performing a perimortem cesarean section

are that the fetus must be viable, the prognosis for the mother's survival must be grave, and the emergency physician must be familiar with the technique. A successful outcome is directly dependent on the rapid delivery of the fetus within 4 to 5 minutes after the maternal cardiac arrest, but the procedure should be performed immediately if any signs of fetal heart activity have been detected. The chance of delivering a healthy infant is excellent if delivered in less than 5 minutes. As minutes pass and fetal anoxia persists, the prognosis for a neurologically normal infant deteriorates rapidly.

Once the decision to go forward with the procedure has been made, the technique is straightforward. Considerations of proper aseptic technique and cosmetic results are not important. During the procedure, cardiopulmonary resuscitation (CPR) should be continued. A midline incision is made from the base of the sternum to the symphysis pubis. All layers of the maternal abdominal wall and peritoneum are incised. When the uterus is encountered, a vertical incision is made on the anterior uterus (Fig. 49.2).

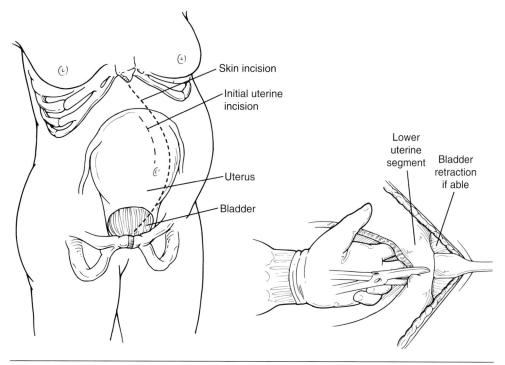

Figure 49.2
Emergent postmortem cesarean section.

If an anterior placenta is encountered when the uterus is opened, it should be rapidly cut through. Care should be taken to avoid fetal injury with sharp instruments. The child should be promptly removed. The nose and mouth of the newborn should be suctioned. The cord should be clamped and cut, and immediate fetal resuscitation begun.

Physical Abuse During Pregnancy

Every clinician who cares for pregnant trauma patients must be aware of the very real possibility that the trauma may be related to physical violence. Often the victim of physical violence does not volunteer the information that she was assaulted. Open and thoughtful questioning sometimes elicits this history. Early identification of women subjected to physical violence and appropriate intervention can potentially reduce the high rate of poor outcomes seen in pregnancies in which physical violence is involved. Physical violence during pregnancy is often directed at the pregnancy. Blows to the abdomen and assaults that result in falls are common mechanisms.

Physical violence during pregnancy has been shown to be associated with preterm labor, low birth weight, kidney infections, maternal smoking, and alcohol abuse. Recognition of physical violence in pregnancy can alert the clinician to some of these other detrimental behaviors. Early intervention by the emergency physician can lead to the possibility of a better outcome in the pregnancy. Physical violence during pregnancy also has been shown to be a predictor of future domestic violence and child abuse. Even if the presenting injury is not severe, questions regarding the circumstances of the injury and appropriate counseling can possibly avert more serious future incidents. All pregnant victims of assault and falls should be interviewed carefully to uncover abuse.

Suggested Readings

American College of Surgeons Committee on Trauma. *Advanced trauma life support manual for physicians.* Chicago: American College of Surgeons, 1997.

Johnson JD, Oakley LE. Managing minor trauma during pregnancy. *J Obstet Gynecol Neonatal Nurs* 1991;20:379–381.

Pearlman MD. Motor vehicle crashes, pregnancy loss and preterm labor. *Int J Gynaecol Obstet* 1997;57:123–126.

Shah AJ, Kilcline BA. Trauma in pregnancy. *Emerg Med Clin North Am* 2003;21:615–629.

Van Hook JW. Trauma in pregnancy. *Clin Obstet Gynecol* 2002;45:414–424.

CHAPTER **50**

Burns

Mary Hancock, MD, FACEP

Chapter Outline

Burn injury constitutes a frequent patient complaint in the emergency department. More than 2.2 million people sustain burns annually in the United States. Although most burns are not life threatening, they are responsible for 12,000 deaths per year. Burns are the second leading cause of accidental death, surpassed only by motor vehicle crashes. Although the number of residential fires has decreased over the last 2 decades, house fires account for the majority of fire-related deaths.

Emergency physicians are responsible for the initial management of most burn patients. Appropriate management of the burn-injured patient in the emergency setting using a structured, multidisciplinary approach is essential for optimal patient outcome. This chapter focuses on thermal injury; however, burns may also occur as the result of exposure to chemical agents, ionizing radiation, and electric current.

Evaluation of the Burn Victim

Prehospital Care

The immediate goal is to remove the victim from the source of the burn. This must be accomplished without endangering rescue personnel.

Immediate causes of death in burn victims are generally coexisting trauma or airway compromise. Rapid primary survey should be performed and any problems with airway, breathing, or circulation corrected promptly.

Constricting clothing or jewelry should be removed to prevent tourniquet effects. Frequently reassess the burn victim for signs of airway compromise or inhalation injury and apply 100% oxygen.

The burning process must be stopped. Remove charred clothing, cool injured tissues, and then place the burn victim in dry, sterile dressings or sheets to avoid hypothermia. When possible, pain control should be initiated.

Emergency Department Evaluation

History

Management of the burn victim varies according to the mechanism of burn injury. Determine the type of burn—flame, scald, chemical, or electrical—and any associated trauma early in the course of evaluation. The victim is more likely to have sustained inhalation injury if he or she was in a confined area with the fire. Determine the duration of exposure as well as possible.

Determination of tetanus status and the information included in the AMPLE mnemonic is also indicated. (See page 395)

Abuse must be considered as a cause of burns, particularly in children and the elderly. Features that may raise suspicion include the following:

Multiple stories of how injury was sustained

Injury attributed to a sibling

Injury claimed to be unwitnessed

Injury incompatible with the developmental level of the child

Pattern burns that suggest contact with an object

Cigarette burns

Stocking, glove, or circumferential burns

Burns to genitalia or perineum

Suspicions of abuse must be reported to the appropriate agencies according to state laws.

Physical Examination

Airway assessment is critical in burn patients to determine potential compromise. Signs of inhalation injury include singed facial and nasal hairs, perioral charcoal, and intraoral charcoal, especially on teeth and gums. Inhalation injury is diagnosed by bronchoscopy. Patients with facial and neck burns often develop massive swelling and airway obstruction. Evaluate for signs of respiratory distress such as rapid, shallow respirations, stridor, wheezing, rales, cyanosis, low oxygen saturation, or cough productive of sooty sputum. Intubate early, before massive edema impairs ventilation.

Breathing adequacy is important to evaluate early and monitor cautiously. Patients in respiratory distress or with suspected inhalation injury should be intubated early.

Note that level of consciousness is NOT a criterion for intubation. A normal mental status does not affect the need to intubate for inhalation injury. Most severely burned patients are quite awake on initial presentation and yet may require intubation. Post-

burn edema of facial tissues and/or inhalation injury occurs quickly; thus, an adequate airway is essential.

Circulation assessment is important. Fluid resuscitation must be adequate to prevent hypovolemia and circulatory compromise.

Determination of the extent and severity of the burn and a thorough secondary survey from head to toe are imperative.

Fluid management and initial treatment options are dependent on accurate assessment of injuries. Identification of associated trauma may guide therapy and destination for treatment as well.

Laboratory Studies

Patients with severe burns require laboratory workup to include the following:

Complete blood cell count

Chemistry profile

Arterial blood gas with carboxyhemoglobin

Creatine phosphokinase and urine myoglobin in electrical injuries or if significant muscle damage

Pulse oximetry may yield a falsely elevated value in burn patients because it measures carboxyhemoglobin as oxyhemoglobin.

Radiographic Studies

Chest x-ray films should be obtained on all patients with a possibility of inhalation injury and on those requiring intubation. The initial chest x-ray film rarely shows significant findings of smoke inhalation because radiographic findings may lag hours behind clinical findings. Findings of inhalation injury may include nodules, consolidations, interstitial edema, and atelectasis. If the history and physical findings suggest trauma, other plain x-ray films and/or computed tomography (CT) scans should be obtained as indicated.

Emergency Department Management

Airway stabilization is the primary initial priority. Airway edema occurs early and intubation should be considered early. Fiberoptic bronchoscopy may be helpful in determining inhalation injury.

Obtain intravenous (IV) access with two large-bore peripheral lines and administer crystalloids. (Lactated Ringer's is preferred by most.) Fluid needs can be calculated using the Parkland formula:

$$(4 \text{ mL crystalloid}) \times (\%\text{TBSA burn}) \times (\text{Body weight in kilograms})$$

where TBSA is total body surface area. One half of this calculated fluid volume is to be given in the first 8 hours from the time of the injury, and the remainder over the subsequent 16 hours.

For example: A 70-kg man with a 40% surface area burn would require $(40) \times (70 \text{ kg}) \times (4 \text{ mL/kg}) = 11,200 \text{ mL}$ of IV fluid in the first 24 hours divided into 700 mL/hour for the first 8 hours, then 350 mL/hour for the remaining 16 hours.

Monitor fluid status frequently; urine output should be maintained at 0.5 mL/kg/hour. Although this formula gives a good starting estimate, the IV drip can be adjusted according to the urine output. This formula may not accurately predict fluid needs in patients with electrical burns or co-existing trauma.

Pediatric patients often need maintenance fluids *in addition* to the replacement fluid calculated. The formula for fluid needs in a pediatric patient is as follows:

Maintenance fluid
  = (100 mL/day for first 10 kg)
  + (50 mL/day for second 10 kg)
  + (20 mL/day for weight in excess of 20 kg)

In a child, some advocate maintenance fluids plus additional fluids at 2 to 3 mL/kg × %TBSA. As with the Parkland formula, one half the volume is given in the first 8 hours postburn and the remainder in the subsequent 16 hours.

Adequate urine output in children is 1.0 to 1.5 mL/kg/hour; in infants, it is 1.5 to 2.0 mL/kg/hour.

Determine the presence of circumferential burns early in the evaluation. Circum-ferential injuries to the neck, chest, and extremities are life or limb threatening. Assess for signs of inadequate perfusion such as warmth, sensation, and range of motion; remember, loss of distal pulses is a late sign of inadequate perfusion. Escharotomy may be necessary in these cases. The eschar is tough and rigid and serves as a tourniquet when circumferential. Escharotomy should be performed along the lateral aspect of the extremity or chest down to the level of the subcutaneous fat (Fig. 50.1). Because deep burns are insensate, no anesthetic is required. Use of electrocautery can reduce bleeding.

Local Burn Care

Most burns in the emergency department are minor. It is important that the patient has adequate follow-up. Table 50.1 sum-

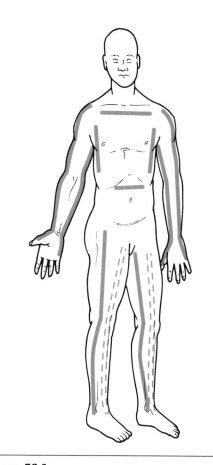

Figure 50.1
Diagrammatic representation of escharotomy sites.

marizes the classification and initial wound management for the patient with burn injury.

First-degree burns do not require any dressings. Nonsteroidal antiinflammatory agents are useful for pain management.

Second-degree burns are treated with topical agents and skin substitutes. Topical antibacterial agents are described in Table 50.2. Table 50.3 summarizes occlusive dressings and skin substitutes.

There is some controversy related to the management of blisters. In general, blisters should be left intact to decrease the likelihood of bacterial colonization. Large or tense blisters can be decompressed by needle aspiration. Open blisters should be débrided. All wounds should then be treated with a topical antibiotic and dressed with gauze and a semielastic bandage. A skin substitute may be chosen in some cases.

Burns to the neck and face are generally treated with topical bacitracin or other antibiotic and left open.

Wounds should be inspected daily or every other day initially.

Table 50.1.

Burn Classification and Initial Wound Management

	First Degree	*Second Degree*	*Third Degree*
Skin depth	Epidermis	Entire dermis, partial dermis; sweat glands, hair follicles intact	Entire epidermis and dermis; +/- subcutaneous tissue, muscle, bone
Cause	Flash flame, UV light	Contact with hot liquids or solids Flash flame to clothing Direct flame Chemicals, UV light	Contact with hot liquids or solids Flame Chemicals Electrical contact
Appearance	Dry, no blisters Minimal or no edema Blanches with fingertip pressure and refills when pressure removed	Moist Large, moist blisters that will increase in size Blanches with fingertip pressure and refills when pressure removed	Dry with leathery eschar Charred with visible vessels Rare blisters No blanching with pressure
Color	Increased redness	Mottled with pink, red, tan, white areas	White, charred, dark tan, red
Sensation	Painful	Very painful	Limited/no pain
Healing time	2–5 days with peeling No scarring May discolor	Superficial: 5–21 days No grafting Deep: 21–35 days if no infection May convert to full thickness and require grafting	No healing potential Requires excision and grafting, depends on extent and location
Topical agents	Lotions, emollients	Bacitracin, Xeroform	Silvadene, Sulfamylon

UV, ultraviolet.

Table 50.2.

Topical Antibacterial Agents

Agent	Advantages	Disadvantages	Comments
Bacitracin	Easy application Good for superficial and facial burns	Rare allergies	Topical antistaphylococcal with no penetrating ability Increases debriding ability of saline wet-to-dry dressings
Mafenide acetate (Sulfamylon)	Penetrates eschar well	Allergy—frequent rashes Metabolic acidosis Painful	Broad-spectrum against gram-negative and some gram-positive organisms NOT a sulfa drug Do not use near eyes
Silver nitrate		Hypotonic solution may leach electrolytes Painful Stains skin Poor eschar penetration	
Silver sulfadiazine (Silvadene)	Good eschar penetration Comfortable application	Transient leukopenia Sulfa allergy Risk of kernicterus (avoid in pregnant and newborns) Retarded healing *in vitro*	Bacterial spectrum similar to mafenide Does not penetrate leathery eschar Developing resistance to gram-negative organisms

UV, ultraviolet.

Moderate to severe burns are very painful and require narcotic analgesia. Narcotics should be given intravenously; intramuscular injection is more erratic and may cause muscle damage. Morphine sulfate is the drug of choice.

For all patients, consider tetanus prophylaxis. Antibiotics are not recommended. Finally, it is important to keep all patients warm, especially those with larger burn surface areas.

Criteria for Burn Center Admission

Burn injuries usually requiring referral to a burn center include those meeting the following criteria:

Third-degree burns greater than 5% TBSA in patients of any age

Second- and third-degree burns greater than 10% TBSA in patients younger than 10 years or older than 50 years

Second- and third-degree burns greater than 20% TBSA in any age group

Second- and third-degree burns involving the face, hands, genitalia, perineum, and major joints

Electrical and lightning injuries

Inhalation injury

Circumferential burns of the thorax or extremities

Significant chemical injury

Coexisting major trauma or significant preexisting medical condition

Pathophysiology of Burn Injury

The skin is the largest organ of the body. It functions to separate us from the environment by allowing for thermal regulation and prevention of fluid loss by evaporation, serves as a barrier to infection, and contains

Table 50.3.

Occlusive Dressings and Skin Substitutes

Occlusive Dressings	Advantages	Disadvantages	Components
Biobrane	Good wound adherence Tolerates external wetting	May increase infection rates	Nylon mesh coated with silastic; Porcine collagen covalently bonded to inner surface
DuoDerm	Greater absorption of fluids	Expense Not for use on deep partial-thickness burns	Hydrocolloids
OpSite, Tegaderm	Easy, frequent wound assessment	Possible fluid retention Not for use on deep partial-thickness burns	Polyurethane films
Xeroform	Good wound adherence Encourages migration of epithelial cells	Must have clean wound surface	Vaseline impregnated gauze with antibacterial chemicals
Scarlet Red	Encourages spread of epithelial cells at accelerated rate	No bactericidal effect	Vaseline impregnated gauze with vital dye (o-Tolylazo-o-tolylazo –β–naphthol)
Xenograft	Temporary protection of wounds free of eschar	Potential for infection Antibodies develop after 7–10 days	Pigskin
Allograft	Temporary closure of wounds free of eschar	Must be stored at 4°C Limited viability (approximately 5 days)	Cadaver skin
Skin Substitutes			
Epidermal	Wide and permanent skin coverage	2–3 week delay Expensive Labor-intensive	Cultured autologous epidermal cells
Dermal	Readily available Use as base Reduce scarring	Need for procurement Potential disease transmission	Allogeneic skin
Dermal	Readily available	Possible need for multiple applications	Fibroblasts on nylon mesh
Combined epi-dermal and dermal	Readily available No need for further autografting	Limited viability and quantity	1. Bovine collagen, allogeneic fibroblasts and epidermal cells 2. Collagen matrix substrate with fibroblasts and epidermal cells

sensory receptors that provide information about our environment. These functions are all compromised somewhat depending on the extent and severity of the burn injury.

The skin is divided into three layers. The epidermis is the outermost layer composed of stratified epithelium. The outermost layers are anucleate cells (stratum corneum), which protects the inner, viable layers (Malpighian layers). The middle layer is the dermis, composed primarily of connective tissue. The nerve endings, nourishing vessels, and hair follicles reside in the dermis. The hypodermis is a layer of adipose and connective tissue between the skin and underlying tissues. This layer varies greatly in thickness and adipose content by body region (Fig. 50.2).

Burn injury severity is dependent on the rate of heat transfer from the heat source to the skin. The temperature of the object and duration of exposure are major components of heat transfer. Exposure to temperatures greater than 45°C leads to cellular damage and protein denaturation.

Burn wounds consist of three regional zones. The central area, or zone of coagulation, is the region of greatest heat transfer.

It consists of dead or dying cells because of coagulation and absent blood flow. The adjacent area is the intermediate zone of stasis, characterized by inflammatory reaction. Tissue perfusion is tenuous in this area and may result in ischemia, converting this zone also to the zone of coagulation over the first 24 to 48 hours. The outermost zone, furthest from the zone of coagulation, is the zone of hyperemia. Circulation to this region is intact, tissue injury is minimal, and spontaneous recovery generally occurs.

Classification of Burn Injury

Determination of the extent and severity of injury is paramount in the care of burns because this determines subsequent management. Accurate assessment of the TBSA affects fluid management and impacts decisions for therapy, including transfer to a burn unit. (See Table 50.1 for a summary of burn classification.)

First-degree burns involve only the epidermis layer of the skin. They present with pain and erythema that blanches with pressure. There are no blisters. Complete healing occurs without scar formation. First-degree

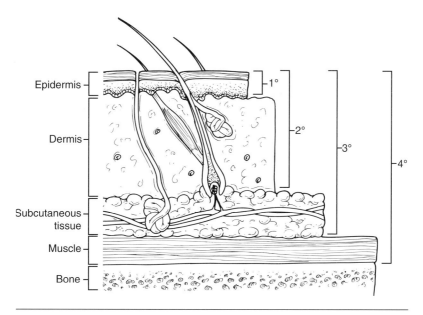

Figure 50.2
Anatomy of the skin relative to levels of injury.

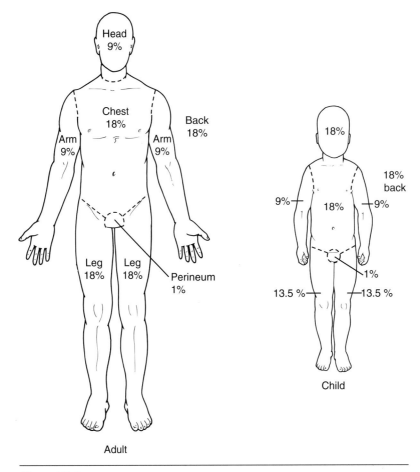

Figure 50.3
Rule of nines for estimating percent of surface area burned.

burns are not included in calculations of the TBSA burned.

Second-degree burns are subdivided into superficial and deep partial-thickness burns. Superficial partial-thickness burns involve the epidermis and the *superficial* dermis. These are very painful and blisters are common. If the blisters are broken, the lesions are moist and erythematous and blanch with pressure. Sensation is intact. These burns heal by reepithelialization from adjacent skin and skin appendages in 2 to 3 weeks with minimal scarring.

Deep partial-thickness burns involve the epidermis and deep structures of the dermis, leaving only few skin appendages intact. These lesions may or may not be painful and may be mottled pink or white.

Deep partial-thickness wounds may be difficult to distinguish from full-thickness burns. They may take 3 to 6 weeks to heal and may be associated with significant scarring and joint contractures.

Third-degree or full-thickness burns involve all layers of the epidermis and dermis and may injure subcutaneous structures. They appear white, gray, tan, or charred, and thrombosed vessels are often seen. The wound is leather-like because of loss of elasticity and insensate because of destruction of nerve endings. These lesions cannot heal spontaneously unless extremely small and are best treated with skin grafting.

Fourth-degree burns involve structures beneath the subcutaneous layer such as muscle, tendon, and/or bone. Myoglobinuria and subsequent renal failure may result from muscular injury.

Estimation of the TBSA is generally based on the "rule of nines" (Fig. 50.3). This is generally adequate for adults but often underestimates TBSA in infants and children. For smaller burns, the "rule of palms" has been used: the size of the child's palm (not including fingers) is approximately 1% of the TBSA. Counting the total number of palm-sized areas of burn totals the percentage of burn. In children younger than 10 years, the proportions of the different body areas vary. Adjustments must be made to accommodate these differences. In the evaluation of smaller burns in children, the palm (including the fingers) best approximates 1% of the TBSA.

Burns are some of the most common injuries encountered in the emergency department. Assessment and management of the airway is the priority in patients with inhalation injury or large burns. Suspect associated trauma in the burned patient and exclude it.

Patients with large burns require aggressive fluid resuscitation; accurate assessment of the severity and extent of the burn is critical to the appropriate management and outcome of the patient. It is prudent to be vigilant for signs of abuse, particularly in patients at the extremes of age.

Suggested Readings

Markovchick V, Pons P. *Emergency medicine secrets*, 2nd ed. Philadelphia: Hanley & Belfus, 1999.

Rosen P, Barkin R, Danzl DF, et al. *Emergency medicine: concepts and clinical practice*, 4th ed. St. Louis: Mosby, 1998.

Stewart C. Emergency care of pediatric burns. *Pediatr Emerg Med Rep* 2000, 5(10);1–3.

Tintinelli J. *Emergency medicine: a comprehensive study guide*, 4th ed. Minneapolis: McGraw-Hill, 1996.

Wald D. Burn management: systemic patient evaluation, fluid resuscitation, and wound management. *Emerg Med Rep* 1998, 19(5),1–8.

Toxicology

CHAPTER 51

Introduction to the Poisoned Patient

K. Sophia Dyer, MD, FACEP, Michelle Fischer Keane, MD

Emergency management of the poisoned patient requires a high index of suspicion, attention to basic emergency medicine principles, and knowledge of the many and varied available poisons. Patients may present with a clear history of ingestion, however in many cases the patient's history may be unobtainable, vague, or completely unknown. Poisoned patients may present with seizure, altered mentation, hypotension, vomiting, delirium and a host of other manifestations. It is incumbent on the emergency physician to maintain a high index of suspicion for poisoning in any unexplained presentation. In this brief chapter we review some basics of toxicology.

History

In any case in which poisoning is either known or suspected, history is essential. Frequently, the patient may not be able to offer any information or may be reluctant; there-fore gathering information from family, friends and pre-hospital personnel is necessary. Obtain any pertinent bottles or paraphernalia. If possible identify the name of the drug, amount consumed, time of exposure and signs and symptoms since the exposure. Try to determine the route of exposure (inhalation, oral, or injection) and route of injection (intravenous, subcutaneous, or intramuscular).

Obtain past medical history, medications and allergies. When there is little or no history available, the clinical presentation of the patient and physical findings become your primary means for identification of the toxin and will guide your intervention and ultimate treatment.

Physical Exam

Physical findings can provide clues to the diagnosis. As with any patient, evaluate airway, breathing, and circulation (the ABCs of emergency management). Note the general appearance of the patient (awake, agitated, stuporous.), the vital signs (pulse, respiratory rate, temperature and blood pressure) and the skin (cyanosis, diaphoresis, flushed, track marks). Are the pupils dilated, constricted, or unequal? Is there evidence of trauma? Is the airway compromised? Note the respiratory examination; some toxins may cause wheezing, or pulmonary edema. Is the abdomen tender? Is there evidence of bowel or bladder incontinence? Perform a complete neurological evaluation. The rectal examination provides information on tone (for the obtunded patient), any foreign materials (body packers), and occult blood in the stool.

It is important to remember that the patient with a suspected or known toxicological etiology of illness still requires the basics of emergency medical management. Attention to airway, breathing and circulation will hopefully keep the patient alive long enough for the alert clinician to start managing the toxicological issues.

Diagnostic Evaluation

Laboratory Tests

After careful history and physical examination, laboratory testing can confirm or rule out toxins in the differential diagnosis. Be reminded that *most* toxins are not readily available on toxicological screening. Although many reference laboratories can test for a wide range of substances, many of these results will not be quickly available to help the clinician. Most hospital laboratories have some toxicological testing available on an emergency basis. The most frequently available toxicological tests are for salicylates, acetaminophen and ethanol. Tricyclic antidepressant levels are readily available in some institutions. Urine can be tested generally for substances such as cocaine metabolites, opiates, barbiturates, benzodiazepines, amphetamines, and marijuana metabolites. It is important that any clinician caring for a patient needing toxicological screening be aware of what is readily available in their laboratory. A statement of "the toxic screens were negative" may have significant differences from one institution to another. It is a better practice to briefly list on the patient's chart what was tested for at your particular institution. Additional caution should be exercised when interpreting negative or positive results on a particular toxicological test result. Some substances (some benzodiazepines) may not be detected on testing. In addition positive results may actually represent a cross-reaction. An example is a positive phencyclidine result from diphenhydramine and dextromethorphan.

Serum or urine testing for pregnancy is important during the evaluation of the woman of childbearing years who is being treated for a potential poisoning. Attempt-ing to abort an unwanted pregnancy is one reason a woman may ingest a substance even if she is not suicidal.

Serum electrolyte testing should also be included in the laboratory evaluation for assessment of anion gap metabolic acidosis (from toxic alcohols, salicylates, iron) and specific electrolyte abnormalities (e.g., hypokalemia from theophylline). Serum osmolality should only be measured by freezing point depression. The values used for the calculated and measured osmolality should be temporally related. Liver and renal function should be assessed if the toxin is known to have end-organ damage to either the liver or kidneys, or if the toxin is unknown.

Electrocardiogram (ECG)

The electrocardiogram (ECG) may be useful in evaluating the poisoned patient. Tricyclic antidepressant toxicity is well known to cause tachycardia and potentially a wide complex tachycardia. Other substances such as digoxin and clonidine can cause bradycardias, giving clues to the substance ingested.

Radiology

Some toxins are visible on plain radiographs. Metals are the most obvious: iron (generally not children's chewable preparations), lead, elemental mercury, and metallic foreign bodies (e.g., button batteries, coins). Potassium and some sustained-release tablets may be visible. Phenothiazines and some chlorinated hydrocarbons can be detected at times. Balloons and other objects may be seen on body packers (individuals who swallow illegal drugs as a method of transport, usually packaged in balloons or plastic). A negative radiograph for these materials does not completely preclude that they have been ingested.

Treatment

Decontamination

For the poisoned patient the D in A-B-C-D represents decontamination in addition to disability. Several modalities are available for decontamination. The most familiar are ipecac, lavage, activated charcoal and whole bowel irrigation. Limitations exist for any form of decontamination. One of the most important points to remember about decontamination is that its effectiveness may be limited by the delayed presentation of the patient to medical care. We briefly review the pros and cons of forms of decontamination.

Ipecac

Ipecac is familiar to both health care professionals and the general public. Ipecac produces its decontamination by inducing vomiting. Ipecac is derived from the plants *Cephaelis ipecacuanha* or *Cephaelis acuminata*. Until 2003, ipecac was recommended for home use, particularly in ingestions in the small child. However, 2003 recommendations of the American Academy of Pediatrics (AAP) removes ipecac as a home treatment. Some general contraindications to the use of induced vomiting include: petroleum distillate ingestion; caustic ingestion; depressed mental status; ingestion that would be expected to cause seizure, depressed mental status, or cardiovascular effects. One of the problems with the use of ipecac is that the emetogenic effects last for 2 hours or longer and may complicate further treatment. In addition it may endanger the patient if vomiting occurs in the presence of decreased mental status.

Orogastric Lavage

Orogastric lavage is another method of gastric emptying. In orogastric lavage a large-bore orogastric tube is placed and the stomach is lavaged, typically with the instillation of activated charcoal after the lavage. A lavage with a standard-bore nasogastric tube (14 to 18 French in adults) will not accomplish significant gastric emptying of pills. Lavage with small nasogastric tubes occasionally is indicated in acid or systemically toxic hydrocarbon ingestions, with care taken to avoid vomiting which could worsen the situation. Pill masses and some sustained release preparations will not be evacuated fully from the stomach. Orogastric lavage should be performed only in a patient who is either fully cooperative or with a controlled airway. Attempting to lavage a patient with a decreased level of consciousness, or who has decreased or absent gag reflex without a controlled airway, can prove hazardous. Orogastric lavage may cause additional esophageal injury in the case of caustic ingestions. In addition, the time of ingestion may limit the usefulness of orogastric lavage. Ingestions that do not slow gastric emptying are lavaged only if the ingestion occurred in the 30 minutes before arrival in the emergency department (ED). Use of the orogastric lavage is usually reserved for life-threatening ingestion such as tricyclic antidepressants, aspirin, and cardiac medications that occur shortly before arrival in the ED.

Activated Charcoal

It is easier to list the substances that are not bound well by activated charcoal, than to list the substances that are bound well by activated charcoal. In general, alcohols, hydrocarbons, metals and caustics are not absorbed well by activated charcoal. The additional concern, with the administration of activated charcoal in the setting of hydrocarbon ingestions, is the propensity to vomit with activated charcoal, which may place the patient at risk for a hydrocarbon pneumonitis. The administration of activated charcoal to a patient who has ingested caustics may make further visualization of esophageal and/or gastric lesions difficult during endoscopy. Futhermore, the propensity to vomit with activated charcoal potentially could re-expose tissue to the caustic agent.

Whole Bowel Irrigation

Another method of decontamination is whole bowel irrigation. Whole bowel irrigation uses an oral polyethylene glycol solution, the solution typically used for bowel preparation before colonoscopy. Whole bowel irrigation can be used when activated charcoal will not bind the toxin, and/or when large amounts of toxin rest in the gastrointestinal tract and the patient would benefit from rapid removal. Examples of situations that might benefit from whole bowel irrigation are large iron ingestions, lithium, and drug packets of cocaine.

Hemodialysis and Hemoperfusion

Hemodialysis and hemoperfusion are the last methods available for elimination of body toxins. Drugs that can be removed by hemodialysis are ethanol, methanol, ethylene glycol, isopropyl alcohol, salicylates, lithium, chloral hydrate, boric acid and bromide. Drugs eliminated by hemoperfusion are carbamazepine, phenytoin, phenobarbital, theophylline, digoxin-Fab fragment complex, chloramphenicol, methotrexate, glutethimide, methaqualone, diquat, paraquat, podophyllum and ethchlorvynol.

Urinary Alkalinization

In addition to dialysis, urinary excretion of some toxins can be enhanced by alkalinization. Urinary alkalinization is accomplished by the addition of 1 to 1.5 mEq/kg of sodium bicarbonate intravenous pyelography (IVP) (2 amps (50mEq/amp) sodium bicarbonate in 1 L D5W) with 20 mEq potassium chloride (Kcl). Salicylates, phenobarbital, isoniazid and phenylbutazone are all toxins in which alkalinization enhances elimination. Urine pH should be above 7.5. Urinary acidification is not recommended.

Summary

The possibility of toxic ingestion should always be considered in the patient in whom a diagnosis may be unclear. In the work up of the poisoned or possibly poisoned patient, history and physical examination are critical. In addition the ABC's of emergency management always come first. Appropriate use of decontamination should be initiated when poisoning is suspected and should not be delayed for toxic screening results. All patients who do not respond immediately to therapy or who have ingestions with late onset effects should be admitted for observation.

Finally, it would be unrealistic to try to remember the details of every human made and natural toxin available. Remember instead that many good text and computer-based resources are available to aid in the management of the poisoned patient. Be familiar with the telephone number for your area poison control center in the United States or Canada.

Suggested Readings

Goldfrank LR, Flomenbaum NE, Lewin NA, et al. Principles of managing the poisoned or overdose patient: An overview. In *Goldfrank's toxicologic emergencies*, 7th ed. Columbus, OH: McGraw Hill, 2002.

Shannon MW, Haddad LM. The emergency management of poisoning. In: Haddad LM, Shannon MW, Winchester JF. *Clinical management of poisoning and drug overdose*. 3rd ed. Philadelphia. Saunders, 1998:2–30.

Smilkstein MJ. Techniques used to prevent gastrointestinal absorption of toxic compounds. In: Goldfrank LR, Flomenbaum NE, Lewin NA, et al, eds. *Goldfrank's toxicologic emergencies*, 7th ed. Columbus, OH: McGraw Hill, 2002.

Toxidromes

Edward W. Boyer, MD, PhD

Toxidromes are constellations of clinical findings that suggest classes of toxins as causative agents. For emergency physicians, the ability to recognize these signs and symptoms is a basic skill. Although each of these conditions can usually be distinguished based on vital signs and physical examination, many exceptions to the toxidromes exist. Moreover, polydrug overdoses can present with a variety of mixed or overlapping toxidromes. The most relevant toxidromes are those from sympathomimetic, sedative-hypnotic, anticholinergic, cholinergic, and opiate agents.

General Evaluation

Vital Signs and Physical Examination

Each toxidrome produces specific patterns of vital sign abnormalities that, when combined with the physical examination, are frequently diagnostic. Pay special attention to the following vital sign abnormalities:

> Respiratory rate greater than 12, or less than 12?
> Cardiovascular: tachycardic and hypertensive, or bradycardic and hypotensive?

> Temperature: hyperthermic or hypothermic?

Physical examination may diagnose a toxidrome in as little as 30 seconds. Although not a substitute for complete physical examination, the clinician must pay particular attention to the following:

> Mental status: awake, agitated, or comatose, appropriately responsive or hallucinating?
> Pupils: pinpoint or enlarged (miosis vs. mydriasis)?
> Oropharynx: dry or moist mucosa?
> Bowel sounds: present or absent?
> Skin: dry or moist?

Table 52.1 illustrates the comparison of physical findings in toxidromes.

General Management

General management principles include supporting the patient's airway, breathing, and circulation and stabilizing vital signs. In addition, most patients should receive activated charcoal to decontaminate the gastrointestinal (GI) tract. Lastly, several drugs produce toxidromes that may, in specific situations, be reversed by antidotes.

Toxidromes

Sympathomimetic Toxidrome

Mechanism

Sympathomimetic agents generate physiological and toxic effect by the following mechanisms:

Table 52.1.

Comparison of physical findings in toxidromes

	Sympathomimetic	Sedative-Hypnotic	Anticholinergic	Cholinergic	Opioid
BP	↑↑	↓	↑ or ↓	Usually ↓	↓↓
HR	↑↑	Ventricular arrhythmia	↑↑	↑	↑ or ↓
RR	↑	↓ or NL	↑	↑	↓↓
Skin	Sweating	NL or cool	Red hot dry	Moist, vasodilated	Pruritus
Temp	↑	↓	↑↑	NL	↓
Pupils	Mydriasis	May be enlarged	Mydriasis	Miosis	Miosis
Mental status	Agitation	Coma	Confusion Hallucination Seizure Coma	Weakness, paralysis	Depressed to coma
Special			Dry mouth Urinary retention Bowel ileus	Lacrimation Diarrhea Urinary incontinence	

BP, blood pressure; HR, heart rate; NL, normal; RR, respiratory rate; Temp, temperature; ↑, increased; ↓, decreased.

Direct stimulation of adrenergic receptors (e.g., albuterol)

Indirect release of norepinephrine from presynaptic neurons (e.g., methamphetamine)

Direct stimulation of α- and β-adrenergic receptors coupled with the release of presynaptic norepinephrine (e.g., dopamine)

Prevention of presynaptic reuptake of norepinephrine, leading to increased synaptic concentration of catecholamines (e.g., cocaine and tricyclic antidepressants [TCAs])

Inhibition of norepinephrine metabolism, using enzyme inhibitors (e.g., monoamine oxidase inhibitors)

Clinical Findings

Regardless of the agent, patients who are intoxicated with the sympathomimetic toxidrome may exhibit the following:

Hypertension and tachycardia

Sweating

Enlarged pupils

Agitation

Seizures

Hyperthermia (either from excessive musculoskeletal activity secondary to agitation or seizures)

Management

In general, the treatment of the sympathomimetic toxidrome can be accomplished by supportive care. In addition to the general principles described previously, patients should receive pulse oximetry and continuous cardiac monitoring. Initial therapy is directed toward patient sedation and control of blood pressure and pulse. Specific modalities are as follows:

Benzodiazepines should be used liberally to control agitation, seizures, and mild to moderate cardiovascular symptoms. Combinations of diazepam and lorazepam are frequently used.

Nitroprusside is used to control blood pressure in intoxicated patients. Because of its short duration of action and ease of titration to desired effect, nitroprusside is effective for rapid blood pressure control.

Paralysis and orotracheal intubation is reserved for severely hyperthermic patients (temperature greater than 105°F) because paralysis interrupts the extreme muscular activity responsible for increased body temperature. Although useful as single therapy, paralysis is especially effective when combined with other cooling therapies, such as cool mist. Clinicians must be careful to obtain an accurate temperature of all hyperpyrexic patients.

Pitfalls

Use of β-blockers should be avoided. Blockade of β-adrenergic receptors may lead to unopposed α-adrenergic effects with attendant hypertension. In addition, failure to provide adequate sedation is a cause of death in severely agitated patients. Any patient who requires physical restraint should receive additional chemical sedation in the form of benzodiazepines and, possibly, paralysis with intubation.

Sedative-Hypnotic Toxidrome

Mechanism

Sedative-hypnotic agents are general central nervous system (CNS) depressants; most stimulate the activity of γ-aminobutyric acid (GABA), an inhibitory CNS neurotransmitter. γ-Hydroxybutyric acid (GHB) is an inhibitory neurotransmitter that also exhibits GABA activity. In general, sedative-hypnotic agents can be divided into barbiturates and nonbarbiturates. Examples of the nonbarbiturates include the benzodiazepines, ethanol, GHB, zolpidem, cyclobenzaprine, and chloral hydrate.

Clinical Findings

Respiratory findings vary with the type of agent used. In general, sedative-hypnotics produce respiratory depression, but they do not produce respiratory rates less than 12 breaths per minute. The notable exceptions are barbiturates. Used clinically in status epilepticus to eliminate CNS electrical activity, barbiturates in overdose may lead to severe respiratory depression. In addition, GHB produces erratic respiratory effort; consequently, patients may be apneic. In contrast, isolated benzodiazepine and ethanol ingestion rarely causes apnea in adults. Although apnea is a very uncommon finding in benzodiazepine overdose, patients may nonetheless require intubation for failure to protect their airway. Typical clinical findings in the patient with a sedative-hypnotic toxidrome include the following:

Ataxia

Coma

Hypotension

Depressed cardiac function (particularly in barbiturate overdose)

Ventricular dysrhythmias (particularly chloral hydrate)

Hypothermia (arises from absence of musculoskeletal activity in a cool environment)

Management

The treatment of the sedative-hypnotic toxidrome is supportive. Patients should receive pulse oximetry and continuous cardiac monitoring. GI decontamination using activated charcoal, although indicated, should be undertaken with caution in a comatose or potentially comatose patient. Phenobarbital overdose may be treated with multiple doses of activated charcoal, but severe poisoning may require dialysis. Specific modalities are the following:

Prevention of aspiration of gastric contents—patients should be positioned so that the risks of aspiration are minimized.

Orotracheal intubation for patients with an inability to protect their airway or apneic patients poisoned with barbiturates or GHB.

β-Adrenergic agonists are used specifically in treating ventricular dysrhythmias from chloral hydrate overdose. β-Blockers have no utility in the treatment of other sedative-hypnotic poisonings.

Pitfalls

Flumazenil, a competitive benzodiazepine antagonist, has been promoted as an antidote to benzodiazepine overdose. Although theoretically useful, flumazenil has several drawbacks that make it unattractive. Flumazenil may create sedative-hypnotic withdrawal, one feature of which is seizures. Patients with flumazenil-induced seizures require urgent treatment with benzodiazepines to terminate seizure activity. Unfortunately, any administered benzodiazepines are inactive because of flumazenil's competitive antagonism of the benzodiazepine receptor. Furthermore, duration of action of flumazenil is far shorter than most sedative-hypnotic agents; therefore, multiple doses of flumazenil are required to maintain reversal. Finally, coma from toxicological causes is well tolerated, and the mortality of sedative-hypnotic poisoned patients who receive adequate medical care is extraordinarily low. If any indication for flumazenil exists, it is for the reversal of excessive conscious sedation in pediatric patients. Even these patients recover rapidly with supportive care alone and, if treated properly, without consequence.

Anticholinergic Toxidrome

The clinical syndrome of anticholinergic poisoning is one of the most common toxidromes. The ability to recognize this toxidrome is a basic emergency medicine skill used in the assessment of poisoned patients.

Mechanism

Anticholinergic agents bind competitively to acetylcholine muscarinic receptors found in the CNS and postganglionic muscarinic parasympathetic fibers innervating the heart, pupils, salivary glands, sweat glands, bladder, and GI tract.

Clinical Findings

The anticholinergic toxidrome is comprised of both central (CNS) and peripheral (muscarinic anticholinergic) signs. The clinical constellation of findings has been described as *blind as a bat, mad as a hatter, red as a beet, dry as a bone, hotter than Hades.* Another version: *can't see, can't spit, can't pee, can't sh . t.*

CNS findings in the patient with the anticholinergic toxidrome include the following:

Confusion

Agitation

Visual hallucinations

Picking and grasping movements

Ataxia

Seizures

Coma

Peripheral muscarinic anticholinergic findings include the following:

Tachycardia

Red, hot skin

Dry oral mucosa

Functional ileus/decreased bowel sounds

Urinary retention

Hypertension

Fever

The central anticholinergic syndrome is a condition characterized by the neurological findings mentioned previously (confusion, agitation, hallucinations, etc.) with no evidence of peripheral toxicity. It may occur at therapeutic dosing of drugs and is found predominantly in the very young, the very old, and those with organic brain syndromes.

Management

Special attention must be paid to stabilizing vital signs. Patients exhibiting the anticholinergic toxidrome may be agitated and combative; in these cases, patients may be severely hyperthermic because of increased musculoskeletal activity and an inability to cool by sweating. Specific modalities include the following:

Sedation: benzodiazepines have been used to sedate those intoxicated with anticholinergic agents. Extremely large doses of benzodiazepines are frequently required, limiting the applicability of this therapy.

Reversal: physostigmine, a cholinergic agent, is used to reverse both central and peripheral anticholinergic signs. Before administering physostigmine, a patient should have an electrocardiogram (ECG), be placed on continuous cardiovascular monitoring, and be placed on oxygen. The normal dose of physostigmine (0.5 to 1.0 mg) should be administered intravenously at a very slow push.

Pitfalls

Physostigmine may lead to increased morbidity and mortality. Several agents, such as TCAs, may produce an anticholinergic toxidrome. In cases in which the QRS duration is greater than 100 msec (as is often seen in TCA poisoning), physostigmine use is associated with cardiac arrest. Therefore, its use should be avoided in these situations. In addition, rapid administration of physostigmine may produce the cholinergic toxidrome, of which bradycardia and increased pulmonary secretions are prominent clinical findings.

Cholinergic Toxidrome

Mechanism

Functionally, cholinergic agents increase the amount of the neurotransmitter acetylcholine or agonize the acetylcholine receptor. Most commonly caused by acetylcholinesterase inhibitors (e.g., organophosphate pesticides and their congeners), the cholinergic toxidrome may also occur from nerve gas agents and naturally occurring alkaloids. In general, there are two types of acetylcholine receptors, the muscarinic and nicotinic receptors, both of which have highly specific clinical effects.

Clinical Findings

The immediate effects of excessive muscarinic stimulation include the following:

Salivation

Lacrimation

Urination

Diarrhea

Abdominal pain (GI distress)

Vomiting

Sweating

Cutaneous vasodilatation

Miosis

Bronchial vasoconstriction

The clinical constellation of findings is often referred to using the SLUDGE mnemonic:

Salivation, Lacrimation, Urination, Defecation, GI distress, and Emesis

Excessive nicotinic stimulation produces the following effects:

Muscle fasciculations

Weakness

Paralysis

Tachycardia

In general, patients with mild to moderate cholinergic intoxication present with SLUDGE findings; those with moderate to severe intoxication present with SLUDGE findings and weakness. Severely intoxicated persons exhibit coma, seizures, paralysis, and SLUDGE signs. Therefore, emergency physicians should rely on muscarinic findings to recognize the cholinergic toxidrome.

Management

Special attention must be paid to stabilization of vital signs. In particular, prevention of hypoxemia secondary to copious airway secretions is needed. Specific modalities are as follows:

Reversal of muscarinic manifestations: atropine is highly effective in blocking the action of excess acetylcholine at muscarinic sites. The goal of therapy is to prevent additional secretions, and atropine is administered until secretions are controlled.

Reversal of nicotinic manifestations: pralidoxime (2-PAM) is effective at removing acetylcholinesterase inhibitors from the enzyme. 2-PAM, if indicated, should be administered early in the course of cholinergic agent poisoning.

Control of seizures: benzodiazepines effectively treat seizures from cholinergic poisoning.

Pitfalls

Acetylcholinesterase chemically reacts with inhibitors such as organophosphates; the product of this reaction is hydrolyzed by 2-PAM. After 24 to 48 hours, however, the enzyme changes shape so that it fails to react with the antidote. This effect is known as "aging."

Opioid Toxidrome

Mechanism

Activation of opiate receptors leads to the inhibition of synaptic neurotransmission in the central and peripheral nervous systems. Opiates (naturally occurring chemicals) and opioids (synthetic derivatives of opiates) bind to and enhance neurotransmission through opiate receptors. Physiological effects of opiates are mediated principally through mu and kappa receptors, which produce analgesia, miosis, respiratory depression, and sedation. Rather than eliminate a painful stimulus, opiates merely decrease the perception of pain or induce euphoria.

Clinical Findings

Opiate toxicity should be expected whenever the triad of CNS depression, respiratory depression, and miosis are present. Clinical findings include the following:

CNS depression, ranging from drowsiness to coma

Respiratory depression with rates as low as 0 to 4 breaths per minute are common in severe intoxication

Miosis

Decreased bowel sounds

Hypotension

Pruritus

Management

Because respiratory depression is the most severe consequence of opioid intoxication, patients require either a chemical or mechanical means to breathe:

Reversal: naloxone is an opioid antagonist with few serious side effects that is highly effective in reversing intoxication.

Mechanical: orotracheal intubation is effective but is expensive and invasive.

Pitfalls

Naloxone has a duration of action of 30 to 60 minutes, whereas heroin may produce intoxication up to 6 hours after use. Consequently, heroin-toxic patients treated with naloxone may have a temporary return to normalcy followed by recrudescence of toxicity once the effect of naloxone has worn off. Therefore, these patients should not be allowed to leave the emergency department even though they possess a normal mental status.

Suggested Readings

Goldfrank L, Flomenbaum N, Lewin N, et al. Vitals signs and toxic syndrome. In: Goldfrank L, Flomenbaum N, Lewin N, et al, eds. *Goldfrank's toxicologic emergencies*, 6th ed. Stamford, CT: Appleton & Lange, 1998: 277–284.

Shannon M. The emergency management of poisoning. In: Haddad L, Shannon M, Winchester J, eds. *Clinical management of poisoning and drug overdose*, 3rd ed. Philadelphia: WB Saunders, Philadelphia, 1998:2–32.

Drugs of Abuse

Michelle Fischer Keane, MD

Mind-altering substances have been used for centuries. Through the years, they have evolved from naturally occurring plants to highly technical chemical substances. All of these substances have some significant impact on the body, ranging from the ravages of long-term addiction to premature death. These substances are constantly changing and new ones continue to appear. This chapter introduces the student to some of the more common and current drugs of abuse.

Cocaine

Cocaine was used as early as 1500 BC by Inca Indians who chewed coca leaves to increase endurance and their ability to work at high altitudes, and for social and religious occasions. The drug was purified in the 1880s by the German chemist Albert Niemann and was used as a tonic or elixir to treat depression, fatigue, hay fever, and asthma, and also as a topical anesthetic on mucous membranes. During this period, co-

caine was also placed in soft drinks, wine, tea, chewing gum, cigarettes, and cigars. In 1906, the Pure Food and Drug Act ended over-the-counter sales of medications containing cocaine, and in 1914 the Harrison Narcotic Act regulated the manufacturing and distribution of narcotics. As a direct result of this legislation, cocaine use dropped until a mid-1970s epidemic, when the drug was rediscovered for recreational use.

In 1985, crack cocaine, a smokeable form, was introduced to the drug scene. Crack was responsible for changing cocaine from a drug of the rich to one of the poor. Prices dropped from $200 a gram to less than $50. Crack cocaine is sold in vials with several "rocks" per vial each costing from $5 to $10. In 1985, there were an estimated 5.7 million frequent users. Cocaine use declined after 1985 but has been on the rise since the late 1990s. From 1999 to 2002, cocaine was the most commonly reported drug in emergency departments in the United States. Common street names for cocaine include coke, nose candy, snow, blow, powder, yahoos, cola, crack, and rock.

Cocaine is produced from the leaves of the coca tree found in areas of South America (Peru, Bolivia, and Colombia). Coca paste (20% to 85% cocaine) is made by dissolving Erythroxylon and coca leaves in kerosene and sulfuric acid. The paste is then mixed with hydrochloric acid, creating cocaine hydrochloride, a water-soluble compound that can be injected or snorted. The coca plant is harvested several times each year. Approximately 300 pounds of leaves are necessary to produce 1 pound of cocaine. By further processing cocaine hydrochloride with baking soda and ammonia or water, a solid smokable base form known as crack is produced. Crack is named for the cracking sound it makes when it is heated. It is colorless and odorless and reaches the bloodstream instantaneously, providing sudden and extreme euphoria lasting 5 to 10 minutes. A smoked dose of cocaine has approximately 60% the potency of an intravenous (IV) dose. When injected IV, cocaine reaches the brain in less than 15 seconds and the high lasts 12 to 30 minutes. Eighty percent to 90% of cocaine use is intranasal. The peak effect is experienced in 2 to 30 minutes and lasts 30 to 60 minutes. However, the effect may be limited by nasal mucosal vasoconstriction. Because of this, a fairly substantial amount is required to obtain euphoria, hence the costliness of snorting cocaine. Recreational users consume 1 to 3 g per week.

Clinical Presentation

The most common effects of cocaine are tachycardia and hypertension (Table 53.1). Serious consequences of cocaine abuse include hyperglycemia, cardiac conduction abnormalities, coronary artery ischemia with vasospasm, ventricular arrhythmias, aortic dissection, myocardial infarction, rhabdomy-olysis, lactic acidoses, hyperthermia, seizures, and strokes. In pregnant users, there is an increased risk of placental abruption, premature delivery, and low-birth-weight infants. More than two thirds of cocaine-dependent patients experience paranoia, often resulting in erratic, violent behavior.

Pathophysiology

Cocaine acts on the central nervous system (CNS) by causing the release of biogenic amines such as norepinephrine and by blocking their reuptake. They act primarily on the dopaminergic portions located in the pleasure centers of the brain. This causes CNS and peripheral nervous system stimulation, local anesthesia, and vasoconstriction. Increased availability of epinephrine causes primarily sympathomimetic effects on the body.

Cocaine is rapidly metabolized into benzoylecgonine. This product is 50 to 100 times more concentrated in the urine, making it a useful metabolite for drug testing. The metabolites can be detected as early as 1 to 4 hours after use and for up to 48 hours. The serum half-life of cocaine is about 1 hour. Cocaine levels do not correlate well with toxicity.

Table 53.1.	
Clinical presentation of cocaine	
Mood-altering	Euphoria, increases self-confidence, increased energy and an increased ability to do work
Neurological	Dizziness, hyperreflexia, tremor, seizures, local anesthesia, paresthesias, headache
Psychiatric	Insomnia, agitation, anxiety, paranoia, delirium, hallucinations, psychosis, labile affect
Eyes	Dilated pupils
Cardiovascular	Hypertension, tachycardia, arrhythmia, palpitations
GI	Nausea, dry mouth, anorexia
Temperature	Elevated
Skin	Diaphoresis

GI, gastrointestinal.

Treatment

The treatment of patients with cocaine intoxication in the emergency department is primarily supportive. Patients require continuous vitals and cardiac monitoring for hypertension, tachycardia, arrhythmias, agitation, and electrocardiographic (ECG) changes. Charcoal is not necessary unless ingestion has occurred. Acute coronary syndrome, which can occur in patients with normal coronary arteries, should be treated the same as one would ordinarily treat myocardial ischemia, except that benzodiazepines (lorazepam 1 to 2 mg IV or diazepam 2.5 to 5 mg IV) should be added to the regimen. In addition, β-blockers are contraindicated because their use would lead to unopposed α-effects. Sodium nitroprusside (0.5 to 10 µg/kg/ minute IV) can be added for hypertension control if sedation is not adequate. Hyperthermia can be treated with rapid cooling. Keep in mind that acetaminophen, salicylates, and dantrolene are not effective. Rhabdomyolysis should be managed with aggressive hydration to maintain adequate diuresis. Remember that in rhabdomyolysis serum creatinine phosphokinase (CPK) should be elevated and urine dipstick will be positive for occult blood, but no red blood cells (RBCs) will be found on formal urinalysis.

Heroin

Heroin was first synthesized from morphine in 1874 by Alder Wright, an English chemist. In 1889, Bayer Chemical in Germany first introduced heroin, taken from the German word *heroisch*, which means "strength." During the early 1900s, heroin, like cocaine, was a common drug in many over-the-counter medications to treat pain, diarrhea, insomnia, and cough. It was not until 1924 that heroin production was outlawed in the United States. Before regulatory legislation, it was estimated that 400,000 Americans in 1900 were narcotic dependent. In 1942, cultivation of the opium poppy was outlawed in the United States; in 1956, the drug was outlawed.

Heroin is produced from morphine, which is an opium derivative. Most of the opium is produced in two regions of the world known at the Golden Triangle (Burma, Laos, and Thailand) and the Golden Crescent (Afghanistan, Pakistan, and Iran). Mexico and Colombia also produce a smaller amount.

Opium is a product of the opium poppies, flowers with a variety of colored petals—red, white, blue, pink, or purple. After the opium poppies ripen, the petals fall off and the poppy pod or capsule is left. Farmers score the poppy capsules, allowing opium to ooze out, dry, and harden. It is then scraped off, collected, and converted in clandestine laboratories to heroin hydrochloride by anhydrous acetylation of morphine.

Heroin carries various street names, such as smack, TNT, white junk, dope, boss, brown sugar, and thing. Its popularity as an abused drug has grown, as evidenced by the number of emergency department visits nationwide, which increased from 42,000 in 1992 to 62,000 in 1993. The last surge of heroin use was in the 1960s. Of the reported 140,000 new users in 1997, 90% were younger than age 26. Users today are more likely to be middle class teenagers who smoke or snort the drug rather than the classic hypodermic needle-using junkie. IV administration is still the preferred method of use among heroin abusers. The purity of heroin available on the street has risen steadily from 2% to 3% in the 1960s to nearly 30% to 50% today. This higher potency permits novices to start with intranasal administration. The onset of euphorigenic action is about 30 minutes after snorting, 15 minutes after subcutaneous injection ("skin popping"), and almost instantaneously after IV injection ("shooting up, mainlining"). The duration of action is 3 to 6 hours. The usual dose is 1 to 25 mg of a 5% concentration. Heroin hydrochloride is always adulterated, or essentially diluted, by the addition of additives like quinine, lactose, mannitol, dextrose, or talc. As of 1998, snorting is the method of choice of heroin experimentation for most American teenagers. This involves heating the insoluble heroin base on aluminum foil and rapidly inhaling the upwardly curling smoke—"chasing the dragon." Heroin's principal effects are that of euphoria, analgesia, and respiratory depression.

Clinical Presentation

Heroin reduces anticipatory anxiety associated with emotional or physical pain, and it alters the person's perception of pain so that discomfort is reduced or eliminated; it also causes somnolence ("nodding off") (Table 53.2). The typical toxidrome of heroin overdose is stupor or coma, miotic pupils, mental clouding, bradypnea, cool, mottled skin, and diminished response to painful stimuli.

Abrupt cessation of heroin use can cause withdrawal symptoms. These symptoms usually occur in any patient with at least 3 weeks of regular use. Withdrawal symptoms develop within 6 to 8 hours after the last dose of heroin, and include agitation, rhinorrhea, lacrimation, yawning, piloerection, diarrhea, abdominal cramps, pupillary mydriasis (dilation), tremulousness, tachycardia, and hypertension. Withdrawal symptoms last from 7 to 10 days and peak at 48 to 72 hours.

Complications of heroin use include respiratory arrest, pulmonary edema, toxic amblyopia, and wound botulism. IV drug users can develop skin abscesses and cellulitis, sep-

tic arthritis, infectious spondylitis or sacroiliitis, Potts disease, vertebral osteomyelitis, and subacute bacterial endocarditis. Sixty percent to 90% of heroin injectors have chronic hepatitis C infection. In addition, sharing needles places users at high risk for human immunodeficiency virus (HIV) disease and hepatitis B.

Pathophysiology

Heroin is believed to possess the highest potential to produce rapidly developing dependence and addiction of any of the common opiate narcotic analgesics. It produces intense euphoria by facilitating direct access to the primitive mammalian reward system. It avidly binds μ, κ, and other stereospecific opiate-receptor binding sites in the locus ceruleus.

Heroin is rapidly deacetylated in microsomes of the endoplasmic reticulum of the liver to 6-monoacetyl morphine (6-MAM). It is then further deacetylated to morphine and excreted in the urine over 30 to 40 hours as free morphine and morphine 3-glucoronide, its major metabolite. A positive urine specimen for morphine, using 300 ng/mL as a cutoff point, can be expected for about 48 hours after the last use. 6-MAM can be examined in some laboratories because it is a metabolite specific for heroin abuse, but the test is costly, and 6-MAM is present for only a few hours after heroin use.

Table 53.2.	
Clinical presentation of heroin	
Mood-altering	Euphoria followed by sedation, somnolence, analgesia
Neurological	Decreased reflexes, slowed comprehension, impaired mentation
Respiratory	Depression, cough suppression
Eyes	Pinpoint or constricted pupils
Cardiovascular	Hypotension, bradycardia, arrhythmias
GI	Nausea, vomiting, constipation
Temperature	Decreased
Skin	Cool, mottled
Genitourinary	Urinary retention

GI, gastrointestinal.

Treatment

A diagnostic trial dose of low-dose naloxone (0.1 to 0.2 mg IV) for suspected addicts clinches the diagnosis. Patients who are somnolent will rouse, respiratory rate will increase, and their pupils will dilate. For nonaddicts, higher doses are indicated (1 to 2 mg). The onset of action of naloxone is within 2 minutes and lasts only 1 to 2 hours. Nalmefene, an opioid antagonist like naloxone, has a longer duration of action (3 to 5 hours) and can also be used. Charcoal should be used for decontamination if ingestion has occurred. Heroin overdose is often associated with pulmonary edema. This can begin almost immediately or be delayed for up to 2 hours (4 hours if taken intranasally). For this reason, the heroin overdose patient should be observed in the emergency department for at least 6 hours.

Treatment for acute opiate withdrawal is primarily supportive because it is almost never fatal. Severe withdrawal symptoms can be treated with clonidine, an α_2-agonist (0.1 to 0.2 mg by mouth [po]), or methadone detoxification (15 to 20 mg/day for 2 to 4 days).

Marijuana (Cannabis)

Although the frequency of marijuana use is decreasing, it is the most common form of illegal drug use in the United States today. For centuries, marijuana has been used for its mind-altering properties. It is estimated that 43 million Americans have tried marijuana and nearly one third of those are regular users. Marijuana today is 5 to 10 times more potent than it was 30 years ago because of fewer contaminants and adulterants. A single marijuana joint has been found to be the equivalent of five tobacco cigarettes. With a high content of carcinogens and long retention time, it may contribute to lung cancer. Interestingly, marijuana has some potential therapeutic uses. Dronabinol (Marinol) is used for relieving nausea caused by chemotherapy. Marijuana also lowers intraocular pressure in glaucoma and is used for stimulating appetite in patients with acquired immunodeficiency syndrome (AIDS).

Marijuana is a naturally occurring cannabinoid from the leaves and flowers of the hemp plant (Cannabis sativa). Its predominant psychoactive substance is delta-9-tetrahydrocannabinol (THC) (4% to 6%). Hashish (20% to 30%), which is more potent than regular marijuana, refers to a dried resin made from the flower tops of the cannabis plant. Sinsemilla is a seedless form of marijuana that is approximately twice as potent as hashish. Marijuana is smoked in "joints," as the common marijuana cigarette. It can also be smoked in "bowls" (miniature pipes) or "bongs" (water- or air-cooled smoking devices that enable the smoker to inhale more with less irritation). Marijuana is deeply inhaled and held for 20 to 30 seconds to increase the amount of active drug absorbed. It can also be ingested or used in a purified IV form. Its effects are noticeable in seconds or minutes, with a peak effect in 10 to 30 minutes lasting 2 to 6 hours.

Clinical Presentation

The most common physical signs of marijuana abuse are tachycardia (one cigarette increases the heart rate 20 to 50 beats per minute) and conjunctival irritation (Table 53.3). A chronic cough and swollen uvula are also common findings. Marijuana inhibits sweating, thus potentially lending to an increase in core body temperature. A multitude of personality changes are seen in marijuana abusers including depression, antisocial characteristics such as isolation and withdrawal, and anxiety. It is important to emphasize that these are secondary to the drug and are not preabuse abnormalities. "Amotivational syndrome" is a classic array of symptoms such as energy loss, decreased ambition, academic underachievement, decreased social relations, and apathy. Long-term effects include decreased plasma testosterone, gynecomastia, oligospermia, and luteinizing hormone (LH) and prolactin suppression leading to sporadic ovulation and irregular menses. There is even a mild immunosuppressant effect caused by marijuana use that results in a lower number of T lymphocytes. Withdrawal symptoms can occur with chronic use but are

Table 53.3.	
Clinical presentation of marijuana	
Mood-altering	Mental relaxation, euphoria, increased sociability and dream-like states
Neurological	Drowsiness, impaired short-term memory, slowed reflexes, ataxia, decreased coordination
Psychiatric	Lapses of attention, poor concentration, speech difficulty, acute panic-anxiety reactions, psychotic episodes
Eyes	Conjunctival injection
Cardiovascular	Tachycardia, orthostatic hypotension
Respiratory	Bronchodilation (low doses), hoarseness, cough, bronchitis
Temperature	Elevated
Skin	Dry

usually mild: irritability, sleep disturbances, tremor, nystagmus, anorexia, nausea, vomiting, and diarrhea.

Pathophysiology

THC binds to anandamide receptors in the brain, causing stimulant, sedative, or hallucinogenic actions depending on the dose and time after consumption. Both catecholamine release and inhibition of sympathetic reflexes may be observed.

THC is metabolized by hydroxylation to active and inactive metabolites with an elimination half-life of 20 to 30 hours. Urine testing is the most effective way to screen for use. The screening test detects marijuana at 20 ng/mL. Because marijuana is highly lipophilic, it has a long half-life and can be detected in the urine 2 to 4 weeks after its use. It is even possible to have a positive screen from passive inhalation of marijuana.

Treatment

In most instances, reassurance and supportive measures are adequate for managing marijuana users. Acute psychotic breaks may be managed with benzodiazepines (lorazepam 1 to 2 mg IV). The tachycardia does not usually require chemical treatment, but if necessary, β-blockers are appropriate. Decontamination is with activated charcoal if ingestion has occurred.

Amphetamines

Until recently, the use of amphetamines has decreased since the 1960s "speed" epidemic. Amphetamines were very popular during the 1940s, 1950s, and 1960s. During World War II, soldiers used amphetamines to counteract fatigue and hunger. During the late 1950s and early 1960s, the drugs were used for weight loss. After the U.S. Food and Drug Administration (FDA) tightened regulations for amphetamine prescriptions, the use of amphetamines dropped. There has been a recent resurgence of use with the introduction of "ice" or "crystal," the smokeable form of methamphetamine (meth). Crystal meth first appeared in Asia in 1985, and by 1988 its use was documented in Hawaii. Other common street names include uppers, speed, black beauties, bennies, whizz, billy, tweak, meth, and white crosses. Because amphetamines are relatively easy to produce and have a longer half-life than cocaine, their popularity has increased while that of cocaine has decreased.

The most common route of administration is oral, but the drugs may also be smoked (crystal methamphetamine), snorted, and injected. Onset of action is approximately 30 minutes after ingestion with the effects lasting up to 14 hours. "Crash," or the immediate appearance of withdrawal symptoms may occur 15 to 30 minutes after heavy dosing.

Clinical Presentation

The toxidrome of amphetamine intoxication includes hypertension, tachycardia, dilated pupils, tremor, cardiac arrhythmias, and increased reflexes. Users seek the effects of euphoria, increased alertness, reduced fatigue, and sense of well-being (Table 53.4).

Overdose can cause coma, circulatory collapse, hypertensive crisis, hyperthermia, or cerebral hemorrhage. Long-term effects of amphetamine abuse include impaired concentration, abrupt mood changes, weight loss, paranoid delusions, and violence.

Withdrawal usually appears 2 to 4 days after last use, but mood disturbance may last several weeks. Symptoms include lethargy, fatigue, depression, anxiety, nightmares, sweating, muscle cramps, abdominal cramps, and hunger.

Pathophysiology

Amphetamines cause direct CNS stimulation through release of presynaptic neurotransmitters, direct stimulation of postsynaptic catecholamine receptors, prevention of reuptake of neurotransmitters, and mild inhibition of monoamine oxidase.

Amphetamines are well absorbed orally and are extensively metabolized by the liver, forming several active metabolites with actions similar to the parent compound. Following deamination and conjugation, the metabolites are excreted primarily in the urine along with 20% to 40% of the unmetabolized parent compound. Excretion of most amphetamines is highly dependent on urine pH, being more rapidly eliminated in an acidic urine.

Treatment

When faced with an amphetamine-toxic agitated patient, use a dark quiet room and benzodiazepines (lorazepam 1 to 2 mg IV, or diazepam 2.5 to 5 mg IV) or haloperidol (5 to 10 mg intramuscular [IM] or IV) for sedation. Hyperthermia is also treated with sedation, but add cooling measures and Dantrolene (1 mg/kg) for malignant hyperthermia. Seizures can be treated with benzodiazepines and phenytoin or phenobarbital. Tachyarrhythmias can be treated with propanolol or esmolol. Charcoal can be administered for decontamination. Renal elimination of the drug can be enhanced by acidification of the urine, but this is not

---

Table 53.4.

Clinical presentation of amphetamines

Mood-altering	Euphoria, increases self-confidence, increased energy and an increased ability to do work
Neurological	Dizziness, hyperreflexia, tremor, seizures, local anesthesia, paresthesia, headache
Psychiatric	Insomnia, irritability, impulsivity, anxiety, panic, hallucinations (visual, tactile, olfactory)
Eyes	Dilated pupils
Cardiovascular	Hypertension, tachycardia, arrhythmia, palpitations
GI	Decreased appetite, dry mouth, nausea, vomiting
Temperature	Elevation
Skin	Diaphoresis

GI, gastrointestinal.

recommended because of the risk of aggravating the nephrotoxicity of myoglobinuria.

Designer Drugs

Designer drugs are drugs produced by a minor modification in the chemical structure of an existing drug, resulting in a new substance with similar pharmacological effects. Because they are slightly different from the illegal parent compounds, they are rendered temporarily immune from the control of the U.S. Drug Enforcement Agency. The most widely used of these designer drugs are the fentanyl analogues and methylenedioxymethamphetamine (MDMA, Ecstasy).

Synthetic opiates are a popular group of designer drugs. Fentanyl analogues were initially developed and marketed in the 1970s as a heroin substitute. They contain the same abilities to block pain and cause euphoria, but are up to 1,000 times as potent as heroin and 200 times more potent than morphine. "China White" is the most frequently used analogue. Users of China White (α-methyl fentanyl) and TMF (3-methyl-fentanyl) have suffered an inordinate number of fatal overdoes either because of its strength or unknown pharmacological properties. They have a 1- to 4-minute onset of action and 30- to 90-minute duration. IV is the most common method of administration. Effects can be reversed with naloxone.

Illicit meperidine use increased during periods when heroin was scarce. Two meperidine analogues appeared on the streets: MPPP (1-methyl-4-phenyl-4-propionoxypiperidine) and PEPAP (1-[2-phenyl-ethyl]-4-acetyloxpiperidine). They were marketed as "new heroin." MPPP was popular among drug users because when it was injected, it produced a euphoria similar to that produced by heroin. An impurity formed during the clandestine manufacture of MPPP, called MPTP (1-methyl-4-phenyl-1,2,3,6-tetrahydropyridine), has been shown to be a potent neurotoxin that causes permanent, rapidly developing Parkinson's disease in patients exposed to this contaminant.

Other designer drugs like 3,4-methylenedioxymethamphetamine (MDMA, Ecstasy, Adam, XTC, E, or X) and 3,4-methylenedioxyethamphetamine (MDEA, M, or Eve) are chemically altered derivatives of amphetamines. They are changed slightly to produce desired mood alterations.

Ecstasy

Ecstasy (MDMA) is an analogue of the stimulant methamphetamine. It shares properties with both amphetamine and hallucinogenic drugs. First synthesized 1914 in Germany, it was used as an adjunct to psychotherapy in the United States until the early 1980s. In 1984, it was made a Schedule I drug. MDMA is a selective serotonergic neurotoxin, hence the long-term deleterious effects. In the United States, the drug has become popular with adolescents at dance halls known as "raves" and on college campuses. The drug appeals to the young, who believe that it enhances empathy, introspection, and closeness to others and induces positive mood states and feelings of intimacy and tranquility.

MDMA is reputedly safe to take as a "recreational" or "therapeutic" drug in a dose of 1 to 2 mg/kg. In the United States, MDMA is available in 100-mg tablets that cost about $20 each. Peak effects occur at 90 minutes and may persist for 8 or more hours. Tolerance to desirable effects and an increase in adverse effects are reported to develop with regular and frequent use.

Clinical Presentation

Physical signs of MDMA ingestion are similar to lysergic acid diethylamide (LSD) ingestion (Table 53.5). The letdown after taking MDMA, which lasts 1 to 3 days, is characterized by drowsiness, muscle aches, jaw soreness, depression, and difficulty in concentrating. Serious adverse effects of ecstasy include serious or fatal heat injury; fluid and electrolyte depletion; and CNS, cardiac, muscular, renal, and hepatic dysfunction, including disseminated intravascular coagulation.

Table 53.5.

Clinical presentation of MDMA

Musculoskeletal	Jaw clenching, muscle spasms, rhabdomyolysis
Mood-altering	Enhances empathy, introspection, closeness to others, induces positive mood states and feelings of intimacy and tranquility
Neurological	Insomnia, nystagmus, difficulty concentrating, seizures, tremors
Psychiatric	Depression, anxiety, paranoia, impulsivity
Eyes	Widely dilated pupils
Cardiovascular	Hypertension, tachycardia, arrhythmia
GI	Nausea, vomiting
Temperature	Elevated
Skin	Diaphoresis, thermoregulation disturbances

GI, gastrointestinal; MDMA, methylenedioxymethamphetamine.

Pathophysiology

MDMA acts in the CNS similar to amphetamines, as discussed earlier. MDMA is metabolized by N-methylation to MDA. Urinary excretion of the parent drug accounts for 65% of the dose. Toxicological screens that test for amphetamines can detect MDMA but at about 50% reduced sensitivity.

Treatment

Treatment includes rapid cooling, rehydration, correction of electrolyte abnormalities, and monitoring for organ dysfunction. This drug has been implicated in at least 53 deaths in the United Kingdom and five more in the United States almost all of which were attributable to profound disturbances in thermoregulation.

Gamma Hydroxybutyrate

Gamma hydroxybutyrate (GHB) was first synthesized in 1960 by French physician Henry Laborit as an alternative anesthetic to aid in surgery. It was shown to cross the blood–brain barrier rapidly to induce a sleep-like state with cardiovascular stability. In 1964, it was introduced as an anesthetic induction agent but was not readily accepted because of the high incidence of vomiting, myoclonus, seizures, and emergence delirium. In the 1970s, GHB was advocated for the treatment of narcolepsy because it increased slow wave sleep and reduced the symptoms of narcolepsy. In 1977, investigators reported that GHB enhanced the effects of steroids and the release of growth hormone. Because of this, body builders started to use the drug to promote muscle development. It was also marketed as an over-the-counter sleeping aid in 1989, but by 1990 was pulled from the shelves because of deaths and serious illnesses. This drug, like ecstasy, has gained in popularity among adolescents in the rave scene.

GHB comes as a clear liquid, looking just like water, or white powder and is sold under a variety of street names including G, liquid E, liquid X, Georgia home boy, fantasy, scoop, and salty water.

Clinical Presentation

After oral administration, GHB is rapidly absorbed within 10 to 15 minutes with a 3-hour duration. GHB produces a state of relaxation with mild euphoria (Table 53.6). An oral dose of 10 mg/kg produces short-term amnesia and hypotonia. Sleep and drowsiness are induced at doses of 20 to 30 mg/kg. IV doses of 50 to 60 mg/kg produce general anesthesia with little analgesia within 5 minutes and lasting 1 to 2 hours. Adverse effects are usually seen within 15 minutes of administration, and spontaneous recovery occurs in 7 hours.

Table 53.6.

Clinical presentation of GHB

Mood-altering	Euphoria, mood elevation, hallucinations, hypnotic tendencies, relaxation state
Neurological	Amnesia, hypotonia, dizziness, vertigo, seizures, anesthesia, coma
Psychiatric	Anxiety, agitation, confusion, emergence delirium
Eyes	Loss of peripheral vision
Cardiovascular	Bradycardia, hypotension
GI	Nausea, vomiting (50%), excessive salivation
Musculoskeletal	Myoclonic muscle movements (jerks)

GHB, γ-hydroxybutyrate; GI, gastrointestinal.

Delirium and generalized seizures are possible. Bradypnea with increased tidal volume is frequently seen. Cheyne-Stokes respiration and loss of airway-protective reflexes occur. Vomiting is seen in 30% to 50% of cases. Incontinence and myoclonus are common findings. Stimulation may cause tachycardia and mild hypertension, but bradycardia is much more common. A withdrawal syndrome can occur with chronic use with symptoms of tremor, paranoia, agitation, confusion, delirium, hallucinations, tachycardia, and hypertension.

Pathophysiology

GHB is thought to be a natural neurotransmitter, a catabolite of γ-aminobutyric acid (GABA), that influences dopamine release in the substantia nigra, producing pleasurable effects such as euphoria, hallucinations, and smooth muscle relaxation. GHB crosses the blood–brain barrier and directly depresses the CNS and causes respiratory depression.

GHB is metabolized to carbon dioxide and water by oxidation via the Krebs cycle with no active metabolites and an elimination half-life of 30 minutes. GHB is usually excreted in the first few hours after its ingestion. The drug is not detectable by routine toxicological tests.

Treatment

Diagnosis is usually suspected clinically in the patient who presents with abrupt onset of coma and recovers rapidly within a few hours. Supportive measures, especially airway control and assistance with ventilations are usually all that is needed. Decontamination with charcoal is helpful if administered soon after ingestion. The withdrawal symptoms of GHB can be treated with benzodiazepines and phenobarbital.

Hallucinogens (Lysergic Acid Diethylamide [LSD] and Other Hallucinogens)

Hallucinogens are defined as drugs that produce visual, auditory, tactile, and olfactory hallucinations. Hallucinogens have been used by many cultures for thousands of years in religious and spiritual experiences. In the 1960s, these drugs became popular through publicity given them by proponents. There are several other important naturally occurring hallucinogens with effects similar to LSD although less potent: psychedelic mushrooms (psilocybin, psilocin), peyote cactus (mescaline), jimson weed *(Daura stramonium)*, nutmeg, and morning glory seeds *(Rivea corymbosa* and *Ipomoea).*

LSD is commonly referred to as acid, dots, cubes, window-pane, or blotter. It is the most potent psychoactive drug known. It is derived from an alkaloid in rye fungus but can be synthesized as well. The usual route of administration is oral, available as tablets or gelatin squares, or applied to pieces of paper known as "blotters." The dose is usually 25 to 100 µg. Onset of action is 30 minutes, with a 2- to 4-hour peak effect and 6- to 12-hour duration of action.

Table 53.7.

Clinical presentation of hallucinogens

Mood-altering	Visual, auditory, olfactory and tactile hallucinations, synesthesia or heightened perception of senses, time distortion
Neurological	Dizziness, paresthesias, hyperreflexia, tremor, ataxia
Psychiatric	Insomnia, irritability, impulsivity, anxiety, panic, hallucinations
Eyes	Dilated pupils, conjunctival injection, lacrimation
Cardiovascular	Hypertension, tachycardia, arrhythmias
GI	Nausea, dry mouth, anorexia
Temperature	Elevation, flushing, piloerection
Skin	Diaphoresis

GI, gastrointestinal.

Clinical Presentation

Acute hallucinogen effects include visual illusions, auditory illusions, "seeing" smells and "hearing" colors (synesthesia), increased tactile sensations, and distortion of time perception (Table 53.7).

Toxic effects of LSD, or a bad trip, include paranoia, depression, anxiety, panic attacks, and fear of disintegration or fragmentation of self. Life-threatening toxicity can occur from intense sympathomimetic stimulation and includes seizures, hypertension, hyperthermia, and cardiac arrhythmias. Chronic effects from LSD include flashbacks, psychoses, depressive reactions, and chronic personality changes.

Pathophysiology

The mechanism of action of hallucinogens, although not exactly known, is probably due to alterations in both the serotonergic and dopaminergic neurotransmitter systems with agonist action on 5-hydroxtryptamine-2 (5-HT$_2$) postsynaptic receptors. These effects are thought to alter the activity of serotonin and dopamine in the brain.

LSD is metabolized by the liver, with subsequent conjugation to glucuronide. Excretion is through the biliary system into the intestinal tract (80% to 90%).

Treatment

Usually, patients having a bad trip or panic reaction can be "talked down" if they are observed in a quiet setting and given gentle reassurance. Phenothiazines should be avoided because of possible synergistic anticholinergic and CNS depressant effects. Benzodiazepines or haloperidol/droperidol may be used. Seizures can be treated with benzodiazepines or phenytoin (Dilantin). Hyperthermia must be addressed and managed quickly to prevent hypotension, coagulopathy, rhabdomyolysis, and multiple organ failure. Decontaminate with charcoal.

Phencyclidine

Phencyclidine (PCP) was first used in the 1960s as a dissociative anesthetic agent but was quickly withdrawn from the market because of emergence delirium—agitation, hallucinations, muscle rigidity, and seizures. The drug is still commonly used in veterinary medicine. Common street names for PCP include angel dust, hog, dust, bromine fluid, and elephant tranquilizer.

PCP is a dissociative anesthetic with analgesic, stimulant, depressant, and hallucinogenic properties. PCP has the ability to interact with many neurotransmitters. Commonly smoked to better titrate the dose, it can also be taken intranasally, orally as a pill, or even intravenously. PCP abuse is not frequent, but it can be an adulterant in other drugs. When PCP is combined with cocaine it is called "space basing." The effects of PCP occur within 2 to 5 minutes if smoked or snorted and 30 minutes if ingested. Peak effect is 15 to 30 minutes if smoked or snorted and 2 to 5 hours if ingested. Duration of action is up to 12 hours. PCP is lipid-soluble and widely distributed to peripheral tissues accumulating in fat. It is secreted into gastric acid and reabsorbed in the intestine (recycling). Because of this phenomenon, PCP has a prolonged half-life of 48 to 72 hours.

Clinical Presentation

The signs and symptoms of PCP intoxication are dose related. PCP intoxication should be the main diagnostic consideration when a patient presents in a comatose state with eyes open, nystagmus, muscle rigidity, and elevated blood pressure and pulse (Table 53.8). The drug is addicting, and with continued use tolerance develops. Withdrawal symptoms occur when the drug is abruptly discontinued and consist of nervousness, anxiety, and depression.

Pathophysiology

PCP has a very complex pharmacology and includes all of the following: CNS stimulation and depression; peripheral autonomic effects; stimulation of opioid receptors; inhibition of reuptake of dopamine, norepinephrine, and serotonin; analgesia; and anticonvulsant activity.

PCP is metabolized in the liver to various hydroxylated derivatives. These are then conjugated with glucuronic acid and excreted in the urine and gastric fluids, both of which are pH dependent.

Treatment

Treatment of intoxication depends on the stage of presentation. Do not try to "talk down" these patients. Benzodiazepines should be used as necessary for sedation or combative behavior. For severe psychosis and agitation, haloperidol may be given (avoid phenothiazine and physostigmine). Use a cooling blanket for hyperthermia to prevent malignant hyperthermia. Nitroprusside, labetalol, or phentolamine may be used for hypertension. Gastric lavage followed by activated charcoal should be administered in severe intoxication to prevent the reabsorption of PCP excreted into the stomach. Acidification of the urine should not be done because it has very little effect on the removal of PCP from the body (it is metabolized in the liver) and may increase risk of rhabdomyolysis. Charcoal should be used for decontamination after ingestion. Patients should be monitored for at least 6 hours.

Ketamine ("Special K")

Ketamine or "Special K" is a short-acting dissociative anesthetic that has psychoactive properties similar to PCP with less dysphoric sequelae. This drug is commercially sold as Ketalar, a powerful anesthetic used

---

Table 53.8.

Clinical presentation of PCP

Mood-altering	Euphoria, decreased inhibitions, feelings of power, altered perceptions of time, space, and body image
Neurological	Lethargy, blank stare, catatonic state, nystagmus, ataxia, stupor, coma with preserved deep pain response, seizures
Psychiatric	Agitation, hostile combative behavior
Eyes	Dilated pupils
Cardiovascular	Hypertension, tachycardia
GI	Increased salivation
Musculoskeletal	Rigidity, twitching
Temperature	Elevation
Skin	Flushed and hot

GI, gastrointestinal; PCP, phencyclidine.

mainly by veterinarians on farm animals. It preserves respiratory drive and muscle tone and augments sympathetic nervous system tone. Available as a liquid, white powder, or pill, it can be inhaled, swallowed, or injected. Induction is complete within 30 seconds and lasts 15 minutes. Analgesia is profound and lasts 40 minutes. The amnestic effect may last for up to 2 hours. Users describe the effects similar to drunkenness but stronger. Others describe a speedy rush within minutes of consuming the drug, followed by powerful hallucinations.

Inhalants

The incidence of volatile substance abuse seems to be stable; the most common abusers are boys younger than 14. Inhalant abuse is highest in urban areas and on North American Indian reservations. The substances are cheap, readily available, and can be obtained legally. The agents are used to "get high." They are first "sniffed," but as the abuse progresses, users start "huffing," which involves soaking a cloth in solvent to increase the amount inhaled. "Bagging" (breathing in and out of a paper or plastic bag containing the volatile substance) is used to intensify the inhalation by more experienced abusers. Tolerance and dependence, with withdrawal symptoms, do develop. When a teenager suddenly collapses while "partying," solvent abuse should be suspected.

Clinical Presentation

Inhalants cause CNS stimulation and excitement progressing to depression (Table 53.9). They may also sensitize the myocardium to the arrhythmogenic effects of catecholamines. Mild irritation of the mucous membranes of the eyes, respiratory system, and gastrointestinal tract does occur.

Overdose can present with respiratory depression, arrhythmia, cardiac arrest, seizure, delirium, stupor, or coma. Sudden sniffing death syndrome is sudden death, probably resulting from a cardiac arrhythmia. Permanent damage to the brain, liver, heart, kidneys, and bone marrow is possible.

Airplane glue (toluene) causes peripheral neuropathies, tremors, and ataxia. Gasoline causes pulmonary symptoms of irritation to the respiratory tract, anemia, neurological problems, visual hallucinations, cardiac arrhythmias, confusion, and renal toxicity. Amyl nitrate ("poppers") causes cardiac problems, hypotension, myocardial ischemia, methemoglobinemia, and even cardiovascular collapse. Inhaled fluorinated hydrocarbons (Freon) can cause cardiac arrhythmias. Typewriter fluid (trichloroethyl-

Table 53.9.	
Clinical presentation of inhalants	
Mood-altering	Euphoria, giddiness
Neurological	Dizziness, headache, ataxia, slurred speech, diplopia, diminished reflexes, drowsiness
Psychiatric	Hallucinations, psychosis, impaired judgment
Eyes	Nystagmus, lacrimation
Cardiovascular	Arrhythmias (tachy and brady)
GI	Nausea, anorexia, vomiting, salivation, diarrhea
Respiratory	Rhinorrhea, mucosal irritation, coughing, choking, tachypnea, wheezing, pulmonary edema, respiratory arrest
Skin	Burns

GI, gastrointestinal.

ene) causes neuropathies, headache, cardiac arrhythmias, renal and hepatic dysfunction, and diffuse CNS symptoms.

Pathophysiology

Abused volatile substances are absorbed rapidly into the bloodstream, are highly lipid soluble, and produce marked CNS effects. The onset of action is immediate and lasts 5 to 15 minutes. Laboratory tests may display any of the following abnormalities: anemia, thrombocytopenia, leukopenia, liver enzyme elevation, proteinuria, or hematuria.

Treatment

Supportive care is usually sufficient, because most inhalant symptoms clear in 4 to 6 hours. Benzodiazepines can be used for seizures and haloperidol for extreme agitation. Always treat patients in a well-ventilated area. Charcoal should be used for decontamination.

Suggested Readings

Cline DM, Ma OJ. *Emergency medicine. A comprehensive study guide. Companion handbook*, 4th ed. New York: McGraw-Hill, 1996.

DiPalma JR, DiGregorio GJ. *Basic pharmacology in medicine,*. 3rd ed. New York: McGraw-Hill, 1990.

Gould Soloway RA. Street-smart advice on treating drug overdoses. *Emerg Nurs* 1993;93(9): 65–72.

Iven VG. Recreational drugs. *Sports Pharmacol* 1998;17:245–259.

Kam PCA, Yoong FFY. Gamma-hydroxybutyric acid; an emerging recreational drug. *Anaesthesia* 1998;53:1195–1198.

Pousada L, Osborn HH, Levy DB. *Emergency medicine*, 2nd ed. Baltimore: Williams & Wilkins, 1996.

Robson P. Cannabis. *Arch Dis Child* 1997;77: 164–166.

Ropero-Miller JD, Goldberger BA. Recreational drugs. Current trends in the 90's. *Toxicology* 1998;18:727–746.

Schultz JE. Illicit drugs of abuse. *Substance Abuse* 1993;20:221–230.

Schwartz B, Alderman EM. Substances of abuse. *Pediatr Rev* 1997;18(6):204–217.

Schwartz RH. Adolescent heroin use: a review. *Pediatrics* 1998;102:1461–1466.

Schwartz RH, Miller NS. MDMA (Ecstasy) and the Rave: a review. *Pediatrics* 1997;100: 705–708.

CHAPTER 54

Cardiovascular Medication Overdose

Mark B. Mycyk, MD

Cardiovascular medications are among the most prescribed drugs throughout the world today, and when used as indicated have proved to be effective in the treatment of many different cardiovascular-related disorders. With increased use naturally comes the potential for increased misuse. Whether ingested accidentally by a toddler who gets into a grandparent's medicine cabinet or ingested intentionally by an adult in a suicide attempt, overdose with cardiovascular medications is the third most common reason for poison-related deaths, according to the data collected annually by the American Association of Poison Control Centers (AAPCC). Poisonings with any of the cardiovascular drugs are always challenging to the emergency physician, and successful outcome depends on early recognition and a systematic approach to management.

Clinical Presentation

Obtaining a history of ingestion is one of the most important steps in the management of these overdoses. It is critical to ask if the ingestion was intentional (i.e., suicidal) or accidental, when the ingestion occurred, and if the patient has any symptoms. Once a history of ingestion of a cardiovascular medication is obtained, immediate attention to the patient's airway, breathing, and circulation (ABCs) is indicated as you continue interviewing the patient. If you are faced with a patient who cannot talk or if history is simply unattainable, any evidence of life-threatening hypotension, bradydysrhythmia, tachydysrhythmia, conduction disturbances, or even congestive heart failure requires you to consider cardiovascular medication overdose in your differential diagnosis. Remember that patients presenting early after an overdose may not have any of these life-threatening signs and may present instead with nonspecific weakness, nausea, vomiting, belly pain, or a depressed mental status.

General Management

The emergency department management for patients poisoned with cardiovascular medications follows the same systematic approach as for any poisoning: addressing the ABCs and providing supportive care early, preventing drug absorption, enhancing elimination, administering antidotal treatment, and providing a safe disposition. Because of the potentially catastrophic nature of cardiovascular drug ingestions, always anticipate life-threatening complications and do not delay in getting the patient on a continuous cardiac monitor, establishing intravenous access, and obtaining a twelve-lead electrocardiogram (ECG) for evaluation. Once these have been done, try to administer activated charcoal as early as possible to absorb any remaining drug in the stomach; preventing the drug from making its way into the bloodstream can save you lots of trouble later. It cannot be stressed enough that appropriate and early supportive care is by far the most important aspect of treating these patients. Remember your advanced cardiac life support (ACLS) principles: if the patient has a low blood pressure, administer a fluid bolus; if the patient has symptomatic bradycardia, administer atropine; if the patient has third-degree heart block, initiate transthoracic pacing.

Any patient who presents with an overdose of a cardiovascular medication requires admission to a monitored bed or intensive care unit after stabilization in the emergency department.

Cardiovascular Physiology and Pharmacological Principles

Treating a patient who has taken a cardiovascular medication overdose requires a firm understanding of where these drugs exert most of their effect. Although cardiovascular medications can be classified into almost a dozen different classes, it is easiest to consider them by their primary site of action: either at the level of the heart or at the level of the blood vessels.

The heart is made up of (a) a specialized conduction system responsible for generating rate and rhythm and (b) the myocardial cells that contract when signaled to do so by the conduction system. A healthy heart depends on the conduction system and the myocardial cells working together. Without a functioning conduction system, the myocardial cells would lack the coordi-

nation needed to initiate the squeeze (inotropy) responsible for circulating blood throughout the body and providing us with a blood pressure. Circulating blood, in turn, provides the conduction system with the oxygen and nutrients necessary for generating a rhythm.

The generation of this electrical rhythm is produced by spontaneous depolarization of the action potential. The five phases (0 to 4) of the action potential are mediated by electrolyte movement in and out of the cell. The ECG is a reflection of that electrolyte movement. The three most important engines that mediate electrolyte movement are the Na-K-ATPase pump, the Na-Ca pump, and the Ca-pump. In the normal heart, spontaneous depolarization occurs fastest in the sinus node, or the pacemaker, and spreads from there through the rest of the conduction circuit down to the individual myocardial cells. Anything that disrupts the generation of this regular, repeated action potential (i.e., anything that disrupts the predictable flux of sodium, potassium, and calcium) prevents a coordinated rhythm from signaling the myocardial cells to contract. In addition to the spontaneously working electrolyte pumps throughout the heart, the myocardial cells contain β_1-sympathetic receptors that initiate cAMP production when stimulated to do so by the sympathetic nervous system: increased cAMP within the cells has the effect of increasing the rate of conduction (chronotropy) or increasing the intensity of the squeeze (inotropy). Therefore, overdose with a cardiovascular medication that works at the level of the heart poisons by interrupting the heart's predictable electrolyte movements or interfering with the signaling capacity of the β-adrenergic cell membrane receptors.

The blood vessels are mainly regulated by the sympathetic nervous system; activity here depends on whether the α-adrenergic or the β-adrenergic receptors are stimulated. α_1-stimulation causes vasoconstriction and an increase in blood pressure, whereas stimulation of the α_2-receptors causes a decrease in blood pressure. Of the β-receptors in the sympathetic system, only the β2-receptors have any significant activity in the blood vessels. When β2-receptors are stimulated, arterioles are relaxed, smooth muscle is dilated, and blood pressure falls. The important point when considering overdose with cardiovascular medications that act at the level of the vessels is this: blocking or antagonizing any of these receptors causes the exact opposite of the receptor's intended effect.

Specific Considerations

Antidysrhythmic Poisoning

Antidysrhythmic drugs are playing an increasing role in the prevention of sudden cardiac death from arrhythmia. Unfortunately, one of the side effects of these medicines is that they can cause arrhythmias from 5% to 15% of the time even in therapeutic doses. The I to IV classification of these drugs is based on a scheme proposed by Vaughan Williams in 1970.

Class I

Class I drugs generally block sodium channels in the myocardium. Class I drugs are divided into three subcategories.

CLASS IA

Class IA drugs include quinidine, procainamide, and disopyramide and work by prolonging the action potential. This mechanism has the effect of lengthening the refractory period, and in overdose this is reflected in the prolongation of the QRS or QT interval. A prolonged QT can lead to torsades de pointes type of ventricular tachycardia and fibrillation. Avoiding drugs that may further prolong the QT, and treating torsades with magnesium sulfate or overdrive pacing are the mainstays of therapy.

CLASS IB

Class IB drugs include lidocaine and tocainide, which slow phase 0 of the action potential, thus shortening the duration of the action potential but prolonging the refractory period. Usually supportive therapy is all that is necessary in these overdoses.

CLASS IC

Class IC drugs include flecainide and propafenone, which depress phase 0 and prolong the QRS, thus prolonging the action potential. Again, supportive therapy is most effective.

Class II

Class II antidysrhythmics consist of β-adrenergic blocking agents. They are among the most frequently prescribed cardiac medicines today, because they are used not only for the treatment of all types of cardiac disorders (ischemia, arrhythmia, congestive failure) but also for treatment of thyroid storm, glaucoma, migraines, and anxiety. Most of these β-blockers cause poisoning at the β1-receptors. By blocking the β-receptors of the heart, cyclic adenosine mono-phosphate (cAMP) concentrations are decreased, which result in slowed conduction (decreased automaticity) and a less intense myocardial squeeze (inotropy). This is helpful in a patient with hypertension, because a slower and less intense squeeze naturally creates a lower blood pressure. Too much β-blockade is problematic, and these patients classically present with bradycardia and hypotension. If the patient continues to have a low blood pressure despite addressing the ABCs and providing adequate fluid administration, several different therapeutic strategies must be considered. Because these overdoses result in blocked receptors, the most effective therapy consists of bypassing these receptors with glucagon administration. Glucagon works, because it bypasses the membrane β-receptors and exerts its effect within the heart where it directly increases intracellular cAMP. An increase in cAMP increases the rate and intensity of squeeze even if the outer membrane receptors are blocked. Pressor agents that stimulate beta activity should also be used to compete for the blocked receptors, but it makes intuitive sense that glucagon is more helpful early on. In addition to glucagon and pressors, atropine is also an option because it blocks parasympathetic activity at the vagal nerve and not at the site of poisoning. If intravenous medical therapy fails, transthoracic cardiac pacing is indicated.

Class III

Class III antidysrhythmics consists of amiodarone and bretylium; they work by prolonging the action potential and prolonging the QT interval. Torsades de pointes is the major sign of poisoning, and treatment is with magnesium or overdrive pacing.

Class IV

Class IV antidysrhythmics include the calcium channel antagonists, the most popularly prescribed antidysrhythmics today, which coincidentally are associated with the most fatalities. Although there are several subclasses of calcium channel antagonists, what is important is that they all have the effect of preventing calcium movement from outside the cell into the cell. Without calcium, the action potential is depressed and the myocytes cannot provide the squeeze necessary for adequate blood pressure. Bradycardia and hypotension is the classic presentation of these overdoses, much like in β-blocker overdoses. In a situation in which you cannot get a history from the patient, it is extremely difficult to distinguish calcium channel poisoning from β-blocker poisoning.

As with the other antidysrhythmics, the cornerstone of treatment is supportive therapy and prevention of absorption with activated charcoal. One of the reasons calcium channel antagonists are associated with so many deaths is that they have a prolonged release from the stomach, so early decontamination with whole bowel irrigation to hasten the elimination of these pills should be considered. Because the site of poisoning is the calcium channel, the primary antidote is high doses of calcium to overcome the blocked channels. Calcium chloride or calcium gluconate should be administered every 10 to 20 minutes as dictated by the patient's blood pressure and heart rate.

Glucagon has also been used to increase intracellular cAMP, but with less success than in β-blockers. Pressor agents and atropine have also been used with limited success. Despite high doses of calcium, glucagon, and pressor agents, the mortality rate in calcium channel antagonist overdose is still quite high. Although there are several reasons for the high mortality rate (increased use, sustained release), some think these agents are particularly deadly because calcium channels are found throughout the body and overdose shuts down many more critical organs than just the heart. For this reason, some recent research suggests that insulin and glucose therapy will one day be the antidote of choice in these overdoses for two important reasons: insulin is a powerful endogenous inotrope, and insulin enables the heart to efficiently use added glucose for energy in situations that have the effect of depriving the heart of energy and oxygen (i.e., shock).

Digoxin Poisoning

Digitalis glycosides have been recognized for centuries as beneficial in the treatment of congestive heart failure. They were first identified in such plants as foxglove, lily of the valley, and oleander; today the most commonly used preparation is the synthetically derived digoxin. Digoxin is beneficial in congestive heart failure, because it acts as an inotrope and increases cardiac output while decreasing elevated end-diastolic pressure. It does this at the myocyte by inhibiting the Na-K-ATPase pump; this has the effect of increasing intracellular sodium and indirectly increasing intracellular calcium, which provides enhanced contractility. Because the Na-K-ATPase is such an important pump, underlying electrolyte abnormalities can precipitate digoxin poisoning, particularly hypokalemia in patients who are chronically on diuretic therapy. Cardiac dysrhythmias are the most important manifestation of toxicity. Classically digoxin depresses myocardial conduction and increases automaticity, thus precipitating various atrioventricular (AV) blocks, junctional rhythms, and frequent premature ventricular contractions (PVCs). There are no pathognomonic rhythms for digoxin poisoning; any rhythm disturbance in the setting of digoxin ingestion is a bad rhythm.

Simply obtaining a history of digoxin ingestion is the most important aspect of diagnosis. If the patient is unstable, antidotal treatment is indicated no matter what the level. However, in the stable patient, a history of the amount of ingestion can help guide antidotal therapy in the acute setting as some consider ingestions of greater than 0.1 mg/kg as reason enough for treatment. Obtaining a digoxin level in the acute setting is also helpful. In addition to the other basic laboratory studies, obtaining a serum potassium level quickly is also critical to the management of these patients. Potassium results return quickly from most laboratories and a high potassium level indicates complete Na-K-ATPase block and probable digoxin poisoning.

Unlike the other cardiovascular medications in which supportive therapy is probably the most important aspect of therapy, there is an antidote for digoxin that is very effective and very safe. Digoxin immune Fab fragments work by binding all of the body's digoxin, inactivating it, and allowing it to be excreted via the kidneys. Specific indications include ingestion greater than 0.1 mg/kg, a 6-hour digoxin level greater than 5.0 ng/mL in adults, greater than 4 mg digoxin ingestion in previously healthy children, a serum potassium level greater than 5.0 mEq/L, or the presence of any life-threatening cardiac dysrhythmia or conduction delay. Clinical results are usually evident in 15 to 30 minutes. After the administration of Fab fragments, obtaining digoxin levels is not helpful because the laboratory assay measures both free digoxin and Fab-bound digoxin; therefore, the reported level will be falsely elevated. Remember, when faced with a patient who ingested digoxin, do not administer calcium to treat the high potassium levels, because a blocked Na-K-ATPase guarantees that there is already too much calcium in the myocytes; therefore, any extra calcium will cause such an intense contraction that the heart will never relax (this is called "stone heart").

Summary

Understanding the basic effects of cardiovascular medications enables the clinician to recognize poisoning with these agents and initiate effective therapy. Consider cardiovascular medication overdose in your differential diagnosis with all unstable patients. Sometimes you will need to correct significant vital sign abnormalities before you identify the medication or before you even get a history of overdose.

Suggested Readings

Abad-Santos F, Carcas AJ, Ibanez C, Frias J. Digoxin level and clinical manifestations as determinants in the diagnosis of digoxin toxicity. *Ther Drug Monitor* 1999;22:163–168.

Antman EM, Wenger TL, Butler VP, et al. Treatment of 150 cases of life-threatening digitalis intoxication with digoxin-specific Fab antibody fragments. *Circulation* 1990;81:1744–1752.

Bosse GM, Pope TM. Recurrent digoxin overdose and treatment with digoxin-specific Fab antibody fragments. *J Emerg Med* 1993;12:179–185.

Love JN, Howell JM. Glucagon therapy in the treatment of symptomatic bradycardia. *Ann Emerg Med* 1997;29:181–183.

Love JN, Litovitz TL, Howell JM, Clancy C. Characterization of fatal beta blocker ingestion: a review of the American Association of Poison Control data from 1985 to 1995. *J Toxicol Clin Toxicol* 1997;35:353–360.

Proprano L, Chiang WK, Wang RY. Calcium channel blocker overdose. *Am J Emerg Med* 1995;13:444–450.

Ramoska EA, Spiller Ha, Winter M, Borys D. A one year evaluation of calcium channel blocker overdoses: toxicity and treatment. *Ann Emerg Med* 1993;22:196–200.

Weinstein RS. Recognition and management of poisoning with beta-adrenergic blocking agents. *Ann Emerg Med* 1984;13:1123–1131.

Yuan TH, Kerns WP, Tomaszewaki CA, et al. Insulin-glucose as adjunctive therapy for severe calcium channel antagonist poisoning. *J Toxicol Clin Toxicol* 1999;37:463–474.

Acetaminophen

Steven Wexler, MD, FAAEM

Acetaminophen (APAP) is a relatively safe and widely accessible drug. It has been used as an analgesic and antipyretic for approximately 90 years. It is safe for the following reasons: lack of interaction with anticoagulants, no increase in serum levels with dehydration, and noncumulative kinetics when metabolized. It is marketed under many brand names in the United States and used in almost 200 combination medications. Because of its availability, APAP has become one of the drugs most commonly used with suicidal intent in the United States.

Epidemiology

The most frequent cause of APAP poisoning is accidental overdose in the pediatric patient. Intentional APAP overdoses among adolescents and adults cause the highest morbidity and mortality of APAP poisonings. There were 111,175 cases of overdose involving APAP reported to poison centers in 1995, with 103 deaths attributed to APAP toxicity. Despite these numbers, the mortality rate is low because of the straightforward treatment with N-acetylcysteine (NAC).

NAC is the most frequently administered antidote in the United States. Continued mortality from APAP overdose occurs primarily from a delay in seeking treatment.

There is no evidence of a decline in the number of overdose cases involving APAP presenting to emergency departments. Emergency personnel must have a high level of suspicion, send serum APAP levels, use all means possible to obtain the drugs ingested and the time of ingestion, and err on the side of overtreating with NAC rather than not treat at all. We are fortunate that the antidote is readily accessible and easy to give. Outside of those patients presenting too late, only errors in not considering the possibility of APAP ingestion can lead to significant mortality and morbidity.

Clinical Presentation

Traditionally the symptomatology of acute APAP overdose is divided into four phases.

Phase 1

The first phase begins shortly after the ingestion and may last 12 to 24 hours. Nausea, vomiting, anorexia, and diaphoresis are the common manifestations, although some patients may be totally asymptomatic during the initial phase.

Phase 2

The second phase begins 24 to 72 hours postingestion and is often called the quiescent period. There are fewer gastrointestinal symptoms while hepatic damage is occurring. Right upper quadrant pain may develop as liver enzymes, prothrombin time (PT), and bilirubin all begin to increase. The kidneys may be affected and oliguria may develop.

Phase 3

The third phase occurs 72 to 96 hours postingestion and is the critical time period in the prognosis of the patient and the extent of the liver failure. The patient suffers from anorexia, nausea, and vomiting. The liver enzymes reach their peak. Experience shows that if the PT continues to rise beyond the third day postingestion, the patient will often require a liver transplant. Liver biopsy at this time reveals centrilobular necrosis. Hepatic encephalopathy may be present.

Phase 4

Phase 4 occurs 4 days after the ingestion. During this time, the patient's liver injury either resolves or proceeds into fulminant liver failure.

Treatment

All overdose or suspected overdose patients should be handled in a systematic way. Airway, breathing, and circulation (ABCs) are always the first priority. While the ABCs are being assessed, the patient should be placed on a cardiac monitor, pulse oximetry should be obtained, an intravenous line established, and an electrocardiogram performed. Management of the patient with an altered level of consciousness should include a bedside blood glucose level and intravenous administration of glucose if necessary. Naloxone and thiamine should be administered if clinically indicated. Blood should be sent to the laboratory for levels of sodium, potassium, chloride, bicarbonate, blood urea nitrogen, creatinine, glucose, alcohol, APAP, and aspirin and serum osmolality; a pregnancy test should also be performed if indicated.

Once the patient has been initially stabilized, a detailed history is obtained including the substances ingested, how much, and at what time the ingestion occurred. Use all potential resources including the patient, family, friends, police, or paramedics to obtain as much information as possible.

Decontamination and treatment now become the focus. Consider oral-gastric lavage if the patient arrives in the emergency department within 30 minutes of a potentially lethal ingestion. Airway compromise and aspiration are significant risks during the procedure; thus, the decision to perform oral-gastric lavage should not be taken lightly. Some would argue that the effective use of NAC as an antidote obviates the need for the risky oral gastric lavage in the overdose patient who has an isolated APAP ingestion. Recent studies support this view.

Activated charcoal should be given within the first hour of ingestion of APAP and may reduce the serum level even after absorption is complete. It has two potential benefits: preventing the absorption of toxic agents in the gastrointestinal tract and enhancing the elimination of agents already absorbed. The standard dosage is 1 g/kg. The use of charcoal before NAC does not reduce the absorption of the antidote sufficiently to affect the patient. Even the use of activated charcoal in the poisoned patient, once considered dogma, has come under question and its total benefit is uncertain.

After the initial stabilization and appropriate decontamination are performed, a 4-hour APAP level should be obtained for the immediate release preparation. If the time of ingestion is unknown, an immediate level should be sent followed by a repeat in 4 hours. The concern is that APAP serum levels do not reach their peak before a 4-hour level. Further consideration must be given to the potential of extended-relief (release) Tylenol and the coingestion of drugs that decrease gastrointestinal motility. Extended-relief preparations reach peak levels between 5 and 14 hours. This is particularly important because the classic approach to APAP overdose was to obtain a 4-hour serum level, and if that level was below the Rumack-Matthew nomogram, then the patient did not need to be treated with NAC.

The Rumack-Matthew nomogram is a plot of serum APAP levels versus time

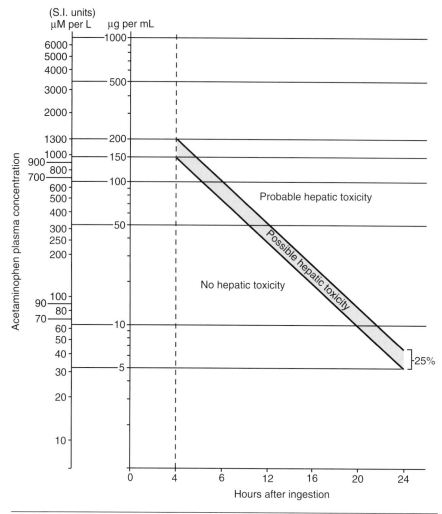

Figure 55.1
The Rumack-Matthew nomogram for acute acetaminophen poisoning. Plasma aceta-
minophen levels are plotted against time after ingestion. (From Rumack BH and Mathew
M. Acetaminophen poisoning and toxicity. *Pediatrics* 55:871, 1986 with permission.)

(Figure 55.1). Any level above this line should be treated with NAC. Levels at or near the nomogram line should be considered for treatment if the following questions are uncertain: Is this a 4-hour level? Is the APAP ingested extended-relief or immediate release? Has the patient taken other substances that may slow the gastrointestinal tract? Does the patient have cirrhosis or liver disease? Is the patient an alcoholic? Does the patient take phenobarbital or isoniazid? Is the patient suffering from starvation or anorexia? Did the patient take multiple doses of APAP at different times?

Alcoholics and cirrhotics have liver glutathione concentrations that are significantly lower than the average population. There have been several reports of alcoholics developing early severe liver damage and nephrotoxicity with APAP levels below the toxic nomogram lines.

The dosage of NAC is 140 mg/kg orally followed by 70 mg/kg every 4 hours for a maximum of 17 doses. NAC has just (2004) been approved for intravenous use in the United Sates but has been used successfully this way in Europe and Canada and is the preferred method of administration. Recent

Table 55.1.
Treatment summary for acetaminophen ingestion

Monitor, IV, pulse oximetry

Laboratory tests: Serum electrolytes, BUN and creatinine, glucose, alcohol, acetaminophen (initial level and a level 4 hours postingestion if time known and immediate-release preparation), aspirin, liver function tests, and serum osmolality; pregnancy test if indicated

Electrocardiogram

Bedside glucose level if altered mentation

Naloxone and thiamine if indicated

Consider activated charcoal 1 g/kg

Determine the need for NAC based on: the Rumack-Matthew nomogram and coingestions, liver disease, acetaminophen sustained-release preparations, alcoholism, starvation, anorexia, phenobarbital or isoniazid medications; give NAC if indicated 140 mg/kg oral or IV load, followed by 70 mg/kg every 4 hours for 17 doses maximum

Serial liver function analysis

BUN; blood urea nitrogen; IV, intravenous; NAC, N-acetylcysteine.

studies suggest that NAC may be given orally for a shorter course of 36 hours and 9 doses, if the patient has not exhibited any evidence of hepatic injury (aspartate aminotransferase/alanine aminotransferase [AST/ALT] greater than 1,000 IU/L) by 36 hours. It has even been suggested that treatment with NAC could stop once the serum levels of APAP have disappeared and there is no evidence of hepatotoxicity, typically less than a 24-hour duration (Table 55.1).

Pathophysiology

Acetaminophen

In acute overdose, the main site of organ injury is the liver. Of these patients, approximately 1% to 10% suffer concomitant renal injury. Renal toxicity is thought to be secondary to the liver failure, and in a few cases renal toxicity has occurred with mild or no hepatic injury. It is theorized that the APAP can be metabolized in the renal medulla, creating toxic reactive metabolites.

APAP is rapidly absorbed in the gastrointestinal tract, reaching a peak plasma concentration within 30 to 120 minutes.

Peak plasma levels are usually reached within 4 hours for the immediate-release preparation but may occur within 30 minutes if APAP syrup is ingested. A toxic ingestion is considered to be 150 mg/kg or greater. APAP has a large volume of distribution within the body because of its lack of binding to serum proteins.

Therapeutic doses of the drug are metabolized in the adult liver by glucuronidation (60%) and sulfation (30%) and an estimated 4% to 7% are eliminated unchanged in the urine. Neither the drug nor the metabolites are toxic. Only a small amount of APAP is converted to the highly reactive intermediate N-acetyl-p-benzoquinoneimine (NAPQI) by the cytochrome P-450 mixed-function oxidase system. Under normal circumstances, reduced glutathione detoxifies NAPQI into harmless cysteine and mercapturate conjugates, which are renally excreted. In the setting of a significant overdose, however, glucuronidation and sulfation quickly become overwhelmed by the amount of APAP present. The drug is then shunted to the cytochrome P-450 system. When approximately 70% of hepatic glutathione is depleted, the toxic metabolite then binds with hepatic cell macromolecules, producing tissue necrosis. Liver pathology consists mostly of centrilobular necrosis with reticulin collapse and almost no inflammation.

There is great variability to the toxic side effects of APAP. Up to 20% of patients with toxic levels do not develop hepatotoxicity. Severe liver damage occurs in approximately 8% without antidotal therapy. Fatal hepatic failure occurs in about 1% to 2% of patients with severe liver damage. Age, diet, nutritional status, metabolic state, and concomitant drug ingestion affect individual changes in cytochrome P-450 activity and susceptibility to hepatotoxicity. Alcoholism, chronic ingestion of drugs that induce hepatic microsomal enzymes, starvation (which depletes glutathione), and ingestion of multiple doses of APAP over time enhance hepatotoxicity. Children are less likely to develop hepatotoxicity because of their relatively high activity of the sulfonation enzyme system.

N-acetylcysteine

NAC is thought to act primarily by replenishing mitochondrial and cytosolic glutathione stores that have been depleted by the highly reactive APAP metabolite NAPQI. NAC may also repair oxidative damage caused by NAPQI either directly or through the generation of cysteine or glutathione. When administered many hours after overdose, NAC, a powerful antioxidant, may protect against further hepatic damage through an action on neutrophils. From retrospective data, it is suggested that treatment with NAC may benefit patients in fulminant hepatic failure induced from APAP. In one study, 37% of patients who received NAC died, compared with 58% who did not receive NAC.

Side effects of NAC include nausea, vomiting, a maculopapular rash, hypokalemia, metabolic acidosis, mild thrombocytopenia,

and precipitation of bronchospasm in asthmatics. There are no data on the teratogenicity of NAC; however, it would appear that the risk of untreated APAP toxicity is a far greater threat to the fetus than NAC treatment. The risk of not treating pregnant women almost certainly far exceeds any potential risk to the developing fetus if a toxic ingestion has occurred.

Suggested Readings

Anker A, Smilkstein M. Acetaminophen concepts and controversies. *Emerg Med Clin North Am* 1994;12:335–349.

Bisovi KE and Smilkstein MJ. Acetominophen. In: Goldfrank LR, Flomenbaum NE, Lewin NA, et. al. eds. *Goldfrank's toxicological emergencies*, 7th ed. Columbus, OH: McGraw-Hill, 2002:480–505.

Cetaruk EW, Dart RC, Hurlbut KM, et al. Tylenol extended relief overdose. *Ann Emerg Med* 1997;30:104–108.

Ellenhorn MJ. *Ellenhorn's medical toxicology: diagnosis and treatment of human poisoning.* Philadelphia: Lippincott, Williams & Wilkins, 1997;180–195.

Henry JA, Hoffman JR. Continuing controversy on gut decontamination. *Lancet* 1998;352:420–421.

Roth B, Woo O, Blane P. Early metabolic acidosis and coma after acetaminophen ingestion. *Ann Emerg Med* 1999;33:452–456.

Rumack BH, Matthew H. Acetaminophen poisoning and toxicity. *Pediatrics* 1974;55:871–876.

Whitcomb DC, Block GD. Association of acetaminophen hepatotoxicity with fasting and ethanol use. *JAMA* 1994;272:1845–1850.

Woo O, Mueller P, Olson K, et al. Shorter duration of oral N-acetylcysteine therapy for acute acetaminophen overdose. *Ann Emerg Med* 2000;35:363–368.

Salicylate Overdose

Brook D. Beall, MD

Salicylates have been used for medicinal purposes since ancient times. Salicylate use was first described in the Ebers papyrus of Egypt more than 3,500 years ago as a treatment for rheumatic conditions. First derived from Myrtle leaves, salicylates later made from (and named after) willow trees were prescribed by Hippocrates. Felix Hoffman, a nineteenth-century German chemist, was the first to synthesize acetylsalicylic acid (modern aspirin), which is now found in hundreds of pharmaceutical preparations. Salicylates come in many forms (including slow release) and are components of Pepto-Bismol, Ben-Gay, Alka-Seltzer, and oil of wintergreen. More than 200 fatalities each year are due to analgesics, usually acetaminophen or aspirin. In 1999, 214,000 analgesic exposures were reported to the American Association of Poison Control Centers (AAPCC).

Half of fatalities resulting solely from aspirin ingestion are among patients 50 or older. Awareness of polypharmacy and liberal use of toxicological screens is important for this population. Coingested substances commonly encountered with salicylate include psychiatric medications, opiates, and acetaminophen. In addition, concurrent use of hypoglycemic agents and anticoagulants increase toxic effects on metabolism and hemostasis.

Pathophysiology of Salicylate Toxicity

The structure and function of acetylsalicylic acid has been known for 30 years. It inhibits the formation of thromboxane, prostacyclin, and other inflammatory mediators, many of which regulate the intravascular environment. Cardiovascular benefits derive from inhibition of platelet aggregation. Maintenance of gastrointestinal (GI) mucosa is altered and may contribute to peptic ulcer disease or bleeding complications. Excluding hypersensitivity reactions, acute ingestion of less than 200 mg/kg of salicylate is rarely toxic. A larger ingestion disrupts oxidative phosphorylation in tissues with higher salicylate concentrations. Loss of aerobic metabolism is a critical mechanism of toxicity with overdose. Anaerobic metabolism of glucose produces less energy, promotes lactic acidosis, and increases the risk of tissue hypoglycemia, which may cause mental status changes and seizures. Acidosis creates an environment in which salicylate toxicity is further magnified by greater tissue penetration (nonionized salicylate concentration doubles as the pH declines from 7.4 to 7.2). Nonionized salicylic acid is the form capable of crossing cellular membranes and entering tissues. Acidosis is self-perpetuating; potentially deadly; and is associated with renal, hepatic, and other organ dysfunction.

Clinical Presentation

Salicylate overdose may be intentional and known but often presents in nonspecific

Table 56.1.

Findings in significant salicylate toxicity

	Early	Delayed/Serious	Critical
Neurological	Excitability or lethargy	Delirium and seizures	Coma and death (possible cerebral edema)
Pulmonary	Hyperpnea or tachypnea	Hyperpnea increases	Respiratory depression (possible pulmonary edema)
Other Systems	Nausea, dehydration, tachycardia	Toxic appearance and fever (pseudosepsis)	Organ failure, cardiac depression (possible multiorgan failure)
Laboratory	Acute level of 30+ mg/dL or any chronic ingestion with symptoms	Levels near 100 mg/dL or acidemia (any amount)	Life-threatening acidemia (± severe electrolyte changes)

ways. Early presentations include vertiginous symptoms, tinnitus, headache, and nausea (sometimes with vomiting and/or diarrhea). Family members and emergency medical services (EMS) personnel should be questioned about pill bottles (over-the-counter and prescription).

Mental status and respiratory pattern are the most important components of the physical examination in salicylate overdose (Table 56.1). Hyperpnea (deep breathing) appears early and is progressive with levels of toxicity. Subtle mental status changes often begin with either excitability or lethargy. Confusion is common in the elderly. Salicylates should be considered for unexplained tachypnea, acidosis, delirium, bleeding, and pulmonary or cerebral edema and for septic-appearing patients without a source. Hyperpyrexia (high temperature) may also be present. Severe toxicity presents with declining mental status progressing to seizures or coma. Therefore, mental status and pH are at least as important as salicylate levels for patient assessment and treatment decisions.

Salicylate ingestion should be considered in children who are febrile, tachycardic, and diaphoretic. Reye's syndrome (which may occur in adults) is a syndrome of fatty infiltration of the liver leading to liver failure with approximately 30% mortality. Vomiting, hypoglycemia, and lethargy progressing to coma are prominent features of this syndrome. It is classically associated with salicylate use in children with concurrent viral infections.

Diagnostic Evaluation

Salicylate levels and the Done nomogram are useful if interpreted within the clinical context. The Done nomogram may help determine severity of ingestion if a level 6 hours after ingestion is obtained. It plots salicylate concentrations at various times after ingestion to allow risk stratification of patients. The nomogram was constructed in 1960 using primarily pediatric data following ingestion of immediate-release salicylates; it should be used cautiously in other contexts. In particular, the nomogram should not be used reflexively to defer aggressive therapy if patients are stratified as "mild" based on their salicylate level and time since ingestion. Chronic ingestion by an older or sicker individual is among the most dangerous, although the measured level may be quite low. Mortality of 25% has been reported for symptomatic salicylate toxicity presenting without an acute ingestion. Salicylate levels between 30 and 130 mg/dL are most commonly reported among patients who die following ingestion. A level greater than 30 mg/dL at any time should be taken very seriously. If aggressive therapy is not undertaken for these patients, they require frequent reevaluation and serial laboratory evaluation. Patients with levels closer to 100 mg/dL must be treated aggressively even if they are healthy and appear well. Damage is thought to correlate with peak serum salicylate level. The time from ingestion is important when interpreting levels, but this information is frequently not available or reliable. Patients with slow-release forms or with any detectable salicylate 30 or more hours after an acute ingestion are at increased risk.

Patients with salicylate ingestion usually require analysis of arterial blood gases (ABGs) because salicylate levels are not reliable predictors of illness shortly after ingestion or when timing is unknown. The classic presentation is an anion gap metabolic acidosis mixed with a respiratory alkalosis (the respiratory component often predominates initially). Acidosis (as salicylate available to penetrate tissues increases) is self-perpetuating, is dangerous in any amount, and should prompt treatment as if the salicylate level were much higher than that obtained. A relative or absolute respiratory acidosis may be due to a coingested substance and if present requires an explanation. Broad toxicology screens must include acetaminophen. Blood chem-istries, a complete blood cell (CBC) count, and clotting times round out the evaluation. An electrocardiogram (ECG) should be obtained unless the patient is young and a second ingestion has been absolutely ruled out. A flat plate x-ray film of the abdomen (KUB) should be obtained to help rule out a large ingestion of enteric-coated slow-release preparations, which may be visible on x-ray film. The term *KUB* (Kidneys, Ureter, Bladder) is technically a misnomer, although the name is often used. It is the x-ray film used to look for kidney stones, and, as such, actually cuts off a portion of the abdomen, which may need to be seen in an abdominal study. A second delayed salicylate level should be obtained within 6 hours of the initial level. Patients whose salicylate levels do not decline or who are at risk for development of acidosis require aggressive management.

Management of Salicylate Toxicity

Management is directed by clinical appearance, degree of acidosis, and amount ingested (known or inferred). Activated charcoal should be used if there is any likelihood that salicylate remains in the GI tract. Intravenous (IV) fluid should be given (unless a patient is already volume overloaded) to maximize urine output and urinary excretion of salicylate. Patients not admitted to the hospital should be observed for at least 6 hours and have a documented decreasing salicylate level. Poison control should be contacted and serum pH checked except in the most benign ingestion with a low salicylate level, alkaline urine, and excellent clinical appearance. More aggressive measures are indicated with any potentially life-threatening ingestion. Treatment of coingested substances (particularly acetaminophen) should always be considered early.

Decontamination with at least 50 g (1 g/ kg in children) of oral activated charcoal (AC) is essential to stop further absorption of salicylate and other toxins. Administration within 2 hours of ingestion is a reasonable goal, but speedy administration is crucial. Bowel obstruction and hematemesis are the only contraindications. Risk of aspiration (inhaling vomited charcoal, thereby injuring the lung) is around 2% and should only enter consideration for patients presenting many hours after ingestion. For those patients with depressed mental status, intubation should be considered before charcoal administration. Some experts recommend repeating charcoal (diluted in water) every 2 to 4 hours, and one small study found decontamination benefits with doses repeated at 4 and 8 hours. Gastric lavage and forced emesis (ipecac) have never proven more useful and carry greater risks than AC. Gastric lavage is only considered for patients presenting shortly after ingestion who are extremely symptomatic or have a clearly life-threatening ingestion. Whole bowel irrigation with isotonic preparations may have a role as an alternative to AC, particularly if all substances ingested are slow-release formulations (e.g., enteric-coated aspirin).

Supportive care involves maintaining or correcting respiratory status, intravascular volume, glucose, and electrolytes while assessing the degree of salicylate toxicity. All patients should be placed on their left side and those with declining or severely altered mental status may require intubation. Although compensatory respiratory alkalosis should not be limited, artificial hypocarbia has not proven beneficial. IV fluids (starting with at least 1 L normal saline [NS]) are used to maximize tissue perfusion with attention to both urine output and other vital signs.

Fluids with 5% dextrose should be used for all patients unless they have a perfect mental status or are already hyperglycemic. Electrolytes should be replaced, with particular attention to potassium and calcium levels. Potassium is often required when large amounts of fluid are given, especially as any acidemia is corrected. Aspirin may worsen any bleeding coagulopathy, but platelets and clotting factors are rarely necessary. Hyperpyrexia related to salicylate ingestion is treated with axillary ice.

Ill patients and those with large or unknown ingestion quantity should be started on a sodium bicarbonate drip and may require more aggressive measures. Bicarbonate infusion is justified with any acidosis, with increasing levels of serum salicylate, or with a salicylate level greater than approximately 30 to 35 mg/dL. For treatment, 50 mEq or more of sodium bicarbonate (approximately 1 mEq/kg) is added to each liter of IV fluid. Typically, 2 to 3 amps of sodium bicarbonate are added to 1 L of D5W. Alkalinization of serum (with aggressive potassium repletion) is primarily directed at removing salicylate rather than correcting acidosis. A therapeutic pH is generally felt to be at least 7.4 to 7.45 and a pH below 7.2 requires aggressive correction. Urinary pH must be kept above 7.5 to 8 to facilitate trapping and elimination of salicylic acid (the ionized form will not be able to escape the renal tubule following filtration). Urinary alkalinization is nearly impossible without potassium repletion. Hypokalemia forces the kidney to produce more acidic urine to reabsorb more potassium. This process limits salicylate excretion and perpetuates acidosis because the nonionized form of salicylate increases in concentration with acidic urine. Forced diuresis is not indicated and does not perform as well as alkalinization for accelerating salicylate excretion.

The most seriously ill patients (especially with levels greater than 100 mg/dL) are admitted to intensive care and considered for hemoperfusion to directly remove salicylate. Standard dialysis may correct acidosis and electrolyte balance but is less efficient at reducing salicylate levels. Indications for dialysis include seizures, coma, deteriorating status, pulmonary edema, and failure of liver or kidneys. In the absence of other indications or significant acidosis, dialysis is generally not considered for salicylate levels below 80 to 120 mg/dL within the first 6 hours. Older patients, especially with chronic toxicity, may be considered for dialysis at lower salicylate levels (40 to 50 mg/dL). Pregnant patients are also candidates for early delivery because salicylates cross the placenta and have been linked to fetal demise.

The sequential treatment options in salicylate overdose are summarized in Table 56.2.

Table 56.2.

Sequential treatment options in salicylate overdose

All	IV fluids (D5 $^1/_2$NS) and activated charcoal (consider WBI if enteric coated)
Most	Maximize urinary output and avoid hypoglycemia or hypokalemia
Some	Bicarbonate therapy and consider ICU admission (goal serum pH > 7.4)
Highest Risk	Hemodialysis (consider hemoperfusion for early presentation of a large ingestion)
Critical	Treat organ failures as needed (intubation, vasopressors, anticonvulsants, blood products)

ICU, intensive care unit; IV, intravenous; NS, normal saline; WBI, whole bowel irrigation.

Patient Disposition

Salicylate toxicity is a part of many differential diagnoses in the emergency department. Treatment is challenging because initial appearance may not predict outcome and coingestion is frequent. Mental status and pH are as important as salicylate levels to determine therapy. If any doubt exists regarding disposition, patients should be admitted because delayed acidosis and hypoglycemia are potentially deadly complications. Discharge from the emergency department necessitates serial laboratory evaluation and clinical reassessment. A patient with a small unintentional ingestion (without other ingested substances) may be appropriate for discharge if the quantity consumed is known without doubt. Psychiatric consultation should be obtained for any patient with an intentional ingestion. By contrast, high-risk features include chronic toxicity, acidemia, suicidal ideation, and comorbid conditions. Supportive therapy, AC, and the maintenance of high urine output (preferably alkaline) are the mainstays of therapy. These principles guide the successful evaluation and management of patients with salicylate toxicity.

Suggested Readings

Anderson RJ, Potts DE, Gabow PA, et al. Unrecognized adult salicylate intoxication. *Ann Intern Med* 1976;85:745–748.

Barone J. Evaluation of the effects of multiple-dose activated charcoal on the absorption of orally administered salicylate in a simulated toxic ingestion model. *Ann Emerg Med* 1988; 17:34–37.

Bond R. The role of activated charcoal and gastric emptying in gastrointestinal decontamination. *Ann Emerg Med* 2002;39:273–286.

Done A. Significance of measurements of salicylate in blood in cases of acute ingestion. *Pediatrics* 1960;26:800–806.

Flomenbaum NE. Salicylates. In: Goldfrank LR, Flomenbaum NE, Lewis NA, eds. *Goldfrank's toxicological emergencies*, 7th ed. Columbus, OH: McGraw-Hill, 2002:507–526.

Juurlink D. Gastrointestinal decontamination for enteric-coated aspirin overdose: what to do depends on who you ask. *J Toxicol* 2000;38: 465–470(abst).

Litovitz T, Klein Schwartz W, White SR, et al. 1999 Annual report of the American Association of Poison Control Centers Toxic Exposure Surveillance System. *Am J Emerg Med* 2000;18:517–574.

Seger D, Murray L. Aspirin, acetaminophen, and nonsteroidal agents. In: Marx J, Hockberger RS, Walls RM, et al, eds. *Rosen's emergency medicine*. St. Louis: Mosby, 2002, 1250–1262.

Environmental

Hyperthermia

Lamont G. Clay, MD

Hyperthermia is defined as an increase in the body's core temperature beyond the normal setpoint. The body is in constant balance between heat gain and heat loss. Hyperthermia is an abnormal increase in heat production either through the environment or metabolic processes or through failure of the body's heat dissipation mechanisms. Heat becomes a problem when the heat that is generated or gained by the body is more than the heat that is lost or dissipated by the body.

Hyperthermia does not affect the hypothalamic setpoint for temperature regulation; instead, the core temperature of the body is raised regardless of the setpoint. Febrile illnesses, on the other hand, increase the thermoregulatory setpoint of the body in response to an environmental stressor, usually infection. The body increases the setpoint to accommodate increased metabolic activity by the immune system to combat infection. In heat-related illness, the mechanisms of the body that promote heat loss are challenged or, in heatstroke, overwhelmed by the amount of heat gain.

Epidemiology

There were more than 7,000 deaths in the United States from 1979 to 1997 attributed to heat illness. The incidence of heatstroke ranges from 17.6 to 26.5 per 100,000 population during heat waves in the United States and is higher in countries that border the equator. This does not accurately depict the true impact of heat illness because many cases go unreported or are misdiagnosed. Unfortunately, the incidence of heat illness has not decreased with improved medical technology. In fact, the incidence may be increasing. As recently as 1995, during a major heat wave in Chicago, more than 700 deaths were attributed to heat illness.

Who is at risk for heat illness? Those living in areas or climates with very high ambient temperatures are at the greatest risk. Also at increased risk are those who cannot protect themselves during heat waves. This includes inner city populations, the elderly, immunocompromised persons, athletes, and those who work in poorly air-conditioned environments or outdoors. It is important to recognize who is at risk because heat illness can be prevented, or at least reduced, by proper planning and education.

Pathophysiology

The human body is set to function at a core temperature of 37°C or 98.6°F. The most common methods for measuring body temperature are the rectal, oral, tympanic, and axillary measurements. Rectal temperature is usually the most accurate measurement, does not depend on patient cooperation, and can be measured very accurately at the extremes of high and low. Oral temperature is usually slightly less than rectal and depends on patients to keep their mouths completely closed and to have had no recent hot or cold beverages or food. The axillary temperature is usually 1° less than oral temperature. Tympanic temperatures depend on correct position of the thermometer in the ear, a clean ear canal, and a patient who has not just stepped in from extreme outdoor temperatures.

Heat is generated, regulated, and removed by the body through certain homeostatic mechanisms. These mechanisms are controlled through the body's neuroendocrine axis, the pituitary and the hypothalamus. The hypothalamus determines the setpoints for the body. These setpoints include acceptable ranges for temperature, volume, osmolality, satiety, and body fat content. Temperature is controlled by the posterior, lateral, and premamillary hypothalamic nuclei of the anterior hypothalamus. These neurons sense a change in the temperature of the blood circulating past them and regulate the appropriate response to the change in temperature. It is important to look at the physiology of how the body gains and loses heat.

Heat Gain

The body gains heat by two major mechanisms: metabolic processes that generate heat as a byproduct and ambient or environmental heat. All metabolic functions in the human body are exothermic reactions that produce heat as a byproduct. The basal metabolic rate determines the heat gained via these metabolic functions. The basal metabolic rate is usually constant but does vary with exercise and with high ambient temperatures. If heat-dissipating mechanisms were not working, then the average 70-kg person would gain 1.1°C per hour.

Heat Loss

Heat loss occurs through heat transfer to the surrounding environment. This is regulated by four major mechanisms: conduction, convection, radiation, and evaporation.

Conduction

Conduction is transfer of heat from warmer to cooler environments through direct physical contact. Air is not a great medium for conduction; therefore, heat loss via conduction is relatively low, accounting for approximately 2% to 5% of heat loss. Immersion in cold water (water is 25 to 30 times more effective than air as a thermal conductor) can result in significant heat loss. This is important in cases of hypothermia but also in cooling a patient that is suffering from hyperthermia.

Radiation

Radiation is heat transfer by electromagnetic waves. Heat energy transfers from higher temperature to lower temperatures. Therefore, if the body core temperature is higher than the ambient temperature, significant heat can be lost to the environment. Up to 65% of heat loss in cool environments can be attributed to radiation. Conversely, when the body core temperature is lower than the ambient temperature, the body can accumulate a significant amount of heat.

Convection

Convection is heat loss to air and water vapors circulating around the body. Convective forces are dependent on several factors. For ambient temperatures much less than the temperature of the skin, ambient cooling can be significant. When ambient temperatures approach that of the peripheral skin, this method is minimal and may lead to further heat gain. The amount and velocity of wind also affects the amount of heat loss by convection. As the wind velocity increases, so does the capability of convection for heat loss. Convection is responsible for 10% to 15% of heat loss on average. Loose-fitting clothing allows for more circulating air currents, which increases convection.

Evaporation

Evaporation is the conversion from a liquid state to a gaseous state or phase. When the ambient temperature is high, evaporation becomes the biggest component of heat loss. This occurs as sweat evaporates from the skin. Evaporation can account for roughly 20% to 25% of heat loss. Evaporation is controlled by cholinergic sympathetic activity and is therefore decreased by anticholinergic medications. Evaporation is also hampered by increased humidity. When the water vapor gradient on the skin is lower, the amount of energy transferred is lower.

Acclimatization

Acclimatization is the process by which the body slowly adjusts to working or exercising in an environment with a high ambient temperature. This process usually takes from 1 to 2 weeks. The physiology is poorly understood but is most likely a constellation of physiological mechanisms mediated by aldosterone. Aldosterone affects the sodium concentration of urine, causing an earlier onset of sweating and creating a greater total sweat volume. It is also postulated that an increase in heat shock proteins, and a decrease in inflammatory mediators, helps to prevent the cascade that leads to severe heat illness. This cascade has been found to be similar to the complicated cascade of sepsis.

Clinical Presentation

The clinical presentation of hyperthermia in a person is a spectrum ranging from mild symptoms of cramps to heatstroke, which ultimately can be fatal. These entities in Table 57.1 are discussed later, from less severe to most severe. The factors that put a patient at higher risk for heat-related illness are listed in Table 57.2.

Table 57.1.

Types of heat related illness

Diagnosis	Symptoms	Treatment
Heat cramps	Muscle cramps	Salt repletion
Heat tetany	Hyperventilation with paresthesias, carpopedal spasms	Oral repletion, support
Heat syncope	Venous pooling leading to loss of consciousness	Rule out other causes of syncope, avoid prolonged standing
Prickly heat	Maculopapular rash on erythematous base	Avoid heat, use loose clothing
Heat edema	Swelling of hands and feet	None
Heat exhaustion	Fatigue, dizziness, lightheadedness, nausea, vomiting, hypotension, tachycardia	Fluid and salt repletion
Heatstroke	Core temperature above 40°C or 104°F, anhidrosis, altered mentation, seizure, coma	Aggressive cooling: ice water immersion, ice packs, cooling blankets, fans

Table 57.2.	
Risk factors for hyperthermia and heatstroke	
Medications/Drugs	*Comorbid Disorders*
Diuretics	Hypertension
β-blockers	Obesity
Anticholinergics	Atherosclerosis
Phenothiazines	CAD
Sympathomimetics	CHF
Thyroid hormone	Gastroenteritis
Calcium channel blockers	Scleroderma
Cocaine	Dermatitis
Ethanol	
LSD	
PCP	

CAD, coronary artery disease; CHF, congestive heart failure; LSD, lysergic acid diethylamide; PCP, phencyclidine.

Heat Cramps

Heat cramps are intermittent cramps, ranging from mild to severe, in large muscle groups. Unlike generalized muscle cramps and heat related-tetany, these cramps occur after the individual is done with work or exercise. Heat cramps are secondary to an underlying salt deficiency in a dehydrated patient. The patient is hypovolemic but has lost more salt than water. The treatment for heat cramps is salt repletion orally or, for more severe or recalcitrant cases, intravenous (IV) repletion. It is important to use caution in the diagnosis of heat cramps rather than the diagnosis of the salt-deficiency form of heat exhaustion.

Heat Tetany

Heat tetany is usually associated with short, intense periods of heat exposure leading to hyperventilation. Many of the symptoms of normal hyperventilation occur, including a respiratory alkalosis and paresthesias. The paresthesias are usually perioral or in the extremities, and the tetany is usually associated with carpopedal spasm. The treatment for heat tetany is largely supportive. Patients should be given oral repletion and cautioned to rest and to avoid hot ambient environments if possible.

Heat Syncope

Heat syncope is associated with decreased venous return and subsequent venous pooling in the lower extremities. This can lead to syncope from decreased cerebral blood flow. This usually affects people standing for prolonged periods who have failed to acclimatize. The treatment for heat syncope is awareness and proper preparation if standing for long periods. Patients are told to flex their knees slightly while standing. There is further benefit in periodically flexing the calf muscles to increase tone and thus venous return. Heat syncope is a diagnosis of exclusion. More serious causes of syncope should be considered and ruled out. Careful history and physical examination are the keys to making the diagnosis. Lack of risk factors for cardiovascular disease, age, and symptoms help to delineate heat syncope from other causes of syncope. Heat syncope is treated with fluid resuscitation and recumbent positioning to allow for redistribution of vascular volume. Avoidance of prolonged standing, if possible, is also recommended.

Prickly Heat (Heat Rash)

Prickly heat is also known as heat rash, lichen tropicus, or miliaria rubra. Prickly heat usually occurs in tropical and humid climates. The usual rash is maculopapular on an erythematous base. The rash is extremely pruritic, and the patient usually presents secondary to the intense itching. The rash is usually present in clothed areas of the body. It results from sweat pores that are blocked by macerated stratum corneum, causing vesicles that manifest in the Malpighian layer of the skin. A keratin plug manifests after 7 to 10 days. This plug can cause further obstruction and a second rupture with deep vesicles formed within the dermis. This has been referred to as the profunda stage and can last for weeks. This stage is much less pruritic and is characterized by white papules, as opposed to the macular papules with the superficial variety. Both the superficial and the deep forms can lead to a chronic dermatitis. The rash is self-limiting; however, bacterial superinfection is common. This cellulitis is frequently caused by *Staphylococcus aureus* and should be treated with appropriate antibiotics when detected. Avoidance of excessive heat and the application of loose clothing when exposed to excessive heat are recommended.

Heat Edema

Heat edema refers to swelling of the hands and the feet, usually in the first few days of heat exposure. Heat edema occurs in patients who are not acclimatized to their environment and is a self-limiting process. The edema usually involves only the hands and the feet. Edema that is pretibial or more extensive should be considered another systemic process. A careful physical examination and history must be done to rule out more serious causes of peripheral edema. The pathophysiology of this edema is poorly understood. No treatment is necessary except assuring the patient that it is a self-limiting process and admonishing the patient of more severe heat illnesses.

Heat Exhaustion

Heat exhaustion occurs when the heat-dissipating mechanisms of the body become fatigued because of dehydration in the setting of heat stress. Heat exhaustion is usually the result of exercise or work in an environment with a high ambient temperature. There are two forms of heat exhaustion: water depletion and salt depletion. Patients with water depletion heat exhaustion have inadequate repletion of fluids lost during heat stress. These patients have a progressing hypovolemia and hypernatremia. Patients with salt depletion heat exhaustion replenish themselves with water but too little salt. These patients have isotonic dehydration as opposed to the hypernatremic dehydration of the water depletion type.

Heat exhaustion is a diagnosis of exclusion. The diagnosis is made more difficult because patients present with a constellation of vague symptoms. These symptoms include fatigue, diaphoresis, dizziness, lightheadedness, nausea, vomiting, orthostatic hypotension, and tachycardia. Core temperature is either normal or mildly elevated. Physical examination and laboratory studies are consistent with underlying dehydration. Patients frequently present with dry mucous membranes, tachycardia, and orthostatic hypotension. Laboratory studies show evidence of prerenal azotemia and hemoconcentration. Treatment consists of aggressive fluid replacement, salt repletion, and rest. It is not necessary to admit these patients unless there is a concomitant illness.

Heatstroke

Heatstroke is a true medical emergency. Heatstroke occurs when the heat-dissipating mechanisms are completely overwhelmed. The body's core temperature rises above 40°C or 104°F, leading to a cascade that affects multiple organ systems. Early heatstroke can be difficult to distinguish from severe heat exhaustion. However, with heat exhaustion the patient presents diaphoretic, and with heatstroke, patients usually present with anhidrosis. The most important factor distinguishing the two disorders is the presence of central nervous system (CNS) symptoms. These symptoms include altered mental status, seizure, and even coma.

It is postulated that heatstroke leads to multiple organ system dysfunction through the production of multiple cytokines. This release of cytokines is referred to as the acute phase response. This response is similar to the systemic inflammatory response syndrome (SIRS) in sepsis. These cytokines cause decreased clotting, increased vascular permeability, and a leukocytosis. Endotoxin is also released as a result of increased vascular permeability and splanchnic vasoconstriction. In addition to intracellular mediators, the natural response of the body to heat stress eventually can work against itself if prolonged exposure occurs. The body responds to heat stress by a profound peripheral vasodilation to maximize heat loss by radiation. This also increases cardiac output two to four times that of normal, placing a strain on patients with cardiovascular disorders or those with muted responses from medications. The other main mechanism for heat dissipation is evaporation. This is dependent on sympathetic nervous response and can also be decreased by medications that block cholinergic response.

A hallmark of heatstroke is CNS dysfunction. This can include seizures, cerebral edema, decerebrate and decorticate posturing, delirium, and coma. CNS dysfunction is universal in patients with body temperature exceeding 42°C or 108°F.

There are two types of heatstroke, classic and exertional. Classic heatstroke is seen in older individuals typically predisposed to heat illness (Table 57.2). This group includes the elderly, those with psychiatric illness, those who live alone, inner city populations without air conditioning, and those with medical conditions or medications that increase risk for heat-related illness. Exertional heatstroke, on the other hand, is seen in younger persons, athletes, military personnel, or persons performing strenuous exercise or work under heat stress conditions.

Differential Diagnosis

Infection

Heatstroke is not always an easy diagnosis to make. Having a strong clinical suspicion can lead to earlier treatment and better patient outcomes. It is important to administer cooling methods before the diagnosis is confirmed, if clinical suspicion is high. The diagnostic challenge is based on the breadth of the differential. Febrile illnesses are a much more common entity than heat illness and therefore must be excluded first. This includes all infectious causes: bacterial, viral, and fungal. A complete history and physical examination are vital to narrowing the differential.

Noninfectious Causes

Medication-Related Causes

Noninfectious causes must also be considered. The patient's medication list and social history can be important in making the correct diagnosis. Patients on antipsychotic medications can present extremely hyperthermic, confused, and rigid. These are hallmarks of neuroleptic malignant syndrome. The treatment for neuroleptic malignant syndrome is very different from heatstroke; however, many of the patients taking these medications are at increased risk for heat illness, making the diagnosis difficult.

Antidepressant medications can also cause a hyperthermic disorder. Serotonin syndrome is a vague constellation of symptoms that can include hyperthermia. Serotonin syndrome should be considered in patients taking antidepressants. This is especially true if the dose has been changed recently or another agent has been added.

Endocrine Causes

Hyperthyroidism can cause hyperthermia along with tachycardia, hair thinning, low energy, and weight loss. Heat illness occurs acutely, whereas symptoms from hyperthyroidism are usually more subacute or chronic. The exception is thyroid storm, which is a medical emergency. The overall presentation of symptoms can exclude this diagnosis, along with confirmatory laboratory tests such as triiodothyronine (T_3), thyroxine (T_4), and thyroid-stimulating hormone levels.

Inherited: Malignant Hyperthermia

Malignant hyperthermia is another cause of hyperthermia. Malignant hyperthermia is an autosomal dominant inherited syndrome that results in severe hyperthermia and abnormal muscular contractions when predisposed patients are exposed to certain anesthetics. These patients are exposed to anesthesia and typically react in the operative or perioperative period.

Diagnostic Evaluation

A complete social history can aid in the diagnosis. Alcohol and illicit drug use place people at increased risk for heatstroke and other heat illnesses. In addition, certain illicit drugs, such as amphetamines and cocaine, can cause severe catecholamine release, causing hyperthermia and tachycardia.

Laboratory testing can augment diagnostic decision making; however, there is no gold standard test for determining heatstroke. Blood should be sent for toxicology screens, along with basic screening laboratory tests such as complete blood cell count, chemistry panel, and liver function tests. Chest x-ray examination should be obtained, along with urinalysis. These tests help to rule out infectious causes and may demonstrate sequelae from heatstroke.

Treatment

If the diagnosis is suspected or confirmed, aggressive cooling techniques should be instituted. First, an accurate rectal temperature should be obtained. If this temperature is greater than 40°C, cooling should begin. The various methods of cooling the patient are based on assisting or augmenting the natural cooling mechanisms of the body.

To augment conduction, or cooling by direct contact, ice water immersion, ice packs, and cooling blankets can be used. To increase evaporation, or cooling by conversion from liquid to the gaseous phase, body cooling units or fans may be used.

Evaporation is the preferred method. Immersion is the most effective method but is generally impractical in the emergency department setting where large water immersion tubs are not available. It is also cumbersome to monitor the patient. The evaporation method of choice is the fanning method. The patient is stripped of all clothing and then sprayed with tepid water. The exposed patient is then placed under a fan or fans to increase evaporation. It may be difficult to have the patient on continuous cardiac monitoring with constant water vapor; however, unlike immersion, it is possible to monitor the patient's temperature rectally. This method is also better tolerated by awake patients and is minimally invasive.

More invasive procedures have been postulated, such as iced peritoneal lavage, gastric lavage, and cardiopulmonary bypass, but have been studied only on animal models.

Cardiopulmonary bypass with a heat exchanger has been used in cases of neuroleptic malignant syndrome and malignant hyperthermia. Cardiopulmonary bypass is not routinely used because it is extremely invasive, and other less invasive techniques are as effective. Cooling measures should be stopped when the patient has a core temperature of 39°C or 102.2°F to avoid hypothermic overshoot.

Treatment should include addressing the possible complications of heatstroke. Heatstroke affects many organ systems. Careful assessment of each organ system for possible complications is important. Autonomic instability is common with heatstroke. Patients are often tachycardic and hypotensive. These patients are hypovolemic from dehydration and should receive fluid resuscitation. High-output heart failure from peripheral vasodilation and dehydration is not uncommon. It is important to evaluate the patient carefully before aggressive fluid resuscitation. Many with heatstroke are elderly patients. These patients may be intravascularly depleted but can quickly go into pulmonary edema if there is a history of congestive heart failure. Moreover, heatstroke could cause pulmonary edema in some patients, which is also worse with IV fluids. In addition, blood pressure may improve with cooling methods. Others will not respond even with cooling, and cautious hydration. It may be necessary to place a pulmonary artery catheter to correctly assess volume status in these patients. Further fluid expansion or the use of vasopressors should be used as needed.

Renal perfusion, like intestinal or splanchnic perfusion, is decreased as more and more of the blood volume is shunted to the periphery. This decreased perfusion can lead to acute renal failure from acute tubular necrosis. In cases of exertional heatstroke, rhabdomyolysis can occur. Rhabdomyolysis can cause renal failure via myoglobinuria. This usually occurs 1 to 2 days following the initial heat stress; however, careful documentation of urine output and urinalysis should be obtained in the emergency department.

Coagulopathies should be treated with replacement by platelets and fresh frozen plasma as needed. Coagulation studies are usually normal on the first day, with changes occurring after 2 to 3 days. Retinal and renal hemorrhages and disseminated intravascular coagulation (DIC) have been reported.

Seizures occur rarely and can be controlled by cooling measures and low doses of benzodiazepines.

Antipyretics have been shown to provide no benefit in heatstroke. Dantrolene, a medication effective in reducing hyperthermia in malignant hyperthermia and neuroleptic malignant syndrome, also has not been shown to be effective in heatstroke. In fact, there are no pharmacological interventions shown to be effective in heatstroke.

Prevention

The most important treatment for heat illness is prevention and awareness. The public must be aware of the dangers of heat waves and must be apprised when a heat wave is approaching. Strenuous activity either via work or leisure should be avoided if at all possible. If unavoidable, precautions should be taken to provide proper hydration and allotting time for rest in a cool environment.

At-risk individuals in inner cities must be identified and followed closely. Cooling centers must be established to allow the elderly and the indigent availability to air conditioning. These centers must be advertised and used by at-risk populations to avoid serious morbidity and mortality from heat illness.

Prevention of heat illness is becoming more important as global warming raises the ambient temperature in moderate climates. As more heat waves hit these moderate climates, it will be increasingly important to avoid heat illness before it strikes.

Suggested Readings

Anonymous. Heat related illness, deaths, and risk factors—Cincinnati and Dayton, Ohio, 1999, and United States, 1979–1997. *MMWR Morb Mortal Wkly Rep* 2000;49:470–473.

Bouchama A, Knochel JP. Medical progress: heat stroke. *N Engl J Med* 2002;346:1978–1988.

Cooper KE. Some responses of the cardiovascular system to heat and fever. *Can J Cardiol* 1994; 10:444–448.

Costrini AM, Pitt HA, Gustafson AB, et al. Cardiovascular and metabolic manifestations of heat stroke and severe heat exhaustion. *Am J Med* 1979;66:296–302.

Dematte JE, O'Mara K, Buescher J, et al. Near fatal heat stroke during the 1995 heat wave in Chicago. *Ann Intern Med* 1978;129:173–181.

Gaffin S, Gardner J, Flinn S. Cooling methods for heatstroke victims. *Ann Intern Med* 2000;32: 678–679.

Heat wave. *Am J Pub Health* 1997;87:1515– 1518.

Kilbourne EM, Choi K, Jones ST, et al. Risk factors for heatstroke: a case control study. *JAMA* 1982;247:3332–3336.

Knochel JP. Heat stoke and related heat stress disorders. *Dis Mon* 1989;35:301–77.

McPhee SJ, Lingappa VR, Ganong WF, et. al. *Pathophysiology of disease, an introduction to clinical medicine*, 4th ed. Columbus, OH: McGraw-Hill, 1997.

Porter M. Exertional heat illness. *Lancet* 2000; 355:1993–1994.

Simon HB. Current concepts: hyperthermia. *N Engl J Med* 1993;329:483–487.

Tek D, Olshaker JS. Heat illness. *Emerg Med Clin North Am* 1992;10:299–331.

Whitman S, Good G, Donoghue ER, et al. Mortality in Chicago attributed to the July 1995 heat wave. *Am J Public Health* 1997;87:1515–1518.

Hypothermia

J. Matthew Sholl, MD, MPH

Hypothermia is defined as a core body temperature less than 35°C (95°F) (normal body temperature is 36.4°C to 37.5°C [97.5°F to 99.5°F]). It can be thought of as a syndrome in which heat loss exceeds heat production. Hypothermia has effects on many different organ systems and, in contrast to frostbite, is a systemic, not focal, cold injury. Hypothermia does not require freezing temperatures. In fact, many cases of hypothermia happen in areas that are commonly thought of as warm, such as the southern United States and the tropics. Hypothermia can occur at any time of the year. The only requirement is exposure to a temperature less than 35°C (95°F).

There were 12,368 deaths in the United States attributable to hypothermia between the years 1979 and 1995 for an annual average of 723. Half of the deaths were in persons 65 years of age or older. Men appear to be affected more than women. This may reflect increased risk-taking behavior in men; men are more apt to be homeless, alcoholics, mountaineers, hikers, and hunters. Racial differences may reflect socioeconomic factors including access to shelter, protective clothing, and adequate home heating. Persons who appear to be most at risk are homeless, elderly, victims of trauma, children, and outdoor enthusiasts.

Hypothermia may be divided into three categories: primary, secondary, and induced. Primary (or accidental) hypothermia is caused solely by exposure to cold temperatures. Heat loss occurs through conduction, radiation, evaporation, and convection; radiation and conduction lead to the majority of heat loss. Exposure to cold water increases conductive heat losses up to 20 times. In contrast, heat production is much more limited and occurs through basic metabolic activities like shivering, release of epinephrine, norepinephrine, and thyroxine and by initiating behavioral changes including seeking warmth, shelter, and clothing. Typical histories involve young, healthy patients engaged in outdoor activities including skiing and snowboarding, hiking and mountaineering, water sports, or hunting. Accidental hypothermia is also frequently seen in urban environments. Risk factors are homelessness, lower socioeconomic class, and extremes of age. The elderly are at risk because of decreased muscle mass and therefore less heat genesis through shivering, and children and infants are at risk because of increased body surface area.

Table 58.1.

Diseases and conditions leading to hypothermia

Metabolic	Hypoglycemia, hypothyroidism, hypopituitarism, hypoadrenalism, DKA
CNS	Head trauma, CVA, spinal cord tumor/injury, sarcoid, tumors, Alzheimer's disease, Parkinson's disease, Wernicke's encephalopathy, neuropathies
Drugs	Alcohol, narcotics, benzodiazepines, barbiturates, phenothiazines, thioridazine (Mellaril), tricyclic antidepressants
Miscellaneous	Sepsis, dermatological diseases, burns, trauma, malnutrition, anorexia nervosa, pancreatitis, extremes of age, mental illness

CNS, central nervous system; CVA, cerebrovascular accident; DKA, diabetic ketoacidosis.

Secondary hypothermia refers to hypothermia resulting from an underlying disorder that predisposes patients to a cold state by increasing heat loss, decreasing heat production, or altering the body's ability to thermoregulate (including altering a patient's ability to initiate behavioral changes). Secondary hypothermia is a syndrome or a final common pathway for multiple injuries, intoxications, and disease states. Table 58.1 lists various conditions that may lead to hypothermia. Two major causes are trauma and substance abuse.

Induced hypothermia is the final category of hypothermia. This is most commonly seen during surgeries such as coronary artery bypass grafting and valve replacements.

Clinical Presentation of Hypothermia

When exposure to a cold environment is obvious, the history of present illness may be simple. In these cases, it is important to determine the ambient temperature the patient was exposed to, the duration of exposure, and any protective measures the patient took (e.g., clothing, attempted shelter). Attention should also be directed toward teasing out potential risk factors as suggested by the location where the patient was found (i.e., urban vs. rural) and the patient's past medical history.

Vital Signs

Perhaps the most important vital sign in hypothermia is temperature. This is a frequently omitted vital sign and should always be requested if missing from the initial vital assessment. Adequate core temperature measurement is essential and is best recorded by rectal probe thermometer. Rectal temperatures are by far the most reliable and reproducible, much more so than tympanic (subject to errors from user variability), oral (which may be affected by ambient air passing through the nasopharynx), and axillary (which does not give a true representation of core temperatures, especially as rewarming is initiated). Care must be taken in ensuring that the thermometer is capable of measuring temperatures as low as 25°C (77°F). Clinical manifestations vary with the stage of hypothermia, defined as mild (35°C to 32.2°C [95°F to 90°F]), moderate (32.2°C to 28°C [90°F to 82.4°F]), and severe (<28°C [<82.4°F]). Important markers during the decline in temperature include loss of shivering at 32°C (90°F), severe changes in mental status at 32°C (90°F), Osborn J waves at 33°C (91.4°F), spontaneous arrhythmias at 32°C (90°F), and spontaneous ventricular fibrillation at 28°C (82.4°F).

After a brief period of tachycardia and tachypnea in mild hypothermia, a linear decrease in pulse, blood pressure, and respiration reliably occurs as hypothermia progresses. If alterations in this pattern are observed, secondary illnesses, injuries, or intoxications are the likely etiology. Pulse and blood pressure may be difficult to obtain because of decreased cardiac output and the patient's cold skin impeding the sense of touch. In these cases, Doppler may be necessary to aid in obtaining vital signs. The profound depression of pulse, blood pressure, and respiration in combination with severe mental status changes and total reduction in metabolic rate may mimic a death-like state leading to the maxim: No patient is dead until they are warm and dead.

The remainder of the physical examination should serve two purposes: (a) to search for risk factors of hypothermia and (b) to build supportive evidence for the diagnosis of hypothermia. Hypothermic patients demand a thorough physical examination looking for evidence of drug abuse (including track marks or works and drugs stashed in the patient's clothes), intoxication, trauma (including head trauma), cerebrovascular accident (CVA), dermatological diseases, frostbite, and the patient's general state of health.

Hypothermia has many effects on various organ systems and attention should be paid to each in detail.

Central Nervous System

As core temperature decreases, mental status diminishes. Mild hypothermia is associated with errors in judgment, confusion, dysarthria, and decreased fine motor skills. This is followed by decreased gross motor skills, hyporeflexia, and further confusion in moderate hypothermia. Interestingly, pupillary reflexes are lost during this stage, which may lead to fixed, or sluggish, and dilated pupils. Profound loss of consciousness, coma, and areflexia generally occur in severe hypothermia at temperatures less than 28°C (82.4°F).

Cardiovascular Effects

As mentioned previously, initial cardiovascular effects include tachycardia and increased cardiac output. Other early cardiovascular abnormalities include peripheral vasoconstriction. As cold stress worsens, bradycardia, hypotension, and decreased cardiac output predominate. Hypothermia has interesting effects on the myocardium, causing multiple electrocardiographic (ECG) changes including PR, QRS, and QT interval prolongation. Spontaneous cardiac arrhythmias occur at temperatures less than 32°C (90°F). Myocardial fragility is further increased at temperatures less than 28°C (82.4°F) with multiple cases of spontaneous ventricular fibrillation generated from presumably minor trauma. One such case occurred as a patient was being transferred from an emergency department gurney to an intensive care unit bed. Care must be taken in handling hypothermic patients!

Renal System

With increases in peripheral vasoconstriction and increased shunting to the core, rates of glomerular filtration increase. This, combined with cold-induced blunting of the tubular response to antidiuretic hormone (ADH) leads to increased urination, commonly called cold diuresis. As hypothermia and hypovolemia worsen, severe oliguria occurs. This may be complicated by rhabdomyolysis and acute tubular necrosis in patents found down for a prolonged time.

Other Manifestations

Many other organ systems are affected by hypothermia. Although tachypnea occurs early in hypothermia, decreased respiratory rates prevail as temperature falls further. This is due to direct depression of central respiratory centers. Other pulmonary manifestations include bronchorrhea and decreased gag reflex, which may lead to aspiration.

Coagulation is directly impaired by hypothermia. The coagulopathy is typically not reflected in the prothrombin time (PT) or partial thromboplastin time (PTT) because the patient's blood is rewarmed to perform these tests, thus abolishing the underlying cold stress. Increases in blood viscosity and increases in bone marrow and hepatic sequestration of platelets may also occur.

Finally, many gastrointestinal manifestations may arise, including ileus, pancreatitis, gastric stress ulcers, and decreased hepatic function. Ringer's lactate should be avoided in volume resuscitation because of the liver's inability to convert lactate to bicarbonate. Normal saline is the fluid of choice for resuscitation in hypothermia.

Diagnostic Evaluation of Hypothermia

Laboratory Evaluation

The following is a list of suggested laboratory tests and studies that should be performed in a hypothermic patient. Further studies should be guided by the patient's clinical picture, physical examination, and past medical history.

The complete blood cell (CBC) count may have several abnormalities. As body temperature drops, hematocrit increases secondary to decreases in plasma volume from cold diuresis (2% for every 1°C fall in body temperature). Low platelets and white blood count are common because of the previously mentioned sequestration by bone marrow and liver.

Multiple electrolyte derangements are possible and are secondary to fluid shifts and shunting during cooling and rewarming phases. Values should be followed serially, especially during the rewarming phase. Elevations of blood urea nitrogen (BUN) and creatinine are very common abnormalities,

resulting in part from hypovolemia. A primary, causative hypoglycemia or a secondary hypoglycemia (from depletion of glycogen stores) may be seen. However, very early in hypothermia, hyperglycemia is common because of catecholamine-induced glycogenolysis.

On arterial blood gas (ABG) analysis, the machine warms the blood before running the assay, so the PaO_2 and PCO_2 will appear higher from the test than they actually are in the patient. The pH on the ABG will be artificially lower than in the patient because of this. Despite rewarming during ABG analysis, correction for temperature is not necessary.

As mentioned earlier, PT and PTT are usually falsely normal because of rewarming of blood during measurement. Coagulopathies, including disseminated intravascular coagulation, are common during and after rewarming; therefore, coagulation factors should be serially monitored.

Electrocardiogram

The electrocardiogram is possibly one of the most important studies in hypothermic patients. Prolongation of the PR, QRS, and QT intervals are common. Osborn J waves are seen at temperatures less than 33°C (91.4°F) (Figure 58.1). These are positive deflections in the left ventricular leads at the junction of the QRS and ST segments and are seen in

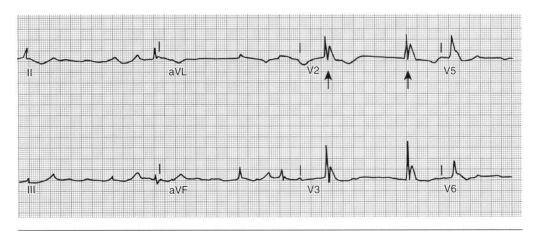

Figure 58.1
Osborne waves in hypothermia.

25% to 30% of patients. Various arrhythmias occur at temperatures less than 32°C (90°F) and spontaneous ventricular fibrillation is seen at temperatures less than 28°C (82.4°F).

Chest X-Ray

Chest x-ray films should be obtained early to rule out aspiration pneumonia, rewarming pulmonary edema, and acute respiratory distress syndrome.

Treatment of the Hypothermic Patient

Aggressive Airway Management and Advanced Cardiac Life Support

Initial management should follow the standard airway, breathing, and circulation (ABCs), as explained in Chapter 2, and advanced cardiac life support (ACLS) protocols with certain exceptions. Aggressive airway management should proceed as usual given the propensity for both mental status changes and aspiration from cold-induced bronchorrhea and reduction of the gag reflex. Multiple studies have confirmed that endotracheal intubation does not induce dysrhythmias. Oral-tracheal intubation is preferred; however, it may be difficult given muscular rigidity and spasm. Neuromuscular blockers are ineffective at temperatures less than 30°C (86°F) and should not be used. Blind nasogastric intubation may be necessary. Cuff pressures should be monitored continually during rewarming, because the volume and pressure will increase.

Respirations and pulses may be very difficult to obtain if bradycardia and bradypnea are severe. Dopplers may help confirm presence or absence of pulse. If no pulses are found or if on cardiac monitoring the patient is found to be in a nonperfusing rhythm, cardiopulmonary resuscitation (CPR) is indicated. CPR may be difficult and may require increased force because of decreased elasticity and compliance of the chest wall.

Cardiac monitoring should be initiated early. Initial treatment of ventricular fibrillation and pulseless ventricular tachycardia follows standard ACLS protocols, and defibrillation should be attempted using standard stepwise increase in joules. Electric cardioversion is frequently ineffective; in these situations, aggressive rewarming modalities should be used, with attempts at defibrillation after every 1°C to 2°C increase in body temperature. Pharmacological therapies are ineffective at temperatures less than 30°C (86°F) and standard doses may lead to toxicity, given decreased hepatic metabolism. These interventions should therefore be avoided until body temperature is greater than 30°C (86°F), at which point the lowest effective dose should be used. Bretylium appears to be the only effective agent at severely cold temperatures; however, effective doses and infusion rates of this and other drugs are unknown.

Multiple cardiac arrhythmias may occur in hypothermia and proper management remains controversial. Many of these arrhythmias resolve with adequate rewarming and do not require therapy. Atrial fibrillation is common and, given low ventricular response rates, usually does not require treatment. Sinus bradycardia is generally considered benign and readily resolves as body temperature increases. Isolated studies suggest transcutaneous pacing may be effective and safe in severe hypothermia with bradycardia.

Supplemental oxygen should be used in nonintubated patients. Peripheral, rather than central, intravenous access should be obtained given fear of inducing arrhythmias from subclavian or internal jugular approaches. Hypotension is common and generally due to volume depletion. Aggressive volume resuscitation should be initiated with normal saline. Vasopressor agents are typically ineffective. Foley catheters should be placed to follow urine output and to help guide volume resuscitation.

Rewarming Techniques

The general principle in the treatment of hypothermia is to halt the underlying process causing heat loss and to encourage rewarming. Removal from a cold environment and transport to the hospital may be the first step to halting the underlying process. Wet clothes must be removed quickly and further heat loss to the environment discouraged by setting the treatment room's thermometer above body temperature. The three basic means of rewarming are passive external rewarming, active external rewarming, and active internal (core) rewarming. Controversy exists in naming the most effective rewarming protocol. Standard treatment practices are reflected in Figure 58.2.

Passive External

Passive external rewarming includes removing the patient from the windy, wet, and cold environment and adding insulating layers. This is a primary treatment modality only in patients who are still shivering (i.e., mild to early moderate hypothermia with temperatures greater than 32°C [89.6°F]) and is considered an adjunct in nonshivering patients. Shivering remains one of the best noninvasive means to rewarm patients, with rates up to 2.0°C per hour.

Active External

Active external rewarming involves adding an external heat source to aid in treatment. These methods have traditionally been used in hypothermic patients who are hemodynamically stable with perfusing cardiac rhythms. Modalities include heat lamps, hot water baths, and forced hot air blankets. The benefits of these rewarming methods include their minimally invasive nature, widespread availability, and rewarming rates up to 2.4°C per hour (using forced hot air blankets at 38°C [100.4°F]). Given these advantages and recent studies using only active external rewarming even in severely hypothermic patients, these methods are gaining popularity.

There has been hesitancy to use these methods in the past for fear of afterdrop or further decrease in core temperature from preferential rewarming of the periphery leading to delivery of cold blood to the core. Some also believe this would exacerbate hypotension. Although early studies confirmed this entity, multiple trials using active external rewarming have not found afterdrop to be of clinical significance.

Active Internal

Active internal rewarming is the most invasive and potentially rapid means of rewarming a patient and includes adding a heat source (usually fluids) to a patient or warming the blood directly by extracorporeal rewarming. Multiple different modalities exist. Warm

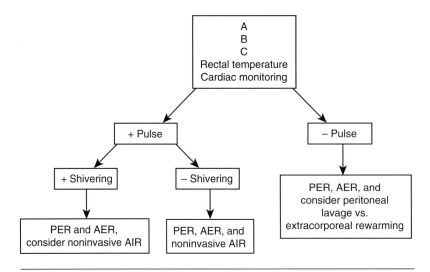

Figure 58.2
Proposed treatment algorithm for hypothermia. A, airway; B, breathing; C, circulation; AER, active internal rewarming; AIR, active external rewarming; PER, passive external rewarming.

humidified oxygen has the theoretical benefit of preferentially rewarming the heart, great vessels, and pulmonary system. Oxygen is warmed to 40°C to 45°C (104°F to 113°F) and administered via a humidified system. In practice, rewarming rates are only 1°C per hour, relegating this modality to an adjunctive treatment.

In warmed intravenous fluid therapy, normal saline is warmed to 40°C [104°F] using standard fluid warmers such as the Level 1 rapid infuser. Rewarming rates of 1.75°C per hour may result. Researchers at Cook County Hospital recently studied the safety and efficacy of centrally administered 65°C [149°F] normal saline. Although rewarming rates of 3.7°C per hour and no intimal injuries noted promise a potential rewarming method, further studies must be performed evaluating the safety in peripheral intravenous delivery.

Warmed gastric, colonic, and bladder irrigation are of insignificant benefit given the small surface areas of each organ. With pleural lavage, 42°C (107.6°F) fluid is infused through a large-bore chest tube in the anterior axillary line of the right chest (to decrease risk of cardiac arrhythmias) and drained through a second chest tube in the posterior axillary line. Although obvious clinical benefits from direct warming of the heart and lungs may exist, no study has adequately studied this technique.

Peritoneal lavage involves infusing liquid heated to 45°C (113.0°F) into the peritoneum via two exchange catheters. Reaching flow rates of 10 to 20 mL/kg (up to 6 L/hour) rewarming rates may reach up to 4°C/hour. This modality has the benefit of being minimally invasive and readily available, and it allows for continued external cardiac massage during implementation. It may also be beneficial in correcting electrolyte abnormalities if dialysate is substituted for normal saline. This technique is popular in many European hospitals and is sometimes used as the primary modality in hemodynamically unstable patients without cardiac arrest.

The final means of active internal rewarming is extracorporeal rewarming. Four methods are available: hemodialysis, arteriovenous (AV) rewarming, venovenous (VV) rewarming, and cardiopulmonary bypass (CPB). Hemodialysis uses a single vessel (preferably the femoral vein) and a two-way catheter and has the advantage of rapid correction of electrolyte abnormalities and removal of dialyzable intoxicants. AV and VV rewarming use a countercurrent heat exchange system.

By far, the most rapid rewarming modality available remains CPB. CPB may be instituted by either femoral-femoral bypass or standard aortic-right atrial bypass and has the advantage of complete circulatory support and maintenance of oxygenation. Rewarming rates may exceed 1°C to 2°C every 3 to 5 minutes. Most studies show 47% to 60% recovery rates with minimal to no neurological impairment. This technique is generally reserved for severely hypothermic patients with hemodynamic instability or ventricular arrhythmias.

Many researchers have proposed several poor prognostic indicators for hypothermic patients, including initial serum pH less than 6.5, initial serum potassium (K^+) greater than 10 mEq/L, and severe coagulopathies. However, several case reports have documented survivors with pH as low as 6.51 and serum potassium of 11.8 mEq/L. Independent risk factors include past medical history and coexistent traumatic injuries or ingestions. There are no valid prognostic indicators of survival, and all patients should be aggressively resuscitated until clinical judgment dictates termination of care.

Disposition

Disposition is determined by the patient's clinical and socioeconomic status. Certainly young, healthy, mildly hypothermic patients who are adequately rewarmed may be discharged to a home or shelter of adequate temperature. In mildly hypothermic homeless patients or patients of poor means who do not have adequate shelter from the elements, admission to a nonmonitored floor is indicated granted they leave the emergency department normothermic. Otherwise, disposition is guided by the patient's past medical history and clinical picture. Patients undergoing active rewarming should be admitted to intensive care settings to ensure continued and adequate rewarming. Once normothermic, otherwise healthy patients with no other comorbidities may be transferred to a nonmonitored floor or discharged.

Suggested Readings

Avidan M, Jones N. Convection warmers—not just hot air. *Anaesthesia* 1997;52:1073–1076.

Braun R, Krishel S. Pearls, pitfalls, and updates—environment emergencies. *Emerg Med Clin North Am* 1997;15:469–473.

Brunette D, McVaney K. Hypothermic cardiac arrest: an 11 year review of ED management and outcome. *Am J Emerg Med* 2000;18:418–422.

Dixon R, Dougherty J. Transcutaneous pacing in a hypothermic-dog model. *Ann Emerg Med* 1997;29:602–606.

Dobson J, Burgess J. Resuscitation of severe hypothermia by extracorporeal rewarming in a child. *J Trauma* 1996;40:483–485.

Epstein D. Preventing hypothermia-related death [Letter]. *JAMA* 1997;278:115–116.

Gilbert M, Busund R. Resuscitation from accidental hypothermia of 13.7°C with circulatory arrest [Research Letter]. *Lancet* 2000;355:375–376.

Greif R, Rajek A. Resistive heating is more effective than metallic-foil insulation in an experimental model of accidental hypothermia: a randomized controlled trial. *Ann Emerg Med* 2000;35:337–345.

Hanania N, Zimmerman J. Environmental emergencies—accidental hypothermia. *Crit Care Clin* 1999;15:235–249.

Handrigan M, Wright R. Factors and methodology in achieving ideal delivery temperatures for intravenous and lavage fluid in hypothermia. *Am J Emerg Med* 1997;15: 350–353.

Josephs J, Farmer C. Hypothermia and extracorporeal rewarming: the journey toward a less invasive, more accessible methodology. *Crit Care Med* 1998;26:1994–1945.

Koller R, Schnider T. Deep accidental hypothermia and cardiac arrest—rewarming with forced air. *Acta Anaesthesiol Scand* 1997;41:1359– 1364.

Larach M. Accidental hypothermia. *Lancet* 1995; 345:493–498.

Lazar H. The treatment of hypothermia [Editorials]. *N Engl J Med* 1997;337:1545–1547.

Mair P, Kornberger E. Accidental hypothermia [Letter]. *Lancet* 1995;345:1048–1049.

Mair P, Kornberger E. Forward blood flow during cardiopulmonary resuscitation in patients with severe accidental hypothermia: an echocardiographic study. *Acta Anaesthesiol Scand* 1998;42: 1139–1144.

Morgan R, King D. Urban hypothermia: many elderly people cannot keep warm in winter without financial hardship. *BMJ* 1996;312:124.

Seigler R, Golding E. Continuous venovenous rewarming: results from a juvenile animal model. *Crit Care Med* 1998;26:2016– 2020.

Sheaff C, Fildes J. Safety of 65 degrees C intravenous fluid for the treatment of hypothermia. *Am J Surg* 1996;172:52–55.

Sim M-M, Kuo Y. Accidental hypothermia in the subtropics [Correspondence]. *Am J Emerg Med* 2000;18:357–358.

Sloan D. Urban hypothermia: number of excess deaths in the winter is large [Letters]. *BMJ* 1996;312:124.

Steele M, Nelson M. Forced air speeds rewarming in accidental hypothermia. *Ann Emerg Med* 1996;27:479–484.

Walpoth B, Walpoth-Aslan B. Outcome of survivors of accidental hypothermia and circulatory arrest treated with extracorporeal blood rewarming. *NEJM* 1997;337:1500–1505.

Submersion Injuries

Edward P. Curcio, III, MD

Submersion injury is one of the more common environmental injuries encountered in emergency medicine. In 1998 4,406 people drowned; one fourth of those were children younger than 15 years. Drowning is the second highest cause of accidental death in the population younger than the age of 44. In children, drowning is the *leading* cause of accidental death. Approximately 6% of all drownings are thought to be due to child abuse. The possibility of abuse should be kept in mind, especially in small children. In all age groups, the exact incidence of near drowning, or those who have survived the initial episode, is thought to be anywhere from 2 to 20 times that number. Their care is complicated by the fact that other injuries are often present, such as trauma and hypothermia.

Definitions

To discuss submersion injuries, we need to have some basic definitions for the terms that are used. *Drowning* is the actual death of a patient who suffocates from submersion in a fluid within 24 hours of the initial event. *Near drowning* implies that the patient has survived the 24 hours after the initial event. *Secondary drowning* refers to death from complications related to a submersion injury, usually from hypoxia, respiratory distress syndrome, or cerebral swelling.

Dry drowning occurs when there is severe laryngospasm, preventing the aspiration of fluid into the lungs. This can occur up to 10% of the time but accounts for up to 90% of all successful resuscitations. *Wet drowning* is when fluid or particulate matter enters the lungs and causes hypoxia.

Role of Alcohol in Drowning

Alcohol plays a large role in drowning victims. One survey in Massachusetts showed that 36% of men involved in aquatic activities had consumed alcoholic beverages. Alcohol contributes to submersion injuries by the obvious effect on judgment and by increasing heat loss and vomiting. However, the effect on judgment probably plays the largest role. Victims misjudge swimming distances and water temperatures. The higher ratio of men who drown than women is believed to be due to men's higher incidence of alcohol consumption and the higher incidence of exposure to the water. Furthermore, 40% to 50% of adolescent victims have been using alcohol.

Pathophysiology

Initial Response to Submersion

Think back to your first cold swim of spring, and remember that first frigid gasp. It is referred to as the "panic gasp" and is a reflex. This first breath can be beneficial or detrimental, depending on whether you are above or below the water. If you are above the water, the panic gasp is quickly followed by hyperventilation in response to the cold immersion and panic. If you are below the water, the gasp results in early inspiration of fluid.

Cold water affects muscle coordination, making it harder to swim. Paradoxically, being a better swimmer reduces the likelihood of survival because the instinct to swim to safety hastens hypothermia. An approximate rule of thumb is that you have a 50% chance of swimming 50 yards in 50° water. A positive predictor of survival time in cold-water immersion is percentage of body fat: a higher percentage provides more insulation and a longer survival time.

Once the victim is below the water's surface and is unable to breathe, carbon dioxide (CO_2) accumulates in the bloodstream from *hypo*ventilation. Paradoxically, the initial hyperventilation from panic has lowered the partial pressure of carbon dioxide (pCO_2), thus blunting the brain's signal to accelerate respiration. Ten percent of victims have severe laryngospasm, which prevents any fluid from entering the lungs. The other 90% aspirate the surrounding fluid and its contaminants. It is common to find sand bronchograms on the initial chest x-ray film.

Mammalian Dive Reflex

Once submerged, cerebral hypoxia develops over 8 to 10 minutes, which is the limiting factor to survival. A small percentage of victims exhibit the mammalian dive reflex, slowing their heart rate and shunting the available blood selectively to the brain and core organs. This response is from the contact of cold water to the victim's face and occurs mostly in children. Heart rates can slow to 8 to 10 beats per minute as the core cools to 30°C. There are reports of survival of drownings for up to 66 minutes of submersion, but there is some debate whether survival was dependent on the dive reflex.

Hypothermia and Prolonged Survival

One of the proposed mechanisms for prolonged survival is the protective property of hypothermia on hypoxic injury to the brain. Surgeons use this philosophy during open-heart surgery, cooling patients to slow their metabolic rate and prolong the time available to operate. However, in the field the brain must be cooled *before* the hypoxic injury occurs. Studies have shown that to be protective, the brain must be cooled at least 7°C in 10 minutes or less. Unfortunately, in 10 minutes of immersion the brain only cools 3°C.

How can we explain the prolonged survival of hypothermic victims? One of the ways would be another method of rapid cooling. Mechanisms proposed have included rapid cooling via swallowing of cold water, aspiration of cold water, and the large surface-to-volume ratio of pediatric patients. What does seem to be evident is that for cold water to be protective, it must be very cold (less than 5°C). In a study in Kings County, Washington, where the water is rarely this cold, the highest rate of survival was seen in patients with core temperatures greater than 34°C, whereas patients with temperatures less than 34°C had a higher incidence of neurological damage. It was unlikely in this population that the protective core cooling temperature was ever reached.

Salt Water and Fresh Water Submersion

In the early 1980s, much was made of salt water versus fresh water submersion and the subsequent electrolyte and blood volume differences that were found. Salt water theoretically could cause increased pulmonary edema because of the diffusion of intravascular fluid into the alveoli and the diffusion of salt water into the bloodstream causing hypernatremia. Fresh water theoretically would diffuse quickly into the bloodstream, causing a dilutional anemia and hyponatremia. In fact, these mechanisms are of little importance. In autopsy reports, less than 150 mL of water were found in the lungs of adult drowning victims. To cause electrolyte abnormalities, at least 20 mL/kg must be aspirated, and for a dilutional anemia, at least 10 mL/kg would need to be aspirated. Thus, a 70-kg male would need to aspirate 700 mL to 1,400 mL of fluid, levels at which survival is rarely seen.

In survivors, contaminants are important. Seawater contains more than 20 known pathogens, including *Pseudomonas putrefaciens, Staphylococcus aureus,* and *Vibrio parahaemolyticus.* There has also been a report of hypercalcemia from a 28-year-old man who fell into oily seawater mixed with drilling fluid. Thus, it is important to keep in mind the exact nature of the fluid in which the patient was found. Regardless of the fluid aspirated, physiologically, all drownings lead to surfactant wash out, ventilation perfusion mismatch, and intrapulmonary shunting, which all result in hypoxia.

Clinical Evaluation and Management

Prehospital

The prehospital care of the submersion victim can be complex with the challenge of a rescue and resuscitation. Issues of rescue are beyond the scope of this chapter, but a word of warning is necessary. Many rescuers have become victims themselves in an attempt to rescue the submersion casualty. The American Red Cross recommendation of "Reach, Throw, Row, then Go" should be heeded to minimize the rescuer's risk. This refers to the recommendation to first try to reach the victim with an object such as a long pole, throw the person a buoyant object, row to the victim in a boat or raft, and if necessary go for help.

Airway, breathing, and circulation (the ABCs of care) should still be followed in prehospital care with the following caveats. In the actual water, it is very difficult to obtain a definitive airway. Instead, emphasis should be placed on getting to safety. Once on land, the patient should be placed horizontally on the beach. Second, there should be a high suspicion for cervical spine injury. Surf, falls greater than 10 feet, diving injuries, and boating incidents all contribute to the high number of concomitant cervical spine injuries. The jaw-thrust maneuver is recommended over the head-tilt method because of this injury pattern. Ventilation should be initiated with adequate cervical spine stabilization. If ventilation is attempted twice and no air is able to pass into the lungs, suspect an obstruction. Current American Red Cross and American Heart Association recommendations include the use of the Heimlich maneuver if there is suspicion of a foreign body or vomitus obstructing the airway. However, there is no role for the Heimlich maneuver in an effort to "squeeze" the water out of the lungs. The amount of water in the lungs is small, and the Heimlich maneuver only increases the incidence of emesis in near-drowning victims.

The optimal airway control is intubation and 100% oxygen (O_2) delivered to the lungs. The next best method of ventilation is to provide positive-pressure ventilation either by bag-valve-mask (BVM) or mouth-to-mask ventilation. Positive-pressure ventilation forces the alveoli open and moves the small amount of water in the lungs into the intravascular space Cardiopulmonary resuscitation (CPR) should also be started as soon as lack of a pulse has been established. Of note in the hypothermic patient, a pulse is often difficult to ascertain; thus, feeling for a minimum of 60 seconds is necessary. Furthermore, it is very difficult to do effective CPR while in the water; thus, every effort should be made to bring the patient to safety.

Prehospital care of the unconscious patient should also include the usual coma protocol regimen of naloxone (to reverse narcotic overdose) and thiamine and glucose (to reverse hypoglycemia). Third, reversing any *hypothermia* should also take precedence. It is unlikely that any field rewarming strategies will add heat to the patient, but removal of cold wet clothes and the addition of warmed blankets, warm packs to the groin and neck area, and warm intravenous (IV) fluids will help stop the continuing loss of heat during transport. Care should be taken not to move the patient too aggressively, because the irritable hypothermic heart can enter into an arrhythmia due to rough handling. Transport to the closest facility should proceed as quickly as possible for all submersion victims.

Emergency Department

On arrival in the emergency department (ED), patients must be divided into three groups from most unstable to most stable: the *unresponsive patient*, the *symptomatic patient* who is awake with some evidence of respiratory insult, and the *asymptomatic patient*.

Unresponsive Patient

PRIMARY SURVEY

The unresponsive victim requires immediate attention. A brief history is obtained from the emergency medical technicians (EMTs) or family members as care is initiated. The history should concentrate on total "down" time (time victim was unconscious and hypoxic) and prehospital care. Airway, breathing, circulation, disability, and exposure (the ABCDEs of patient care) should be followed, concentrating on the airway first. It is not uncommon for submersion victims to have foreign bodies such as sand, debris, and vomitus in the airway. Clear the airway with suction or McGill forceps, always preserving cervical spine immobility. If a definitive airway is needed but is not present, an endotracheal tube (ETT) should be placed immediately. Be aggressive with initial airway management; there is *no* evidence that intubation of the hypothermic patient predisposes to arrhythmias. After the ETT tube is placed, the ventilator setting should be 100% oxygen with early use of

positive end-expiratory pressure (PEEP). The addition of PEEP helps keep the alveoli open, which have a tendency to collapse secondary to surfactant wash out. In addition, warmed humidified oxygen should be used for its slight effect in warming hypothermic patients. Arterial blood gas levels should be obtained to guide ventilation and evaluate the presence of hypoxia. A postintubation chest x-ray film establishes correct ETT placement and the presence of pulmonary injury. Check for other injuries including pneumothorax, foreign bodies, and early acute respiratory distress syndrome.

With airway and breathing controlled, it is time to turn to circulation. Hypotension should be addressed per advanced cardiac life support (ACLS) protocols with a bolus of warmed IV fluid attempted first. Remember that the interstitial fluid present in the lungs is secondary to permeability damage and is not due to pump failure. Vasopressors such as dopamine and dobutamine may be needed if IV fluid does not bring an improvement in the blood pressure.

SECONDARY SURVEY

Disability should be assessed next with special attention to the initial care of the cerebral hypoxic injury. Unfortunately, 12% to 27% of all drowning victims have subsequent neurological damage. Most of this damage has occurred before arrival at the ED. The role of the ED physician is to prevent any further hypoxia, which would worsen the patient's outcome. There remains some debate on the use of hyperventilation and steroids for reduction in intracranial pressure secondary to cerebral edema. Cervical spine fractures also need to be assessed. A portable lateral cervical spine x-ray film should be obtained, followed by definitive imaging once the patient is stabilized.

Assessment of exposure is next, starting with an accurate temperature. Temperature is best obtained via a low-reading rectal thermometer, because this has been shown to correlate closely with actual body core temperature. Both active external and internal warming measures should be started on the hypothermic patient, which are discussed in Chapter 58. If the patient is normothermic and comatose on arrival, a poor outcome is usually the rule. Finally, a detailed secondary examination should be completed to look for any evidence of further trauma.

DIAGNOSTIC EVALUATION

Ancillary testing includes portable lateral cervical spine and chest x-ray films; electrocardiogram (ECG); and initial laboratory testing including a complete blood cell count, electrolytes, blood urea nitrogen, creatinine, and type and crossmatch. An arterial blood gas level can also be helpful in guiding therapy after intubation. An orogastric tube and a Foley catheter should be placed. Computed tomography (CT) scan of the head can also be helpful if head trauma or stroke is suspected in the comatose patient.

DISPOSITION

Admission should be to the appropriate intensive care unit, with a pulmonary consult to help manage the patient.

Symptomatic Patient

PRIMARY SURVEY

The symptomatic awake patient often arrives with evidence of respiratory insult including dyspnea, cough, or chest pain. Initial approach should still follow the ABCs of care, with an oxygen saturation obtained as a part of the other normal vital signs. A nonrebreather oxygen mask should be placed, and a rapid targeted physical examination completed. Remember to assess for any cervical trauma! A patient who walks into the ED can have a cervical spine injury, especially if the mechanism of injury is a diving, falling, or a surfing injury. If there are any signs of trauma, (e.g., tenderness along the cervical spine), the spine must be immobilized.

If there are any signs of pulmonary instability, a portable chest x-ray film should be ordered, and an arterial blood gas level obtained for an accurate measure of hypoxia. Guidelines for intubation include inability to maintain a partial pressure of oxygen, arterial (PaO_2) above 60 mm Hg with 100% oxygen or increasing partial pressure of carbon dioxide, arterial ($PaCO_2$). Continuous positive airway pressure (CPAP) can also be helpful to avoid intubation. The CPAP works by keeping the alveoli open. Nebulized albuterol, a β_2-agonist, can also be helpful in controlling bronchospasm secondary to inhaled submersion irritants. Intubation should be performed in any patient with other indications for airway protection such as altered mentation, persistent oxygen desaturation, or loss of gag reflex.

Circulation should be maintained with IV fluids, and if necessary vasopressors also can be used. Disability should be addressed, as with the unconscious patient. Supportive care of oxygenation, ventilation, and warming the hypothermic patient is the best way to treat any cerebral insult.

SECONDARY SURVEY

After the patient is stabilized, an accurate history must be obtained. First, the amount of time the patient was submerged and the type and temperature of the water in which the patient was immersed must be established. Of note, witnesses are notoriously inaccurate both in overestimating and underestimating the amount of time a victim was submerged, so consider times given as rough estimates. Second, the presence of prehospital care, including CPR, should be established because patients have a higher level of survival with early intervention. Third, the mechanism of injury should be established because this will help the search for associated injuries, specifically whether any trauma occurred. Finally, a complete history including medications, allergies, and the use of any alcohol or drugs should be obtained.

A thorough physical examination should be completed looking for any evidence of trauma and extent of pulmonary insult. Respiratory rate, oxygen saturation, and an accurate rectal temperature all need to be recorded. Ancillary testing includes a chest x-ray film; complete blood cell count; ECG;

and levels of electrolytes, blood urea nitrogen, creatinine, and arterial blood gas.

DISPOSITION

Disposition of all symptomatic patients is fairly simple with overnight admission to a ward with continuous pulse oximetry monitoring available. Most respiratory distress manifests within 6 hours, but observation in the hospital is prudent.

Asymptomatic Patient
PRIMARY SURVEY

In the asymptomatic patient with a history of submersion, the ABCs of care should be followed. Initial vital signs should include oxygen saturation. Oxygen via facemask at 8 to 10 L/minute should be instituted until a comprehensive evaluation has been completed.

SECONDARY SURVEY

The history should include the time the patient was submerged, circumstances regarding the submersion, temperature of the water, prehospital care, and presence of respiratory complaints. A full history should be obtained including past medical history, medications, allergies, past surgical history, and the use of any alcohol or drugs. Vital signs are important, as always, with an accurate rectal temperature to assess for hypothermia. Pay particular attention to the lung examination, starting with the respiratory rate and oxygen saturation. Listen carefully for any evidence of rales, crackles, wheezes, or evidence of pulmonary insult. The best care is supportive care with oxygen, CPAP, and the use of nebulized albuterol to help open the airways. Look closely for any evidence of trauma, including a detailed cervical spine and abdominal examination.

Ancillary testing includes a chest x-ray, ECG (if the patient is hypothermic or has a history of heart disease), and an arterial blood gas level on room air. This will establish a baseline and give an accurate PaO_2 measurement that will help guide disposition.

DISPOSITION

The disposition of asymptomatic patients has changed recently. Initially it was recommended to admit all submersion patients for observation because of the risk of sudden decline in pulmonary function even with a normal initial examination, so-called *secondary drowning*. However, more recent studies suggest that all patients who subsequently decline can be identified with a careful initial examination and observation in the ED for 6 hours. These patients all need close follow-up with a repeat examination within 24 hours. If this is not possible, the patient should be admitted overnight for observation.

Predicting Outcome

One area of controversy in the care of submersion victims is predicting patient outcome. Survival of submersion victims seems to be dichotomous in nature, with either complete recovery or death. Ten percent of all victims survive with lasting neurological damage. Unfortunately, no rules exist to help us predict who will survive neurologically intact, despite presenting in extremely grave condition, including coma. Factors that seem to be associated with a good outcome include alert on admission to ED, hypothermia, older child or adult, brief submersion time, good response to initial resuscitation, and on-scene CPR. Hypothermia can be both protective and detrimental at the same time, with protective effects occurring if the brain is cooled before the hypoxic injury. Remember, there is no hard and fast rule, so from an emergency medicine viewpoint all patients should be resuscitated.

Poor outcomes are usually associated with age younger than 3 years, fixed dilated pupils in the ED, submersion longer than 5 minutes, no resuscitation attempts for longer than 10 minutes, preexisting chronic disease, pH of 7.10 or less, or coma on admission to the ED.

Suggested Readings

Conn AW, Barker GA. Fresh water drowning and near-drowning—an update. *Can J Anaesth* 194; 31:538–544.

DeNicola LK, Falk JL, Swanson ME, et al. Common issues in pediatric and adult clinical care submersion injuries in children and adults. *Crit Care Clin* 1997;13:477–500.

Gooden BA. Why some people do not drown. Hypothermia versus the diving response. *Med J Aust* 1992;157:629–632.

Graf WD, Cummings P, Quan L, et al. Predicting outcome in pediatric submersion victims. *Ann Emerg Med* 1995;26:312–319.

CHAPTER **60**

Electrical and Lightning Injuries

John M. Swanson, MD, FACEP

Electrical and lightning injuries represent unusual, but not uncommon, presentations to the emergency department. Despite underreporting, there are more than 1,000 fatalities (0.5 per 100,000 population) from electrical injuries alone each year, and more than 5,000 emergency department visits in the United States for these injuries. Electrical injuries account for 5% of all burn center admissions. Thirty-three percent of all electrical injuries are occupational, with 5 in 100,000 miners or electrical workers dying yearly.

Lightning injuries cause approximately 250 fatalities a year and are responsible for another 1,500 serious injuries. In deaths attributed to natural disasters, lightning injuries are second only to flash flooding. Lightning injuries are more commonly seen in mountainous areas and around large bodies of water. In the United States, Florida and Texas report the greatest number of deaths from lightning yearly.

Management of electrical and lightning injuries requires knowledge of basic science and injury-specific pathophysiology both in the field and in the emergency department. A well-trained emergency physician is in the unique position to combine knowledge of both advanced trauma life support and advanced cardiac life support to manage patients found in cardiopulmonary arrest. This chapter introduces the reader to caring for both the electrical- and lightning-injured patient.

Electrical Injuries

Pathophysiology

Electricity causes human injuries through a multitude of mechanisms. The electric current can cause damage to body tissues, and the conversion of electrical energy to thermal energy can cause burns, both superficial and deep. Muscle contractions, or the loss of controlled muscle function, can also cause injuries such as falls.

Consolidated Edison employed scientist W.B. Kouwenhoven in the early 1900s to heighten worker safety by detailing risks within the electrical injury. He described six variables that affect the extent of electrical injuries (Table 60.1).

Voltage (V) is the electrical pressure or difference between two objects that causes electrons to flow. Electrical injuries have been classified artificially as either high or low voltage, with 1,000 volts as the cutoff.

Resistance (R) is difficult to quantify in human injuries because it is altered by the type of tissue affected, contact area, presence of moisture, and duration of contact. In general, resistance of muscle, blood vessels, and nervous tissue is lower than that of skin, bones, fat, and tendons. Electrons preferentially flow across tissues with low resistance. Hence, critical internal structures are often injured with little apparent injury to tissues with higher resistance. The presence

Table 60.1.
Kouwenhoven's injury variables
Voltage (V)
Resistance (R)
Amperage (I)
Current type (alternating vs. direct)
Contact duration
Pathway across tissues
Kouwenhoven's injury variables are the strongest determinants of the extent of an electrical injury.

of water, or even perspiration, markedly reduces tissue resistance.

Amperage (I), or current, is the flow of electrons measured in amperes (A). Current flow is directly related to the voltage and indirectly related to resistance. (Ohms law describes the relationship as follows: amperage = voltage/resistance.)

There are two basic types of current: alternating current (AC) and direct current (DC). In AC, electrons flow back and forth, in both directions (alternating). In DC, electrons flow in a single direction. AC is responsible for most electrical injuries and is more dangerous than DC of the same voltage. DC tends to cause a single muscle contraction, often throwing the victim from the source of current, whereas AC causes repeated muscle contraction. In the case of a handheld object, strong forearm flexors tend to overpower wrist extensors, causing tetany and prolonged contact with the current. Low-voltage AC has a narrow margin of safety before reaching amperage dangerous to humans. Tetany may occur with 20 mA, and respiratory arrest occurs at 30 to 40 mA. Ventricular fibrillation can occur at 50 to 100 mA.

The pathway of current is also critical in determining the extent and nature of injuries. Entry and exit sites more correctly should be called source and ground. If the pathway between the source and ground includes tissues of the central nervous system, muscles of respiration, the heart, or a gravid uterus, a life-threatening injury may occur. Contrary to previous beliefs, it recently has been shown that a vertical current through the body is more dangerous than a horizontal current, as exhibited by the scalp and calf electrodes used in electrocution.

The duration of contact affects the tissues by two primary mechanisms. First, as tissue damage occurs, resistance is lowered, furthering more tissue damage. Second, electrical energy is converted to thermal energy. Joules law states that $H = I^2RT$, where H is heat, I is amperage, R is resistance, and T is time. Heat is then accompanied by burns, from temperatures as high as 3,000°C with high-voltage exposure.

Electrical Injuries

Electrical injuries are commonly occupational injuries. Data indicate that 33% of all electrical injuries occur on the job. It is also well accepted that underreporting of these injuries is common. Fifty percent of injuries are secondary to direct contact with power lines, and another 25% are caused by contact with electrical tools. Eighty percent of those injured are adults. Electrical injuries in children have a bimodal distribution, both in age and in type of current encountered. Children are injured by low-voltage AC 45% of the time and high-voltage DC 55% of the time. Children younger than 6 years are most commonly affected by household AC sources, and teenagers are more commonly injured by exposure to high-voltage power line sources.

Prehospital providers, and well-meaning bystanders, need to make sure that the scene of the injury has been secured before attempting to provide care to the injured. One must shut off power to all high-voltage sources and approach even low-voltage sources with caution, especially if conditions are wet. Water, or even sweat, decreases the resistance to electrical currents dramatically.

Victims are often unable to provide history of the event and must be treated with the standard precautions afforded to all trauma victims. Spinal immobilization should be provided, and triage of these patients should be urgent, given the possibility of unrecognized traumatic injuries or arrhythmias.

Cardiopulmonary arrest is a common presentation in electrical injuries. Classically,

AC injuries initially cause ventricular fibrillation and respiratory paralysis, which, if left untreated, will progress to asystole resulting from hypoxia. DC injuries more classically induce asystole. All arrhythmias should be approached according to advanced cardiac life support (ACLS) guidelines. Extremity injuries can include fractures from either forceful muscle contraction or falls caused by the initial shock. Injuries to the skin may include large thermal burns from heat formation. However, small punctate burns with underlying damage that is difficult to appreciate initially are more likely. Skeletal muscle injury may cause rhabdomyolysis. Children often suffer specific injuries: 25% of children's burns are oral commissure burns caused by sucking on electrical cords. Damage can occur immediately to the orbicularis oris muscles and even to developing dentition. Delayed bleeding can occur when the scab separates from the lips, avulsing the labial artery.

Electrical Injury Management

Emergency department management should consist of attention to airway, breathing, and circulation (the ABCs) and then focus on the multitude of injuries found during a careful secondary survey. Further management is based partly on initial findings. In general, electrocardiograms (ECGs) should be obtained on all adults suffering from high- or low-voltage injuries. Asymptomatic adult victims of low-voltage injuries also should have an evaluation for myoglobinuria. With no signs of arrhythmias or rhabdomyolysis, asymptomatic adult victims may safely be discharged with outpatient follow-up.

Victims of high-voltage (arbitrarily defined as greater than 1,000 V) mandate a more exhaustive workup: cardiac monitoring, basic blood work, and hospital admission. Most advocate telemetry monitoring because of the rare arrhythmia that has been described in patients who suffer these high-voltage injuries.

Recently, studies have been performed to suggest that cardiac monitoring or even ECGs may not be necessary in a subset of pediatric victims. Pregnant mothers warrant special considerations; ultrasonography and fetal monitoring should be part of their initial evaluation. Involvement of the consulting trauma surgeon early in the emergency department workup is advisable in facilitating the management, admission, and follow-up for these patients.

Lightning Injuries

Lightning Formation

From prehistoric times, humans have been fascinated with lightning, which has been represented in primitive art worldwide since 2000 BC. Much of lightning's mystique remains even today. In evaluating and treating lightning injuries, the first step is to understand lightning formation.

The study of storm clouds and lightning formation is both markedly complex and even controversial in some aspects to this day. A simplified explanation is included here. Storm clouds form when a cold air, high-pressure system moves into a warm air, low-pressure system. Moisture from the warm air system condenses, releasing energy. This energy is distributed unevenly within the cloud, leaving charge differences between layers within the cloud and between the cloud and the ground. When the differentials are high enough, lightning formation occurs to equalize them.

Initially, an indiscernible "leader stroke" travels from the cloud to the ground. An ionized pathway is formed with both negative and positive charges. As the leader stroke heads toward earth, the charge differential between the cloud and the earth forces numerous "pilot strokes" to head from the now relatively positively charged earth upward. When one of these pilot strokes contacts the leader stroke, the charge differential between the cloud and the earth dissipates in a highly visible "return stroke" that we see as lightning. One to 30 return strokes may occur in one channel, which is responsible for the flickering of lightning we often appreciate. Lightning has been measured reaching 8,000°C and has a diameter of

Table 60.2.

Mechanism of lightning injuries

Direct strikes
Contact injury
Splash injury
Step voltage
Shock wave

roughly 7 cm. The super-heating and super-cooling of air that occurs around lightning is responsible for the thunder heard after the charge dissipates. The differential may be as great as 100 million to 2 billion volts.

Lightning Injuries

Lightning may cause injuries by five primary mechanisms (Table 60.2). Direct strikes occur when a person is out in the open and is struck by lightning. Contact injuries occur when an item held by a person is struck. Side splashes occur when current "splashes" from the object hit to one of less resistance. A group of people or a herd of livestock may be injured simultaneously by this mechanism. Step voltage occurs as the electrical charge dissipates through the ground, or even water, that it has struck. Current may pass up one leg and down the other of a potential victim if a large differential exists between the two legs! This mechanism of injury also may produce mass casualties. The last mechanism of injury is that afforded by the explosive shock wave that occurs when lightning strikes nearby.

Most of the current transferred in lighting frequently flashes over patients. Therefore, it has been called a "flashover." Charges delivered internally are magnitudes of power less than the potential found within lightning. This allows for a much higher survival rate than the lay public would expect; current mortality estimates range from 25% to 32%.

Lightning Injury Management

Initial management may commonly involve more than one victim; 30% of all lightning strikes injure two or more people. Medical providers should provide care to those in cardiopulmonary arrest first. This runs contrary to medical care rendered in most mass casualty incidents, in which mortally wounded individuals must be denied care. In lightning injury, respiratory arrest is seen more frequently than cardiac arrest. Respiratory arrest is a central paralysis, caused by an electrical disruption of the medullary respiratory center. The initial cardiac arrest typically results in asystole, which is often followed by some form of organized cardiac activity resulting from the heart's innate automaticity. It is crucial to provide prolonged respiratory support to all those initially apneic to avoid secondary anoxic cardiac arrest.

Neurological injuries range from mild to severe. They include skull fractures, intracranial bleeding, seizures, amnesia, coma, blindness, dysesthesias, and delayed neuropsychological changes. Patients may experience these injuries from both the electrical and blunt trauma that occurs with many lightning strikes. Many victims experience a phenomenon known as Charcot's paralysis, leaving affected limbs appearing blue and pulseless. Symptoms include pain, pulselessness, paresis, and sensory changes that are caused by autonomic and peripheral nerve damage and malfunction. Usually these symptoms clear in a matter of hours. Two thirds of patients are affected in the lower extremities and one third in the upper extremities.

Up to 89% of lightning strike victims suffer from cutaneous burns. Unlike high-voltage injuries, the brief flashover effect spares victims from most major burns. Four major types of burns are associated with lightning injuries: feathering burns, linear burns, punctate burns, and thermal burns. Feathering burns, also known as Lichtenberg figures, are pathognomic of lightning strikes. They represent electron showers tracking over the skin. Linear burns are first- and second-degree burns that are thought to be caused by sweat vaporization, because they occur over body areas with high sweat presence. Punctate burns appear similar to cigarette burns and often occur in groups. They can be full thickness but range only from a millimeter to a centimeter in diameter. Clothing can either be ignited or heated by lightning strikes, causing thermal burns. Metal buckles and coins have caused such burns.

Other injuries are commonly described. Typically, 30% to 50% of all victims have ruptured tympanic membranes, and more than half of those injured have ocular injuries including cataracts, hyphemas, vitreous hemorrhage, and uveitis. Treatment of these patients requires a complete secondary survey and appropriate referral. Admission criteria have not been proposed, although monitoring and observation would seem warranted for all but those completely asymptomatic patients.

Suggested Readings

Bailey B, Gaudreault P, Thivierge RL, et al. Cardiac monitoring of children with household electrical injuries. *Ann Emerg Med* 1995;25: 612–617.

Cooper MA. Lightning injuries. In: Rosen P, Barkin R, Hayden SR, et al, eds. *Emergency medicine: concepts and clinical practice*, 4th ed. St. Louis: Mosby, 1998:1010–1022.

Cooper MA, Andrews CJ. Lightning injuries. In: Auerbach P, ed. *Auerbach's wilderness medicine: management of wilderness and environmental injuries.* St. Louis: Mosby, 1995:261–289.

Einarson A, Bailey B, Innocencion G, et al. Accidental electric shock in pregnancy: a prospective cohort study. *Am J Obstet Gynecol* 1997;176:678–681.

Fontanarosa PB. Electrical shock and lightning strike. *Ann Emerg Med* 1993;22:378–387.

Garcia CT, Smith GA, Cohen DM, et al. Electrical injuries in a pediatric emergency department. *Ann Emerg Med* 1995;26:604–608.

Graber J, Ummenhofer W, Herion H. Lightning accident with eight victims: case report and brief review of the literature. *J Trauma Injury Infect Crit Care* 1996;40:288–290.

Jain S, Bandi V. Electrical and lightning injuries. *Crit Care Clin* 1999;15:319–331.

Milzman DP, Moskowitz L, Hardel M. Lightning strikes at a mass gathering. *South Med J* 1999;92:708–710.

Ore T, Casini B. Electrical fatalities among U.S. construction workers. *J Occup Environ Med* 1996;38:587–592.

Purdue GF, Hunt JL. Electrocardiographic monitoring after electrical injury: necessity of luxury. *J Trauma Injury Infect Crit Care* 1986;26: 166–167.

Rai J. Electrical injuries: a 30 year review. *J Trauma Injury Infect Crit Care* 1999;46:933–936.

CHAPTER 61

Bites and Stings

Robert L. Hood, MD, PhD, FACEP, Nicholas J. Jouriles, MD

The subject of bites and stings comprises a huge array of topics. Some of these are quite common, such as dog bites. Some, such as octopus bites, are highly unusual. The emergency physician is the specialist most likely to see the majority of these cases. Although we cannot present all types of bites and stings in this book, we have attempted to give the student a taste of this fascinating area of emergency medicine. Topics covered in this chapter include animal bites, bee stings, marine envenomations, snakebites, and arthropod bites.

Animal Bites

Because most states do not legally require the reporting of animal bites, the true inci-dence is unknown. Animal bites remain a very common problem for emergency de-partments across the country. Dog bites ac-count for most animal bites; children and young adults are the most common victims. Most fatalities occur in children younger than 10 years. The dog most commonly as-sociated with a fatal injury is the pit bull.

Bite attacks by animals may result in both blunt and penetrating trauma. Injuries include extensive soft tissue damage, frac-tures, neurovascular injury, and secondary infections. The organisms found in dog bite wounds are numerous. Up to 60% of in-fected wounds grow more than one organ-ism. *Staphylococcus*, *Streptococcus*, *Klebsiella*, and *Pseudomonas* species are all common. The risk of infection is related to location, severity of injury, associated foreign body, time until treatment, and patient factors such as age and underlying illnesses. Animal bites should also be considered tetanus-prone wounds. Cat bites are important for the association of *Pasteurella multocida*, which is found in approximately 80% of healthy cats. Antibiotics (penicillin, amoxi-cillin/clavulanate, cefuroxime, or doxycy-cline) should be administered. Cephalexin, commonly ordered for skin infections, does not work against *Pasteurella multocida*.

Rabies

Rabies is an enormous health problem in the Third World and approximately 35,000 peo-ple die from the disease every year. In the United States, human rabies is extremely rare. It is nonexistent in Hawaii. On average one or two cases per year are reported in the

United States. Currently, most cases result from exposure while traveling outside of the United States or from interaction with bats, skunks, foxes, or raccoons.

Transmission Through Animals

Rabies is caused by an RNA rhabdovirus. Animals that acquire the virus become sick and die. Animals are capable of transmitting rabies once they start secreting virus in saliva. Most, but not all, animals with rabies will be sick before they begin to excrete the virus. When symptoms initially begin in animals, rabies may be very difficult to diagnose. Symptoms may include aggressive behavior, ataxia, irritability, anorexia, lethargy, or excessive salivation. An unprovoked bite from a domestic animal may be a sign of rabies.

Once the animal is bitten, the rabies virus replicates in the muscle cells near the site of the bite and ascends through peripheral nerves to the central nervous system. The incubation period from bite to disease in humans ranges from 30 to 90 days. The human prodrome is nonspecific and misdiagnosis often occurs. Clinical suspicion, especially with a history of possible rabies-contaminated bite, is the key to the diagnosis. Once the disease is fully manifested and easy to diagnose, rabies is almost always fatal. Death occurs within 3 to 10 days.

Treatment

No specific or effective rabies treatment currently exists. Only three patients have ever been known to survive rabies, and all received some sort of preexposure or postexposure treatment. Currently the most effective form of treatment is to offer postexposure immunization and treatment for patients who are bitten by animals at risk for carrying rabies. Bites to the head or neck have a higher mortality rate than those to the legs.

If the patient is at risk for rabies, postexposure prophylaxis should be started. If the animal is a stray and is caught, it should be sacrificed and examined for rabies. If rabies is not found, the postexposure prophylaxis can be discontinued. If the patient is bitten by a domestic animal, the animal can be observed for 10 days; if it does not become sick, postexposure prophylaxis can be discontinued. If the animal does become sick, it should be sacrificed and examined pathologically.

Rabies treatment consists of three steps: wound care, passive immunization, and active immunization. All three are required. Treatment should begin within 24 hours. Rabies is easily killed by sunlight, soap, or drying. Current recommendations of the Centers for Disease Control and Prevention (CDC) include washing the wound with soap and water as quickly and thoroughly as possible. Swabbing the wound with a soap solution is essential. Immunization should begin immediately with human rabies immune globulin (HRIG). The dose is 20 IU/kg, with half infiltrated at the local site and the other half given intramuscularly (IM). Human diploid cell rabies vaccine (HDCV) should also be given on the first day, followed by four required injections on days 3, 7, 14, and 28. HRIG and HDCV should be given at different sites and never mixed in the same syringe. There are reports of treatment failure when the rabies immunization has been given in the gluteal muscles. It is currently recommended that these shots be given in the deltoid muscle.

Human Bites

Human fight bites are commonly seen when a patient punches someone, catches his or her teeth with a closed fist, and suffers a laceration over a metacarpal-phalangeal (MCP) joint on the dominant hand. The laceration is infected with common skin flora and oral anaerobes. Any MCP laceration after a fight should be considered infected. Such a wound should be thoroughly explored. Any evidence of fracture, tendon injury, or joint involvement should be evaluated by an orthopedist or hand surgeon. These wounds should be irrigated extensively and left open. The patient should receive local wound care, tetanus prophylaxis, and antibiotics (penicillin, amoxicillin/clavulanate, or clindamycin).

Arthropods

Hymenoptera

Hymenoptera is an order of arthropods composed of bees, wasps, hornets, yellow jackets, and ants. Bees and wasps have modified ovipositors that protrude from the abdomen and act as a hypodermic needle in administering the venom. They both have barbed stings. In the bee, the entire stinging apparatus is pulled from the bee after stinging a victim, resulting in the death of the bee. The wasp may inflict many stings without damaging its stinging apparatus. The most common enzymes deposited by these stings include the peptides phospholipase A and hyaluronidase. These cause toxicity by activating low-molecular-weight inflammatory substances such as bradykinin, acetylcholine, histamine, and serotonin. There are also many antigenic substances that account for the induction of a hypersensitivity reaction.

Bee stings can cause an immediate life-threatening allergic reaction. More people in the United States die of bee stings than any other form of bite. The anaphylactic shock that results should be treated immediately with supportive care (e.g., airway management and intravenous fluids) as well as antiallergy care (epinephrine, antihistamines such as diphenhydramine, and steroids). If in shock, the patient should receive intravenous epinephrine immediately.

Those patients susceptible to life-threatening allergic reactions to bee stings should be counseled about outdoor activities (avoiding bees nests, not wearing colorful, flower-like clothing) and prescribed an epinephrine syringe and instructed on its use. The epinephrine syringe should be readily available at all times, and patient self-administration may prove life saving. Those patients with less than life-threatening allergic reactions may be treated with antiallergic therapy, tetanus prophylaxis, and local wound care. Analgesics are frequently needed.

Ticks

Ticks belong to the class Arachnida, which includes the spiders and scorpions and are found in almost all habitats throughout the United States. As vectors for disease-causing organisms, they are second only to mosquitos worldwide, and account for the leading cause of vector-borne diseases in the United States.

Hard ticks (Ixodidae) are responsible for all tick-borne diseases in the United States, with the exception of relapsing fever (soft ticks, Argasidae). Ticks feed on the blood of animals including mammals, birds, and reptiles. After contact with the host, they bury their feeding parts into the flesh and often produce a cement-like substance to secure their position. Most produce an anticoagulant, which aids in the acquisition of the blood meal.

Many tick-borne diseases are found in the United States. The most common of these are babesiosis, Colorado tick fever, Lyme disease, Rocky Mountain spotted fever, relapsing fever, ehrlichiosis, and tularemia (Table 61.1).

In addition to diseases produced by microorganisms carried by ticks, humans may develop tick paralysis after being bitten. The exact mechanism of this disease is not fully understood but seems to be through the production of a toxin that affects peripheral nerves. Symptoms occur 4 to 5 days following a bite and usually begin with a bilateral ascending paralysis of the lower extremities. If not treated, this can lead to respiratory failure and death. Removal of the tick reverses symptoms.

Management of the diseases caused by tick bites may be extensive and exceeds the scope of this work. Basic principles start with prevention of the tick bite. Measures to be taken include avoidance of tick-infested areas; wearing suitable protective clothing; using insect/tick repellants; and carefully examining all parts of the body, including the scalp, axillae, and groin, for the presence of ticks.

When a tick is found, the method of removal is important. Although there are many anecdotal methods (hot match head, finger-

Table 61.1.

Tick-borne diseases found in the United States

Disease	Organism	Tick Vector
Babesiosis	Babesia microti	Ixodes scapularis (deer tick)
Colorado tick fever	Orbivirus	Dermacentor andersoni (wood tick)
Lyme disease	Borrelia burgdorferi	Ixodes scapularis Ixodes pacificus (deer tick)
Rocky Mountain spotted fever	Rickettsia rickettsii	Dermacentor andersoni (wood tick) Dermacentor ariabilis (dog tick)
Relapsing fever	Borrelia hermsii	Ornithodoros hermsi
	Borrelia turicatae	Ornithodoros turicata
	Borrelia parkeri	Ornithodoros parkeri
Ehrlichiosis	Ehrlichia chaffeensis	I. scapularis (deer tick) Amblyomma americanum (Lone Star tick)
Tularemia	Francisella tularensis	A. americanum (Lone Star tick)

nail polish, alcohol), none of these has proved superior to simple traction and extraction. Grasp the tick near the buried head, preferably with forceps, and pull out at 90 degrees to the skin. Avoid squeezing the body so as not to inject additional material into the bite site. The tick should be dropped into a bottle of alcohol or flushed down the toilet.

Marine Envenomations

The sea contains a vast number of organisms from many genera and several different phyla. In the following section, the evaluation and treatment of envenomations from the following groups are discussed: coelenterates (jellyfish), cephalopods (octopus), vertebrates (lion and stonefish), and echinoderms (sea urchins and sea cucumbers). Although this list is somewhat limited, the principles of diagnosis, evaluation, and treatment provide a solid foundation for the practicing clinician.

Coelenterates

Members of the phylum Coelenterata, which includes the jellyfish, account for more envenomations in humans than any other group. There are approximately 9,500

species in this group, of which approximately 100 are toxic to humans. Members of this phylum are characterized by having only two germ layers, the ectoderm and endoderm, separated by an acellular matrix referred to as the mesoglia. They characteristically have stinging cells or *cnidocysts*, which produce the envenomation effect. These stinging cells contain highly sophisticated structures, which act as hypodermic needles to inject toxin directly into the skin.

The phylum Coelenterata contains four medically important groups: class Hydrozoa (Portuguese man-o-war and fire corals), class Scyphozoa (true jellyfish), class Cuboza (box jellyfish), and class Anthozoa (sea anemones).

Pathophysiology

The pathophysiology of envenomation by coelenterates involves the injection of venom into the skin by the firing of the cnidocysts. These cells are located both on the body surface and along the tentacles of these animals. Although these function naturally in the capture and killing of prey, accidental contact by humans produces painful and occasionally deadly results. Coelenterate toxin contains several groups of substances including histamine, fibrolysins, kinins, hyaluronidases, phospholipases, and various cardiogenic and neurotoxic substances.

Most often coelenterate envenomations occur in people vacationing at the beach when there are large numbers of jellyfish in the surf. Although most U.S. envenomations are from nondeadly species and produce mild irritation, there are occasionally more severe cases such as those caused by *Physalia physalis* or the Portuguese man-o-war.

Clinical Presentation

The clinical presentation varies from pain to life-threatening anaphylaxis. The patient may have dermal evidence of the sting, with areas of swelling and erythema, which may be linear when there was contact with tentacles. When ocular contact occurs, there may be signs of conjunctivitis and periorbital edema. Some lesions eventually may become hemorrhagic, ulcerated, or secondarily infected.

Treatment

Very often either the patient or a concerned bystander has initiated some form of treatment on scene. Although these efforts are well intentioned, unless the appropriate treatment has been initiated, the symptoms may actually worsen. If the patient is washed off with fresh water, the osmotic effect on the remaining, unfired cnidocysts will cause them to fire, resulting in additional envenomation.

Hospital treatment varies according to the severity of the envenomation. Initial efforts should be directed at inactivating any remaining cnidocysts followed by removing any visible tentacles. The patient should be completely undressed. The affected areas should be flushed with copious amounts of normal saline. In the case of envenomation by the box jellyfish or sea wasp (*Chironex fleckeri*) and Portuguese man-o-war (*Physalia*) a dilute solution (5%) of acetic acid neutralizes the toxin.

Envenomation by the box jellyfish has been noted in some cases to cause fairly rapid mortality. In patients who survive to the hospital, a specific antivenin is available and should be used. This species is found primarily in the Pacific waters around Australia and is not generally found in U.S. waters.

After the application of normal saline or acetic acid solution, remove the remaining cnidocysts and tentacles by applying shaving cream and scraping with a common table knife. Tetanus prophylaxis should be administered if indicated, but antibiotic therapy is not indicated unless secondary infection occurs.

Pain control may be achieved with parenteral narcotics, and pruritus is usually controlled satisfactorily with antihistamine medications such as diphenhydramine or hydroxyzine. Laboratory studies are not generally helpful except in extreme and severe cases of envenomation requiring hospitalization.

Cephalopods

Octopus bites are extremely rare because most of these animals are shy and reclusive by nature. However, when caught or harassed, they may bite and cause minor local injury. The exception to this general rule occurs with the deadly envenomation by the blue-ringed octopuses *Ilapalochlena luminata* and *Hapalochlena maculosa*.

The blue-ringed octopuses are found in the tide pools and coastal waters of Australia. They are small animals with a total length rarely exceeding 20 cm and are brown with blue rings on the tentacles. When the animal is agitated or upset, the rings glow with an impressive blue fluorescent color. Although they excrete their venom into the surrounding water to paralyze prey, most human envenomations arise from a bite from their parrot-beak-like mouth.

Pathophysiology

The toxins produced by octopuses and stored in their salivary glands are varied in chemical content but include the neurotoxin *tetrodotoxin*. This toxin has been shown to affect sodium channels in the cell membrane, blocking peripheral nerve conduction, which leads to paralysis and respiratory failure. Tetrodotoxin is also found in puffer fish (Fugu) and may cause nausea and vomiting, paresthesias, miosis, diabetes insipidus, and depressed cortical activity. The venom of the blue-ringed octopus also has been shown to contain hyaluronidase, tyramine, 5-hydroxy-tyramine, acetylcholine, and dopamine.

Treatment

Appropriate prehospital treatment includes rapid evaluation and intervention by paramedics to ensure airway control and intravenous access. Although not essential, a positive identification of the offending animal is useful. Because respiratory failure is a real possibility, rapid transport to an appropriate health care facility is mandatory. When possible, immediate irrigation of the wound site is advisable. Pressure immobilization is also recommended.

Treatment for octopus envenomation is primarily supportive. Airway control is paramount and may require endotracheal intubation. Effects of the venom usually wear off in 12 hours and survival to this time generally ensures a good outcome. Tetanus prophylaxis should be accomplished when indicated. No antivenin currently exists for

blue-ringed octopus bites, but there have been anecdotal reports of success in treating muscular weakness from tetrodotoxin using neostigmine and edrophonium. Four-amino pyridine, a drug used in patients with multiple sclerosis, has been shown to be useful in animals given tetrodotoxin.

Lionfish and Stonefish

Members of this group belong to the family Scorpaenidae and include the lionfish, the stonefish, zebra fish, scorpion fish, sculpin, and bull trout. These fish all possess the ability to envenomate humans by virtue of specialized spines attached to venom glands (Fig. 61.1). These animals are responsible for more envenomations than any other fish except for stingrays.

The taxonomic classification of these fish is confusing, but there are three genera recognized as containing the poisonous varieties: *Pterois*, long spines with a small venom glands (e.g., lion fish); *Scorpoena*, short, thick spines with more potent sting (e.g., scorpion fish); and *Synanceia*, highly developed venom glands capable of producing human

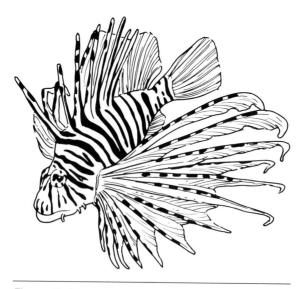

Figure 61.1
The lionfish with specialized spines attached to venom glands.

fatality (e.g., stone fish). Although most species are located in subtropical waters, a significant number of these fish are found off U.S. waters. Most envenomations reported in the literature are from the lionfish and are due to aquarium enthusiasts carelessly handling these fish. In addition, there are reports of fishermen and people wading in shallow water being envenomated by members of this group. Severity of envenomation increases from members of *Pterois* to *Scorpoena* to *Synanceia*, with the stonefish representing the most severe and potentially lethal attack.

Pathophysiology

The venom apparatus in members of the Scorpaenidae consists of several dorsal, ventral, and anal spines, which are covered by a thin membrane. Envenomation occurs when the membrane is pushed back over the spine, compressing the venom glands at the base of the spine. The venom then travels along grooves in the spine and is injected into the victim. Generally, the pectoral fins (spines) do not contain venom sacs.

The venom is composed of several heat-labile proteins of high molecular weight. Treatment is based on the heat-labile nature of the toxins.

Treatment

As with all potentially lethal envenomations, attention should be focused on airway, breathing, and circulation (the ABCs of resuscitation). Spines should be removed gently when possible and bleeding controlled. If possible, the affected limb can be immersed in hot water (upper limit 114°F [45°C]) to help inactivate the toxin.

Administration of analgesia should be considered with appropriate orders from medical control and rapid transport to an appropriate medical facility should be accomplished. If possible, identification of the species involved may be helpful but should not delay care or transport of patient.

After the primary survey, secondary survey, and stabilization of vital signs have been

accomplished, pain control should be addressed. Most envenomations by members of the Scorpaenidae are extremely painful. Stonefish envenomation produces excruciating and often incapacitating pain, which may involve the entire limb as time passes. Use of local anesthetics (e.g., lidocaine) is usually effective, but occasionally parenteral narcotic agents may be required. Mild to moderate pain may persist in the affected area for days to weeks.

On physical examination, puncture wounds may be surrounded by darkened, necrotic tissue. Visible spines should be removed and the possibility of embedded spines should be explored. Plain film x-rays occasionally show a portion of the bony spine in the tissue, but ultrasound scan of the wound site should be considered. When a foreign body is detected, surgical removal and débridement is recommended.

The wound should be irrigated extensively with normal saline, and hot water immersion should be done, keeping the water temperature below 114°F (45°C). Tetanus prophylaxis is recommended. Use of antibiotics initially is controversial. Some experts suggest withholding antibiotic therapy until infection occurs. Other authors suggest giving antibiotics to cover the appropriate marine bacteria, including *Vibrio* species.

In cases of severe stonefish envenomation with life-threatening systemic symptoms, the use of stonefish antivenin may be considered. This is available from Australia's Commonwealth Serum Laboratories (CSL). As with all antisera developed from hyperimmunized equine serum, the risk of allergic reaction is very real and must be weighed against the clinical situation. In cases of serious envenomation, hospitalization with appropriate consultations should be considered.

Echinoderms

The phylum Echinodermata contains a large, diverse group of organisms divided taxonomically into four classes: Asteroidea (starfish), Ophiuroidea (brittle stars), Holothuroidea (sea cucumbers), and Echinoidea (sea urchins). They are characterized by the presence of pentamerous symmetry (five-sided body symmetry) and a hard calcific outer shell. In addition, these animals all have one or more of the following: sharp spines protruding from the body, pedicellaria (small grasping organs with miniature "jaws" at their ends), and tentacles. Only a few species of Asteroidea, Ophiuroidea, and Holothuroidea are capable of causing significant envenomation in humans.

Crown-of-Thorns Starfish

Within the Asteroidea group, the Crown-of-Thorns starfish *(Acanthaster planci)* causes the most serious envenomation in humans. This creature populates the Indo-Pacific regions ranging from the coast of East Africa and Madagascar to the coast of Central America. It is unlike other starfish in that it contains more than five separate arms (up to 20) and has thick, long spines on the aboral surface. If the spines are stepped on or handled roughly, numerous toxins are released into the victim.

Following envenomation by *Acanthaster,* there is often excruciating, intense burning pain at the puncture site. Divers may become disoriented after envenomation and as-cend too rapidly, risking serious injury. Other systemic symptoms reported include nausea, vomiting, headache, arthralgias, paresthesias, and muscular paralysis.

Sea Urchins

Envenomation from sea urchins (Echinoidea) occurs from contact with either the spines or the pedicellaria, depending on the species. Long-spined sea urchins such as *Echinothix* species release toxin into the victim when the integument overlying the spines is ruptured or from venom canals located in the spines when they are broken off in the victim's skin. Sea urchins such as *Toxopneustes pileolus* have pedicellaria, which are characterized by the presence of venomous fangs located on the delicate jaw-like tips of the pedicellaria. These produce the most serious envenomations in the sea urchin group and may continue to release toxin even after the pedicellaria have broken away from the animal.

Short-spined sea urchins such as *Phormosa* species cause envenomation when stepped on, disrupting the overlying integument. Other members in this group, such as *Astheriosoma* species and *Araesoma* species can deliver a severe sting from venom glands at the tip of the spines without actual puncture by these spines (Fig. 61.2).

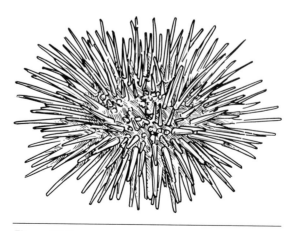

Figure 61.2
The sea urchin causes envenomation when stepped on.

Sea Cucumber

Sea cucumbers (Holothuroidea) are the least toxic of the echinoderms, unless ingested. Some species produce a toxin associated with the organs of Cuvier (thin, white on pink, tubular structure extruded from the anus when the animal is disturbed). The toxin causes skin irritation and may result in serious inflammation of the conjunctiva when the material gets into the eyes. This has occurred in divers trying to clear their masks in the presence of a disturbed sea cucumber.

Clinical presentation includes puncture wounds, which may manifest bleeding, ecchymosis, or surrounding erythema. In more severe cases, systemic symptoms may be present including nausea and vomiting, generalized weakness, respiratory distress, and paresthesias. Cardiac dysrhythmias and deaths resulting directly from echinoderm envenomation have not been documented, but there is at least one report of drowning secondary to the incapacitating pain produced by the sting of the flower sea urchin *(Toxopneustes pileolus)*.

Treatment

Prehospital treatment includes the administration of appropriate analgesia for the intense pain produced by various envenomations. Hot water immersion (temperature not to exceed 114°F [45°C]) has proven useful in echinoderm envenomations. Pressure immobilization, a technique for slowing circulation of a toxin while maintaining adequate blood flow to an extremity, may be attempted in cases of anaphylaxis.

After appropriate stabilization methods are used, care should be directed at appropriate pain control measures and wound care considerations. Puncture wounds often require débridement to assure removal of any foreign body. X-ray films may be useful to identify and locate radio-opaque foreign bodies such as spines, but occasionally ultrasound scans may be necessary. Copious irrigation and tetanus prophylaxis are always indicated. Long-term sequelae of echinoderm envenomation may include chronic pain, granuloma formation, wound infection, and wound tattooing from echinoderm pigment.

In the rare occurrence of ocular injury from the organs of Cuvier in holothuroids, a thorough slit lamp examination is warranted to rule out corneal injury or keratitis. Obtaining emergent ophthalmological consultation is recommended when evidence of eye injury is confirmed.

Snake Envenomation

Few other animals in nature evoke such emotion in humans as snakes. Throughout history they have been feared, taunted, and exploited. Some human cultures historically worshipped snakes and several religious groups continue to make snake handling an integral part of their services. The snake was symbolized as the embodiment of evil in the book of Genesis in the Bible and continues even in present time to fascinate and terrify human beings, especially with the thought of being bitten.

Historically, snakebite has been treated in many ways. Often, the results of treatment proved much more deleterious than the bite. Therefore, successful management of poisonous snakebites relies on a broad knowledge of these animals, including their venom, behavior, and natural history.

Epidemiology

There are approximately 45,000 to 50,000 snakebites reported annually in the United States. Of these, about 8,000 (17%) are from poisonous species and result in between 9 and 15 fatalities per year.

Throughout the world there are approximately 3,000 species of snakes including 400 that are considered poisonous. Poisonous snakes native to the United States are divided into two groups: the Crotalidae or pit vipers, and the Elapidae or coral snakes. The Crotalidae are represented by three genera: *Crotalus* and *Sistrurus* (rattle snakes), which include approximately 15 species, and *Agkistrodon*, which includes the copperhead (*Agkistrodon contortrix*) and the cottonmouth moccasin (*Agkistrodon piscivorus*). The Elapidae includes only two genera: *Micrurus* (North American coral snake) and *Micruroides* (Sonoran coral snake).

The highest bite rates are in North Carolina, Arkansas, Texas, Mississippi, and Louisiana, and most of these bites occur, as might be expected, between April and October. The incidence of snakebite is much higher in males with most of these bites occurring in the 18 to 28-year age group. The location of snakebite is most commonly on the extremities, with 80% on the finger or hand and approximately 15% on the ankle. Several reports have been published describing poisonous snakebites to the face and neck. In most of these, complications were severe, resulting in high morbidity. At least 40% of bites are a direct result of purposely handling the snakes and are thus classified as nonaccidental.

Identification of Poisonous Snakes

There are four identifying characteristics of the Crotalidae. These include vertical pupils, triangular-shaped heads, facial pits, and a single row of subcaudal scales. In addition to these characteristics, certain genera of Crotalids have distinctive rattles (*Crotalus* and *Sistrurus*). These are interlocking segments formed at the tail whenever the snake molts. Because many snakes molt several times per year, the number of rattles does not correlate necessarily with the age of the snake. The well-known buzzing sound produced by the rattlesnake occurs when the tail is vibrated from 20 to 85 cycles per second.

Identification of the members of the Elapidae native to the United States is relatively easy because they have bright yellow and red colors interrupted by black stripes. The sequence of these colors is important in identification, because the coral snakes always have red bordering on yellow, and "false coral snakes" such as the Mexican milk snake or king snake have red bordering on black. The saying "red touch yellow kill a fellow, red touch black, venom lack" is useful for remembering this sequence.

Snake Venom

Approximately 90% to 95% of the dry weight of snake venom is protein and is remarkably resistant to drying, temperature changes, and drugs. It contains enzymes and both toxic and nontoxic proteins. Included in these toxins are hydrolases, neurotoxins, cardiotoxins, and myotoxins.

Generally, the toxins are directed at immobilizing and killing the prey quickly, so that it cannot escape beyond the reach of the snake. Most toxins contained in snake venom produce their effect on the nervous system, thus paralyzing the prey, or on the cardiovascular system, causing cardiac arrest or hemorrhaging.

Pathophysiology

One of the predominant effects of snake venom in humans is related to the cytotoxic properties of the toxins on human endothelial cells and the resultant fluid leak secondary to this damage. In addition, snake venom acts directly on the coagulation system, resulting in platelet aggregation and affecting the clotting pathways involving fibrinogen.

Although venom-induced myonecrosis has been observed, this is usually not clinically significant because most human envenomations are subcutaneously delivered. Most human envenomations do not result in appreciable neurological effect. One exception to this is found in Mojave rattlesnakes (*Crotalus scutulatus scutulatus*) specific to certain geographical locations in the Southwest United States. Certain components of the venom of this snake have a direct effect on the presynaptic site of the neuromuscular junction, causing neuromuscular blockade.

Venom from the coral snakes is primarily neurotoxic, with fewer local effects than the Crotalid venom. Symptoms may be delayed for several hours and include weakness, fasciculation, cranial nerve abnormalities, and bulbar paralysis.

Fortunately, very few venomous snake bites in North America result in death. In fact, in one review of deaths in California, more people were killed by Hymenoptera species (i.e., bees, wasps) stings than by snakebites.

Clinical Presentation

The most common initial response of the victim is panic and fear. This often results in physical signs and symptoms not directly related to the envenomation, such as nausea, vomiting, tachycardia, diaphoresis, and extreme agitation. By far, the most common initial symptom is burning pain at the bite site accompanied by swelling and the development of ecchymosis.

Determining bite location and obtaining a complete history are important. Generally, bites on more distal parts of the body have less serious outcomes than those on the more proximal areas. In addition, children and elderly patients have worse outcomes.

The type of snake and biting mechanism are important. Pit vipers generally strike quickly with a single bite. Coral snakes, on the other hand, often chew at the bite site, thus injecting more venom. In as many as 25% of snakebites, there may be no envenomation, resulting in a "dry bite."

Other factors also must be considered, including the species of snake and the size of the snake. Larger snakes generally inject more venom, and the toxicity of venom varies with the species of snake. Generally, Elapid venom results in very little local effects but causes systemic neurotoxicity. Crotalid bites more often result in local tissue necrosis and hemorrhage.

Treatment

An accurate evaluation of snakebite severity is paramount in developing a treatment plan. Historically, the two most common methods of grading snakebite severity included the minimal-moderate-severe scoring method, and the Grade I to IV scoring method. Both methods are easily used and can estimate accurately the amount of antivenin required for treatment. In addition to these scoring methods, others with both clinical and research value have been developed, such as the Snakebite Severity Score.

Infection may complicate snakebites and requires the use of appropriate antibiotics. Pathogens found in the mouths of snakes include *Clostridium*, *Pseudomonas*, and *Staphy-lococcus* species. Several other complications have been reported to accompany snakebites including anaphylaxis, Guillain-Barré syndrome, cerebral infarct, and acute myocardial infarction.

Prehospital

Historically, venomous snakebite has been treated by various methods including electroshock, incision and suction devices, ice application, and tourniquets. Although use of a suction device such as the Extractor has shown some success in animal models, none of these methods have been shown to be of benefit in humans, and most actually increase morbidity. If prolonged transport time to an appropriate treatment facility is anticipated, the use of a mild constriction band may be used. It is generally placed 5 cm above the snakebite site and only occludes lymphatic flow while allowing arterial and venous blood flow to continue. This method has been widely accepted for certain Elapid snakebites in Australia and New Guinea.

In 1984, the American Association of Poison Control Centers and the American College of Emergency Physicians set forth a set of guidelines for the initial field treatment of poisonous snakebites. It was recommended that the patient be kept warm, comfortable, and reassured while the area of the bite was immobilized and placed below the level of the heart if possible. One should avoid stimulants (e.g., caffeine and alcohol) and be sure to remove all constrictions in the area (e.g., rings). Rapid and timely transport to the closest appropriate medical facility should then be arranged. Identification of the species of snake should be carried out, if possible.

Emergency Department

Following primary and secondary survey in the emergency department, the physician must determine if envenomation has occurred and must document the physical findings at the time of presentation. These include the area and level of swelling, including measurements of the limb circumference. The presence of any systemic signs and symptoms should also be noted.

Assuming evidence for envenomation is present, intravenous access should be established and baseline blood samples should be sent. This should include a complete blood cell count, electrolyte panel, blood urea nitrogen, creatinine, prothrombin time, partial thromboplastin time, fibrinogen, fibrin split products, urinalysis, and blood type and crossmatch. If the envenomation is potentially severe, a second intravenous line should be started with a large-bore catheter to facilitate the delivery of blood products or fluid boluses. An electrocardiogram should be done on all victims older than 40 years.

The state-of-the-art treatment for moderate to severe snakebite envenomation remains the use of antivenin and more recently Crofab. Because antivenin is prepared from horse serum, a major concern with its use is acute hypersensitivity reaction often leading to outright anaphylaxis. Even with a negative skin test, the initial dose should be diluted 1:4 or 1:5 in 5% dextrose/water and infused at only 50 to 75 mL/hour for the first 10 minutes. If no reaction develops, the remainder of the vials of antivenin are given intravenously over the next 2 to 4 hours. If the initial skin test is positive, and the administration of antivenin is required because of the severity of the bite, the patient should receive the antivenin in an intensive care unit equipped to treat anaphylaxis.

Antivenin is most effective if given within 4 hours of the bite. It is usually less effective after 12 hours but has been shown to reverse ongoing coagulopathy as far out as 24 hours. The amount of antivenin administered has varied over the last several decades, but the most recent recommendations are 5 vials for mild envenomation, 10 vials for moderate envenomation, and 15 or more vials for severe envenomation. Antivenin acts on a molecule-for-molecule basis; therefore, the same amount should be used in pediatric bites, because the amount of venom per bite would most likely be similar. Recently Crofab, crotalidae polyvalent immune FAB, has been approved for use in snake bites. It has fewer complications and

greater ease of administration. In many institutions it is replacing antivenin.

Although there has been at least one case of abruptio placenta complicating the administration of antivenin to a pregnant woman following snakebite, antivenin is not specifically contraindicated in pregnancy. If an allergic reaction does develop, however, 25 to 50 mg of ephedrine should be administered intravenously rather than epinephrine, which decreases uterine blood flow.

Finally, general wound care should be undertaken with consideration given to antibiotic prophylaxis and tetanus immunization status. Fasciotomy remains controversial in the treatment of snakebites. Because snake venom often may result in myonecrosis as a direct toxic effect, it can be difficult to distinguish between this effect and compartment syndrome secondary to swelling. Most of the studies have led to the belief that fasciotomy should be avoided unless there is objective evidence for compartment pressures exceeding 30 mm Hg persisting for longer than 1 hour.

In conclusion, principles guiding the appropriate management of venomous snakebite should center on early recognition of the signs of significant envenomation and the early use of antivenin when appropriate. Prehospital care should be limited to general support measures, avoidance of ice application, tourniquet application, and incision and suction of the wound. Continuous evaluation of the bite area and recognition of systemic signs and symptoms are paramount to successful management.

Spider Bites

The class Arachnida, which includes the spiders and scorpions, contains the largest number of venomous organisms known. Of the approximately 20,000 species of spiders, only a few produce any significant envenomation in humans and only two are of any importance in the United States. These are the black widow spider *(Lactrodectus mac-*

tans) and the Missouri fiddle-back spider or brown recluse *(Loxosceles reclusa)*.

Black Widow Spider

There are many species of *Latrodectus* throughout the world, but the predominant black widow species in the United States is found in all states except Alaska. The female is glossy black in color with the familiar red "hour-glass" shape on the ventral side. The male *L. mactans* is not poisonous, is much smaller in size, and is brown in color.

Black widows are generally reclusive and shy and bite only when disturbed or agitated while guarding egg sacs. The venom of the black widow consists of systemic toxins including a mammalian neurotoxin and latrotoxin, which induces release of neurotransmitters from nerve terminals.

Clinical Presentation

Patients with black widow bite may complain of local pain at the time of the bite or may not know they have been bitten. There may or may not be local erythema and tenderness at the bite site. In cases of moderate to severe envenomations, systemic symptoms appear within 30 to 60 minutes after the bite with severe muscle spasms, primarily involving the abdomen and back. There may also be generalized weakness, ptosis, fasciculations, salivation, priapism, agitation, diaphoresis, nausea, and vomiting.

Abdominal pain may mimic appendicitis, and a careful history is important. In extremely rare cases, symptoms may progress to respiratory muscle paralysis and death. Most symptoms resolve within 4 or 5 days, although muscle pain may persist for weeks.

Treatment

Treatment includes the liberal use of muscle relaxants (benzodiazepines). The use of calcium gluconate has historically been recommended, although at least one recent study of 163 cases showed no beneficial effect. Latrodectus antivenin is available for extremely serious cases but is rarely recommended.

Brown Recluse Spider

The brown recluse spider is a small venomous spider found primarily in the Midwest and southeastern parts of the United States. Almost never producing fatal envenomations, the brown recluse bite often results in local and occasionally severe tissue necrosis. The adult spider measures only 0.25 to 0.5 inches in length and has a distinctive fiddle-shaped design on the dorsal surface. They are active at night and live in dark warm recesses of old buildings, basements, and garages. They too are shy, and bite only when disturbed or pressed against the body.

Clinical Presentation

Venom from the brown recluse spider contains eight or nine major factors, including hyaluronidase and various cytotoxins. Patients bitten by the brown recluse usually have immediate local symptoms characterized by a stinging sensation at the bite site that may last for hours. The area quickly becomes red and swollen and develops a dark violaceous-centered lesion and subsequent necrosis. After 2 or 3 weeks the eschar sloughs, leaving a necrotic based crater at the envenomation site.

Systemic involvement can result in hemolysis and rhabdomyolysis. In very rare cases, thrombocytopenia, disseminated intravascular coagulation, renal failure, and death have been reported.

Treatment

Treatments have historically been many and varied, including electroshock therapy, hyperbaric oxygen (HBO), steroids, and surgery. In fact, reviewing the care of 112 patients, brown recluse bites do well with only routine wound care, with no deaths or serious complications.

Suggested Readings

Auerbach PS. Marine envenomations. *N Engl J Med* 1991;325:486–493.

Auerbach PS. *Wilderness medicine: management of wilderness and environmental emergencies,* 3rd ed. St. Louis: Mosby-Year Book, 1995: 1346–1350.

Clark RF, Wethern-Kestner S, Vance MV, Gerkin R. Clinical presentation and treatment of black widow spider envenomation: a review of 163 cases. *Ann Emerg Med* 1992;21:728–787.

Cunningham P, Goetz P. *Venomous and toxic marine life of the world,* 2nd ed. Houston: Pisces Books, 1996:77–91.

Gold BS, Barish RA. Venomous snakebites: current concepts in diagnosis, treatment, and management. *Emerg Med Clin North Am* 1992;10:249–267.

Halstead BW, Auerbach PS. *Dangerous aquatic animals of the world: a color atlas: with prevention, first aid and treatment.* Princeton: Darwin Press, 1992:45–49.

Owenby C. Pathology of rattlesnake envenomation. In: Tu AT, ed. *Rattlesnake venoms.* New York: Marcel Dekker, 1982:163–209.

Russell FE, Carlson RW, Wainschel J. Snake venom poisonings in the United States: experiences with 550 cases. *JAMA* 1975;233: 341–344.

Sullivan JB, Wingert WA, Norris RL. North American venomous reptiles. In: Auerbach PS, ed. *Wilderness medicine.* St. Louis: Mosby-Yearbook, 1995:680–709.

Williamson JA, Fenner PJ, Burnett JW. *Venomous and poisonous marine animals: medical and biological handbook.* Sydney, AU: NSW University Press, 1996:88–97, 106–117, 312–325.

Wright SW, Wrenn KD, Murray L, Seger D. Clinical presentation and outcome of brown recluse spider bite. *Ann Emerg Med* 1997; 30:28–33.

The Laboratory in Emergency Medicine

Laboratory Medicine

Peter W. Emblad, MD, FACEP

Up to 85% to 90% of medical diagnoses are made on the basis of history and physical examination alone. To help confirm diagnoses and to help with unknown diagnoses, we rely on ancillary tests, including laboratory tests and imaging modalities. The utility of these tests is dependent on the person ordering and interpreting the results. Occasionally, the laboratory tests reveal a result that makes the diagnosis easy (i.e., a K^+ of 7.4); however, this seems to be the exception rather than the rule. Usually, the results deviate from the normal parameters only slightly (if at all) and are helpful only if the person interpreting the results is knowledgeable enough to extract the relevant information. The causes of laboratory abnormalities are legion, and a complete discussion is beyond the scope of this book. However, a basic understanding of laboratory medicine is as vital for the emergency physician as any other topic and can aid not only in the diagnosis of disease entities but also in guiding therapy appropriately. You are encouraged to consult a comprehensive book on laboratory medicine for a more complete understanding when necessary.

Complete Blood Cell Count

White Blood Cell Count

An increase in the white blood cell (WBC) count is usually seen with infection and inflammation. Leukocytosis, an increase in the number of total WBCs, is more commonly seen with bacterial rather than viral infection but remains nonspecific. Acute bacterial infection may lack leukocytosis in 10% to 45% of the cases in normal hosts and much more commonly in individuals that are immunocompromised (i.e., human immunodeficiency virus [HIV]-positive or diabetic individuals).

In addition to an increase in the total neutrophil count, there is often an increase in the number of immature cells, most notably the band and early segmented neutrophils. This is known as a "left shift," after the maturation diagram by Schilling in which the more immature cells were on the left and the more mature cells on the right. There is a large variation between technologists' interpretation of band counts; one study of 15 technologists reading the same smear on two different occasions showed a band count that varied from 3% to 27%. There is still debate about which is a more reliable sign of infection, an elevated neutrophil count or an elevated total WBC count. One study found that total neutrophil count was elevated more often than WBC count in documented urinary tract infections (UTIs) and bacteremia, whereas the reverse was true for appendicitis and acute cholecystitis.

Causes of leukocytosis (increased WBC count) include the following:

- Infections (both localized and generalized)
- Inflammation (i.e., vasculitis)
- Myeloproliferative disorders
- Tissue necrosis (i.e., burns, myocardial infarction [MI])
- Physiological stress (e.g., exercise, emotional stress, pain)
- Medications (especially steroids)

Causes of leukopenia (decreased WBC count) include the following:

- Infection (especially overwhelming sepsis or viral)
- Underlying hematopoietic disease (aplastic anemia, agranulocytosis)
- Immunosuppression
- Medications (antibiotics, chemotherapeutic agents)

White Blood Cell Differential

The relative percentages of the different subtypes of WBCs allow the clinician to further narrow the differential diagnosis. A *lymphocytosis* is most commonly seen with viral infections but can also be seen with certain chronic medical conditions (Crohn's disease, ulcerative colitis, vasculitis, Addison's disease, and thyrotoxicosis). A *monocytosis* is more frequently seen in association with disseminated tuberculosis (TB), subacute bacterial endocarditis (SBE), lymphomas and carcinomas, and certain infections not commonly seen in the United States (typhoid fever, malaria, and leishmaniasis).

Eosinophilia can be seen with allergic conditions (asthma, hay fever), parasitic infestations (roundworms, flukes), skin diseases (pemphigus, psoriasis), and some chronic medical conditions (Hodgkin's disease, polyarteritis nodosa, and sarcoidosis) and in people undergoing peritoneal dialysis.

Red Blood Cell Indices and Anemia

For the emergency physician, the hemoglobin (Hg) and hematocrit (Hct) are the most useful of the red blood cell (RBC) indices, because they are often more indicative of an acute process than are the other indices. Generally, a hypochromic, microcytic anemia is probably from iron deficiency, and macrocytic anemia is from vitamin B_{12} or folic acid deficiency or drug-induced bone marrow toxicity. A normochromic, normocytic anemia is likely from acute blood loss (what most emergency physicians are mainly concerned with), hemolytic anemia, and anemia of chronic disease. Patients with an acute hemorrhage can have a marked drop in their RBC count but may have a normal Hct. Remember that the Hct measures only the relative percentage of blood volume that is composed of erythrocytes. In an acute bleed, the percentages do not change, only the whole volume. With time, as cell production increases, and if patients are given crystalloid fluids, the Hct can change dramatically.

Hematocrit and Hemoglobin

Some physicians speak in terms of Hg, some in terms of Hct. Which is better, and what is the difference? Hg is the amount of Hg in a given volume of whole blood. Hct is the percentage of blood volume that is composed of erythrocytes. The Hct is usually about three times the value of the Hg. Disproportions occur primarily when the cells are markedly abnormal in size or shape.

Platelets

Platelets are found throughout the vascular distribution and are used for clot formation. Low platelet levels (thrombocytopenia) can be caused by either decreased production (i.e., myeloproliferative disorders) or increased destruction. Increased destruction can be seen in the following conditions:

- Infections (SBE, HIV, septicemia, mononucleosis)
- Drug-induced destruction (penicillins, heparin, sulfonamides, quinine)
- Idiopathic thrombocytopenic purpura (ITP)
- Thrombotic thrombocytopenic purpura (TTP)
- Disseminated intravascular coagulation (DIC)
- Systemic lupus erythematosus (SLE)
- Toxemia of pregnancy
- Renal insufficiency

An increase in the number of platelets (thrombocythemia) can be caused by many conditions including the following (percentage of cases are given in parentheses):

- Myeloproliferative diseases (13%)
- Malignancy (13%)
- Infections (31%)
- Recent surgery (especially splenectomy) (19%)
- Chronic inflammation (i.e., irritable bowel syndrome [IBS], collagen disease)
- Trauma, massive hemorrhage, thrombus

In addition, up to 50% of people with new onset thrombocythemia were later found to have malignancy.

Electrolytes

In the strictest sense of the word, electrolytes refer to sodium, potassium, and chloride only. When most medical personnel refer to electrolytes, they mean the previous three in combination with carbon dioxide (CO_2), blood urea nitrogen (BUN), creatine, and glucose (occasionally with calcium, magnesium, and phosphate as well). The electrolyte panel offers a wealth of information about the homeostatic mechanisms occurring in the human body.

Sodium

Sodium is the most abundant cation in the extracellular fluid and a major contributor to serum osmolality. Sodium is needed for regulation of serum osmolality, acid-base regulation, and maintenance transmembrane electronic potential. The kidneys are the primary control point of sodium homeostasis. Hyponatremia can present with any or all of the following: muscle cramps, agitation, nausea, depressed sensorium, hypothermia, seizures, Cheyne-Stokes respirations, and depressed deep-tendon reflexes. Hyponatremia is further classified as hypovolemic, euvolemic, and hypervolemic. Hypovolemic hyponatremia is seen in vomiting, diarrhea, burns, hypoaldosteronism, and hyperglycemia, among others. These patients often manifest signs and symptoms of dehydration. Syndrome of inappropriate secretion of antidiuretic hormone (SIADH), hypothyroidism, glucocorticoid deficiency, or drug side effects (i.e., diuretics, narcotics, acetaminophen, nonsteroidal antiinflammatory drugs [NSAIDs], and chlorpropamide) most commonly cause euvolemic hyponatremia. Hypervolemic hyponatremia is the most common form of hyponatremia and is usually due to congestive heart failure (CHF), cirrhosis, nephrotic syndrome, renal failure, and psychogenic polydipsia.

Hypernatremia is less common than hyponatremia but is associated with significant mortality. Patients with hypernatremia commonly present with neurological symptoms ranging from restlessness to hyperreflexia and, ultimately, death. As with hyponatremia, patients with hypernatremia can be hypovolemic, euvolemic, or hypervolemic. Hypovolemic hypernatremia is commonly seen when patients have high fluid losses (i.e., from sweating) and replace the lost fluid with hypotonic solution. Euvolemic hypernatremia is seen in diabetes insipidus. Hypervolemic hypernatremia is usually iatrogenic from intravenous (IV) infusions of hypertonic solutions.

Potassium

Potassium is the major intracellular cation and is important in regulating excitability of nerves and muscles. For the emergency medicine physician, this is one of the most important electrolytes because minor fluctuations, in either direction, can affect the cardiovascular system. Potassium is regulated chronically by the kidneys (via aldosterone stimulated secretion) and acutely by hydrogen ion and potassium ion countertransport. This means that as the pH of the intravascular space decreases, hydrogen ions are shuttled into the cells and potassium ions out of the cells. This also explains why bicarbonate is effective in treating hyperkalemia.

Hypokalemia can occur from intracellular shifting (as explained previously) or from increased total potassium loss from the body. The more common causes include alcoholism, anorexia, vomiting, diarrhea, diuretics, corticosteroids, and Cushing's syndrome. Patients with hypokalemia present with electrocardiographic (ECG) changes (and possible associated arrhythmias), cramps, and weakness.

Hyperkalemia is most commonly caused by renal failure (and the ensuing loss of excretion), potassium intake, cell lysis (true or laboratory error), Addison's disease, and acidosis. Patients commonly present with muscle weakness (if early or mild) or cardiac rhythm disturbance, hypotension, and cardiac arrest (if high or late).

Chloride

Chloride does not play a very active role in physiological homeostasis. As the most abundant extracellular anion, it neutralizes positive charges. It also helps maintain osmolality by following sodium passively. Chloride values are also affected by bicarbonate concentrations because of the bicarbonate-chloride exchange that occurs in the proximal renal tubules, such that there is a net excretion of chloride in metabolic acidosis. Chloride values can thus be used to confirm fluid and acid-base abnormalities.

Hypochloremia commonly occurs secondary to increased gastric losses (emesis, nasogastric suction, histamine-2 [H_2] blockers) or to metabolic acidosis with the resultant shift. Hyperchloremia is seen in dehydration

and renal failure. The signs and symptoms of hyperchloremia and hypochloremia are those of dehydration or acid-base abnormalities, rather than from the alteration of the actual chloride.

Blood Urea Nitrogen

BUN is one of the more useful parameters in the electrolyte panel. One can assess renal function, hydration status, and level of catabolism using the BUN level. Although the acronym is for *blood* urea nitrogen, it is actually the serum level that is measured not the amount in the RBCs. Urea is filtered through the glomerulus, after which about 50% is reabsorbed. This is dependent on the rate of flow through the renal system, such that the slower the filtration (i.e., in dehydration and hypotension), the more time is available for reabsorption and the higher the BUN. Generally speaking, a low BUN is usually only seen in dilutional (i.e., acute fluid overload) states, although severe malnutrition or liver failure may also depress the level. A high BUN (i.e., azotemia) has numerous causes, which are best categorized as prerenal, intrarenal, or postrenal.

Prerenal causes are either because of decreased renal perfusion (as in CHF, shock, hypovolemia) or increased protein breakdown (i.e., gastrointestinal [GI] bleed, burn, muscular injury, increased protein intake). Intrarenal causes of a high BUN include acute renal failure and chronic renal dysfunction (from entities such as glomerulonephritis, diabetes, pyelonephritis). Postrenal causes of azotemia refer to obstruction anywhere along the urinary tract. Certain drugs also have been known to affect the BUN, either via interrupting protein breakdown (corticosteroids, tetracycline) or via nephrotoxicity (NSAIDs, cyclosporine, aminoglycosides, nitrofurantoin, and others).

Creatinine

Creatinine is formed from the breakdown of creatine in muscle and is freely filtered through the kidneys with no reabsorption (a small amount is actively secreted, although that amount is negligible). Serum creatinine level is thus a good approximation of the glomerular filtration rate (GFR). The creatinine level reflects alterations in normal kidney function, although it takes time to reach a new steady state. For example, a patient with renal artery thrombosis will effectively decrease the kidney function by 50% and will reach a new steady-state serum creatinine level (double normal) in about 1 day. A sudden decline in renal function by 90% would take 4 days to reach steady-state level. Generally, the maximum rate of increase of serum creatinine is 1 to 2 mg/dL/day. Generally, an increased serum creatinine level reflects a decreased GFR. This, in turn, can be caused by decreased blood flow (dehydration, low output states), decreased excretion (obstruction or intrinsic renal dysfunction), or increased creatinine production (i.e., vigorous exercise, hyperthyroidism, muscular dystrophy, ingestion of roasted meats). Some drugs can also increase the creatinine level by inhibiting tubular secretion (especially cimetidine, aspirin, trimethoprim, and spironolactone). Other substances that can falsely elevate the creatinine level include cefoxitin, cephalothin, dopamine, levodopa, lidocaine, and ketones. An elevated glucose level can also elevate the creatinine level, although this can be corrected for by subtracting 0.5 mg/dL from the creatinine level for every 100 mg/dL elevation in the plasma glucose.

Blood Urea Nitrogen-to-Creatinine Ratio

The BUN-to-creatinine ratio can be used, in combination with the isolated BUN and creatinine values, to give a more complete insight into the underlying disease process. A normal ratio is 12 to 16 in healthy individuals. Often, a BUN/Cr ratio greater than 20:1 suggests prerenal causes, whereas a ratio from 10:1 to 20:1 is more suggestive of a renal dysfunction. An increased ratio with a normal creatinine is seen in prerenal azotemia (often dehydration, CHF, or blood loss), increased muscle catabolism, GI hemorrhage, and high protein intake. An increased ratio with a high creatinine level is

seen in postrenal azotemia (especially obstructive uropathy). A decreased ratio with a decreased BUN is observed in acute tubular necrosis, starvation, liver disease, SIADH, pregnancy, and after dialysis. A decreased ratio with an increased creatinine is seen in rhabdomyolysis and in renal failure in muscular individuals. Aberrant or inappropriate ratios are seen in patients with diabetic ketoacidosis (DKA) and with cephalosporin therapy.

Glucose

Hypoglycemia is diagnosed by not only the glucose level but also by the presence of signs and symptoms suggestive of hypoglycemia, with improvement with administration of glucose. Postprandial (or reactive) hypoglycemia is common and can be seen in healthy persons. Other causes of low glucose level include liver failure, CHF, renal disease, diabetes, certain drugs (especially insulin, sulfonylureas, aspirin, alcohol) and endocrine tumors. Hyperglycemia is most commonly seen in association with diabetes but can also be seen as a result of stress (i.e., acute MI, sepsis) or dehydration (hyperosmolarity), as a side effect of drugs (especially steroids), and with certain genetic disorders (e.g., cystic fibrosis).

Liver Function Tests

The term *liver function test* (LFT) is a misnomer, because it really consists of those tests that are more indicative of biliary tract disease and hepatic inflammation rather than a measurement of the true function of the liver. To accurately measure the liver function, it is necessary to examine the products that are produced by the liver, namely albumin, fibrinogen, proteins, and vitamin K-dependent clotting factors. The most sensitive of these tests is the prothrombin time (PT). This is a measure of the vitamin K-dependent clotting factors. Hence, any drug (e.g., warfarin) or disease (e.g., malabsorption) that interferes with vitamin K uptake and its utilization influences this variable. In the absence of these conditions, a prolonged PT is indicative of liver failure and carries a poor prognosis.

Alkaline Phosphatase

Alkaline phosphatase (AP) is found in many tissues, including the liver, bone, WBCs, intestines, placenta, and kidneys. Thus, the AP level would be expected to be higher in pregnancy (from the placenta), during an adolescent growth spurt, in patients with neoplasia, or in patients with a healing fracture (from osteoblastic activity). In the presence of cholestasis, the liver actually synthesizes more AP, and this is released into the blood because it cannot pass through the bile. Hence, AP level can be used as a confirmatory test of biliary system obstruction and hepatic inflammation but is not very specific to the liver. Generally, the degree of AP elevation is reflective of the severity of the obstruction. In fact, elevation *less than* three times normal is evidence against complete extrahepatic obstruction, and most likely represents intrahepatic obstruction. It is possible to measure isoenzymes of AP for greater specificity, but this is usually time intensive and is not commonly done in the emergency setting. It should be noted that oral contraceptive pills could cause a cholestatic picture with elevated levels of AP and gamma-glutamyl transpeptidase (GGT) but with normal levels of aminotransferases. This usually resolves quickly with cessation of the pills. AP concentration rises transiently for the first 2 to 3 hours after a fatty meal, which may give an erroneous result.

Gamma-Glutamyl Transpeptidase

In contrast to AP, GGT is not found in bone or placental tissues and hence is specific to the liver. GGT is an enzyme found in the biliary tree. It is often elevated with alcoholic liver disease and is usually elevated with pancreatitis, both acute and chronic. For reasons that are not entirely clear, GGT level can be elevated 4 to 5 days after an acute MI. This is the most sensitive screening test for alcoholism. GGT is markedly elevated in chronic active hepatitis (often greater than seven times normal), more so than in acute hepatitis.

Aminotransferases

Although both of the aminotransferases (aspartate aminotransferase [AST], formerly serum glutamic oxylate transaminase [SGOT], and alanine aminotransferase [ALT], formerly serum glutamic pyruvate transaminase [SGPT]; also known as transaminases) are found primarily in the liver, AST is not as specific as ALT. AST is found in lung, cardiac, pancreatic, hepatic, and renal tissues. Thus, AST levels may be elevated in nonhepatic injury, such as acute MI, pulmonary embolus, muscular injury, and hemolysis. Nevertheless, the aminotransferases are very sensitive in reflecting hepatic inflammation and necrosis. Very high concentrations are often seen with acute viral hepatitis and drug or toxin reactions. AST levels may be falsely elevated in diabetic ketoacidosis and with certain drugs (erythromycin, ampicillin, and methyldopa). The level of ALT, in addition to being a marker of hepatic inflammation, is often slightly elevated in obesity.

The ratio of AST/ALT can be used to determine etiology, because a ratio greater than 1.5 is suggestive of alcoholic liver disease or intrahepatic cholestasis. Acute viral hepatitis usually presents with a ratio of less than 0.65, and a ratio much higher than that is a sign of poor prognosis.

Lactate Dehydrogenase

Lactate dehydrogenase (LDH) is found in most human tissues and therefore is not very specific to the liver or biliary tree. However, elevated concentrations are observed in hepatitis, biliary obstruction, and hemolysis. The total LDH level can be fractionated to isoenzymes that are more specific for liver, cardiac, muscle, or brain disease. This fractionation is time consuming and hence is not useful for the emergency physician. In many hospitals, routine LFTs do not include LDH.

Bilirubin

The Hg from destroyed RBCs is converted in the spleen to unconjugated (indirect) bilirubin. Unconjugated bilirubin is carried by albumin to the liver, where it is conjugated with glucuronic acid to become conjugated (direct) bilirubin. This, in turn, is excreted into the gut, where it is converted into urobilinogen, some of which is reabsorbed and excreted either back into the gut or into the urine, accounting for the color of both materials. Obstruction of this process can lead to an increase in the total bilirubin count. Determination of which is more elevated, direct or indirect bilirubin, can clarify the point of obstruction. Clinical jaundice is visible when total bilirubin concentration is 2 to 4 mg/dL and higher. In infants, a high level of unconjugated bilirubin can lead to kernicterus (bilirubin encephalopathy). An elevated unconjugated bilirubin level is seen in hemolysis, congenital abnormalities (Gilbert's syndrome and Crigler-Najjar), and hepatic or posthepatic jaundice. An elevated conjugated bilirubin is not very specific in identifying the point of obstruction. Nevertheless, if the conjugated bilirubin makes up the majority of the elevated bilirubin level, the obstruction is more likely posthepatic. Similarly, if the conjugated bilirubin makes up a smaller percentage of the total bilirubin level, the obstruction is probably hepatic.

Ammonia

Protein is digested in the intestinal tract where it is converted to ammonia. This, in turn, is absorbed into the bloodstream and transported to the liver, where it is converted to urea. Ammonia has been postulated to be the toxin responsible for hepatic encephalopathy. Although it is often elevated in patients with cirrhosis and mental status changes, it is not entirely clear if this is the only responsible toxin (if at all). Nonetheless, an elevated ammonia level is associated with hepatic encephalopathy, Reye's syndrome, inborn disorders of the urea cycle, high-protein diets, and use of the drug valproic acid.

Amylase

Amylase is an enzyme secreted by the pancreas and salivary glands to break down starch into individual glucose molecules. Serum levels increase within 2 to 6 hours after the onset of pancreatitis, peak after 12 to 30 hours, and usually return to normal within 3 to 5 days. An increase lasting longer than 7 to 10 days suggests a pancreatic cancer or pseudocyst. An increased amylase level (but less than three times normal) is seen in acute alcoholic intoxication (10% to 40%) and acute abdomen resulting from perforation or ischemia. An elevated amylase level can also be seen in the following conditions: penetrating ulcers, gallstones, alcoholism, hypercalcemia, hypertriglyceridemia, vasculitis, infections, and pregnancy. In addition, many drugs can cause pancreatitis, including cimetidine, estrogens, furosemide, methyldopa, metronidazole, nitrofurantoin, ranitidine, steroids, thiazides, and valproic acid.

Lipase

Lipase is a pancreatic enzyme used to digest fats into triglycerides and fatty acids. Lipase is predominantly of pancreatic origin; therefore, an elevated lipase level is more specific than an elevated amylase level to the diagnosis of pancreatitis. The sensitivity and specificity of lipase for acute pancreatitis is 86% and 99%, respectively (compared with 95% and 88% for amylase). The onset, rate of rise, and decline mimic that of amylase.

Suggested Readings

Bakerman S, Bakerman P, Strausback P. *Bakerman's ABC's of interprertive laboratory data*, 3rd ed. Myrtle Beach, SC: Interpretive Laboratory Data, 1994.

Ranson, JHC. Etiological and prognostic factors in human acute pancreatitis: a review. *Am J Gastroenterol* 1982;77:633–638.

Ravel R, ed. *Clinical laboratory medicine.* St Louis: Mosby, 1995.

Traub S, ed. *Basic skills in interpreting laboratory data*, 2nd ed. Bethesda, MD: American Society of Health System, 1996.

Wallach J. *Interpretation of diagnostic tests*, 6th ed. Boston: Little, Brown and Company, 1992.

Wynn TE. Identification of band forms, *Lab Med* 1984;15:176.

CHAPTER **63**

Arterial Blood Gases

Peter W. Emblad, MD, FACEP, Corey M. Slovis, MD, FACP, FACEP

Chapter Outline

The arterial blood gas (ABG) test can be an extraordinarily important and useful blood test. A great deal of data, including acid-base status, oxygenation, ventilation, and more, can be gleaned from this single test. Evaluating the results may create anxiety in the student because of the complexity of data. This chapter gives you an easy-to-use and logical approach to analyzing the ABG result. This chapter is not meant to be all-inclusive but will enable you to tackle the basics of analyzing an ABG result with confidence.

The Three-Step Approach

Step 1: Acidosis or Alkalosis

This is the easiest part. If the pH is 7.35 or lower, the primary disease component is an acidosis. If the pH is 7.45 or higher, the primary disease is an alkalosis.

Step 2: Metabolic or Respiratory

There are two ways to determine whether the primary disease is metabolic or respiratory. The easiest way to memorize it is based on whether the partial pressure of carbon dioxide (pCO_2) and pH change in the same or opposite direction.

Look at the pCO_2. A normal pCO_2 is about 40 mm Hg. If the pCO_2 moves in the same direction as the pH (i.e., both are elevated, or both are depressed), then the disturbance is primarily metabolic. If the pCO_2 moves in the opposite direction as the pH, the disturbance is primarily respiratory. For example, if the pH is 7.15 and the pCO_2 is 60 mm Hg, the patient has a respiratory (the pH and pCO_2 are in opposite directions) acidosis (the pH is below 7.35). So far, this is pretty easy, right?

Now that you memorized the "same way = acidosis and opposite way = alkalosis" rule, a better way to understand the concept is as follows: If the pCO_2 drives the pH, it is respiratory, if not, then it is metabolic. Thus, if the pCO_2 drives the pH, then as the pCO_2 goes down, the pH should rise (respiratory alkalosis); if the pCO_2 rises, then it should drive the pH down (respiratory acidosis). In metabolic processes, the pCO_2 follows the pH in the same direction.

Step 3: If Respiratory, Is It a Pure Process?

Memorize this: For every 10 points that the pCO_2 changes, the pH should move 0.08 (±0.02) in the opposite direction. Close your eyes and repeat this a couple of times until you know it. Thus, if the ABG reveals a pH of 7.24 and the pCO_2 is 60 mm Hg, you have an acidosis (see step 1), which is respiratory (see step 2), and it is a pure process (the pCO_2 is elevated by 20 mm Hg, and the pH is depressed by 0.16 [2 × 0.08]). Now, look at this result and figure out the underlying disturbance (cover the area below it with paper so you cannot cheat): pH = 7.58 and pCO_2 = 20 mm Hg.

This is a pure respiratory alkalosis. If you did not get that, go back and think it through again. If you did, congratulations; you are well on your way.

If it is not a "pure process," then clearly some other disturbance must exist. Therefore, if the pH is lower than it "should be" in a pure process, a metabolic acidosis also exists. If the pH is higher than it should be, then a metabolic alkalosis must also exist.

Try to analyze another result: pH = 7.16 and pCO_2 = 60 mm Hg.

This is a respiratory acidosis with a metabolic acidosis. The pH should be 7.24 because the pCO_2 is elevated by 20 mm Hg; hence, the pH should be depressed by 0.16 (2 × 0.08). It is lower than that; thus, another acidosis must be present.

Applying Steps 1 to 3: Test Examples

Does this make sense so far? Let us do some examples. Work these out rather than skipping ahead, as it will reinforce the concepts; remember, you want to have to read this chapter only once. Cover the text below each problem.

1. pH is 7.58 and pCO_2 is 20 mm Hg

This is an alkalosis (pH greater than 7.45); it is respiratory (pH and pCO_2 move in opposite directions); and it is a pure process (pCO_2 down by 20 mm Hg, pH should go up by 0.16 ± 0.2).

2. pH is 7.16 and pCO_2 is 70 mm Hg

This is a pure respiratory acidosis. Let us go step by step: (a) acidosis, (b) the elevated pCO_2 drove the pH down, and (c) the pCO_2 is up by 30 mm Hg (from 40 mm Hg) and should push the pH down by 0.24 (3 × 0.08), and it did!

3. pH is 7.50 and pCO_2 is 20 mm Hg

This is a primary respiratory alkalosis with a primary metabolic acidosis: (a) alkalosis; (b) pCO_2 is down, which drove the pH up (respiratory); (c) pCO_2 down by 20 mm Hg should equal pH up by 0.16 to 7.56; however, note that it is only up to 7.50. Another way to say it is that the pH is lower than it should be if only the elevated pCO_2 was involved. Therefore, there must be a metabolic acidosis bringing the pH down from expected.

4. pH is 7.55 and pCO_2 is 30 mm Hg

This is an alkalosis that is both respiratory and metabolic. The pH should be 7.48, but it is higher, so there is a concomitant metabolic alkalosis. Let us go step-by-step: (a) alkalosis; (b) pCO_2 down drove the pH up (respiratory); (c) however, it should go to 7.48; thus, it is more alkalotic than it should be, and, therefore, a metabolic alkalosis is also present.

When you have both an ABG sample and a set of electrolytes values (basic metabolic profile [BMP], sequential multiple analysis [SMA-7]), you can do more calculations, for example, to see if a patient is hyperventilating enough in the face of an acidosis and check for a "hidden process."

The 5 Steps to Metabolic Acid-Base Disorders

Step 1: Check All Basic Metabolic Profile Values (Not Just What Is Abnormal)

Step 2: Calculate the Anion Gap

So far, we have covered the respiratory part of the ABG. If in the second step of the ABG analysis, you find that you have a metabolic disturbance, then you will need to look at the electrolytes (or BMP) to calculate the anion gap (AG). The AG is easily calculated (memorize this):

$$AG = Na - (HCO_3 + Cl)$$

where Na is sodium, HCO_3 is bicarbonate, and Cl is chloride. A normal gap should be 12 ± 2, although there is some variation between laboratories, depending on technique.

An elevated AG means there is a metabolic acidosis, regardless of the pH or HCO_3 level.

What causes a metabolic acidosis? By now you should know this as a reflex. If not, time to learn it. The causes of AG acidosis can be remembered by the mnemonic MUDPILES:

M = Methanol (in windshield washing fluid)

U = Uremia (usually AG above 100)

D = Diabetic ketoacidosis (DKA) and alcoholic ketoacidosis (AKA)

P = Paraldehyde (not used anymore for seizures)

I = Iron or isoniazid (INH)

L = Lactic acidosis

E = Ethylene glycol (in antifreeze)

S = Salicylates

While we are at it, let us learn the causes of "normal gap" or hyperchloremic metabolic acidosis. They can be remembered by the mnemonic HARDUP:

H = Hyperventilation

A = Acids (given intravenously to reverse metabolic alkalosis), Addison's disease, or carbonic anhydrase inhibitors

R = Renal tubular acidosis (RTA)

D = Diarrhea

U = Ureterosigmoidostomy

P = Pancreatic fistula or drainage

Step 3: Apply the Rule of 15

This rule is for metabolic acidosis, as are the rules that follow. If a metabolic acidosis exists, the HCO_3 + 15 (±2) mEq/L should equal both the pCO_2 and the last digits of the pH (±0.07). For example, if the HCO_3 is 12 mEq/L, the pCO_2 should be 27 (12 + 15) mm Hg and the pH should be 7.27. The rule of 15 allows you to predict what the respiratory compensation should be and what the pH and pCO_2 should be if pure respiratory compensation exists. If the numbers do not add up this way (i.e., the rule of 15 is broken), then a second process other than respiratory compensation exists.

Another way to think of this is as a new "set-point" for seeing whether the patient's pCO_2 is

1. Appropriately depressed because of compensation only

2. Too low (i.e., a secondary respiratory alkalosis exists)

3. Too high (there is a secondary primary respiratory acidosis)

For example, take the following ABG: pH = 7.35, pCO_2 = 35 mm Hg, and HCO_3 = 20 mEq/L.

This is an acidosis, it is a primary metabolic (pCO_2 and pH move in the same direction), and it is appropriately compensated by the respiratory alkalosis (20 + 15 = 35).

Let us try another: pH = 7.14, pCO_2 = 32 mm Hg, and HCO_3 = 10 mEq/L

This is a metabolic acidosis as the primary disorder (both the pH and pCO_2 go in the same direction). The expected pCO_2 is 25 (±2) mm Hg (HCO_3 of 10 + 15 = 25 ± 2 mEq/L), but the pCO_2 is higher than it should be, meaning there is a superimposed primary respiratory acidosis (or lack of enough hyperventilation). This could be an old person who is septic and is starting to tire out from hyperventilating so long. This person could go into respiratory failure and need emergent intubation. This ABG result gives you early life-saving information before a patient deteriorates and "crashes."

Let us do one more: pH = 7.32, pCO_2 = 20 mm Hg, and HCO_3 = 10 mEq/L

The expected pCO_2 is 25 (±2) mm Hg, but the patient's pCO_2 is too low according to the rule of 15; thus, this patient is hyperventilating more than should be seen from compensation. Thus, this is a primary metabolic acidosis plus a primary respiratory alkalosis.

The rule of 15 is obviously very effective, but it does not work if the HCO_3 is below 10 mEq/L. In these situations, the pCO_2 should be expected to go only to 15 mm Hg by the time the HCO_3 has fallen to 5 mEq/L. Stated differently: As the bicarbonate falls below 10 mEq/L and approaches 5 mEq/L, the pCO_2 should go to 15 mm Hg.

Let us do an example of this: pH = 7.04, pCO_2 = 20 mm Hg, and HCO_3 = 5 mEq/L.

This is obviously a primary metabolic acidosis because the pH is way down and so is the CO_2 (See how easy this is?). However, the pCO_2 should not be 20 (5 + 15) mm Hg as in the previous examples; it should be 15 mm Hg because the HCO_3 is significantly below 10 mEq/L. Therefore, this is a metabolic acidosis and a respiratory acidosis.

Step 4: Check the Delta Gap

The delta gap (also known as the "gap of the gaps") checks for a "hidden metabolic process." It looks to see if a second nongap metabolic acidosis exists or if a superimposed metabolic alkalosis exists. The delta gap is basically this: The fall in bicarbonate should be equal to the rise in the AG.

For example: Na = 140, Cl = 102, HCO_3 = 19 mEq/L

Here the AG is 19, and the HCO_3 is 19 mEq/L. The AG has gone from an absolute upper limit of normal of 14 (remember, normal is 12 ± 2) to 19, or a change of 5. The HCO_3 has gone from a normal 24 to 19 mEq/L, or a change of 5 mEq/L. The change of AG to bicarbonate is 5:5 = 1:1. Thus, there is no hidden process. Beware, because the AG is ± 2 and the change in HCO_3 is ± 2 mEq/L, only call a second process if the bicarbonate is more than 4 mEq/L different than it should be (e.g., 5 mEq/L or more).

Let us do an example: Na = 141, Cl = 110, and HCO_3 = 9 mEq/L.

The AG is 22 (141 − (110 + 9) = 22), and that is 8 above the upper limit of normal (22 − 14 = 8). Therefore, the bicarbonate should be 8 mEq/L below normal, but it

is not (24 − 9 = 15 mEq/L). It is much lower than that. Now think, what could make the bicarbonate lower than it should be? The answer is another metabolic acidosis. Thus, there is both a wide-gap metabolic acidosis and a normal-gap metabolic acidosis.

One last example, and then you can relax your brain: Na = 145, Cl = 100, and HCO_3 = 20 mEq/L.

Here the AG is 25; thus, the change from upper limit of normal is 11 (25 − 14 = 11). The HCO_3 is only 4 mEq/L below normal. It should have fallen by 11 mEq/L to about 13 mEq/L. Thus, the HCO_3 is too high for this gap. Thus, there must be a wide-gap metabolic acidosis and a superimposed normal-gap metabolic alkalosis.

Step 5: If There Is an Unexplained Metabolic Acidosis Check the Osmolar Gap

Generally, an elevated osmolar gap indicates that there has been an ingestion of a toxic alcohol (i.e., methanol or ethylene glycol). It is calculated as follows:

$$Osmolarity = 2 \times Na + Glucose/20 + BUN/3 + ETOH/4.$$

You also have to send blood for a calculated osmolarity. The osmolar gap is the difference between the calculated and the measured. It would not be prudent to send an osmolarity on every intoxicated patient in the emergency department just to check for coingestions, because they are relatively rare. However, because you checked the delta gap on the patient and found an underlying hidden process, your suspicion went up, you ordered the test, made the diagnosis, instituted treatment, and saved a life.

Oxygen Saturation

Now you are done with the hard part of ABGs, figuring out the acid-base disturbances. The rest of the information that is given in the ABG result is the pO_2 and the oxygen (O_2) saturation, both of which can give a tremendous amount of information if used correctly. You ask, why not just use the pulse oximeter? Before answering that question, let us review some basic respiratory physiology.

Oxygen is carried in the red blood cells (RBCs) from the lungs tightly bound to hemoglobin (Hg) and dissolved in the plasma. The amount of oxygen that is dissolved in the plasma is directly proportional to the partial pressure of the oxygen (Henry's law). Thus, when we give someone 100% oxygen, the partial pressure increases and more O_2 is dissolved in the blood. However, most of the oxygen is still bound to Hg. How tightly the Hg binds the O_2 is dependent on how saturated the Hg already is and where the oxygen saturation curve is. Remember that increased temperature, acidosis, and increased pCO_2 shift the curve to the right, causing the O_2 to be less tightly bound to the Hg (easier to unload). This is as it should be, considering that as the RBCs get to the peripheral tissues, the pCO_2 is higher, resulting in early unloading of the oxygen to the tissues.

Conversely, the curve shifts to the left in the face of alkalosis, low pCO_2, and hypothermia, causing the Hg to hang on more tightly to the O_2. Now we can answer the question of how the pulse oximeter helps us.

Pulse Oximetry

The pulse oximeter works by emitting light at two wavelengths and measuring how much of that light is absorbed. Deoxygenated blood absorbs more light at 660 nm, and oxygenated blood absorbs more light at 940 nm. The pulse oximeter is accurate to ±2% when the saturation level (sat) is above 70% to 80%, after which it becomes less reliable. In patients with reduced blood flow from anemia or shock, the pulse oximeter does not detect as much blood, and hence is less reliable.

Percent Oxygen

Percent oxygen is the value obtained from an ABG sample. This is a calculated rather than measured value, based on the partial pressure of oxygen (pO_2) (which is calculated based on the 1% to 2% of the oxygen dissolved in the plasma in normal states). Therefore, the pulse oximeter is theoretically better than the percent O_2 obtained from an ABG sample, in a normal patient.

Special Clinical Situations

The previous information applies to most patients. However, you should be aware of some special situations that make interpretations difficult.

Carbon Monoxide Poisoning

Carbon monoxide (CO) binds to Hg much more tightly than oxygen and displaces oxygen. All CO is bound to Hg not circulating in the plasma. When CO binds to Hg, carboxyhemoglobin is formed. Carboxyhemoglobin absorbs maximally at the same wavelengths as oxyhemoglobin. This means that the pulse oximeter reading will be erroneously high, as will the percent oxygen in the ABG sample (because it is calculated from the dissolved oxygen). The only true way to measure the amount of CO in the blood is by co-oximetry, which uses four wavelengths instead of two and is able to distinguish CO from O_2.

Anemia

The pulse oximeter is accurate until the hematocrit (Hct) is below 20. After that, use the values obtained from an ABG sample.

Hypotension and Shock

The readings on the pulse oximeter may be falsely low because of poor arterial pulsation and vasoconstriction. This also applies to hypothermic patients for the same reason.

Asthma

The pulse oximeter is an accurate reflection of the amount of oxygen in asthmatic patients, but that should not give you false security. The problem in asthma is not oxygenation but rather with ventilation with possible CO_2 retention. As the asthmatic patient tires, CO_2 rises, but oxygen is still high. This is especially deceptive because most asthmatics are being treated with β-agonists through a nebulizer assisted by supplemental oxygen. In these patients, the pulse oximeter reading may be normal until they go into respiratory arrest. These patients must be monitored clinically not via pulse oximeter.

Arterial Versus Venous pH

ABG samples hurt more, are harder to get, and cause more adverse outcomes than venous blood gas (VBG). However, we still do them for many situations. If you are monitoring a patient's pH, a VBG may be just as effective.

In normal patients:

The normal pH by ABG is 7.40 ± 0.02

The normal pH by VBG is 7.38 ± 0.02

Thus, Venous pH = Arterial pH – 0.02

However, in hypotensive patients, there is an increased venous versus arterial pH difference.

In sick, acidotic patients who are not in shock:

Venous pH = Arterial pH – 0.03 to 0.05

Therefore, in most cases in which pH is the main clinical indicator of concern, including DKA and AKA, a venous gas is just as effective. However, in cases of severe hypotension and shock, an ABG sample is more reliable.

A good rule of thumb is as follows: If you merely want pH, and the patient is not in shock, just use a venous pH. You should use venous pH values in following the pH of patients with DKA, AKA, or alcohol intoxication. You can also use the venous pH values for carbon monoxide poisoning, because arterial equals venous for CO. Never use the venous gas to follow ventilation (pCO_2) or oxygenation (pO_2), because the arterial and venous results can be very different.

Summary

Be systematic, and you will be a star.
For ABGs: acidosis or alkalosis.

Metabolic or respiratory

If respiratory, for every 10 pCO_2 units is the pH up or down by 0.08?

For BMPs: Check the numbers.

Check the gap.

Apply the rule of 15.

Check the delta gap.

Consider calculating the osmolar gap.

Suggested Readings

Breen PH. Arterial blood gas and pH analysis. Clinical approach and interpretation. *Anesthesiol Clin North Am* 2001;19:885–906.

Ventriglia WJ. Arterial blood gases. *Emerg Med Clin North Am* 1986;4:235–251.

Wilson R, Barton C. Blood gases: pathophysiology and interpretation. In: Tintinalli JE, Kelen GD, Stapczynski JS, et al, eds. *Emergency medicine: a comprehensive study guide*, 4th ed. New York: McGraw-Hill, 1985:108–117.

64

Culturing Fluids

Kevin G. Wheeler, MD

Cultures are often used to diagnose diseases caused by bacteria, viruses, fungi, or parasites. Bacterial, fungal, and parasitic cultures are especially useful in guiding antimicrobial treatments. This chapter covers the common types of cultures obtained in emergency medicine and their indications and usefulness.

Blood Cultures

Indications

It is the standard of care to obtain blood cultures in any ill-appearing patient who has a fever with no readily identifiable source. Fever is defined differently in different institutions, but in general, a temperature higher than 101.5°F (38.5°C) is considered a fever. When there is a readily defined source of the fever, such as pharyngitis, otitis media, or an obvious viral syndrome, cultures are usually not necessary. However, for the febrile patient in whom you suspect a systemic bacterial infection, blood cultures are useful. The utility of blood cultures varies depending on the source. For example, in pneumonia, blood cultures may be the only method of identifying an organism and have a rela-

tively high yield, making them useful, particularly in very ill patients. Conversely, in cellulitis, an organism is identified in fewer than half the cases. In pyelonephritis, blood cultures are often positive, but the information can be obtained simply by a urine culture, making blood cultures unnecessary. Blood cultures are especially useful in patients who cannot localize symptoms, such as the very young or the very old.

Methods

Blood cultures should be drawn by peripheral phlebotomy from two separate locations. The skin should be sterilized with povidine iodine (Betadine) and allowed to dry before obtaining the blood specimen. The phlebotomist should use sterile technique. Two bottles are inoculated with each blood sample, one bottle for aerobic bacteria and one bottle for anaerobic bacteria. The bottles are then incubated for 24 to 72 hours, and any colonies of bacteria are identified. Sensitivities to common antibiotics are also performed to help guide antibiotic administration. Fungal cultures are drawn in the same manner, but usually only one tube is required. Viral blood cultures and parasitic blood cultures are used only in rare circumstances.

Results and Clinical Implications

Any growth of pathogens from a blood culture is abnormal. Blood cultures can be positive for virtually any organism, but the most commonly isolated organisms include *Strep-*

tococcus species, *Staphylococcus* species, *Enterococci*, *Salmonella*, *Candida*, *Pseudomonas*, *Bacteroides*, *Clostridia*, and *Haemophilus influenzae.*

Positive blood cultures and the subsequent sensitivities guide the choice of which antibiotic is most useful for a patient. However, it is important to realize that blood cultures may be falsely positive, especially for skin contaminants such as *Staphylococcus epidermidis.* The overall clinical picture and the likelihood that a patient is bacteremic should be considered in all positive blood cultures.

Patients who inject intravenous (IV) drugs or who have indwelling IV catheters (e.g., pic lines or central lines) deserve special mention. These patients are at much higher risk of contracting blood infections from skin flora such as *Staphylococcus* species. Fever and significant illness in these patients should be treated as bacteremia until proven otherwise. *Staphylococcus* bacteremia in any patient places that patient at high risk of endocarditis (infection of the heart valves), but this subset of patients is at especially high risk. A positive blood culture for *Staphylococcus* species or any other organism in these patients should be treated with extended IV antibiotics, often for weeks at a time.

Urine Cultures

Indications

A urine culture should be obtained in any acutely ill patient complaining of dysuria, in patients with pyelonephritis, or those with complex medical problems. A culture may also be useful in patients with fever and no obvious source of infection who cannot localize their own symptoms, such as infants or elderly patients with dementia.

Methods

Urine cultures are obtained by "clean catch" or by catheterization. Clean-catch samples are obtained by wiping the opening to the urethra (from front to back) in women, or the tip of the penis in men, three times with three separate sterile wipes. The first few milliliters of urine are then discarded, and a midstream specimen is deposited in a sterile cup. A catheter specimen is obtained by inserting a catheter into the bladder using sterile technique. A clean-catch urine has a higher rate of false positives than a catheterized specimen.

Results and Clinical Implications

A growth less than 10,000 organisms per milliliter is considered a negative result. Any growth greater than 10,000 organisms per milliliter is considered positive. Urine cultures may be used to guide antibiotic treatment. Although most outpatient urinary tract infections are treated empirically with a broad-spectrum antibiotic, inpatient infections, those from indwelling catheters, and infections in patients who are immune compromised are often more complicated; knowing the specific pathogenic organism and its sensitivities can be useful. Antibiotic-resistant *Escherichia coli* and *Enterococcus* species are extremely common, especially in institutionalized patients; therefore, cultures and sensitivities are extremely important in guiding therapy for these patients. Rarely, a fungal species such as *Candida* may grow from a urine culture. When *Candida* or bacteria that usually grow on the skin (normal skin flora) grow from a urine culture, it is up to the clinician to decide the clinical significance of the culture result.

Cerebrospinal Fluid Cultures

Indications

Cerebrospinal fluid (CSF) from virtually all lumbar punctures (LPs) is sent for bacterial cultures. Except in special cases, most LPs in the emergency department are performed to rule out meningitis or subarachnoid hemorrhage. If the patient shows signs of meningitis, treatment is initiated immediately with broad-spectrum antibiotics. Culture results serve only to confirm the diagnosis and guide subsequent treatment. An LP with cultures should be performed on any patient with fever and neck stiffness, change in mental status, or unexplained headache.

Methods

CSF cultures are obtained by performing an LP in the usual sterile manner. The back is prepared with povidine iodine solution, which should be allowed to dry before performing the procedure. A needle is then inserted into the space surrounding the spinal cord, and CSF is obtained. Bacterial cultures are routinely obtained, and viral and fungal cultures can be requested (see Chapter 72).

Results and Clinical Implications

Any patient with suspected meningitis should be treated immediately with empiric broad-spectrum IV antibiotics. CSF cultures are used to guide later therapy and prognosis. CSF cultures are also used to differentiate among bacterial, viral, or fungal meningitis.

Oropharynx Cultures

Indications

Oropharyngeal cultures are obtained to differentiate between bacterial and viral throat infections. A culture may be indicated for any patient with complaints of a sore throat and fever who has signs of bacterial pharyngitis and for whom the clinician would like to differentiate bacterial from viral throat infection.

Methods

To obtain a throat culture, a swab is taken from the both sides of the posterior oropharynx. Some institutions use "rapid *Strep* screen." This is a specific type of culture that informs the clinician quickly, usually in minutes, whether a throat infection is caused by Group B streptococci. The rapid screen is useful when positive; however, it has a high false-negative rate and does not rule out streptococcal pharyngitis. A full throat culture grows any organism found on the swab.

Results and Clinical Implications

Throat cultures are most often positive for *Streptococcus* species if they are positive at all. Streptococcal infection is treated with oral or parenteral penicillin. Other culture results may be treated according to the type of organism and its sensitivities.

Urethral and Genital Cultures

Indications

Urethral cultures in men and cervical cultures in women are obtained for any patient in whom there is a suspicion for a sexually transmitted disease (STD). In men, these diseases may manifest as dysuria or penile discharge, or they may be asymptomatic. In women, there may be vaginal discharge, dysuria, pelvic pain, or no symptoms. It is imperative to culture anyone for whom there is suspicion of an STD, because treatment is necessary to stop the spread of these diseases and to minimize the risk of complications.

Methods

In men, a culture is obtained by inserting a small swab into the urethra. In women, the culture is obtained from the cervical os. The cultures take 24 to 72 hours to grow.

Results and Clinical Indications

A normal result is no growth whatsoever. Most positive cultures grow out *Neisseria gonorrhea* or *Chlamydia trachomatis*. In any patient who has a high suspicion of an STD, treatment for these two organisms should be started empirically, before the culture results are final. If the cultures are negative and the clinical suspicion is low, treatment is not necessary.

Suggested Readings

Barker L, Burton JR, Ziere PD, et al. *Principles of ambulatory medicine*, 4th ed. Baltimore: Williams & Wilkins, 1995.

Barton S, ed. *Clinical evidence*, Issue 5. London: BMJ Publishing Group, 2002.

Braunwald E, Fauci AS, Kasper DL, et al. eds. *Harrison's principles of internal medicine*, 15th ed. Columbus, OH: McGraw-Hill, 2001.

Fischbach F. *A manual of laboratory and diagnostic tests*, 7th ed. Philadelphia: Lippincott, Williams & Wilkins, 2003.

Roberts JR, Hedges JR. *Roberts: clinical procedures in emergency medicine*, 4th ed. Philadelphia: WB Saunders, 2003.

Tintinall JE, Kellen GD, Stapczynski JS, et al. eds. *Emergency medicine: a comprehensive study guide*, 5th ed. Columbus, OH: McGraw-Hill, 1999.

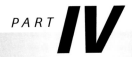

Procedures in Emergency Medicine

CHAPTER **65**

Pain Management, Analgesia, and Sedation

Amy Kontrick, MD

Pain is defined as an unpleasant sensation associated with actual or potential tissue damage that is mediated by specific nerve fibers to the brain, where its conscious appreciation may be modified by various factors. Pain is one of the most common reasons patients present to the emergency department (ED). In addition, many patients experience pain in the ED during the performance of common therapeutic and diagnostic procedures. Therefore, treating a patient's pain in a timely and safe fashion should be a primary goal of the emergency physician.

The goal for managing pain involves all levels of the health care team. Treatment should begin at triage and continue throughout the patient's treatment course. The goals of treating pain are simple; however, they often are not met.

The goals of pain treatment in the ED are as follows:

Choose a safe and effective agent.

Choose the appropriate dose, route, and frequency.

Choose an agent with a rapid onset.

Choose an agent that is easy to administer in the ED.

Choose an agent that is effective and appropriate for discharge.

Despite the simplicity of these goals and the frequency of the complaint of pain, significant failure in its treatment exists. In a study published by Wilson and Pendleton in the *American Journal of Emergency Medicine,* 56% of patients with acute pain of various etiologies received no pain medication in the ED. Of those who did receive pain medication, almost 70% waited more than an hour and nearly 40% waited more than 2 hours. This and many other studies illustrate the inadequate and untimely attention given to pain control.

The reasons for inadequate analgesia are multifactorial: lack of objective measures of pain, relying on inappropriate measures of pain, fear of creating addiction, and fear of obscuring a diagnosis. In addition, ethnicity, age, and other patient characteristics may lead to inadequate treatment of pain.

Central Nervous System Pain Transmission and Perception

To choose an effective and appropriate treatment, one must understand how pain is transmitted, perceived, and modified at the brain and spinal cord level of the central nervous system (CNS). Figures 65.1 and 65.2 illustrate the essential pathways.

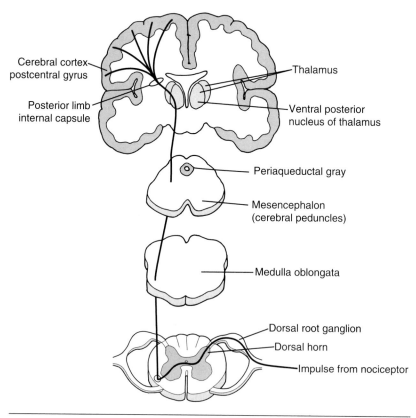

Cerebral cortex-postcentral gyrus

Thalamus

Posterior limb internal capsule

Ventral posterior nucleus of thalamus

Periaqueductal gray

Mesencephalon (cerebral peduncles)

Medulla oblongata

Dorsal root ganglion

Dorsal horn

Impulse from nociceptor

Figure 65.1
The lateral spinothalamic tract carries pain stimuli to the brain.

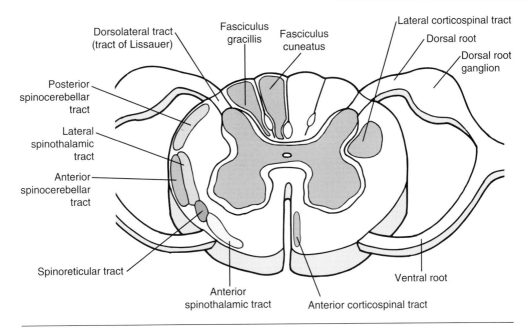

Figure 65.2
Cross section of the spinal cord showing all the major tracts.

Pain Receptors

The transmission of a painful stimulus begins when the threshold of pain is surpassed in specialized free nerve endings of sensory nerves. These specialized peripheral pain receptors are often referred to as nociceptors. These nerve fibers begin the transmission of pain by converting noxious stimuli into electrical activity that can then be transmitted by afferent neurons. A noxious stimulus can be thermal, chemical, or strong mechanical pressure. Tissue damage is believed to cause the release of chemical mediators. These mediators include prostaglandins, leukotrienes, bradykinin, serotonin, substance P, thromboxanes, and platelet-activating factors. These mediators can initiate pain transmission and can cause the sensitization and recruitment of other nerve fibers.

Each sensory neuron has a cell body located in the dorsal root ganglia and a receptor located in the periphery. These receptors are located in dermatomes specific to that neuron. Painful stimuli are transmitted from the periphery to the spinal cord via A-delta and C fibers. The A-delta fiber is a finely myelinated fiber that is responsible for the transmission of fast, localized sharp pain sensation. The C fibers are unmyelinated and conduct more slowly than the A-delta fibers. They are responsible for producing a more continuous pain sensation. These fibers then synapse in the dorsal horn of the spinal cord.

Afferent Sensory Fibers of the Spinal Cord

The dorsal horn of the spinal cord is the gray matter located in its posterior aspect. It is composed of six layers called lamina. Each lamina receives specific afferent sensory and central input and therefore is involved not only in integration of pain stimuli but also its modification and relay. After synapsis in the dorsal horn, pain information is relayed to the brain via the spinothalamic and spinoreticulothalamic tracts.

The spinothalamic tract and the spinoreticulothalamic tracts carry information from the contralateral side. The spinothalamic tract has synapses in the thalamus with third-order neurons continuing to the somatosensory cortex. It is responsible for information regarding the location, quality, and intensity of pain. The spinoreticulothalamic tract synapses in the reticular formation and then the thalamus and some neurons ultimately end in the cortex. It is unclear whether there are distinct differences in function and pain transmission between the two tracts, but it is postulated that the spinoreticulothalamic path may transmit noxious stimuli from deep, visceral structures and it is also perceived as diffuse pain.

Efferent Sensory Fibers of the Spinal Cord

The sensation of pain is modified by actions controlled by certain descending systems. This may occur in the periventricular areas and in parts of the medulla. It is believed that serotonin and norepinephrine play a role in modification.

Pain Perception

Although the threshold needed to initiate nociception is the same in everyone, the perception and reaction to pain is unique. Pain perception is influenced by many factors. The factors studied and found to have the greatest influence on perception are psychological, physiological, and sociological makeup. Therefore, ethnicity, age, and previous experiences all play a part in the makeup of the patient and therefore his or her unique pain experience.

Physiological Effects of Pain

Pain causes many physiologic derangements that may have potentially severe consequences on the patient. These include sympathetic and endocrine stimulation. Sympathetic stimulation leads to increases in systolic and diastolic blood pressure, stroke volume, and oxygen consumption. This can cause problems for patients with limited cardiovascular reserves. Splinting can occur with abdominal and chest pain, leading to a decrease in tidal volume, vital capacity, functional residual capacity, and ultimately resulting in atelectasis. Pain also causes a decrease in gastrointestinal (GI) motility. The endocrine system can mount a "flight or fight" response in which excess cortisol and epinephrine are secreted. Poorly treated pain also leads to muscle spasm, which can further exacerbate pain. In addition, poorly treated or untreated pain can

cause sleep disturbances and anxiety. It is now also believed that some changes that occur during an episode of acute pain, if untreated, may lead to the development of chronic pain.

Clinical Assessment of Pain

Assessing a patient's pain is a difficult and often subjective task. The pain experience is different for each patient and is mediated not only by the anatomic physical nature of the stimulus but also by complex psychosocial aspects. These can include previous pain experiences, cultural background, and the patient's psychosocial makeup. No test or physiological parameter can objectively assess a patient's degree of pain or pain relief.

Attempts to use vital signs including blood pressure, pulse, and respiratory rate as ways of measuring pain have not proven useful. Changes and/or initial derangements in vital signs, facial expressions, or body position do not adequately assess the degree of the patient's pain or the degree to which the patient may feel pain. They also do not adequately reflect the degree of relief a patient may or may not feel following treatment.

Pain Scales

Because the patient's reporting of pain is considered the most accurate form of assessment, many tools and scales are available to the physician as aids. Several aids are depicted in Figure 65.3. A simple descriptive scale can be used. Here the patient is asked simply to describe the pain, ranging from none to the worst possible pain. This may be limited by age and/or language barrier.

Numeric Pain Scale

A numeric pain scale can be presented to the patient at the bedside. The patient is asked to quantify his or her pain on a scale of 0 to 10, with 0 being no pain and 10 being the worst pain possible. The patient may give a verbal response, mark a chart, or if necessary communicate with fingers. Although not as

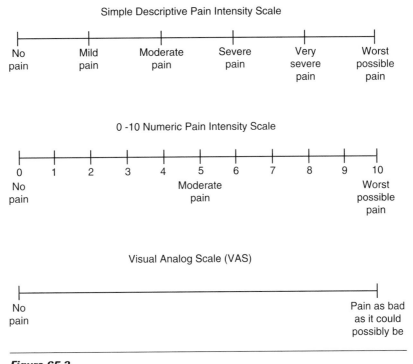

Figure 65.3
Pain assessment scale. (Reproduced with permission from Hinnant DW. Psychological evaluation of testing. In: Tollison, CD, ed. *Handbook of pain management*, 2nd ed. Baltimore: Williams & Wilkins, 1994:25.)

accurate as the visual analog scale (VAS), the numerical rating scale is a simple bedside test that is easy to use.

Visual Analog Scale

The VAS is a 10-cm line on which one end represents no pain and the other represents the worst pain imaginable. The patient is asked to rate pain by either pointing to the line or making a mark on the line. Frequent reassessments can be done by having the patient make new marks on the line in response to treatment. This method has advantages over others in that it is rapid and easy to use, is reproducible, can be used at the bedside, and can be used in children age 6 and older.

Although scales provide a good aid to pain assessment, the only truly accurate measurement of a patient's pain and its response to treatment is the patient's own report. Therefore, frequent reassessments must be performed during the course of treatment. Documentation of assessment and

reassessment provides important data for success of or implementation of new protocols.

Pharmacological Treatment of Pain

Opioid Analgesia

The history of the use of opium and its derivatives dates back to the Babylonians. Derivatives of opium came to be known as opiates. Recently, however, with the development of synthetic and semisynthetic compounds, the term *opioid* is used to describe any substance, natural or synthetic, with morphine-like effects.

Morphine is the prototype of the opioids and is often the "gold standard" against which other analgesics are measured and studied. Today there exist natural, semisynthetic, and synthetic opioids. The phenanthrenes include morphine, codeine, hydromorphone, oxycodone, and hydrocodone. Phenylheptylamines include methadone and

Table 65.1.

Opioid receptor subtypes and their actions

Receptor	Agonist	Antagonist	Physiological Actions	Pharmacological Effects
Mu$_1$	Normorphine	Naloxone	Analgesia, temperature control	
Mu$_2$	Morphine Sufentanil	Naloxone	Respiratory depression, constipation, growth-hormone release	Miosis, bradycardia, hypothermia, indifference to environment
Delta	Enkephalins		Euphoria, brain reward	
Kappa	Metenkephalin B-endorphin Dynorphin		Stimulation, ataxia, locomotor activity	Miosis, sedation
Epsilon	B-endorphin		Heat-related anti-nociception	
Sigma	Pentazocine Phencyclidine Ketamine	Haloperidol	Psychomimetic effects	Mydriasis, respiratory stimulation, tachycardia, delirium

Reproduced with permission from Solomon GD. Analgesic medications. In: Tollison, CD, ed. *Handbook of pain management,* 2nd ed. Baltimore: Williams & Wilkins, 1994:156, 158.

propoxyphene. The phenylpiperidines include meperidine, fentanyl, alfentanil, and sufentanil.

Pharmacology of Opioids

All opioids produce analgesic effects by binding to certain receptors: μ, κ, and δ. Table 65.1 lists the receptor subtypes. The μ-receptor is responsible for analgesia, euphoria, respiratory depression, and physical dependence. The δ- and κ-receptors produce analgesia at the spinal level. All three receptors are found throughout the brain and spinal cord. They are found in high concentration in the dorsal horn of the spinal cord.

By binding to these receptors, opioids cause presynaptic voltage-gated calcium (Ca) channels to close, which decrease transmitter release. Postsynaptically, they cause the opening of K$^+$ channels, thereby decreasing function of the nerve. At the spinal cord level, opioids inhibit release of excitatory neurotransmitters from primary afferents and inhibit dorsal horn pain transmission neurons. Therefore, opioids can alter pain transmission and perception at all levels.

The opioids are ideal agents for management of moderate to severe pain in the ED. They are available via multiple routes and have a rapid onset and relatively predictable side effect profile. These agents can be administered intravenously (IV), intramuscularly (IM), orally (PO), rectally (PR), subcutaneously (SC), transdermally, and transmucosally. They are absorbed rapidly. Many oral forms are subject to significant first-pass effect in the liver, which decreases their potency somewhat. Morphine-equivalent doses of commonly used opioids are shown in Table 65.2. Most opioids are converted to "polar metabolites" and then excreted renally. This may lead to higher levels in patients with renal disease. They are highly lipophilic and may accumulate in fatty tissue, which can cause prolonged elevated levels after repeated dosing.

The hemodynamic effects of opioids require some specific attention. All opioids have sympatholytic effects, potentially causing bradycardia and hypotension. Patients with underlying hypovolemia may be more susceptible to this effect. In addition, some opioids cause the release of histamine that may contribute to their cardiovascular effects.

Adverse Effects

All opioids are capable of causing many of the known side effects. Some agents produce

Table 65.2.

Morphine equivalent dose of opioids

Drug	Dose (mg) IM	Dose (mg) PO	Duration (hours)
Morphine	10	30	4–5
Hydromorphone	1.5	7.5	4–5
Codeine	130	200	4–6
Hydrocodone	–	5–10	4–8
Methadone	10	20	4–5
Levorphanol	2	4	4–5
Oxycodone	15	30	4–5
Oxymorphone	1	6	4–5
Meperidine	75	300	1–3
Pentazocine	60	180	
Nalbuphine	10	–	
Butorphanol	2	–	
Buprenorphine	0.4	0.3 (sl)	

IM, intramuscular; PO, by mouth; sl, sublingual.
Reproduced with permission from Solomon GD. Analgesic medications. In: Tollison, CD, ed. *Handbook of pain management*, 2nd ed. Baltimore: Williams & Wilkins, 1994:158.

certain side effects to a greater or lesser extent and are noted with that specific agent. Opioids exert their effects on the GI system, leading to decreased motility and constipation. They can increase smooth muscle tone, which can lead to biliary tract spasm. Increased smooth muscle tone in the genitourinary (GU) system can lead to ureteral spasm and increased bladder tone. They can cause nausea and vomiting through activation of brainstem chemoreceptors. All opioids have the ability to cause respiratory depression through brainstem receptors. This may be more pronounced and significant in patients with underlying lung disease.

Parenteral Opioids

MORPHINE

Morphine can be administered IV, IM, PO, and SC. IV administration is probably the most useful route in the ED as it allows for rapid onset, easier titration, and painless repeat dosing. When administered IV, its onset of action occurs within a few minutes and lasts approximately 3 to 4 hours. Dosing guidelines for morphine and other common opioids are shown in Tables 65.3 and 65.4. It

is metabolized by the liver to an inactive metabolite that is then excreted renally. Morphine does not have a direct cardiodepressant effect but does cause histamine release. Histamine release can lead to hypotension, urticaria, and bronchospasm in susceptible patients. The hypotension caused by histamine release is secondary to arteriolar and venous dilatation and is nonimmunological.

By increasing tone throughout the GI tract and decreasing the force of peristalsis, morphine can cause delayed gastric emptying and constipation. In addition, morphine has also been postulated to increase sphincter of Oddi tone, which can exacerbate biliary colic. If clinically significant, this can often be overcome by higher doses of morphine.

MEPERIDINE

Meperidine is a synthetic opioid. Meperidine has become one of the most commonly used and misused opioids. Despite its obvious disadvantages when compared with morphine and other opioids, it is still widely used. Meperidine has one eighth of the potency of morphine and has a shorter duration of action (approximately 2 to 3 hours).

Table 65.3.

Dosing guidelines for parenteral opioids

Drug	Route[a,b]	Dosage	Comments
Morphine	IV	Titrate 2–5-mg increments q3–10 min	Preferred first-line agent in
		Peak analgesia in 10–20 min	most situations
		Average = 10 mg q3–4h	
	IM/SC	Average = 10 mg q3–4h	
Fentanyl	IV	Titrate 25–50 µg increments q2–3 min	Ideal for short procedures
		Peak analgesia in 3–5 min	No histamine release
		Duration 30–60 min	
	IM/SC	Not suitable for the emergency department	
Meperidine (Demerol)	IV	Titrate 12.5–50.0-mg increments	Risk of unique CNS toxicity with repeated dosing
		Peak analgesia in 5–10 min	
		Average = 100 mg q2–3h	IM/SC injection is very irritating to tissue
	IM/SC	Average = 100 mg q3h	
Hydromorphone (Dilaudid)	IV	Titrate 0.5–1.0-mg increments	High solubility benefits SC injection
		Peak analgesia in 5–15 min	
		Average = 1.5 mg q3–4h	
	IM/SC	Average = 1.5 mg q3–4h	
Butorphanol (Stadol)	IV	Titrate 0.5–2.0-mg increments	Mixed agonist-antagonist
		Peak analgesia in 4–5 min	May be preferred in bilary colic
		Average = 2 mg q3–4h	
	IM/SC	Average = 2mg q3–4h	

Note: Intervals are approximate. Individual patients may require dosing either more or less frequently.
Caution: Dosing may need to be adjusted in the elderly patients weighing less than 50 kg and those with renal or hepatic insufficiency.
[a] CNS, Central nervous system; IM, intramuscular; IV, intravenous; SC, subcutaneous. Intravenous route is preferred for faster onset and ability to titrate to effect; q, evenly.
[b] Rapid administration increases incidence of respiratory depression, hypotension, nausea, and itching; IV administration should be slow (over 4–5 minutes), with the patient recumbent.
Reproduced with permission from Rozenzveig S. Acute pain management. In: Harwood-Nuss A, ed. *The clinical practice of the emergency physician.* Philadelphia: Williams & Wilkins, 2001:1751.

It is often administered at too small a dose and too infrequently.

The side effect profile of meperidine is similar to that of morphine with a few exceptions. It has less effect on smooth muscle tone, which theoretically results in less spasm of the ureter and the sphincter of Oddi. This theory has not been verified in clinical studies. It has significant anti-muscarinic effects that can cause tachycardia. Meperidine also has some negative inotropic effects. It also possesses an active and toxic metabolite, normeperidine. Normeperidine is CNS toxic and can cause symptoms ranging

from anxiety to seizures and psychosis. Normeperidine has a half-life that is four times that of meperidine. Patients with renal disease are more susceptible to the buildup of normeperidine. A unique and potentially fatal interaction can occur when meperidine is administered to patients taking monoamine oxidase (MAO) inhibitors. The reaction can lead to agitation, hyperpyrexia, and death.

FENTANYL

Fentanyl is a synthetic opioid. It is available in intravenous, transdermal, and transmucosal

Table 65.4.

Pediatric dosing guidelines for drugs for pain management

Drug	Route	Dosage (mg/kg/dose)
Morphine	IV	0.1–0.2
Meperidine	IV/IM	1.0–1.5
Fentanyl	IV	0.001–0.003
	Oral/Transmucosal	0.005–0.015
Codeine	Oral	0.5–1.0 q4–6h
Acetaminophen	Oral/rectal	10–15 q4–6h
Ibuprofen	Oral	5–10 q6–8h

Reproduced with permission from Rozenzveig S. Acute pain management. In: Harwood-Nuss A, ed. *The clinical practice of the emergency physician*, 3rd ed. Philadelphia: Lippincott, Williams & Wilkins, 2001:1750.

preparations; however, the intravenous form is most useful in the ED. The dose of fentanyl is 1 to 3 µg/kg titrated in 25 to 50-µg increments. It has a rapid onset of action (within 1 to 2 minutes), and its duration of action is 30 to 60 minutes. The rapid onset and short duration of action make it an ideal agent in the ED for procedures. In addition, fentanyl has no effect on cardiac contractility and does not cause the release of histamine; thus, it is the most cardiovascularly stable opioid. Fentanyl has also been noted to cause a decrease in intracranial pressure, which makes it useful in the head-injured patient. A large dose of fentanyl when given by rapid intravenous push can lead to chest wall rigidity. The rigidity usually requires doses in excess of those recommended and can be reversed with naloxone or muscle relaxants.

HYDROMORPHONE

Hydromorphone can be administered IV, IM, PO, and PR. It is a cogener of morphine. Hydromorphone has a rapid onset of action and duration of action of 4 to 5 hours. The metabolism of hydromorphone is less affected by hepatic and renal disease than other opioids. This leads to decreased accumulation in patients with hepatic or renal disease and in the elderly who may have subtle dysfunction.

BUTORPHANOL

Butorphanol is a unique opioid that has agonist-antagonist properties. It has rapid onset of action that peaks in about 30 minutes. The half-life is approximately 3 hours. The usual dose is 2 to 4 mg. Butorphanol can lead to an increase in both peripheral and pulmonary artery pressure, which may limit its use in patients with significant cardiovascular disease. Butorphanol has the ability to cause sedation and psychomimetic effects.

Oral Opioids

OXYCODONE

Oxycodone is a phenanthrene derivative. It has potent analgesic effects equal to morphine. It is often combined with aspirin or acetaminophen to augment its analgesic potential. Dosing information for oxycodone and other oral opioids are shown in Table 65.5. Oxycodone can cause significant euphoria; therefore, it has high potential for abuse.

CODEINE

Codeine is probably the most commonly prescribed oral opioid. It is available alone but is often prescribed in combination with acetaminophen. Despite numerous studies demonstrating codeine's weak analgesic properties, it is still widely used. Many studies have demonstrated its analgesic effects to be no better than placebo or acetaminophen alone. Codeine causes less euphoria than other opioids, which decreases its abuse potential. It can cause significant GI side effects including nausea and vomiting and constipation.

Table 65.5.

Oral opioid dosing information

Drug	Analgesic Equivalence[a]	Usual Starting Dose[b]	Usual Interval
Morphine (MSIR, Roxanol, others)	30 mg	15–30 mg[c]	3–4 h
Morphine; sustained release, (MS contin, Oramorph-SR)	30 mg	30 mg[c]	8–12 h
Meperidine (Demerol)[d]	300 mg	50–100 mg	2–3 h
Codeine (in Tylenol#3, others)[e]	200 mg	30–60 mg	3–4 h
Oxycodone (Roxicodone, also in Percocet, Percodan, Tylox, others)	20–30 mg	5–10 mg	3–6 h
Hydrocodone (in Lorcet, Lortab, Vicodin, others)	30 mg[f]	5–10 mg	3–6 h
Hydromorphone (Dilaudid)	7.5 mg	4–8 mg[c]	2–3 h

Note: Addition of a nonopioid may allow lower dosing of an opioid. In using combination products, be careful not to exceed the allowable dose of the nonopioid constituent.

Note: Intervals are approximate individual patients may require dosing either more or less frequently.

Caution: Dosing may need to be adjusted in the elderly patients weighing less than 50 kg and those with renal or hepatic insufficiency.

[a] Doses equianalgesic to intravenous morphine 10 mg and intravenous meperidine 100 mg.

[b] Doses in this column are not equianalgesic.

[c] Usually reserved for chronic, severe pain.

[d] Meperidine has a unique central nervous system (CNS) toxicity with repeated dosing and is not recommended as a first-line agent. See text page 548.

[e] Doses greater than 60 mg are not recommended.

[f] Limited data available.

Reproduced with permission from Rozenzveig S. Acute pain management. In: Harwood-Nuss A, ed. *The clinical practice of the emergency physician.* Philadelphia: Williams & Wilkins, 2001:1753.

HYDROCODONE

Hydrocodone is another potent oral opioid. It is a semisynthetic agent. Often prescribed in combination with acetaminophen and recently with ibuprofen, it is a useful analgesic agent for patients with moderate pain being discharged from the ED. Its analgesic effects are greater than that of codeine and its GI side effects seem to be less.

PROPOXYPHENE

Propoxyphene is a stereoisomer of methadone. It has limited analgesic potential. Some studies have shown it to have minimally greater effect than placebo. It is usually prescribed in combination with aspirin or acetaminophen. Propoxyphene has a narrow therapeutic window, and overdoses can lead to seizures that may be refractory to treatment. Despite its weak analgesic effect and narrow therapeutic window, it is still commonly prescribed; therefore, one should have knowledge of the risks.

Nonopioid Analgesics

Nonsteroidal Antiinflammatory Drugs

Nonsteroidal antiinflammatory drugs (NSAIDs) are an extremely common medication prescribed by emergency physicians for a variety of painful conditions including headache, minor fractures, muscle strains, joint sprains, ureteral calculi, and dysmenorrhea. NSAIDs are ideal for use in the ED because of their potent analgesic, antiinflammatory, and antipyretic effects. They also possess fewer concerning side effects than the opioid analgesics. They lack respiratory depression and CNS depression and are not habit forming. Despite these benefits, NSAIDs do have serious potential side effects that must be considered when prescribing them.

When acute tissue injury occurs, an acute inflammatory response is initiated including the release of proinflammatory mediators. Figure 65.4 demonstrates the cascade. Chronic inflammation involves the

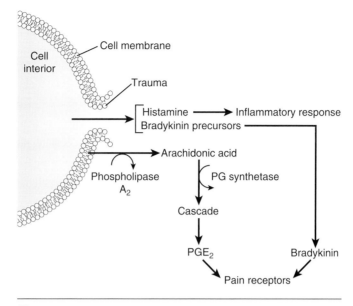

Figure 65.4
Peripheral pain mechanism. (Reproduced with permission from Honig SM. Nonsteroidal anti-inflammatory drugs. In: Tollison, CD, ed. *Handbook of pain management*, 2nd ed. Baltimore: Williams & Wilkins, 1994:167.)

release of inflammatory mediators that are different from those involved in the acute response. NSAIDs act through inhibition of prostaglandin synthesis. Prostaglandin synthesis is inhibited by blocking the enzyme cyclooxygenase (COX), either reversibly or irreversibly (in the case of aspirin). Prostaglandins are chemical mediators involved in inflammation, pain production, and fever. They act in concert with other mediators including histamine, bradykinin, and serotonin to sensitize pain receptors and produce erythema, edema, and hyperalgesia. The analgesic effects seem to result from the inhibition of prostaglandin E_2 (PGE_2) synthesis in the periphery. Antipyretic effects arise from the central inhibition of prostaglandin I_2 (PGI_2). Although the various NSAIDs vary in their structure, duration of action, and side effect profile, they exert their effects in about the same manner. Table 65.6 lists the commonly used nonopioid analgesics, dosages, and cost.

Side effects of the NSAIDs include GI effects ranging from upset to ulceration and bleeding. Renal failure can develop in patients, usually on a prolonged course of

NSAIDs. Elderly patients may also be more susceptible to this effect. All NSAIDs, but especially aspirin, have antiplatelet effects. In addition, hypersensitivity reactions can occur with urticaria, bronchospasm, and anaphylaxis.

Unique Nonsteroidal Antiinflammatory Drugs

Two unique NSAIDS deserve mention and are discussed in the following sections. The first is ketorolac, which is the first parenteral NSAID. The second unique class of NSAIDs is the newly marketed COX-2 inhibitors.

KETOROLAC

Ketorolac is the first parenteral NSAID and can be given IV, IM, or PO. Initial studies put forth its superiority to other NSAIDs and even to some opioids; however, this has been questioned in recent studies that have shown its efficacy to be no greater than other NSAIDs. One unique property it may have is the ability to inhibit both the pathway to synthesize prostaglandins and arachidonic acid, which may give it slightly more

Table 65.6.

Dosing information for nonopioids

Drug	Dosage	Comments	Cost ($)[a]
Acetaminophen (Tylenol)	650 mg q4h 1,000 mg q6h	No antiinflammatory activity	Retails: 0.48/0.72
Aspirin	650–975 mg q4h		Retail: 0.12/0.60
Choline magnesium trisalicylate (Trilisate)	1,000–1,500 mg bid	Available as liquid Minimal antiplatelet activity	1.01/1.40
Diflunisal (Dolobid)	1,000 mg load; then 500 mg bid,		2.88/3.24
Etodolac (Lodine)	200–400 mg q6–8h		NA/2.87
Fenoprofen (Nalfon)	200 mg q4–6h		1.07/1.94
Ibuprofen (Motrin and others)	400 mg q4–6h, or 600 mg q6–8h or 800 mg q8h	Available as liquid	Retail OTC: 0.60/1.08 By Rx: 53/1.12
Indomethacin (indocin)	25–50 mg tid	FDA approved only as an antiinflammatory Frequency of adverse effects higher than other NSAIDs Available as a suppository	0.26/1.16
Ketoprofen (Orudis)	25–75 mg q6–8h		1.38/2.42
Ketorolac, oral (Toradol)	10 mg q6–8h	Not recommended for more than 5 days use	NA/3.20
Ketorolac, parenteral	30–60 mg initially or 15–30 mg initially then 15–30 mg q6h IM or IV	Use the lower dose in patients <50 kg or older than 65, or with renal impairment	NA/28.97
Naproxen (Naprosyn, Aleve)	500 mg then 250 mg q6–8h, or 375 mg bid to tid	Oral liquid available.	NA/2.83
Naproxen sodium (Anaprox)	550 mg then 275 mg q6–8h		NA/2.85

bid, twice a day; COX-2, cyclooxygenase-2; FDA, Food and Drug Administration; IM, Intramuscular; IV, Intravenous; NA, not available NSAID, nonsteroidal antiinflammatory drug; OTC, over the counter; tid, three times a day.
Cost for 24 hours of therapy. Average wholesale price is quoted unless otherwise noted. For many drugs, the generic price is given first, followed by the brand-name price. When a range of doses is available, the cost of the smallest one is recorded.
Reproduced with permission from Rozenzveig S. Acute pain management. In: Harwood-Nuss A, ed. *The clinical practice of the emergency physician,* 3rd ed. Philadelphia: Lippincott, Williams & Wilkins, 2001:1740.

antiinflammatory activity. The main advantage of ketorolac in the ED is its use in patients who cannot take oral medications.

CYCLOOXYGENASE-2 INHIBITORS

There are two forms of COX, COX-1 and COX-2. COX-1 is found in all tissues except red blood cells and is constitutively expressed in the stomach, kidneys, platelets, and endothelial cells under normal states. The COX-2 form is constitutively expressed in brain and kidney but is found in other tissues only when active inflammation is occurring. COX-1 is involved in prostacyclin production, which protects gastric mucosa; therefore, when it is inhibited, the gastric mucosa may develop erosions and ulcerations. Therefore, the selective inhibition of COX-2, which is expressed only at sites of inflammation, would allow the protection of the gastric mucosa and hopefully eliminate some of the major side effects of NSAIDs. Celecoxib is the COX-2 inhibitor marketed now. Celecoxib is currently approved for the treatment of osteoarthritis and rheumatoid arthritis. Celecoxib should not be given to patients with allergies to sulfonamides. Celecoxib has been shown to have significantly fewer GI side effects including erosions and ulceration in studies that compared it with traditional NSAIDs.

Acetaminophen

Acetaminophen is probably the most common medication used to treat mild to moderate pain. It can be found in numerous over-the-counter preparations, and it is also commonly combined with opioids for added analgesic effects. It has both analgesic and antipyretic effects equal to that of aspirin, but, unlike aspirin and the other NSAIDs, it lacks antiinflammatory properties. Its effects have also been linked to the inhibition of COX. It is believed that these effects are more centrally mediated and that it lacks significant antiinflammatory activity because it is relatively inactive in peripheral tissues.

Acetaminophen is available in both oral and rectal forms. It is rapidly absorbed and has an onset of action within about 30 to 60 minutes. It has a half-life of 2 to 4 hours in a normal adult. The half-life is prolonged in neonates and those with hepatic disease. The normal dose of acetaminophen is 10 to 15 mg/kg in children and either 325 to 650 mg every 4 to 6 hours in adults or 1 g every 6 hours. It is recommended for the treatment of headache, myalgias, and other mild pain syndromes. It can be used in combination with an opioid for added analgesia. Acetaminophen is the agent of choice for those with a history of peptic ulcer disease, hemophilia, aspirin allergies, and renal disease that would limit the use of NSAIDs.

Metabolism of acetaminophen occurs in the liver through glucuronidation to an inactive metabolite. A small amount may be converted to a reactive metabolite that has hepatotoxic effects, usually less than 4% of the dose. However, those who take an overdose, have underlying liver disease, or have chronic alcohol use may shunt more drug down the toxic pathway, leading to an accumulation of this metabolite. Accumulation of the metabolite can lead to hepatic necrosis (Chapter 55). Chronic alcohol use may lead to stimulation of hepatic microsomal enzymes that can cause accumulation of toxic metabolites even at therapeutic doses. Other potential side effects from acetaminophen are rare but may include pancytopenia and leukopenia. Allergic reactions such as rash and drug fever are possible but extremely rare. Large doses of acetaminophen over a prolonged time may slightly potentiate the effects of warfarin.

Local Anesthesia

Knowledge of the use of local and regional anesthesia through topical anesthetic agents, local infiltration, and regional blocks is an important part of the practice of emergency medicine. These techniques have application to clinical practice on a daily basis because they facilitate laceration repair, incision and drainage of abscesses, central line placement, lumbar puncture, and many other procedures performed in the ED. Knowledge of the agent's use, including appropriate clinical scenarios, combined with knowledge of side effect profiles is crucial. This section reviews pathophysiology of pain transmission and common local anesthetics used in emergency medicine. Appropriate use of local anesthetics improves patient outcome, decreases the need for pain medication, and allows procedures to be performed with greater ease for the physician.

Peripheral Nervous System Pain Transmission

Peripheral nerves are responsible for the transmission of pain from the pain receptors to the spinal cord. At its most basic level, the nerve fiber consists of an axon and its surrounding Schwann cell sheath. Unmyelinated nerve fibers consist of several axons surrounded by a single Schwann cell. Myelinated nerve fibers consist of a single axon and its Schwann cell

sheath that wraps itself around several times, thus creating the myelin sheath.

Nodes of Ranvier are junctions between myelin sheaths that contain the sodium channels required for depolarization of the nerve. These sodium channels are actually protein channels that, when excited, open up and allow for the intracellular flux of sodium. Following stimulation, cutaneous pain receptors cause sodium channels in the nerve ending to open, which depolarizes the nerve and allows for signal transmission. Following depolarization, repolarization allows for the resting transmembrane potential to be reestablished.

Local anesthetics act by binding to the protein channels and blocking the influx of sodium, thereby inhibiting depolarization. Inhibition of depolarization is the basis for blocking the conduction of the nerve impulse. Local anesthetics penetrate unmyelinated or lightly myelinated fibers much quicker and easier than myelinated fibers. This accounts for the lack of motor blockade with full sensory blockade of the area.

Table 65.7.

Characteristics of commonly used local anesthetics

Infiltration Anesthetic	Concentration	Lipid Solubility	Relative Potency	Onset of Action (minutes)	Duration (minutes)	mg/kg	mL/kg
						Maximum Allowable Dose	
Procaine (Novocain)	1%	0.6	1	5–10	60–90	7–10	0.7–1
Lidocaine (Xylocaine)							
—without epinephrine	1%	2.9	2	2–5	50–120	4–5	0.4–0.5
—with epinephrine (1:200,000)	1%	2.9	2	2–5	60–180	5–7	0.5–0.7
Mepivacaine (Carbocaine)	1%	0.8	2	2–5	90–180	5	0.5
Bupivacaine[a] (Marcaine)	0.25%	27.5	8	5–10	240–480	2	0.8

[a]some authorities do not recommend bupivacaine for use in children younger than 12 years.
Reproduced with permission from Lewis LS, Stephan M. Local and regional anesthesia. In: Hentretig FM, King C, eds. *Textbook for pediatric emergency procedures*. Baltimore: Williams & Wilkins, 1997:469.

Local Anesthetic Agents

Local anesthetic characteristics are listed in Table 65.7.

Lidocaine

Lidocaine is an amide anesthetic and is probably the anesthetic most frequently used in the ED. It is available in solutions with concentrations of 0.5%, 1%, and 2%. Lidocaine has an onset of action from 2 to 5 minutes and duration of action of 1 to 2 hours. It is also available in a viscous form, cream, jelly, and spray that vary in concentrations from 2%, 4%, and 10% for the spray. Because it is metabolized hepatically, patients with hepatic failure and decreased hepatic blood flow may develop high plasma levels, leading to systemic toxicity. In addition, lidocaine can be combined with epinephrine to prolong its effect and with bicarbonate to decrease the pain of injection.

Bupivacaine

Bupivacaine is an amide local anesthetic that is supplied in 0.25% concentration. It has a longer duration of action than lidocaine, 4 to 6 hours. Because of its prolonged duration of action, it is commonly used for painful procedures that require a longer time to perform or if postprocedural anesthesia is needed. Bupivacaine is more cardiotoxic than lidocaine and injection may be more painful. It is also not recommended for children younger than the age of 12.

Procaine

Procaine is an ester local anesthetic. It is available in a 1% concentration for injection. It has duration of action of 15 to 45 minutes. It can be used for patients with an allergy to an amide agent.

Tetracaine

Tetracaine is an ester local anesthetic. It has a longer half-life than most local anesthetics and its most common use is as a topical anesthetic. The side effect potential of tetracaine is higher than that of many of the other agents, and significant cardiovascular side effects may develop without the classic preceding neurological symptoms.

Prilocaine

Prilocaine is also an amide local anesthetic. It is supplied in a 4% solution. Its onset of anesthesia is within 2 to 5 minutes and its duration of action is 30 to 60 minutes. It has the lowest cardiotoxic profile of all the local anesthetics. Large boluses of prilocaine (usually doses in excess of 600 mg) have been noted to cause methemoglobinemia.

Topical Anesthetics

Topical anesthetics can be used in a variety of procedures performed in the ED. In addition to making painful procedures more comfortable for the patient, they can dramatically improve the ability of the physician to perform the procedure. These agents are useful for nasogastric tube placement, Foley catheter placement, laceration repair, intravenous placement, and lumbar punctures and can help with the examination of the eye in certain circumstances. The major limitation to these agents is the barrier to absorption provided by intact skin. However, they do penetrate the mucous membranes more easily. The rapid absorption that is possible from mucosal surfaces and the cornea can lead to systemic toxicity if the recommended dose is exceeded. The risk of toxicity is greater in children.

Lidocaine

Lidocaine is available in cream, viscous, jelly, and spray varying in concentration from 2% to 4% for the viscous and jelly forms to up to 10% for lidocaine sprays. Commonly, the 2% to 4% lidocaine jelly can be used for nasogastric tube placement. Viscous lidocaine can be used for analgesia of the throat and pharynx under certain circumstances. It is also commonly added to the "GI cocktail." The 2% form of lidocaine jelly can be used for the placement of Foley catheters and lubrication of endotracheal tubes. It also can be used topically before scrubbing of skin embedded with dirt and road rash. Lidocaine spray can be used to facilitate the placement of a naso-tracheal tube in awake patients.

Eutectic Mixture of Local Anesthetics Cream

Eutectic mixture of local anesthetics (EMLA) cream can be used in the ED for procedures including intravenous placement, lumbar puncture, and ulcer débridement. EMLA cream contains 2.5% lidocaine and 2.5% prilocaine in an oil-and-water emulsion. Dosing is done in grams of cream. A dose of 2.5 g, or 1 premade disc can be applied to the site of venipuncture or lumbar puncture. It requires 1 to 2 hours of application time and the duration of action is approximately 30 minutes. An occlusive dressing placed over the area increases penetration. EMLA cream has been used and studied extensively. The main limitation to its use is its variable absorption through intact skin and the length of time required to achieve anesthesia. This can be overcome by longer application time or larger dose. Depth and duration of anesthesia is also increased in thinner or inflamed skin. Like prilocaine used for injection anesthesia, EMLA cream can cause methemoglobinemia resulting from the metabolite of prilocaine.

Cocaine

Cocaine is an excellent topical anesthetic for mucous membranes. However, its use has been limited by the potential side effects. Cocaine has significant vasoconstrictive effects on the mucosa; it provides excellent analgesia and also shrinks the mucosa. These effects can be very helpful to the emergency physician treating epistaxis. The potential side effects must be recognized and include hypertension, vasoconstriction, and seizures. Therefore, it should not be used in patients with known coronary artery disease.

Lidocaine, Epinephrine, and Tetracaine Solution

A solution of lidocaine, epinephrine, and tetracaine (LET) in a mixture of 4% lidocaine, 1:1,000 epinephrine, and 0.5% tetracaine is used commonly as an anesthetic agent for wound closure. It also can be used as premedication for wound infiltration. It has some advantages over local infiltration in that it is painless, does not distort wound edges, and provides hemostasis. LET can be applied directly to the wound and then applied to a cotton ball and taped to the wound. Anesthesia should occur after approximately 20 minutes. Application to fingers, toes, mucous membranes, nose, ear, and penis should be avoided.

Procedural Sedation

In addition to managing pain, the emergency physician needs up-to-date knowledge of agents used to relieve anxiety and produce sedation during the performance of procedures in the ED. Certain procedures, such as complex laceration repair, incision and drainage (I&D) of abscesses, and joint and fracture reductions, can be done more easily with judicious use of sedating drugs in combination with analgesics. Before proceeding with further introduction of such agents, it is imperative that certain terms be understood to facilitate selection of agents and combinations of agents used for procedural sedation.

Definitions

Analgesia: a condition in which nociceptive stimuli are perceived but are not interpreted as pain

Anesthesia: a state characterized by loss of sensation

Anxiolysis: a state of decreased apprehension concerning a situation without changing the patient's level of awareness

Amnestic: an agent characterized by its ability to disturb the ability of information to be stored

Procedural sedation and analgesia: a technique of administering sedatives, analgesics, and/or dissociative agents to induce a state that allows the patient to tolerate unpleasant procedures while maintaining cardiorespiratory function

Light sedation: drug-induced depression of consciousness in which the patient remains able to respond purposefully to commands. The airway remains patent and protective airway reflexes are maintained. Ventilatory status remains adequate

Deep sedation: drug-induced depression of consciousness in which the patient is not easily aroused but responds purposefully to painful stimulation. Patients may have difficulty maintaining a patent airway and may also have a depressed level of ventilation

Dissociative sedation: a trance-like state induced by a dissociative agent characterized by analgesia and amnesia. Protective airway reflexes and spontaneous respiration are preserved

American Society of Anesthesiologists Patient Classification for Sedation

Performing procedural sedation requires significant preparation, including appropriate patient selection, medication selection, monitoring capabilities, and observation of the patient to recovery. The use of American Society of Anesthesiologists' (ASA) classification assists the physician with patient selection.

Class 1: Healthy patient, no medical problems

Class 2: Mild systemic disease

Class 3: Severe systemic disease, but not incapacitating

Class 4: Severe systemic disease that is a constant threat to life

Class 5: Moribund, not expected to live 24 hours irrespective of operation

In general, elective procedures under sedation in the ED should be reserved for patients in ASA class 1 or 2.

After careful patient selection, the choice of medication or combination of medications must be made. Ideally, the agent or agents would be easily titrated, produce an expected level of sedation, and allow a rapid recovery with few or minimal side effects. Although no single agent provides all of these, many come close. Before selection of the medication, the physician must know advantages, disadvantages, and potential adverse effects.

Procedural sedation should be performed by physicians who have adequate knowledge of the agents used and are skilled in airway management. Procedural sedation should be done in a setting that allows for the management of complications. The patient should be monitored with the use of cardiac monitor, pulse oximetry, blood pressure monitoring, and, in some institutions, end-tidal CO_2 monitoring. Although costly, the use of end-tidal CO_2 monitoring seems promising in detecting hypoventilation during sedation before desaturation. The patient's vital signs should be monitored every 3 to 5 minutes during the procedure and at least every 15 minutes after the procedure until the patient has returned to baseline functioning.

In addition to appropriate personnel and setting, all necessary airway equipment should be readily available at the bedside. This includes supplemental oxygen, bag-valve-mask, and suction and intubation equipment. Reversal agents (flumazenil and naloxone) should be at the bedside if benzodiazepines or opiates are being used.

Anxiolytic Medications Used in Sedation

Benzodiazepines

MIDAZOLAM

The benzodiazepine of choice for procedural sedation in the ED is midazolam. It is a sedative-hypnotic that has anxiolytic, amnestic, and muscle-relaxant effects. It exerts its effects on the CNS by its interactions with the inhibitory neurotransmitter receptor, namely the γ-aminobutyric acid (GABA) receptor. Its actions are indirect through modulation of the receptor and not direct activation. The modulation enhances the inhibitory function of the GABA receptor.

Midazolam meets many of the criteria of an ideal agent: It has a relatively rapid onset of action and a short duration, and it is reversible. Multiple routes including intravenous, intramuscular, rectal, and nasal can be used. Most commonly, midazolam is administered via an intravenous line, where it can be titrated to the desired effect. The initial dose is 0.02 to 0.1 mg/kg IV for an adult and 0.05 to 0.15 mg/kg in a child. The onset of action if administered IV is 2 to 5 minutes. Its duration of action is 20 to 40 minutes. The half-life is 1 to 4 hours. Midazolam is metabolized by the liver and is excreted renally. It may have a prolonged half-life in patients with renal and hepatic disease. Midazolam has twice the potency of diazepam. It produces its desired effects in a dose-dependent manner with anxiolysis first, followed by amnesia and then sedation. The amnesia produced is both anterograde and retrograde.

The major adverse effects of midazolam include hypotension and respiratory depression. Hypotension is often produced with rapid administration of the drug IV. This effect is potentiated in patients who are already hypotensive and if used in combination with other agents that may cause hypotension (i.e., opiates). Respiratory depression is dose dependent and is also potentiated by concomitant use of other respiratory depressants. It is felt to arise from blunting the hypothalamic response to hypercapnia.

In addition, it must be remembered that midazolam provides no analgesia and therefore must be combined with an analgesic for painful procedures. The most common combination used in the ED is midazolam and fentanyl.

Ketamine

Ketamine is an analogue of phencyclidine (PCP) and has sedative and anesthetic properties. It produces dissociative anesthesia characterized by analgesia, amnesia, and catatonia. However, the patient has the ability to protect his or her airway. This makes it an ideal agent for use in the ED under appropriate conditions. It is believed that ketamine exerts its effects through blockade of the membrane effects of the excitatory neurotransmitter glutamic acid at the N-methyl-D-aspartate (NMDA) receptor.

Ketamine is highly lipophilic and rapidly redistributed. Ketamine can be given IV or IM. The dose is 1 to 2 mg/kg IV or 2 to 4 mg/kg IM. The effects last between 15 and 30 minutes. It is metabolized in the liver and excreted in urine and bile. In addition to its anesthetic effects, ketamine also has other characteristic effects and side effects that must be considered when determining its appropriate use. It produces cardiovascular stimulation through central sympathetic stimulation. This leads to an increase in cardiac output, blood pressure, and heart rate. Ketamine should be used with caution in patients with cardiovascular problems.

Ketamine causes an increase in cerebral blood flow and intracranial pressure that could be harmful to the head-injured patient, and it should not be used in these circumstances. Ketamine also acts as a potent bronchodilator through vagolytic and smooth muscle relaxation, which makes it a safe agent for patients with reactive airways disease. It is contraindicated in children younger than 3 months old.

Ketamine has been noted to produce an emergence phenomenon. This has been characterized by disorientation, sensory and perceptual illusions, and often vivid disturbing dreams. It is more common in adults and patients with a history of psychiatric illness. Use of a benzodiazepine in conjunction with ketamine and decreasing external stimuli during the arousal period may help decrease the emergence phenomenon.

Barbiturates

The most effective barbituric drug is methohexital, a fast-acting derivative of barbituric acid. It can be administered IV, IM, or PR. The dose of intravenous methohexital is 0.75 to 1 mg/kg. If given PR, the dose is 20 to 30 mg/kg. It has a rapid onset (usually less than a minute) and duration of action between 4 and 7 minutes if administered IV. Rectal administration induces sleep within 10 minutes, lasting approximately 45 minutes. Methohexital is cleared rapidly relative to the other barbiturates secondary to its rapid clearance from the brain to other tissues. Methohexital is believed to cause an increase in CNS responsiveness to GABA. The resulting decrease in neural activity inhibits ascending conduction to the reticular formation. It is metabolized by the liver and excreted renally. Methohexital is highly protein bound, and states of low plasma protein may lead to a higher level of action of the drug.

Advantages of methohexital include its rapid onset of action and very short duration. It does cause a state of unconsciousness with protective airway reflexes usually maintained. In fact, airway reflexes may be enhanced, which can cause cough and hiccoughs and, in rare instances, laryngospasm. Methohexital provides a profound amnestic effect during its brief duration of action. It must be remembered that methohexital provides no analgesia and must be combined with an analgesic agent for painful procedures.

The major complications associated with use of methohexital are hypoventilation and/or apnea. One study noted brief periods of apnea in as many as 10% of study patients. No patient required intubation; desaturation was not less than 90%, and patients were managed with brief bag-valve-mask assistance. Despite the rapid clearance of this drug, apnea is a major potential complication and must be considered and planned for. Methohexital also should not be used in patients with seizure disorders, because it has been shown to induce epileptiform activity.

Short-Acting Sedative-Hypnotic Agents

Propofol

Propofol is an ultra short-acting sedative-hypnotic agent. Pharmacologically, it acts similarly to barbiturates. It exerts its effect through potentiation of GABA binding in the CNS. It is given IV at a dose of 1.0 to 2.5 mg/kg as a bolus, followed by an infusion of 25 to 125 μg/kg/minute. Its onset of action is less than 1 minute, and it has a duration of 4 to 8 minutes. Propofol is subject to a high clearance rate, thus rendering it short duration of action despite a rather long half-life. Children

may require a higher initial dose and infusion rate compared with adults because of an age-related decrease in volume of distribution. Propofol is highly protein bound and is metabolized by the liver. It provides no analgesia and is not a potent amnestic.

The main complications with propofol are hypotension, dose-dependent sedation, and potential for deep sedation and apnea. The hypotension is more profound than that seen with barbiturates and is secondary to both vasodilatation and a decrease in myocardial contractility. Propofol may also be directly vagotonic. Apnea can result from propofol use, but it is more common with concomitant use of opioid analgesics.

Although propofol has many promising qualities that may make it an ideal agent for use in the ED, it has not been studied as extensively as other sedation medications. The most serious complication is apnea, but most studies have documented it as brief and without significant clinical desaturation. In addition to the fact that fewer study data are available, no set dosing regimen exists.

Etomidate

Etomidate is a nonbarbiturate imidazole-derivative sedative-hypnotic agent. The sedative actions of etomidate are thought to be through enhanced GABA activity. It has been used extensively in the ED as an induction agent before rapid-sequence intubation. It has a rapid onset of action and short duration, thus making it an ideal agent for potential use during procedural sedation. It is administered IV at a dose of 0.1 to 0.4 mg/kg, and its onset of action is usually around 30 seconds. The duration of action is approximately 4 to 8 minutes. The half-life is approximately 1 to 3 hours.

Etomidate has minimal analgesic effect; thus, it should be combined with an opiate or other analgesic during the performance of painful procedures. Etomidate gained widespread use in the ED for induction because of its cardiovascular stability relative to other agents commonly used.

Etomidate may induce hiccoughs. It has a higher incidence of nausea and vomiting than other agents. It has minimal respiratory effects, and these are found to be transitory. It can also cause myoclonus, which can be problematic during the performance of certain procedures. Etomidate has been found to suppress the adrenocortical stress response, but this is likely insignificant for a one-time dose for sedation. It has not been approved for use in children younger than age 10. Although clearly a promising drug, etomidate also has limited prospective study data when compared with other medications and also lacks clear dosing guidelines.

Benzodiazepine Reversal Agents

The most frequently used agent is flumazenil, a benzodiazepine derivative that antagonizes the effect of benzodiazepines at the GABA receptor. Flumazenil competitively and reversibly binds the GABA receptor, thus allowing for its reversal effects. The dose of flumazenil is 0.2 mg to a maximal dose of 1 mg. The effects are usually seen within 1 minute of injection, and it has a half-life of 40 to 80 minutes. Flumazenil does not directly treat the hypoventilation but does reverse the sedation and psychomotor effects of benzodiazepines. Risks associated with its use are seizure, precipitation of benzodiazepine withdrawal, and resedation. Seizures may occur in patients taking benzodiazepines for their seizure disorder. Withdrawal can be precipitated in patients taking benzodiazepines chronically for other conditions (e.g., anxiety). Because of its short duration of action, resedation may occur. Patients should be monitored for at least 40 minutes after administration to avoid this potential complication. If benzodiazepines with longer half-lives are used, the monitoring time would need to be extended.

Conclusion

Patients present to the ED with a variety of painful conditions and complaints and are often subjected to painful diagnostic and therapeutic procedures. Therefore, it is incumbent on the emergency physician to be knowledgeable about all the potential agents that are available to treat patients' pain and anxiety and to facilitate the performance of diagnostic and therapeutic procedures. The physician must be knowledgeable about the potential adverse reactions and events that may occur with any medication or combination of medications and must be skilled in the emergency management of these conditions before any medication is administered to a patient.

Suggested Readings

Avramov MN, White PF. Methods for monitoring the level of sedation. *Crit Care Clin* 1995; 11:803–826.

Barr J, Donner A. Optimal intravenous dosing strategies for sedatives and analgesics in the intensive care unit. *Crit Care Clin* 1995; 11:827–842.

Bauman LA, Kish L, Baumann RC, Politis GD. Pediatric sedation and analgesia. *Am J Emerg Med* 1999;17:1–3.

Berman D, Graber D. Sedation and analgesia. *Emerg Med Clin North Am* 1992;10:691–704.

Blackburn P, Vissers R. Pharmacology of emergency department pain management and conscious sedation. *Emerg Med Clin North Am* 2000;18:803–826.

Bonica JJ. Anatomic and physiologic basis of nociception and pain. In: Bonica JJ, ed. *The management of pain*, 2nd ed. Philadelphia: Lea & Febiger, 1990:28–94.

Bonica JJ. History of pain concepts and therapies. In: Bonica JJ, ed. *The management of pain*, 2nd ed. Philadelphia: Lea & Febiger, 1990:2–17.

Bouckoms AJ. Pain relief in the intensive care unit. *J Intensive Care Med* 1988;3:32–51.

Chudnofsky CR, Lozon MM. Sedation and analgesia for procedures. In: Marx JA, Hockberger R, Walls R, et al, eds. *Rosen's emergency medicine concepts and clinical practice*, 5th ed. St. Louis: Mosby, 2002: 2577–2590.

Colaric KB, Overton DT, Moore K. Pain reduction in lidocaine administration through warming and buffering. *Am J Emerg Med* 1998; 16:353–356.

Colburn KK, Flores R, Rambharose J. The role of COX-2 inhibitors in emergency and acute care medicine. *Emerg Med Rep* 2000;21: 23–34.

Dickinson R, Singer AJ, Carrion W. Etomidate for pediatric sedation prior to fracture reduction. *Acad Emerg Med* 2001;8:74–77.

Ducharme J. Acute pain and pain control: state of the art. *Ann Emerg Med* 2000;35:592–602.

Ducharme J, Barber C. A prospective blinded study on emergency department pain assessment and therapy. *J Emerg Med* 1995; 13:571–575.

Dursteler BB, Wightman JM. Etomidate-facilitated hip reduction in the emergency department. *Acad Emerg Med* 2000;7:1165–1166.

Ernst AA, Marvez-Valls E, Nick TG, Weiss SJ. LAT (lidocaine-adrenaline-tetracaine) versus TAC (tetracaine-adrenaline-cocaine) for topical anesthesia in face and scalp lacerations. *Am J Emerg Med* 1995;13:151–155.

Furst DE. Nonsteroidal anti-inflammatory drugs; disease modifying antirheumatic drugs; non-opioid analgesics; drugs used to treat gout. In: Katzung BC, ed. *Basic and clinical pharmacology*, 7th ed. Stamford, CT: Appleton & Lange, 1998:578–602.

Green SM. Propofol for emergency department procedural sedation—not yet ready for prime time. *Acad Emerg Med* 1999;6:975–978.

Green SM. Procedural sedation terminology: moving beyond "conscious sedation." *Ann Emerg Med* 2002;39:433–435.

Hall JL. Anatomy of pain. In: Tollison CD, ed. *Handbook of pain management*, 2nd ed. Baltimore: Williams & Wilkins, 1994:11–17.

Havel CJ Jr, Strait RT, Hennes H. A clinical trial of propofol vs midazolam for procedural sedation in a pediatric emergency department. *Acad Emerg Med* 1999;6:989–997.

Hinnant DW. Psychological evaluation and testing. In: Tollison CD, ed. *Handbook of pain management*, 2nd ed. Baltimore: Williams & Wilkins, 1994:18–35.

Honig SM. Nonsteroidal anti-inflammatory drugs. In: Tollison CD, ed. *Handbook of pain management*, 2nd ed. Baltimore: Williams & Wilkins, 1994:165–172.

Hostetler MA, Auinger P, Szilagyi PG. Parenteral analgesic and sedative use among ED patients in the United States, combined results from the National Hospital Ambulatory Medical Care Survey. *Am J Emerg Med* 2002;20: 139–143.

Hostetler MA, Barnard JA. Removal of esophageal foreign bodies in the pediatric ED: is ketamine an option? *Am J Emerg Med* 2002; 20: 96–98.

Jackson R, Carley S. Towards evidence based emergency medicine: best BET's from the Manchester Royal Infirmary. Use of propofol for sedation in the emergency department. *Emerg Med J* 2001;18:378–379.

Jones JS, Johnson K, McNinch M. Age as a risk for inadequate emergency department analgesia. *Am J Emerg Med* 1996;14:157–160.

Kehlet H. Pain relief and stress management. In: Cousins MJ, Phillips GD, eds. *Acute pain management*. New York: Churchill Livingstone, 1986:49–76.

Keim SM, Erstad BL, Sakles JC, Davis V. Etomidate for procedural sedation in the emergency department. *Pharmacotherapy* 2002;22:586–592.

Lang JD. Pain: a prelude. *Crit Care Clin* 1999; 15:1–16.

Lerman B, Yoshida D, Levin, MA. A prospective evaluation of the safety and efficacy of Methohexital in the emergency department. *Am J Emerg Med* 1996;14:351–354.

Lewis LS, Stephan M. Local and regional anesthesia. In: Henretig FM, King C, eds. *Textbook of pediatric emergency procedures*. Baltimore: Williams & Wilkins, 1997:469, 471.

Liebelt E, Levick N. Acute pain management, analgesia, and anxiolysis in the adult patient. In: Tintinalli, JE, ed. *Emergency medicine: a comprehensive study guide*. New York: McGraw-Hill, 2000:251–268.

Martin JJ, Moore GP. Pearls, pitfalls, and updates for pain management. *Emerg Med Clin North Am* 1997;15:399–415.

Miller RD. Local anesthetics. In: Katzung BC, ed. *Basic and clinical pharmacology*, 7th ed. Stamford, CT: Appleton & Lange, 1998: 425–433.

Miner JR, Heegaard W, Plummer D. End-tidal carbon dioxide monitoring during procedural sedation. *Acad Emerg Med* 2002;9:275–280, 2002.

Miner JR, Krieg S, Johnson C, et al. Propofol vs methohexital for procedural sedation for fracture and dislocation reduction. *Acad Emerg Med* 2002;9:364–365.

Murphy MF. Sedation. *Ann Emerg Med* 1996; 27:461–463.

Murray MJ, deRuyter ML, Harrison BA. Opioids and benzodiazepines. *Crit Care Clin* 1995;11: 849–872.

Muse DA. Conscious and deep sedation. In: Harwood-Nuss A, Wolfson AB, Linden CH, et al, eds. *The clinical practice of emergency medicine*, 3rd ed. Philadelphia: Lippincott, Williams & Wilkins, 2001: 1758–1762.

Orlinsky M, Dean E. Local and topical anesthesia. In: Roberts JR, Hedges JR, eds. *Clinical procedures in emergency medicine*, 3rd ed. Philadelphia: WB Saunders, 1998:454–473.

Paris P, Stewart R, eds. *Pain management in emergency medicine*. Stamford, CT: Appleton & Lange, 1988.

Paris P, Stewart R. Pain management. In: *Emergency medicine concepts and clinical practice*, 4th ed. St. Louis: Mosby, 1998:276–300.

Phillips GD, Cousins MJ. Neurological mechanisms of pain and the relationship of pain, anxiety and sleep. In: Cousins MJ, Phillips GD, eds. *Acute pain management*. New York: Churchill Livingstone, 1986:21–48.

Pomeranz ES, Chudnofsky CR, Deegan TJ, et al. Rectal methohexital sedation for computed tomography imaging of stable pediatric emergency department patients. *Pediatrics* 2000; 105:1110–1114.

Powell CV, Kelly AM, Williams A. Determining the minimum clinically significant difference in Visual Analog Pain Score for children. *Ann Emerg Med* 2001;37:28–31.

Priestley SJ, Taylor J, McAdam CM, Francis P. Ketamine sedation for children in the emergency department. *Emerg Med* 2001;13:82–90.

Proudfoot J. Analgesia, anesthesia, and conscious sedation. *Emerg Med Clin North Am* 1995;13: 357–374.

Rosenzweig S, Mines D. Acute pain management. In: Harwood-Nuss A, Wolfson AB, Linden CH, et al, eds. *The clinical practice of emergency medicine*, 3rd ed. Philadelphia: Lippincott, Williams & Wilkins, 2001: 1747–1753.

Ruth WJ, Burton JH, Bock AJ. Intravenous etomidate for procedural sedation in emergency department patients. *Acad Emerg Med* 2001; 8:13–18.

Scarfone RJ, Jasani M, Gracely EJ. Pain of local anesthetics: rate and buffering. *Ann Emerg Med* 1998;31:36–40.

Sedik H. Use of intravenous methohexital as a sedative in pediatric emergency departments. *Arch Pediatr Adolesc Med* 2001;155:665–68l.

Selbst SM, Clark M. Analgesic use in the emergency department. *Ann Emerg Med* 1990; 19:1010–1013.

Shafer A. Complications of sedation with midazolam in the intensive care unit and comparison with other sedative regimens. *Crit Care Med* 1998;26:947–954.

Shields RE. A comprehensive review of sedative and analgesic agents. *Crit Care Nurs Clin North Am* 1997;9:281–287.

Skokan EG, Pribble C, Bassett KE, Nelson DS. Use of propofol sedation in a pediatric emergency department: a prospective study. *Clin Pediatr* 2001;40:663–671.

Smith DW, Peterson MR, DeBerard SC. Local anesthesia: topical application, local infiltration, and field block. *Postgrad Med* 1999; 106(2):57–66.

Solomon GD. Analgesic medications. In: Tollison CD, ed. *Handbook of pain management*, 2nd ed. Baltimore: Williams & Wilkins, 1994: 155–164.

Swanson ER, Seaberg DC, Mathias S. The use of propofol for sedation in the emergency department. *Acad Emerg Med* 1996;3: 234–238.

Todd KH, Deaton C, D'Adamo AP, et al. Ethnicity and analgesic practice. *Ann Emerg Med* 2000; 35: 11–16.

Turturro MA, Paris PM, Yealy DM, et al. Hydrocodone versus codeine in acute musculoskeletal pain. *Ann Emerg Med* 19910;20: 1100–1103.

Vinson DR, Bradbury DR. Etomidate for procedural sedation in emergency medicine. *Ann Emerg Med* 2002;39:592–598.

Wahlgreen CF, Quiding H. Depth of cutaneous analgesia after application of a eutectic mixture of the local anesthetics lidocaine and prilocaine (EMLA cream). *J Am Acad Dermatol* 2000;42:584–588.

Way WL, Fields HL, Way EL. Opioid analgesics & antagonists. In: Katzung BC, ed. *Basic and clinical pharmacology*, 7th ed. Stamford, CT: Appleton & Lange, 1998:496–515.

Wilson JE, Pendelton JM. Oligoanalgesia in the emergency department. *Am J Emerg Med* 1989; 7:620–623.

Yealy DM. Safe and effective . . . maybe: etomidate in procedural sedation/analgesia. *Acad Emerg Med* 2001;8:68–69.

ABCs

Airway Management

Keith S. Boniface, MD

Management of the airway is an essential skill for the emergency physician. Emergent airway management in the ill or injured patient can be particularly challenging. Patients may be hemodynamically unstable or profoundly hypoxic. They may have impending mechanical airway obstruction or an airway blocked by secretions, vomit, or blood. They may be combative or seizing or they may have a suspected cervical spine injury. Furthermore, the environment may be chaotic and noisy. In addition to these challenges, the emergency physician must be prepared for complications of airway management and have multiple means available to definitively secure the airway.

Initial Steps in Airway Management

In the unresponsive patient, the most common cause of airway obstruction is the patient's tongue, which slips posteriorly to occlude the oropharynx. One of two maneuvers can be used to anteriorly displace the tongue from the posterior wall of the pharynx.

If there is any possibility of a cervical spine injury, it is vital to avoid manipulation that may cause motion to the head and neck. In this situation, the **jaw-thrust** (Fig. 66.1) maneuver is used to open the airway. The physician grasps the angles of both mandibles by the fingers, with thumbs braced against the maxilla (or face mask if the patient is being ventilated). The airway is opened by anteriorly displacing the jaw with the fingers of both hands, while the hands maintain cervical spine immobilization.

If there is no risk of a cervical spine injury, the **head tilt-chin lift** (Fig. 66.2) maneuver is used. The palm of one hand is placed against the patient's forehead and gentle downward pressure is applied, while the fingers of the other hand are placed under the chin, to lift, slightly extending the head on the neck and anteriorly displacing the jaw.

Tongue obstruction of the airway is the simplest and most easily treated cause of airway obstruction. Treatments for other causes of airway obstruction may be simple (e.g., suctioning or removal of foreign mater-

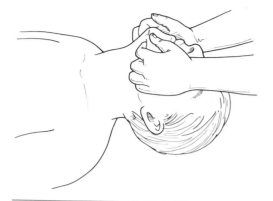

Figure 66.1
The jaw thrust maneuver opens the airway while protecting the cervical spine.

ial) or complex (e.g., a surgical airway). The rest of this chapter focuses on the techniques that may be needed in advanced airway management.

Oral and Nasopharyngeal Airways

Oral and nasal airways are adjuncts to help maintain an adequate airway. They are also important devices for improving bag-valve-mask ventilation of a patient.

Oral airways are rigid plastic devices designed to extend from the teeth to the back of the tongue (Fig. 66.3). The presence of a gag reflex is a contraindication to the use of an oral airway, because these patients may

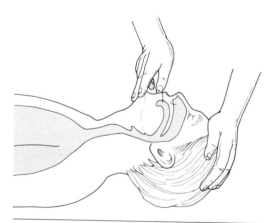

Figure 66.2
The head tilt-chin lift maneuver is used when cervical spine protection is not needed.

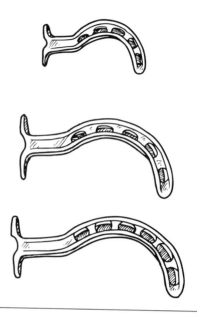

Figure 66.3
Oral airways are inserted to keep the tongue from obstructing the posterior pharynx. They are also used to protect endotracheal tubes from being bitten.

vomit and aspirate. To properly size an airway, it should extend from the corner of the mouth to the earlobe. To insert, the mouth is opened using a spreading scissors-like motion of the thumb and index finger, with the thumb resting on the bottom teeth and the finger resting on the top teeth (Fig. 66.4). After the mouth has been opened as far as possible, being careful not to injure the palate, the airway is inserted upside-down until it meets the hard palate, then it is rotated 180 degrees while advancing, until the rim is at the patient's teeth and the tip is pointing down the patient's throat. Alternatively, the airway may be inserted right-side up, using a tongue blade to push the tongue anteriorly.

When an oral airway is contraindicated, either by an intact gag reflex or severe oral trauma, a nasopharyngeal airway may be used (Fig. 66.5). Patients with an intact gag reflex usually tolerate nasal airways. They are contraindicated in patients with extensive nasal trauma or suspected basilar skull fracture. An airway is chosen that is slightly smaller in diameter than the nostril and is sized for length by measuring from the tip of the nose to the

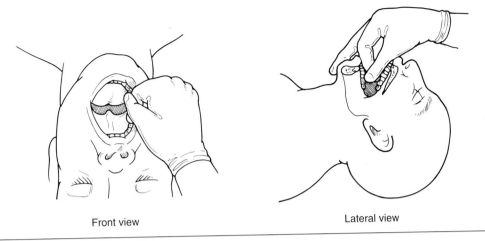

Front view   Lateral view

Figure 66.4
Proper technique for opening the airway involves a scissor-like motion of the thumb and index finger.

earlobe. After application of water-soluble lubricant, it is placed in the larger nostril with the bevel facing the septum and gently advanced along the floor of the nostril (not upward toward the top of the head) until the flange is seated against the nostril.

Orotracheal Intubation

Indications for intubation include inadequate oxygenation or ventilation, decreased mental status with inability to protect the airway, increased intracranial pressure (ICP) requiring hyperventilation, and sedation and control of a combative patient who may require radiological or other studies. Placement of an endotracheal tube entails certain risks, and these risks should be considered in every situation before proceeding with intubation.

Airway Assessment

Airway assessment in the emergency department is limited because of the urgency of patient presentation and level of acuity of illness. However, a few brief observations can identify patients who will prove difficult to intubate. The mnemonic MOUTHS summarizes physical features that can complicate intubation, as follows:

Mandible: Is the distance from the symphysis of the mandible to the hyoid bone less than 6 cm?

Opening: Does the mouth open less than 3 cm?

Uvula: Assess the modified Mallampati score by opening the mouth maximally and noting which posterior structures (uvula, soft and hard palate, tonsillar pillars) are visible (Fig. 66.6).

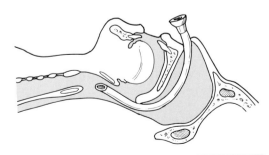

Figure 66.5
A nasal airway can be used when an oral airway is contraindicated.

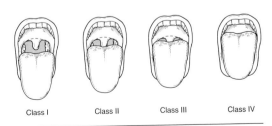

Class I   Class II   Class III   Class IV

Figure 66.6
Ease or difficulty of the airway can be assessed using a scoring system based on the Mallampati classes.

Teeth: Are prominent central incisors present? Is there loose dentition? Is there a receding chin or overbite?

Head: Is the patient able to approach the sniffing position?

Silhouette: Are there any abnormalities (e.g., kyphosis, goiter, or traumatic swelling) that will make intubation difficult?

Identification of a patient with a potentially difficult airway allows for anticipation of difficulties and may prompt consideration of maneuvers other than rapid-sequence intubation.

Equipment and Monitoring

Emergency department personnel who will be using the airway equipment should check it at the beginning of every shift. Suction must be set up and working with tonsil tip attachment. Oxygen should be available via non-rebreather mask and bag-valve-mask apparatus with a variety of masks available. A laryngoscope handle and variety of sizes of Miller (straight) and MacIntosh (curved) blades should be available, and the lights should be tested. Endotracheal tubes in an assortment of sizes should be available, with stylets. A 10-mL syringe is needed for cuff inflation. An end-tidal CO_2 detector is used to assist in confirmation of tube placement. Oral and nasal airways can make the difference between a "cannot intubate, cannot ventilate" situation and adequate mask ventilation. Monitoring equipment includes electrocardiogram (ECG), blood pressure, and pulse oximeter monitors.

Alignment of Axis

Direct laryngoscopy for the purpose of endotracheal intubation can be conceptualized as attempting to align three tubes in a straight line, to enable visualization of an object (glottic opening) at the other end (Fig. 66.7). Extension of the head on the neck and flexion of the neck at the lower cervical spine (in patients without c-spine injury) to attain a "sniffing position" assists in aligning the oral, pharyngeal, and laryngeal axes to

permit visualization of the glottis. Rolled sheets beneath the occiput and external manipulation of the larynx may be helpful in producing alignment of structures and visualization of the laryngeal inlet.

Direct Laryngoscopy

The mouth is opened fully using the fingers of the right hand in a scissors technique. The laryngoscope blade (curved = Macintosh, straight = Miller), held in the left hand of the intubator, is introduced into the right side of the patient's mouth and advanced posteriorly, sweeping the tongue to the left. If the Macintosh blade is used, it is inserted in the vallecula and the epiglottis is retracted indirectly by pressure on the vallecula, exposing the glottis. If the Miller blade is used, it is advanced past the epiglottis, and the epiglottis is then retracted directly. (See Fig. 66.9 on page 571.) The force on the laryngoscope handle should be a steady upward motion along the axis of the handle, NOT a levering-type force, because this can damage dentition. External manipulation of the larynx by the intubator's right hand (mnemonic BURP: backward [posterior], upward [cephalad], rightward pressure] may help to bring the vocal cords into the field of view. Upward retraction of the upper lip by an assistant aids in exposure of the cords. Once the cords are seen, the tube is advanced under direct visualization between the cords and then 3 to 4 cm farther. The stylet is immediately removed, the balloon filled, and placement confirmed by listening over each axilla for breath sounds and over the stomach for air. In addition, a confirmatory chest x-ray film is obtained to view the endotracheal tube's position relative to the carina.

Rapid-Sequence Induction Intubation

Rapid-sequence induction (RSI) is the cornerstone of emergency department airway management. It was adapted from the anesthesia literature based on the assumption that all patients presenting to the emergency department have full stomachs and present

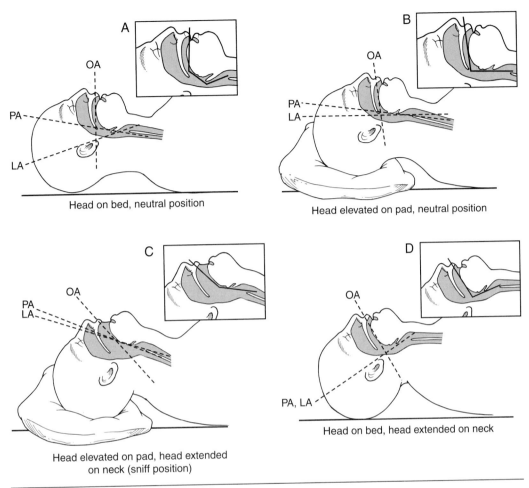

A   Head on bed, neutral position

B   Head elevated on pad, neutral position

C   Head elevated on pad, head extended
on neck (sniff position)

D   Head on bed, head extended on neck

Figure 66.7
Proper positioning of the head aligns the airway and posterior pharynx for ease of intubation.

an increased risk for aspiration. RSI combines intravenous (IV) sedation in combination with a short-acting neuromuscular blocker, usually succinyl choline. The succinyl choline causes loss of muscle tone in about 1 minute, with return of muscle function in about 5 minutes. While the patient is iatrogenically paralyzed, endotracheal intubation is facilitated by the flaccidity of the patient's muscles. During RSI, the patient will have no respiratory effort; therefore, intubation must proceed rapidly, or the patient will require bag-mask ventilation. The steps of RSI can be remembered as 9 Ps:

1. Prepare equipment
2. Preoxygenate
3. Position the patient
4. Premedication
5. Prime (induction agents)
6. Pressure (cricoid)
7. Paralytics
8. Pass the tube through the cords
9. Placement is confirmed

Preparation of Equipment

All equipment should be checked before any medication administration or intubation attempt. Two endotracheal tubes, of the size anticipated and one-half size smaller, should be prepared with stylets, ensuring that the stylets do not protrude from the end of the endotracheal tube. Preparation also includes removing dentures; placing two IV lines in the patient; connecting the patient to ECG, O_2 saturation, and blood pressure monitors; and notifying respiratory therapy that a ventilator will be needed. If RSI is planned, weight-appropriate medications should be drawn up in clearly labeled syringes.

Preoxygenation

As soon the decision to intubate has been made, place the spontaneously breathing patient on 100% oxygen by nonrebreather mask. This facilitates the "wash out" of nitrogen stores and the buildup of an oxygen reservoir. Administering 100% oxygen does not mean ventilating the patient with the bag-valve-mask. Ideally, RSI is performed in the spontaneously breathing patient without any positive-pressure ventilation until the endotracheal tube is passed. This minimizes insufflation of the stomach and subsequent risk of aspiration. If the patient is not spontaneously breathing, positive-pressure ventilation with bag-valve-mask is instituted.

Position

If the patient can tolerate the supine position, place the patient toward the head of the bed. Next, fold a sheet (or sheets) under the patient's head to put it in the sniffing position (if no cervical spine injury is present). Then, raise the bed so the patient is at a comfortable height for the intubator.

Premedication

Premedication includes lidocaine in patients with head injury and increased ICP (minimizing an increase in ICP brought on by laryngoscopy) or bronchospasm (minimizing further spasm induced by airway manipulation). Pancuronium is administered in a defasciculating dose in patients with head injury or any other conditions in which the muscle fasciculations of succinylcholine would be detrimental. Atropine is administered to pediatric patients to prevent bradycardia during laryngoscopy.

Prime

Priming medications, or induction agents, are used before paralytic agents to prevent the patient from being aware of the paralysis. The main agents used are ketamine, midazolam, thiopental, and etomidate. Ketamine is used in status asthmaticus, because it is a bronchodilator; it is also useful in trauma with hypotension because it has minimal blood pressure effects. Ketamine should be avoided in head trauma, because it raises ICP. Midazolam should be used with caution in the hypotensive patient because hypotension occasionally is associated with its use. Thiopental is used in patients with head trauma because it lowers ICP; however, it also causes hypotension. Etomidate has the beneficial properties of lowering ICP and not causing hypotension, so it is useful in trauma. These medications should be given a sufficient time before administrating paralytics.

Pressure

Cricoid pressure, or Sellick's maneuver, is pressure placed on the cricoid ring by an assistant to occlude the esophagus and thereby to decrease the risk of aspiration (Fig. 66.8). The pressure is not meant to interrupt emesis, and attempting to do so may result in esophageal injury. In the vomiting patient, cricoid pressure should be released and the patient log-rolled onto the side as the mouth is suctioned. Cricoid pressure should be instituted before the paralytics are administered and held until the endotracheal tube cuff is inflated and the tube position is confirmed.

Paralytics

Paralytics used in RSI ideally have a very rapid onset and a short duration of action (in case the patient is unable to be intubated and spontaneous respirations become desirable). The medication that comes closest to ideal is the depolarizing paralytic succinylcholine. The onset of action is 30 to 45 seconds, and most patients begin to regain respirations after about 5 minutes. The drawback to succinylcholine is that it causes fasciculations of the muscles. Consequently, it causes

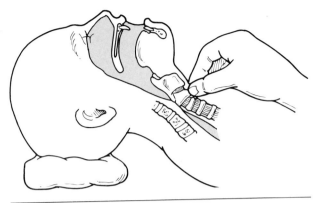

Figure 66.8
Pressure placed on the cricoid ring by an assistant occludes the esophagus, thereby decreasing the risk of aspiration. (Reproduced with permission from Benumof JL. *Principles and procedures in anesthesia and intensive care.* Baltimore: JB Lippincott, 1992.)

increase in intragastric, intraocular, and ICP and hyperkalemia. It should be avoided in patients with preexisting paralysis or severe burns more than 12 hours old (higher risk for hyperkalemia) and in patients with penetrating injuries to the eye. It may be used in patients with head trauma if premedication and priming medications are used to blunt the increase in ICP. Other nondepolarizing agents include pancuronium and vecuronium, which have a longer onset and duration of action.

Passing the Tube

Using direct laryngoscopy, the endotracheal tube is passed through the vocal cords. To perform laryngoscopy, the mouth is opened fully using the fingers of the right hand in a scissors technique. The laryngoscope blade (curved = Macintosh, straight = Miller), held in the left hand of the intubator, is introduced in the right side of the patient's mouth and advanced posteriorly, sweeping the tongue to the left. If the Macintosh blade is used, it is inserted in the vallecula and the epiglottis is retracted indirectly by pressure on the vallecula, exposing the glottis. If the Miller blade is used, it is advanced past the epiglottis and the epiglottis is then retracted directly (Fig. 66.9). The force on the laryngoscope handle should be a steady upward motion along the axis of the handle, NOT a levering-type force. External manipulation of

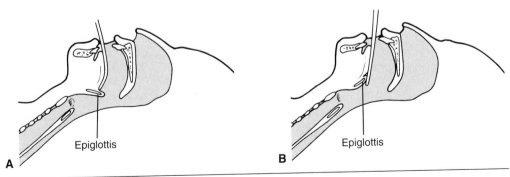

A   B

Figure 66.9
Placement of curved (A) and straight (B) laryngoscope blades. (Reproduced with permission from Benumof JL. *Principles and procedures in anesthesia and intensive care.* Baltimore: JB Lippincott, 1992.)

the larynx by the intubator's right hand may help to bring the vocal cords into the field of view. Once the intubator has visualized the cords, the tube is advanced under direct visualization as it passes between the cords and then 3 to 4 cm farther.

After the tube is observed to pass between the cords, the endotracheal tube is stabilized, the laryngoscope is withdrawn, the stylet is removed, the balloon is inflated with 10 mL of air, and the bag-valve apparatus and end-tidal CO_2 detector is attached.

Placement

Tube placement is confirmed in the trachea by multiple means. The best confirmation is the intubator's clear visualization of the tube passing through the vocal cords. In addition, or when visualization is not certain, there are several other steps to confirm correct placement. First, several breaths are given via bag-valve apparatus, and breath sounds are examined in both axillae and over the epigastrium. Diminished breath sounds on the left indicate probable right mainstem intubation, and the cuff should be deflated as the tube is withdrawn 2 cm, listening for return of breath sounds on the left, at which point the cuff is reinflated and the tube is secured. Prominent sounds over the epigastrium, diminished breath sounds bilaterally, and inadequate rise and fall of the chest are all indicative of esophageal intubation, and the tube should be removed and the patient ventilated via bag-valve-mask. A color change on the end-tidal CO_2 detector is a good indicator of tracheal intubation. An increase in oxygen saturation to 100% is another indicator of endotracheal placement. A chest x-ray film is taken immediately after intubation to determine exact depth of intubation; the tip of the endotracheal tube should lie within 3 cm of the carina. However, the x-ray film cannot differentiate between esophageal and tracheal intubation, because both tubes lie in the center of an anteroposterior x-ray. It is important to note that no one method for confirmation of tube placement is fail-safe, and multiple methods should routinely be used. After placement is confirmed, the endotracheal tube is secured and an orogastric tube is placed to decompress the stomach.

Alternate Methods of Intubation

Most patients requiring intubation in the emergency department are intubated using RSI. The main contraindications to RSI are any conditions that prevent intubation or preclude ventilation with a bag-valve-mask; these conditions are screened for in the preintubation airway assessment. Several alternate means of tracheal intubation exist, and the emergency physician must be skilled in these techniques to be prepared to manage the anticipated or unanticipated difficult airway.

Awake Oral Intubation

The technique for awake oral intubation combines liberal local airway anesthesia with judicious IV sedation. It is useful in cases of blunt or penetrating airway trauma (where bag-valve-mask ventilation could result in insufflation of subcutaneous tissues and distortion of airway anatomy) and any anticipated difficult airway. Airway anesthesia consists of 5 mL of 4% lidocaine, nebulized over 5 to 10 minutes, if time permits. If time is an issue, 10% lidocaine topical spray to the oropharynx or hypopharynx will allow laryngoscopy. (Exercise caution with topical benzocaine, because it is associated with methemoglobinemia.) Local anesthesia, combined with 1 to 2 mg of midazolam intravenously and explanation of the procedure to the patient, permits laryngoscopy and intubation without abolishment of spontaneous respirations.

Blind Nasotracheal Intubation

The technique for blind nasotracheal intubation involves blind passage of the endotracheal tube from the nares past the glottis into the trachea, using the sounds of respiration through the tube as a guide. Because breath sounds are essential to blind passage of the tube, apnea is a contraindication to this technique. Other contraindications include coagulopathy, extensive midface trauma or suspected basilar skull fracture, upper airway foreign body or epiglottitis, blunt or penetrating neck injury, and prosthetic heart valves (relative contraindication because of the small risk of transient bacteremia).

Nasal intubation is a useful tool for the anticipated difficult airway in the spontaneously breathing patient with no suspicion of a cervical spine injury or in situations in which paralytics are unavailable.

First, the nostril is prepared using topical anesthetics and vasoconstrictors. Cocaine 4%, or a combination of phenylephrine or oxymetolazone, and 10% lidocaine spray to nares and pharynx can be used. An endotracheal tube 0.5 to 1.0 size smaller than that for oral intubation is chosen and lubricated. The patient is then positioned in the sniffing position, the bevel of the tube is placed facing the septum, and the tube is advanced directly posteriorly during inspiration. As the tube passes from the nasopharynx to the oropharynx and hypopharynx, the intubator listens carefully to the sounds of respiration at the end of the tube. As the glottis is approached, breath sounds will become louder. Tracheal intubation occurs at a depth of 26 to 28 cm and is preliminarily indicated by fogging of the tube, breath sounds from the tube, coughing with passage of tube through glottis, and lack of vocalization. Smooth passage of the tube and loss of breath sounds indicates esophageal intubation. In this situation, withdraw the tube until breath sounds are heard again, then increase head extension and apply cricoid pressure as tube is readvanced with inspiration. Tube placement is subsequently confirmed as usual. Complications of this procedure include bleeding (moderate to severe in 6% of patients) and infection (bacteremia, retropharyngeal abscess, and sinusitis).

Fiberoptic Intubation

Most anesthesiologists in the United States favor fiberoptic intubation as the initial approach to the anticipated difficult airway. The technique is similar to fiberoptic naso-pharyngoscopy, a procedure familiar to emergency physicians, and consequently it is used more frequently in the emergency department.

The first step in fiberoptic intubation is topical anesthesia—identical to blind nasotracheal intubation if planning a fiberoptic nasal intubation or to awake oral intubation if planning a fiberoptic oral intubation. If the intubation is to be oral, a bite block is recommended to protect the scope from damage. An appropriately sized endotracheal tube is then "loaded" onto the scope, the patient's airway is suctioned thoroughly, and the scope/endotracheal tube is advanced either orally or nasally past the glottis to the level of the carina. At this point the endotracheal tube is advanced carefully off the scope to the appropriate depth (26 to 28 cm if nasal, 21 to 23 cm if oral), and the endoscope is removed. Tube placement is confirmed using conventional means.

Digital Intubation

Digital intubation is ideally suited to the prehospital environment because it can be performed in close quarters using only a tube and stylet. The patient must be deeply unconscious, and a bite block should be used to protect the fingers of the intubator. The stylet is inserted into the endotracheal tube, taking care to ensure that the stylet does not protrude from the end of the tube. A 90-degree bend is placed a few centimeters proximal to the balloon. If available, an assistant may help by grasping the patient's tongue with gauze and exerting gentle traction. The intubator's nondominant hand is then inserted in the patient's mouth, the middle finger reaches for the epiglottis and elevates it (functioning much like a Miller blade), and the index finger helps direct the tube anteriorly through the glottis. Backward upward pressure on the larynx may help in passage of the tube. Placement of the tube is then confirmed as usual. Disadvantages of this procedure include the risk of injury if the patient bites down on an unprotected hand; moreover, it is useful only in a limited subset of patients.

"Cannot Intubate, Cannot Ventilate"

The emergency physician must have a pre-existing plan for the unanticipated difficult airway. Most patients can be intubated with RSI by using different laryngoscope blades, multiple attempts, and multiple laryngoscopists. However, a small percentage of patients cannot be intubated by conventional means. If the patient can be ventilated via bag-valve-mask, then there is time to summon assistance or try other techniques (i.e., fiberoptic). If the patient cannot be ventilated, then he or she will soon die without rapid intervention. These interventions can be separated into adjunct ventilatory devices (laryngeal mask airway [LMA], Combitube, and transtracheal jet ventilation [TTJV]) and surgical cricothyrotomy.

Laryngeal Mask Airway

The LMA was designed to fill the gap between mask ventilation and endotracheal intubation. It is placed blindly in the hypopharynx, where its contours form a seal against the glottis and enable more efficacious ventilation than with mask ventilation. The drawback is that it does not afford the airway protection that a cuffed tube in the trachea provides; thus, its usefulness is limited in the emergency department (where everyone is assumed to have a full stomach and subsequently at risk for aspiration) to the "cannot intubate, cannot ventilate" situation. The LMA is contraindicated in patients with airway problems at or below the level of the epiglottis (upper airway foreign body, epiglottitis, tracheal or laryngeal trauma, anaphylactic laryngeal edema, or periglottic hematoma or abscess).

When the LMA is inserted correctly, the tip occupies the entire hypopharynx and rests against the upper esophageal sphincter behind the cricoid cartilage. The LMA is prepared for insertion by checking the cuff for leaks and then deflating while pressing it flat against the table to create a "floppy shovel" shape. The posterior (not the glottic) aspect of the mask is lubricated with water-soluble lubricant. The LMA is grasped at the tube just proximally to the mask by the thumb and forefinger of the dominant hand, and the lubricated surface is placed against the hard palate (with the mask opening facing the tongue). The index and middle fingers maintain cephalad pressure as the LMA is advanced from the oropharynx to curve into the hypopharynx until resistance is encountered. The LMA is then stabilized while the other hand is removed. The cuff is then inflated, adequacy of ventilation is assessed, and the tube is secured (Fig. 66.10). Because this does not protect sufficiently against aspiration, an endotracheal tube should be placed as soon as possible to definitively secure the airway. This can be accomplished by passing a fiberoptic scope loaded with a lubricated endotracheal tube through the LMA, by blindly passing an endotracheal tube through an intubating LMA (in either case leaving the LMA in place subsequently but deflating the cuff), or by enlisting the assistance of anesthesiology.

Transtracheal Jet Ventilation

TTJV, also called needle cricothyrotomy, is a procedure that can provide not only life-saving oxygenation but also ventilation for prolonged periods when performed properly. Contraindications include significant laryngeal injury or total airway obstruction (because this can lead to barotrauma). The equipment necessary includes a jet ventilator (either commercially available or assembled from supplies readily available in the emergency department), an oxygen source, a 14-gauge over-the-needle IV catheter, and a 5-mL syringe with 2 mL of saline.

The key landmark for the procedure is the cricothyroid membrane, which is located in the depression between the thyroid cartilage ("Adam's apple") superiorly and the cricoid cartilage inferiorly. The skin is prepped with povidone-iodine solution. The needle is attached to the syringe with saline and advanced at a 45-degree angle caudally through the inferior portion of the cricothyroid membrane. Aspiration of air bubbles confirms entry into the larynx, and the cannula is advanced off the needle until its hub is snug against the skin. At this point, the jet ventilator is secured to the catheter and to the wall oxygen source opened maximally. The patient

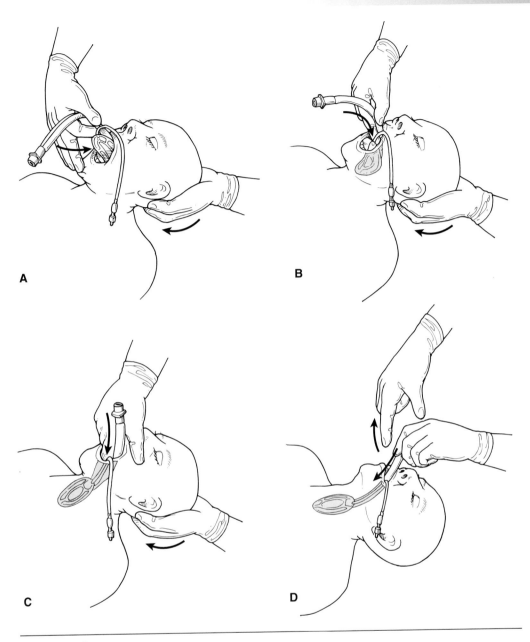

Figure 66.10
Insertion and positioning of the laryngeal mask airway. (Reproduced with permission from Barash PG, Cullen BF, Stoelting RK. *Clinical anesthesia,* 3rd ed. Philadelphia: Lippincott, Williams & Wilkins 2000.)

is ventilated at a rate of 20 breaths per minute (use the thumb to cover the hole in the oxygen tubing for 1 second for inspiration, then release the thumb for 2 seconds for passive expiration). The catheter is then secured in place using sutures or ties, and oxygenation is monitored with oximetry.

The most frequent complication of TTJV is subcutaneous emphysema, occurring 2% to 10% of the time. This can be minimized by firmly securing the hub of the catheter to the neck. Other complications include tracheal mucosal ulceration, bleeding, and vocal changes.

Surgical Cricothyrotomy

Surgical cricothyrotomy is the approach of choice for the patient who cannot be intubated or ventilated by any other means in a timely fashion (Fig. 66.11). Relative contraindications include age younger than 5 years (TTJV is recommended in these patients) and bleeding diathesis; absolute contraindications include significant damage to the cricoid cartilage or larynx.

After locating the cricothyroid membrane, the anterior neck is quickly prepped with povidone-iodine and the larynx is stabilized with the nondominant hand. A 3-cm to 4-cm vertical incision is made in the midline, followed by a 1-cm horizontal stab incision in the inferior portion of the cricothyroid membrane (to avoid the cricothyroid arteries). The scalpel handle is then inserted through the incision and rotated 90 degrees to enlarge the opening. Alternatively, the spreading tips of Mayo scissors may be used to widen the space. A number 5 or 6 Shiley tracheostomy tube is then inserted into the larynx, the cuff is inflated, the tube secured, and placement is verified by multiple means. If a tracheostomy tube is not available, an endotracheal tube may be used temporarily.

Complications of surgical cricothyrotomy can be divided into early and late. Early complications include failure to place tube

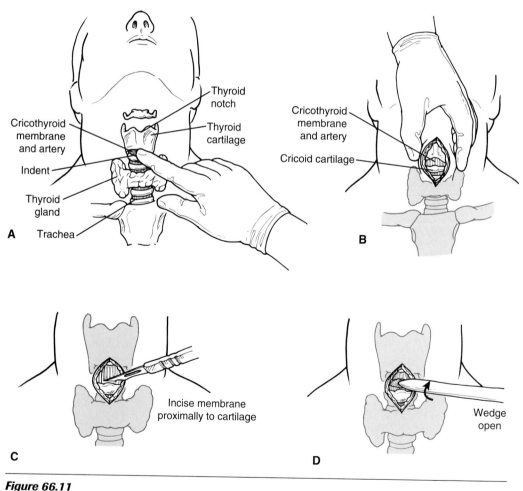

Figure 66.11
Surgical cricothyrotomy. (Reproduced with permission from Barash PG, Cullen BF, Stoelting RK. *Clinical anesthesia*, 3rd ed. Philadelphia: Lippincott, Williams & Wilkins 2000.)

or prolonged procedure time, bleeding, sub-cutaneous emphysema, and infection. Late complications include voice changes, laryngeal stenosis, and tracheomalacia.

Suggested Readings

American Society of Anesthesiologists Task Force on Management of the Difficult Airway. Practice guidelines for management of the difficult airway. *Anesthesiology* 1993;78:597–602.

Benumof JL. Management of the difficult adult airway. *Anesthesiology* 1991;75:1087–1110.

Benumof JL. Laryngeal mask airway and the ASA difficult airway algorithm. *Anesthesiology* 1996;84:686–699.

Benumof JL, Scheller MS. The importance of transtracheal jet ventilation in the management of the difficult airway. *Anesthesiology* 1989;71:769–778.

Chang RS, Hamilton RJ, Carter WA. Declining rate of cricothyrotomy in trauma patients with an emergency medicine residency: implications for skills training. *Acad Emerg Med* 1998;5:247–251.

Criswell JC, Parr MJA. Emergency airway management in patients with cervical spine injuries. *Anaesthesia* 1994;49:900–903.

Crosby ET, Cooper RM, Douglas MJ, et al. The unanticipated difficult airway with recommendations for management. *Can J Anaesth* 1998;45:757–776.

Delaney KA, Hessler R. Emergency flexible fiberoptic nasotracheal intubation: a report of 60 cases. *Ann Emerg Med* 1988;17:919–926.

Gausche M, Lewis RJ, Stratton SJ, et al. Effect of out-of-hospital endotracheal intubation on survival and neurological outcome. *JAMA* 2000;283:783–790.

Gerardi MJ, Sacchetti AD, Cantor RM, et al. Rapid-sequence intubation of the pediatric patient. *Ann Emerg Med* 1996;28:55–74.

Hastings RH, Marks JD. Airway management for trauma patients with potential cervical spine injuries. *Anesth Analg* 1991;73:471–482.

Mallampati SR, Gatt SP, Gugino LD, et al. A clinical sign to predict difficult tracheal intubation: a prospective study. *Can Anaesth Soc J* 1985;32:429–434.

McAllister JD, Gnauck KA. Rapid-sequence intubation of the pediatric patient. *Pediatr Clin North Am* 1999;46:1249–1284.

Stewart RD. Tactile orotracheal intubation. *Ann Emerg Med* 1984;13:175–178.

Tintinalli JE, Claffey J. Complications of nasotracheal intubation. *Ann Emerg Med* 1981;10:142–144.

CHAPTER **67**

Peripheral Intravenous Access

Patricia Mather Harrison, RN, MS, ACNP, CCRN, CEN

Chapter Outline

Peripheral intravenous (IV) cannulation is the most common invasive procedure performed in the emergency department (ED). Professionals at many levels are trained to perform IV access: physicians, nurses, prehospital providers, technicians, and medical students. This chapter describes the indications and contraindications of peripheral IV access, preparation and equipment, site selection, cannulation technique, and complications.

Indications

IV access is commonly initiated in the ED for a wide variety of reasons: (a) fluid therapy, (b) delivery of medications, (c) phlebotomy, and (d) short-term nutrition administration. Peripheral lines are also placed in anticipation of a patient's condition suddenly worsening, which may require quick action using the IV access for treatment. The use of a saline lock catheter system is preferable when limited IV fluid administration is anticipated and access is needed for medication delivery. This is especially useful in patients with renal, cardiac, or hepatic failure.

Contraindications

Peripheral lines should not be attempted in any extremity with a traumatic injury, burns, massive edema, or phlebitis because of the potential for fluid extravasation or inadequate flow. Caution should also be taken with patients who have indwelling fistulas or shunts. Because of an increased risk of infection or thrombosis, the opposite arm should be used for access if at all possible. In addition, patients who have undergone a mastectomy should have their IVs placed in the opposite arm.

Preparation and Equipment

Organization is essential in preparing for IV access, especially if performing the procedure alone. The necessary items are IV catheter and needle, gloves, povidone-iodine solution or 70% alcohol to clean the skin, a tourniquet to occlude the venous blood flow, and sterile gauze pads to wipe away any excess cleaning solution and to stop any bleeding from the site after withdrawal of a catheter. An IV solution and tubing or saline lock should be assembled before catheter insertion. Items such as tape, topical antibiotic, and dressings are also required.

Each hospital has a policy and procedure specific to their institution regarding site preparation and care. Universal precautions are taken on all patients requiring any venipuncture. These include at minimum wearing gloves at all times and preferably eye protection to avoid contact with splashing materials containing blood. Special attention for patients with latex allergy should be followed regarding preparation and equipment.

Many types of catheters are available for peripheral access: a plastic catheter over a hollow steel needle, a hollow steel needle, a plastic catheter, or a plastic catheter inserted through a hollow steel needle. The catheter

Table 67.1.

Size of Angiocatheter	Indications for Use
16 gauge	Profound volume loss, usually hemorrhagic
18 gauge	Any trauma with the potential for serious injury
	Patients requiring blood transfusions
	Patients in shock, or severely volume depleted
20 gauge	Any patient who is stable and does not require large volumes of fluid or blood. Can be used in blood transfusions if necessary
22 gauge	Patients with difficult access and limited need for intravenous access
	Pediatrics
24 gauge	Pediatrics only

over the needle is the most common type used for peripheral access (Table 67.1).

Site Selection and Catheter Insertion

The veins of the upper extremity are usually chosen to initiate IV lines because of the many sites available and their relative comfort. The most distal vein should be attempted first, so that in the event of an unsuccessful attempt, the more proximal site is available, and proximal fluid leakage from the previous stick is avoided. The volar aspect of the forearm and veins of the hand are the preferred sites. The antecubital space is preferred by many clinicians, despite the need to immobilize the arm to prevent kinking of the catheter. The external jugular is a site often used as a last resort to avoid central venous catheterization in patients without suitable arm veins.

Once the site has been selected, apply a tourniquet proximal to the site. Prepare the skin and pull it taut to help stabilize the vein. Sometimes tapping the vein with your fingers flat causes the vein to engorge and become more visible. Hold the IV catheter in your dominant hand and puncture the skin rapidly with a sterile catheter, at a 30-degree angle, bevel up, and parallel to the vein (Fig. 67.1). Once inside the vein, advance the needle and catheter as a

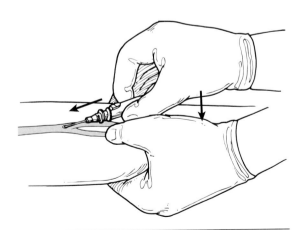

Figure 67.1
Proper position of the intravenous (IV) catheter relative to the skin, with a 30-degree angle, bevel up, and parallel to the vein.

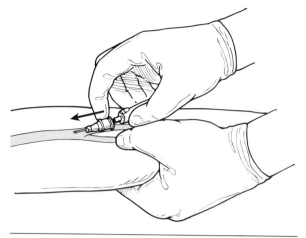

Figure 67.2
The needle is stabilized while the catheter is advanced
over the needle into the vein, to the hub of the catheter.

unit until blood is seen in the flash chamber. Then, hold the needle stable, and advance the catheter over the needle into the vein to the hub of the catheter (Fig. 67.2). Stabilize the catheter and place direct pressure on the proximal vein over the catheter tip to prevent blood from flowing through the open catheter once the needle is removed (Fig. 67.3). Finally, remove the needle.

Most new IV needles have a safety device to retract the needle into a plastic case to avoid needlestick injuries. The needle should be discarded immediately into an appropriate sharps container. Never stick a used needle into a mattress, even in an urgent situation. A Vacutainer or syringe can then be connected to the hub of the catheter for collecting blood (phlebotomy) (Table 67.2). The institution may have a special procedure for prevention of hemolysis if blood sampling is obtained in this manner. The IV tubing is then attached to the hub of the catheter, the tourniquet is released, and the regulating clamp is adjusted to the desired flow rate. If a saline lock is desired, the intermittent device is flushed with saline and connected at the catheter hub. A sliding clamp on the tubing is then pushed

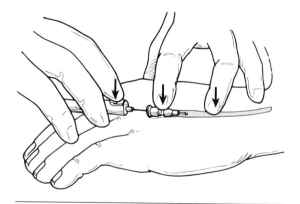

Figure 67.3
The catheter is stabilized and compressed to prevent
blood from escaping, while the needle is removed and
retracted.

Table 67.2.

Types of blood tubes routinely used to draw blood during IV insertion

Purple top	CBC, sedimentation rate
Blue top	PT, PTT, INR
Red top	Type and cross, electrolytes, glucose, BUN, creatinine
Green top	Cardiac enzymes
Tiger top or yellow top	Liver function tests

BUN, blood urea nitrogen; CBC, complete blood cell count; INR, international normalized ratio; IV, intravenous; PT, prothrombin time; PTT, partial prothrombin time.

to occlude blood backflow. This needleless device system is now the standard of care for preventing accidental needlesticks by medical personnel. The site of insertion is usually dressed with an antibiotic ointment and an adhesive bandage or other sterile dressing applied. All waste that contacted the patient's blood should be disposed of into hazardous waste containers.

If circumstances require you to draw blood from the same extremity in which the IV is infusing, do not forget to do so below the infusion site; otherwise, you may dilute the serum chemistry levels with some of the fluid you are infusing.

Complications

Phlebitis may occur in up to 75% of hospitalized patients. Leaving the catheter in the vein for a prolonged time, large catheter size, and infusion of irritant solutions all increase the risk of phlebitis. Methods to decrease this risk include changing the IV site after 3 days (sooner if placed prehospital), dissolving irritant medications with a larger volume of fluid, and checking the insertion site for tenderness and swelling. If phlebitis is suspected without infection (cellulitis), application of warm moist heat and elevation of the extremity are helpful. Observation of blood in the flash chamber when inserting the catheter, along with checking for swelling, tenderness, pain, and flow from the

drip should prevent accidental infusion of IV fluid into the subcutaneous tissue. Although this is usually not dangerous, it is painful to the patient and, simply put, is bad form.

If infiltration occurs, you can attempt to aspirate some fluid using a 3-mL syringe attached directly to the IV catheter. If you feel resistance, remove the catheter. If blood is obtained, discard the blood and flush the catheter carefully with a sterile saline flush. The major complication of flushing an infiltrated IV line is central embolism.

Air embolism occurs rarely when air enters into the patient's bloodstream through the catheter or through IV tubing when the IV bag has been allowed to empty. Attention should be paid to ensure that IV bags do not run dry and that there is no air in the IV lines. A tremendous amount of air must reach the heart to cause an air embolism. In most cases the IV setup must be left open to the air and unattended for a prolonged time for enough air to enter the vein. A stray bubble in the IV tubing is no cause for you to become anxious about an air embolism.

Suggested Readings

Brunner L, Suddarth D. *Lippincott manual of nursing practice*. Philadelphia: Lippincott Williams & Wilkins, 2000:97–99.

Smith S, Duell D. *Advanced nursing skills*. Philadelphia: Lippincott Williams & Wilkins, 2001:850–853.

CHAPTER 68

Central Catheter Insertion

L. Kristian Arnold, MD, FACEP

Indications for cannulating the central circulation arise frequently in emergency medicine. The common reasons are to administer high-volume resuscitation, obtain peripheral venous access, or perform an intervention such as implanting a temporary pacemaker or central pressure monitor.

Access is usually accomplished via direct "blind" percutaneous venipuncture of large-caliber proximal tributary veins: the internal jugular (IJ), subclavian (SC), or femoral veins. Each route of access has distinct advantages and disadvantages.

Methods of accessing the central circulation via peripherally inserted catheters (PIC lines) are more commonly reserved for long-term access and are not covered in this chapter. Techniques of insertion using ultrasound or Doppler-guided needles are not covered separately in this chapter because they both require the same understanding of the anatomy, use the same approaches covered here, and require additional setup time and equipment not always available in the emergency department.

The choice of the IJ versus SC vein is dependent on several variables: foremost is which procedure you are most comfortable performing. In addition, several factors may influence the choice of SC versus IJ. For example, unlike the IJ vein, the SC vein cannot be compressed externally. In any patient with a coagulopathy, the IJ vein would be the best choice to avoid bleeding complications. The SC approach may also be complicated by puncture of the pleural space, creating a pneumothorax. The IJ may be difficult in patients with poor anatomic landmarks, for example, the morbidly obese. The IJ puncture is also difficult to perform in patients who cannot lie flat with the head held in an extended and rotated position. Various authors have proposed different techniques for accessing either the SC or IJ vein, implying that there is no single "correct" method.

Anatomy

These procedures must be done blindly, relying on the operator's knowledge of the relationships between surface and regional subcutaneous anatomy, including the location, caliber, and course of the veins. Therefore, this chapter focuses on developing an understanding of the regional anatomy and the relationship of the access technique to anatomic features.

Subclavian Vein

The course of the SC vein is demonstrated in Fig. 68.1.

The SC vein generally passes under the clavicle at the junction of the middle and medial thirds on the right and slightly more medially at approximately the junction of the medial and second fourths on the left. The vein courses slightly cephalad while the clavicle in its medial third assumes a more transverse direction. The vein passes over the superior border of the first rib in a fossa. It then joins with the IJ vein to form the innominate or brachiocephalic vein. The pleural dome is located medial and posterior to this confluence by only a few millimeters.

Internal Jugular Vein

The anatomy of the IJ vein is demonstrated in Fig. 68.2.

From its original relationship slightly lateral and posterior to the carotid artery, the IJ courses in a straight line toward its junction with the SC vein behind the cephalad border of the clavicle just as it starts to broaden at its medial end for articulation with the first rib and sternum. As the two vessels course toward the thoracic outlet, the jugular moves more anterior and diverges slightly laterally. The IJ vein and carotid are wrapped in a common fascia, the carotid sheath. This is directly attached to the fascia on the underside of the sternocleidomastoid muscle, thus making attempts at retraction of the muscle to expose the vein not only futile but also probably counterproductive because they are likely to distort the anatomy of the vein. The vagus and phrenic nerves course adjacent to the IJ and have been injured in cannulation attempts.

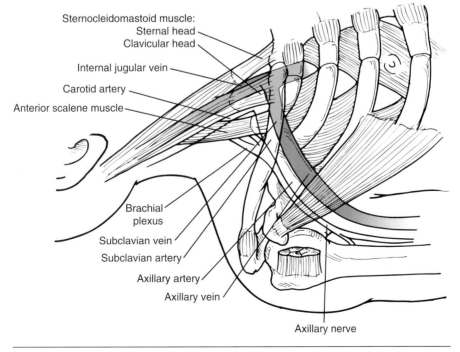

Figure 68.1
Anatomy of subclavian vein.

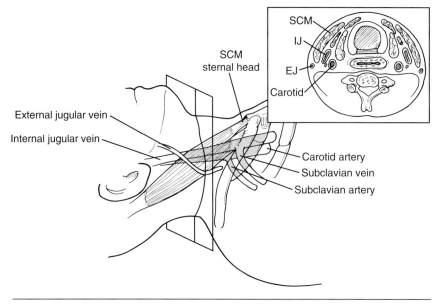

Figure 68.2
Anatomy of internal jugular vein.
SCN, Sternocleidomastoid muscle.

Femoral Vein

The femoral vein is located medial to the artery as they pass through the femoral triangle. The mnemonic NAVEL (Nerve, Artery, Vein, Empty space, Lymphatics— progressing from lateral to medial) describes the relation of the contents of the femoral triangle. The vein and artery pass under the inguinal ligament in a direction effectively toward the umbilicus of a slender abdomen.

If the femoral arterial pulse is not palpable, you may locate the vein using surface landmarks. The femoral artery reliably lies below the inguinal ligament at the midpoint between the inferior border of the anterior superior iliac spine and the midpoint of the symphysis pubis. The vein lies 1 cm (approximately one fingerbreadth) medial to this.

Patient Preparation

Psychological Preparation

If time permits for the awake patient, you should briefly explain the reason for the procedure and describe its possible complications. Generally, it is advisable to obtain written consent, although this topic is in active discussion in the medical literature at the time of this writing. Extremely agitated or anxious patients may require medication to calm them, thus improving the odds for easy success and lowering the potential for risks to both you and the patient. If sedation is necessary, you must use precautions for monitoring a sedated patient covered by drapes.

Patient Positioning

The patient should be in 15 to 20 degrees of Trendelenburg for the SC and IJ approaches. Trendelenburg positioning has been shown to aid dilatation of the IJ vein. Trendelenburg positioning also increases the intrathoracic venous pressure, decreasing the likelihood of air being aspirated into the circulation during the procedure.

For the SC approach, the patient's shoulders should be in neutral position, with the arms along the side of the body and the head in neutral position, facing forward. For the IJ approaches, the patient's head should be turned 30 to 45 degrees toward the opposite side from that being accessed. This slightly accentuates the positioning of the IJ slightly anterior to the carotid. If the patient's head is turned too far, it may impede access because the sternocleidomastoid muscle tends to pull over and cover the IJ. Some authors have favored an anterior IJ approach with the head facing forward.

Skin Prep and Drape

All efforts should be undertaken to adhere to strict aseptic technique, because most line infections stem from a breach in this part of the procedure.

In preparing for either the SC or IJ approach, prep the skin covering both sites. If your initial approach is unsuccessful, you can switch to the other site without having to completely reprep the patient. Most of the central venous access kits include a fenestrated drape to create a small sterile field. A minimum of three drapes is necessary to create the recommended sterile field. A lower rate of catheter infection has been associated with the use of formal surgical draping technique as opposed to using the "eye drape."

Operator Preparation

It is imperative for you to protect yourself from blood or body fluid exposures. At a minimum, wear a surgical mask and eye protection in addition to sterile gloves. Ideally, you should wear a sterile gown as well.

Equipment Setup

It is most efficient to set up the opened access kit on the side of your dominant hand. When reaching for additional materials, you will not have to transfer them from hand to hand nor will one hand have to cross the other to reach for materials. Do NOT recap needles! This is a very common mistake that ends in a needlestick injury to the operator.

Finder Needle

A 23-gauge, 3-cm needle can be used initially rather than the 16-gauge cannulation needle to locate the vein. When you see that you are in the vein, withdraw the "finder" needle just to the point where it can no longer aspirate blood. Commit to memory the direction of the finder needle. Take the 16-gauge cannulation needle-syringe complex with your dominant hand and bring it into a parallel position to the finder needle complex. Continue to watch the field while withdrawing the finder needle and placing it back to your tray safely. Now, insert the cannulation needle complex, attempting to follow the same trajectory as the finder needle.

Central Vein Access Technique

Subclavian Vein

Infraclavicular Approach

The needle should pass under the clavicle at the junction of the middle and medial thirds of the bone. Typically, the vein lies directly behind the clavicle at this point; therefore, the most appropriate direction for the needle is toward the superior border of the clavicle at the edge of the sternal notch. It is important to enter the skin far enough away from the clavicle to allow the subcutaneous tissue to be compressed in a manner that the needle can be advanced under the clavicle on as flat a plane as possible relative to the coronal (frontal) plane of the patient. Direction of the SC needle is demonstrated in Figs. 68.3 and 68.4. The needle should be advanced until it strikes the clavicle. Gradually "walk" the needle tip by carefully repositioning the needle more inferiorly. Once the needle passes under the clavicle, a small amount of negative pressure should be applied in the syringe. The needle should enter the vein within 1 to 1.5 cm of advancing past the border of the clavicle.

Supraclavicular Approach

Several authors have advocated the supraclavicular approach to the SC vein as being simpler and safer than infraclavicular approaches. The technique starts with the skin puncture lateral to the lateral margin of the clavicular insertion of the sternocleidomastoid muscle and one fingerbreadth above and behind the clavicle. The needle is directed anteriorly approximately 15 degrees and at an angle of approximately 45 degrees to the sagittal and horizontal planes, toward a point approximately halfway between the

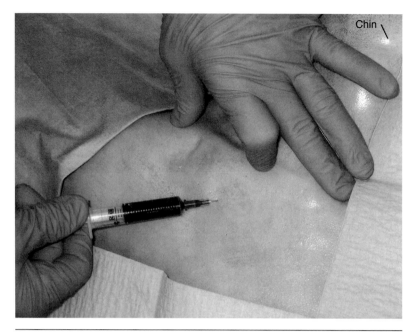

Chin

Figure 68.3
Subclavian needle is directed toward the superior border of the clavicle at the edge of the sternal notch.

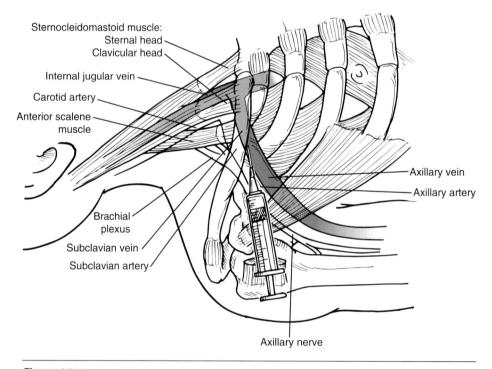

Sternocleidomastoid muscle:
Sternal head
Clavicular head
Internal jugular vein
Carotid artery
Anterior scalene
muscle

Axillary vein
Axillary artery

Brachial
plexus
Subclavian vein
Subclavian artery

Axillary nerve

Figure 68.4
Anatomic view of the subclavian needle direction.

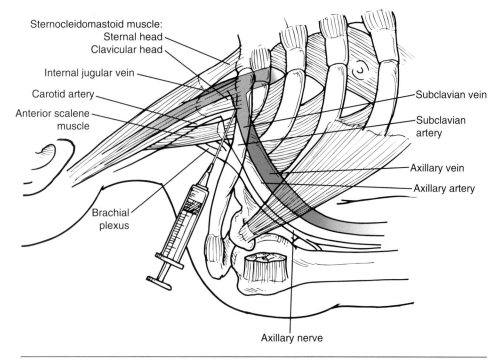

Figure 68.5
Anatomic view of the supraclavicular approach to the subclavian vein.

location of the contralateral nipple and the midline of the sternum on a slender male torso. The vein should be entered within 2.0 to 3.0 cm from skin entry. A perceived advantage of this approach is that the needle is entering the body in a direction relatively away from other critical structures in the region: the SC artery, located posteriorly, and lung, located below the plane described earlier. The supraclavicular approach to the SC vein is illustrated in Fig. 68.5.

External Jugular Vein

The central circulation can be cannulated via the external jugular (EJ) vein using the "J" tip of the guidewire. This route has been advocated because of its lower complication rate with comparable rates of proper catheter placement. Some central venous access kits contain a needle-catheter complex that looks like a standard intravenous catheter. This is used to cannulate the EJ. The needle is withdrawn and the guidewire is advanced through the short catheter.

Internal Jugular Vein

Although some authors have advocated the left IJ approach, most sources recommend choosing the right over the left to avoid the complication of cannulating or lacerating the thoracic duct.

Posterior Approach

The posterior approach is accomplished from the posterior border of the sternocleidomastoid muscle just cephalad to where the EJ vein crosses the posterior border of the muscle. If the EJ vein is not visible, the point of skin entry is approximately at the junction of the middle and lower thirds of the aspect of the sternocleidomastoid muscle. Recall again the anatomy (the vein courses along the posterior aspect of the sternocleidomastoid muscle); the needle must be directed upward from the posterior border of the muscle to follow a path along the undersurface of the muscle. To accomplish this, the operator's hand is lowered 15 to 20 degrees from the coronal plane prior

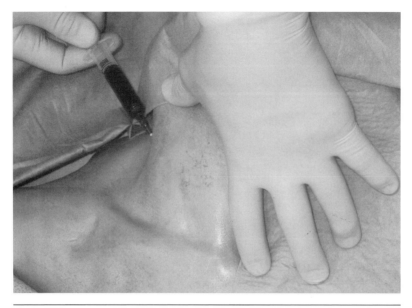

Figure 68.6
The posterior internal jugular (IJ) vein, anterior view, enters the skin at the
point where the posterior external jugular (EJ) vein crosses the posterior aspect
of the sternocleidomastoid (SCM) muscle and directs the needle toward the
contralateral nipple at a 45-degree angle to the horizontal and sagittal plane at
the supraclavicular area.

to skin puncture. The needle should be directed along a line 45 degrees from the horizontal and sagittal planes. The needle should enter the vein within a maximum of 1 to 2 cm from skin entry. The anterior approach to the posterior IJ vein is illustrated in Fig. 68.6. The lateral approach to the posterior IJ vein is illustrated in Fig. 68.7.

Anterior Approach

The anterior approach to the IJ is accomplished from the medial border of the sternocleidomastoid muscle at the level of the cricoid cartilage. The pulse of the carotid is palpated with three fingers of the nondominant hand placed side by side to give linear orientation. The fingertips are moved slightly back and forth over the pulse of the carotid so that you can appreciate the contour of the artery and point of maximal impulse (PMI) of the pulsations. These fingers should remain lightly palpating the carotid pulse over the PMI until the vein has been entered. Recalling the anatomy, the skin should be entered between the fingers palpating the

arterial pulse and the medial border of the sternocleidomastoid muscle. The needle is directed along a plane from the point of entry toward the location of the ipsilateral nipple on a slender male chest. The needle is directed into the neck at an angle of 45 to 60 degrees to the frontal plane. Entry into the vein should occur within 2 cm from skin entry. If the vein is not entered on the first pass, the needle should be withdrawn to the skin and redirected slightly more laterally. The frontal approach to the anterior IJ is illustrated in Fig. 68.8. The lateral approach is shown in Fig. 68.9.

Central Approach

The central approach is accomplished by entering the skin at the apex of the angle created by the divergence of the sternal and clavicular heads of the sternocleidomastoid muscle. This approach should be reserved for the right side only to avoid injury to the thoracic duct. This point can be located by asking the patient to lift his or her head from the table while his or her head is

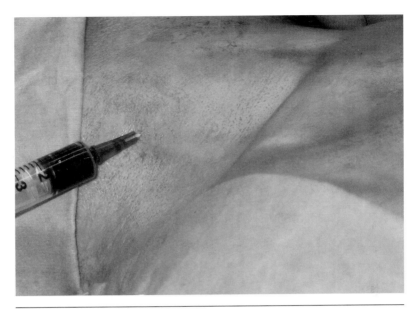

Figure 68.7
The lateral view to the posterior internal jugular (IJ) vein illustrates the 15- to 30-degree angle of the needle in relation to the sternocleidomastoid (SCM) muscle and external jugular (EJ) vein.

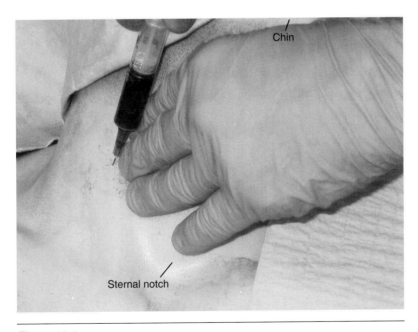

Figure 68.8
The anterior internal jugular (IJ) vein, frontal approach, illustrates the needle directed toward the ipsilateral nipple.

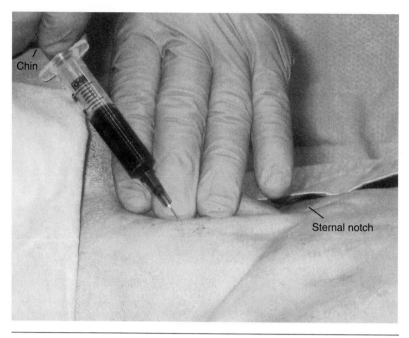

Figure 68.9
The anterior internal jugular (IJ) vein, lateral approach, shows the 45- to
60-degree angle of the needle to the skin and the placement of the fingers on
the carotid pulse.

turned 45 degrees away from the side of entry. In a patient unable to assist in location, the point of entry should be approximately two fingerbreadths (2.0 to 2.5 cm) above the clavicle between the two heads of the sternocleidomastoid muscle. The needle complex is angled at 45 to 60 degrees to the frontal plane and directed toward the point where the nipple would be on a slender male torso. The vein should be entered within 1.0 to 1.5 cm from skin entry This approach presents a particular problem in a significant number of patients, in whom the IJ vein overlays the carotid artery at the upper part of the angle. Figure 68.10 illustrates the frontal approach to the central IJ vein. The lateral approach is shown in Fig. 68.11.

Femoral Vein

To locate the femoral vein, start by locating the femoral arterial pulse, if present; otherwise, locate the midpoint of the line between the inferior border of the anterior superior spine and the midpoint of the symphysis pubis. From either of these points, the vein should lay approximately one fingerbreadth medially.

Place the long finger over either the point of maximal arterial pulse, or the midpoint between the anterior superior iliac spine and the symphysis pubis at the inguinal ligament, with the orientation of the finger in the long axis of the artery with the other fingers in extension. The vein should be located under the finger that is the next more medial to the long finger.

Catheter-Over-Wire Technique

The catheter-over-wire technique is also known as the Seldinger technique after the physician who developed it. It involves passing a flexible spring-coil "wire" through the vein access needle, dilating the subcutaneous tract, passing the desired catheter over the wire to the appropriate depth, and ultimately removing the wire. The operator should pay attention at all times to the whereabouts and control of the end of the guidewire not being passed through the needle to be sure that it remains sterile.

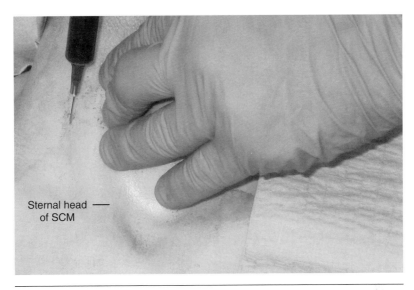

Figure 68.10
The central internal jugular (IJ) vein, frontal approach, places the needle at the apex of triangle created by the two heads of the sternocleidomastoid (SCM) muscle. The needle is directed toward the ipsilateral nipple.

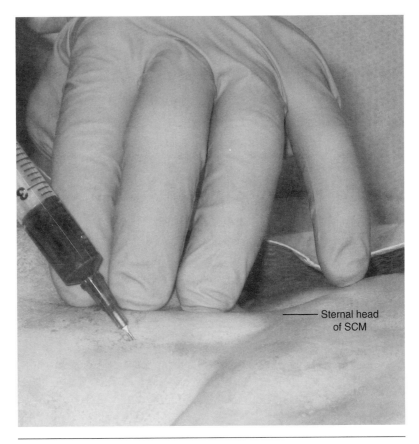

Figure 68.11
The lateral approach of the central internal jugular (IJ) vein shows the angle of the needle at 45 to 60 degrees.

Anchoring and Bandaging

Once the catheter is in place, it must be secured. Suturing, the traditional method, is a high-risk part of the procedure for the operator. If the straight needle provided in many kits is used for suturing, proceed with extreme caution. In fact, because straight needles have more potential for operator injury, it may be safer to supply your own curved needle. Most catheters have small tabs on the hub with holes in them. A stitch should be placed in the skin under one of the tabs and tied to itself to create a loop. Then the needle should be passed, dull end first, through the hole in the tab and three knots tied. The initial skin loop prevents the tab from being pulled tightly enough against the underlying skin to cause ischemia.

The skin around the entry site should be cleaned of any blood using moistened sterile gauze. Additional application of antiseptic ointment at the catheter entry point may decrease migration of bacteria to the subcutaneous tissue. Application of a transparent occlusive bandage allows observation for signs of cellulitis at the entry site and decreases the incidence of catheter contamination.

Complications

Numerous patient complications have been documented with each of the approaches to the central circulation. The most commonly cited complications of SC and IJ vein catheterization are arterial puncture and pneumothorax. Although relatively rare, air embolism is of real concern in the SC and IJ approaches. Other reported complications of accessing the SC have included laceration or cannulation of the thoracic duct on the left or the lymph duct on the right, brachial plexus injury, and SC vein thrombosis. Accessing the IJ vein has been associated with phrenic nerve damage, intrathecal catheter placement, and tracheal puncture. The femoral vein has a higher incidence of thrombophlebitis reported compared with the SC and IJ veins. Shearing of the guidewire has been observed with all approaches. Several authors have documented that complications are higher when the procedure is performed by less experienced operators.

Failed Attempts

In the event that the SC or IJ vein cannot be cannulated after several attempts, the site should be abandoned. The patient's vital signs should be checked, with particular attention to respiratory rate. An alternate route should be selected on the same side. If both the SC and IJ routes are unsuccessful on one side, a chest x-ray film should be obtained before commencing attempts on the opposite side.

Wrap-up

Once bandaging is completed, all sharps should be disposed of in an appropriate safety container. For SC and IJ catheterizations, a postprocedure chest x-ray film should be obtained to verify the lack of pneumothorax and the position of the catheter tip. The tip should be lying in the superior vena cava, seen on chest x-ray film as adjacent to the patient's right side of the vertebral bodies at the level of the fourth thoracic vertebra. If the catheter was placed via the left SC vein, attention should be directed to the catheter tip on x-ray film to be sure it does not appear to impinge on the wall of the vena cava.

Suggested Readings

Jesseph JM, Conces DJ Jr, Augustyn GT. Patient positioning for subclavian vein catheterization. *Arch Surg* 1987;122:1207–1209.

Kavic SM, Atweh N, Ivy ME. Image of trauma. *J Trauma* 2000;49:569.

Land RE. Anatomic relationships of the right subclavian vein. *Arch Surg* 1971;102:178–180.

Schwartz AJ, Jobes DR, Levy WJ, et al. Intrathoracic vascular catheterization via the external jugular vein. *Anesthesiology* 1982;56:400–402.

Sterner S, Plummer DW, Clinton J, Ruiz E. A comparison of the supraclavicular approach and the infraclavicular approach for subclavian vein catheterization. *Ann Emerg Med* 1986;15:421–424.

Sulek CA, Gravenstein N, Blackshear RH, Weiss L. Head rotation during internal jugular vein cannulation and the risk of carotid artery puncture. *Anesth Analg* 1996;82:125–128.

Willeford KL, Reitan JA. Neutral head position for placement of internal jugular vein catheters. *Anaesthesia* 1994;49:202–204.

Wu X, Studer W, Erb T, et al. Competence of the internal jugular vein valve is damaged by cannulation and catheterization of the internal jugular vein. *Anesthesiology* 2000;93:319–324.

Wound Care

CHAPTER **69**

Anesthesia: Local Agents and Regional Blocks

Andreas Dewitz, MD

Patients presenting to the emergency department (ED) with soft tissue problems that will ultimately require wound repair or minor surgical intervention make up a significant proportion of all ED encounters. Minimizing the pain of the wound repair or surgical intervention while achieving optimal results remains a constant goal of good wound management. The regional anesthetic techniques discussed here, including both infiltration anesthesia and regional nerve blocks, have an excellent safety profile and are frequently used in the ED to achieve this goal.

History

Topical and subcutaneous anesthetic agents have been in use for more than 100 years beginning with the use of topical cocaine solutions for eye surgery described by Koller in 1884. Halsted and Hall described subcutaneous nerve blocks with cocaine in 1885. By 1894, local anesthetic infiltration techniques were used clinically to block specific nerve groups. Procaine (Novocain) was first synthesized in 1905 and was the primary local anesthetic agent used for many decades. Lidocaine first came into clinical use in 1948 and remains the primary local anesthetic agent in use in the ED today.

Definitions

Topical anesthesia refers to local anesthetic agents applied either directly to mucous membranes or to open abraded skin where the anesthetic agent can be readily absorbed and subsequent superficial cutaneous anesthesia can occur (see Chapter 65). (Some agents such as EMLA—a combination of prilocaine and lidocaine—have the advantage of being absorbed through intact skin.)

Infiltration anesthesia, also known as "field block" or "barrage block," refers to the deposition of anesthetic solutions in the subcutaneous tissue in the general course of a given group of subcutaneous nerves.

Peripheral nerve block refers to the deposition of local anesthetic solutions in close proximity to specific nerve bundles with subsequent local anesthesia of the sensory territory served by that individual nerve.

Local Anesthetic Agents

Pharmacology and Physiology

Structurally, local anesthetics consist of an aromatic lipophilic group of atoms bound to a hydrophilic group with an intermediate group of carbon atoms in either an ester linkage (procaine, benzocaine) or an amide linkage (lidocaine, prilocaine, bupivacaine). Physicochemically, these agents are weak bases with pH greater than 7.4. They are usually prepared as hydrochloride salts with a pH of 4 to 7 and are highly ionized and water soluble. In tissue, body buffers raise the pH of the anesthetic agent, thereby increasing the lipid-soluble free base, which subsequently crosses the axonal membrane. Once the drug is in the more acidotic intracellular milieu, a shift to the more ionized and active form of the drug occurs.

The local anesthetic agent's mechanism of action consists of sodium (and possible calcium) channel blockade resulting in a nondepolarizing conduction block of the nerve fibers in contact with the anesthetic agent. Metabolism of the ester group of local anesthetic agents (procaine, prilocaine, benzocaine, and cocaine) occurs predominantly by way of plasma pseudocholinesterases, whereas metabolism of the amino-amide group of local anesthetic agents (lidocaine and bupivacaine) occurs by way of liver microsomal enzymes. Elimination is renal.

Toxicity

Toxicity to the local anesthetic agents routinely used in the ED is fortunately rare given the usually relatively low drug dosages used. However, several categories of toxicity are worthy of review.

Nervous System Toxicity

All local anesthetic agents cross the blood–brain barrier, and central nervous system (CNS) toxicity is related to the intrinsic potency of the anesthetic agent, the degree and rapidity of absorption, and arterial pH (acidosis worsens the toxicity). Signs and symptoms can include lightheadedness, circumoral numbness, drowsiness, disorientation, slurred speech, muscle twitching, seizures, and respiratory arrest. Treatment includes oxygen, diazepam, and correction of any acidosis. Local neurotoxicity is rare except with intraneural injection, in which the mechanical pressure of the anesthetic solution within the nerve sheath can cause a compression neuropraxia.

Cardiovascular Toxicity

Cardiovascular toxicity is related to the fact that all local anesthetics except cocaine are vasodilators. Cardiovascular depression can occur at high blood levels of the local anesthetic agent. However, this toxicity threshold is three to four times higher than that for CNS toxicity. Signs and symptoms may include pallor, diaphoresis, hypotension, and bradycardia. Treatment includes the usual advanced cardiac life support (ACLS) resuscitative measures.

Allergic Reactions

Allergic reactions to amino amides such as lidocaine and bupivacaine are extremely rare. Amino esters such as procaine (Novocain) and benzocaine are metabolized to para-aminobenzoic acid (PABA) derivatives, which, in turn, are responsible for most true allergic reactions. The preservatives methylparaben or metabisulfite used in multidose vials also have been implicated as a cause of allergic reactions to local anesthetic agents. Ultimately, however, most untoward reactions to local anesthetic agents encountered in the ED are due to patient anxiety or to vasovagal reactions from the overall wound care process.

Vasoconstrictors

The addition of a vasoconstrictor agent such as epinephrine to the local anesthetic agent offers potential advantages. It slows absorption of the drug, reduces systemic toxicity, and most importantly, can prolong block duration by 50% to 100%. In addition, the local hemostatic effects of an epinephrine containing anesthetic solution are frequently used to advantage in a wound with ongoing bleeding.

However, specific contraindications for vasoconstrictor use should be noted; these break down into anatomic and medical categories. End-arterial beds (fingers, toes, ears, penis, nose—all the appendages) should not be exposed to solutions containing epinephrine because of potential adverse tissue ischemia. Medical contraindications include severe hypertension, coronary artery disease, peripheral vascular disease, thyrotoxicosis, and use of monoamine oxidase (MAO) inhibitors. Some authors have suggested that the local vasoconstriction associated with the use of local anesthetics containing epinephrine carries with it a possible increased risk of wound infection.

The epinephrine concentration typically used for local anesthesia in the ED is a 1:100,000 solution. It should be stressed that plain anesthetic solutions are usually adequate for most ED wound repairs. However, the use of an epinephrine-containing anesthetic solution can be helpful in situations in which no anatomic or medical contraindications exist and (a) when hemostasis is desirable (e.g., a scalp laceration with ongoing poorly controlled bleeding or oozing) or (b) when a complicated or prolonged wound repair is anticipated and an extended anesthetic effect would be desirable. In the latter setting, alternatively, one could use a longer acting agent such as bupivacaine.

Factors Affecting Conduction Blockade

Numerous factors affect the duration of the local anesthetic conduction blockade: (a) the volume, type, and concentration of the agent used; (b) inherent penetrating and diffusing characteristics of the local anesthetic agent; (c) the distance between the nerve and the local anesthetic agent; (d) the diameter of the nerve being blocked; and (e) adjacent tissue characteristics, such as fat content and local tissue pH. Low pH of the surrounding tissue (frequently encountered in the setting of a subcutaneous abscess needing incision and drainage) adversely affects the formation of the lipid-soluble free base form of the anesthetic agent. Without this transition, little of the drug can cross the axonal membrane and local anesthetic efficacy is significantly decreased. To overcome this barrier when draining an abscess, one should try to deposit the local anesthetic agent in the healthier, less inflamed surrounding tissues where the block will be more effective. Often, the addition of intramuscular or intravenous analgesia, or even conscious sedation, may be necessary to achieve adequate patient comfort for the planned procedure.

Local Anesthetic Agent Formulations

Lidocaine is commonly available in 1% and 2% solutions for infiltration (plain, or with epinephrine); a 4% solution for topical use; 2% gel, viscous, or jelly formulations for topical use; and a 10% lidocaine spray for topical use. Bupivacaine is commonly found in 0.25% and 0.5% solutions, either plain or with epinephrine. Benzocaine is available as a 20% spray for topical use.

Dosing Limits and Duration of Action

Local anesthetic dosing guidelines typically recommended for lidocaine set a 4 mg/kg limit for plain solutions and a 7 mg/kg limit for solutions containing epinephrine. Because of its increased potency, the dosing limit for bupivacaine is set at 2 mg/kg for plain solutions and 3 mg/kg for epinephrine-containing solutions. Remember that a 1% solution contains 10 mg of the anesthetic agent. For example, a 15-mL injection of a plain 2% lidocaine solution (an amount that might be used for adequate chest wall anesthesia before inserting a chest tube) would represent a dose of 300 mg of lidocaine, or slightly more than the 4 mg/kg recommended limit in a 70-kg person. Therefore, use of an epinephrine-containing solution would be recommended in this setting (with its 7 mg/kg dosing limit). When using high volumes of anesthetic agent, it is particularly important to observe dosing limits to avoid drug toxicity.

The duration of action of a given local anesthetic agent is quite variable and a function of the many variables noted previously. In general, plain lidocaine solutions provide a local anesthetic effect lasting for 1 to 2 hours; with epinephrine added, the local anesthetic effect can extend to 2 to 4 hours. Plain bupivacaine solutions provide a local anesthetic effect lasting for 5 to 7 hours with 10 to 12 hours or longer of local anesthesia when epinephrine is added. However, because of the wide variability in clinical duration of action, it is much more useful to assess the patient and provide additional local anesthesia if the patient states that the block's effect has worn off.

Technical Considerations

The maximal local anesthetic drug dosages allowed for a given patient should be calculated before the procedure, and one should observe appropriate dosing limits. Lower drug concentrations may be used for field blocks, and higher drug concentrations used for nerve blocks where there is often a somewhat larger diameter nerve to penetrate. From a procedural standpoint, it is wise *always* to aspirate before drug injection to avoid the possibility of an intravascular injection. Slow injection of the anesthetic agent is also advised, and it is important to wait for the block to take effect before cleaning or suturing begins. Be aware of and watch for signs and symptoms of toxicity when using high doses of local anesthetic agent or when injecting in very vascular areas. After the procedure, instruct the patient to avoid mechanical or thermal trauma to areas of sensory block and state how long this may last. In addition, please remember that an oral analgesic agent may often be required after the block has worn off.

Techniques to Decrease Pain of Injection of Anesthetic Agent

Techniques reported to decrease pain on injection include the following: (a) skin desensitization by brisk rubbing or pinching before injection, (b) slow injection speed, (c) use of a smaller rather than larger gauge needle, (d) limiting the number of needlesticks by using a longer needle to reach more of the wound edge with a given needle stick, (e) injection through the open wound edges rather than through the surrounding intact skin, (f) addition of 1 mL of 4% sodium bicarbonate to 9 mL of anesthetic agent, and (g) warming the anesthetic solution. Avoid use of multidose vials in the ED because the risk of cross contamination is great. Note that all of the blocks described later can be performed with a 5- or 10-mL syringe and a 25-gauge 5/8-inch or 22-gauge 1 1/2-inch needle.

Regional Anesthesia of the Scalp and Face

The three branches of the trigeminal nerve (ophthalmic, maxillary, and mandibular divisions) make up the sensory supply of the face. As a useful reference landmark, note that the foramina where the supraorbital, infraorbital, and mental nerves exit all line up on a vertical axis roughly in line with the patient's mid-position pupil (Fig. 69.1). This anatomic alignment becomes helpful in knowing where to deposit the anesthetic solution for the facial blocks discussed later.

Forehead Anesthesia

Clinical Utility

Forehead anesthesia is used in repair of lacerations and/or foreign body removal in the mid forehead region extending to the vertex of the scalp.

Nerves to be Blocked

Nerves to be blocked include the following: (a) medial and lateral branches of the supraorbital (frontal) nerve and (b) supratrochlear nerve. A bilateral block is required for midline injuries.

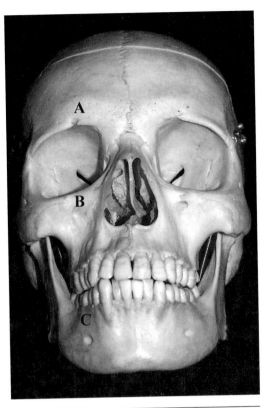

Figure 69.1
The foramina through which the supraorbital (**A**), infraorbital (**B**), and mental nerves (**C**) exit all lie on a sagittal plane that includes the midposition pupil of the ipsilateral eye.

Area of Anesthesia

The area of anesthesia is illustrated in Fig. 69.2. The area extends from the lateral eyebrow to the midline forehead, beginning at the supraorbital rim and extending posteriorly to the vertex of the scalp. A bilateral block covers from lateral eyebrow to lateral eyebrow extending to the vertex of the scalp.

Block Technique

Block technique is demonstrated in Figs. 69.3A and B. Locate the supraorbital rim by palpation. The supraorbital nerve branches exit at the supraorbital foramen in vertical alignment with the pupil at midline gaze. The supratrochlear nerve is located more medially along the supraorbital rim below the medial aspect of the eyebrow. Using a 25-gauge 5/8-inch, needle aim superiorly *away* from the globe with the goal of depositing 2 to 3 mL of 1% to 2% lidocaine solution just *above* the supraorbital rim in a supraperiosteal location as close to the branches of the supraorbital and supratrochlear nerves as possible. Midline injuries require a bilateral block for adequate central anesthesia.

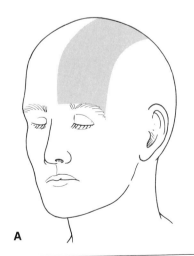

A

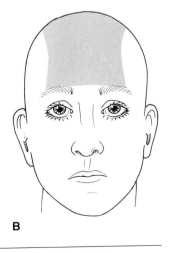

B

Figure 69.2
Supraorbital and supratrochlear nerve blocks. Area of anesthesia with (**A**) unilateral and (**B**) bilateral block.

A
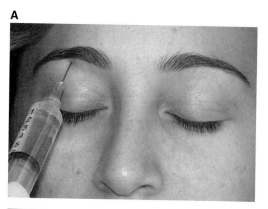

B
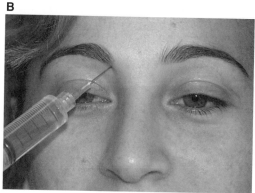

Figure 69.3
Supraorbital (**A**) and supratrochlear (**B**) nerve block technique.

Comments

Injection directly into the thick skin of the forehead is often difficult, and the block is more easily accomplished by using the supraperiosteal injection technique at the orbital rim as described previously. It is advisable to keep a finger along the inferior border of the supraorbital rim during injection to prevent ballooning of the anesthetic agent into the upper eyelid. Always aim up, *above* the supraorbital rim and away from the globe!

Upper Lip Anesthesia

Clinical Utility

Upper lip anesthesia is used in laceration repair of the upper lip region.

Nerves to be Blocked

The superior labial and lateral nasal branches of the infraorbital nerve are blocked in upper lip anesthesia.

Area of Anesthesia

Ipsilateral block covers the ipsilateral upper lip and nasal ala to the midline philtrum (Fig. 69.4). Occasionally, inferior palpebral branches are reached with this block as well. Midline lesions require a bilateral block.

Block Technique

The best approach is via the intraoral route using a supraperiosteal infiltration technique (Fig. 69.5). The entry point for injection is at the mucobuccal fold (the sulcus formed

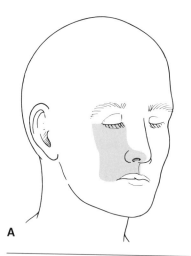

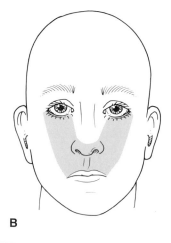

A   B

Figure 69.4
Infraorbital nerve block: area of anesthesia with (**A**) unilateral and (**B**) bilateral block.

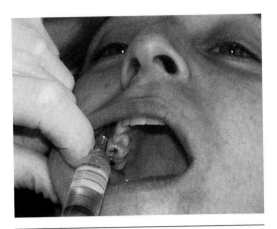

Figure 69.5
Infraorbital nerve block technique.

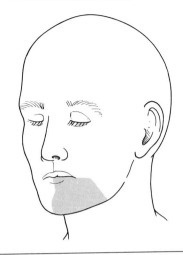

Figure 69.6
Mental nerve infiltration: area of anesthesia.

where the intraoral cheek mucosa folds around toward the gums) between the first and second upper premolars. One should first apply a small amount of a topical anesthetic agent on the oral mucosa (10% lidocaine spray or 20% benzocaine). The injection needle is aimed toward the ipsilateral infraorbital foramen, which is located several centimeters below the globe in vertical alignment with the mid-position pupil. Using a 25-gauge, 5/8-inch needle, 3 to 4 mL of 1% to 2% lidocaine solution are deposited in a narrow fanlike fashion in a supraperiosteal location.

Comments

Use a 5/8-inch needle to ensure that you will always be distant from the globe. Keep a finger below the infraorbital rim to prevent ballooning of the anesthetic agent into the lower eyelid. In edentulous patients, direct the needle by estimating where the foramen should lie by virtue of its approximate vertical alignment with the midposition pupil.

Lower Lip Anesthesia

Clinical Utility

Lower lip anesthesia is used in laceration repair of the lower lip and mental region.

Nerves to be Blocked

The inferior labial and mental branches of the mental nerve are blocked.

Area of Anesthesia

The lower lip and anterior mental region are illustrated in Fig. 69.6. Midline lesions require a bilateral block.

Block Technique

The mental nerve infiltration technique is similar to that used for upper lip anesthesia (Fig. 69.7). Topical anesthesia is first applied at the mucobuccal fold between the first and second lower premolars. Using a 25-gauge, 5/8-inch needle, 3 to 4 mL of 1% to 2% lidocaine solution are deposited in a narrow fanlike fashion in a supraperiosteal location aiming in the direction of the mental foramen. Given the close proximity of

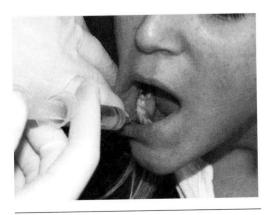

Figure 69.7
Mental nerve infiltration technique.

the facial and mental arteries, it is important to aspirate first to avoid the possibility of an intraarterial injection. Distribution of anesthesia is the ipsilateral lower lip and anterior chin; central lip injuries require a bilateral block.

Comments

Always aspirate before this block. For edentulous patients, estimate the location of the mental foramen as noted previously.

Regional Anesthesia of the Hand

A patient with either a hand injury or hand-related pathology represents a clinical scenario frequently encountered in most EDs. The detailed knowledge of hand anatomy essential for appropriate care and repair of this complicated region is beyond the scope of this chapter. However, many injures are superficial and require little more than irrigation and appropriate wound closure. Of the local anesthetic techniques discussed in this chapter, the nerve blocks of the hand are undoubtedly the most frequently used of the regional block techniques.

The superficial radial nerve, the median nerve, and the dorsal and palmar branches of the ulnar nerve make up the sensory supply of the hand. Figure 69.8 illustrates the sensory territory supplied by each of these nerves in the hand and should be committed to memory. Dorsal and palmar digital nerves provide sensation of the individual digits. The location of these nerves in cross section at the level of the proximal portion of the proximal phalanx (where the digital block is performed) is demonstrated in Fig. 69.9.

Selective blockade of portions of the hand or isolated fingers depends on the nature and location of the clinical problem being addressed. Some injuries are adequately anesthetized with a single block, whereas others require deposition of the local anesthetic agent at multiple sites for effective anesthesia.

Finger Anesthesia

Clinical Utility

Finger anesthesia is used during laceration repair of the digits, nail bed repair, ingrown nail removal, paronychia or felon drainage, foreign body removal, and reduction of finger fractures and dislocations.

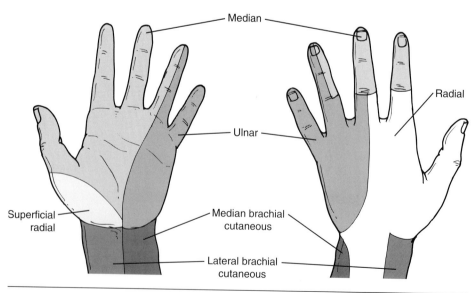

Figure 69.8
Sensory map of the hand.

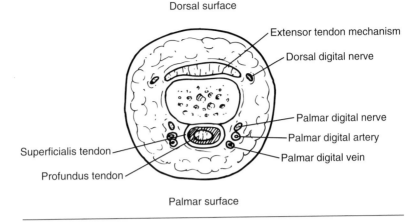

Figure 69.9
Cross-sectional anatomy of the digit at the level of the proximal portion of the proximal phalanx.

Nerves to be Blocked

Digital nerves and dorsal and proper palmar digital branches are blocked during finger anesthesia. Note again, the location of the dorsal and palmar digital nerves on the cross-sectional anatomy diagram at the level of the proximal portion of the proximal phalanx.

Area of Anesthesia

The entire digit, from the level of the proximal digital crease to the fingertip, is included in the area of anesthesia.

Block Technique

Block technique is demonstrated in Figs. 69.10A, B, and C. This approach is essentially an inverted U-shaped field block of the digit. With the 12 o'clock position representing the dorsal midline, the needle entry points are on the dorsal surface of the hand at the 2:30 and 10:30 o'clock positions at the level of the proximal portion of the proximal phalanx. The needle entry location is based on the cross-sectional location of the digital nerves to be blocked.

Using a 25-gauge 5/8-inch needle, a skin wheal is raised and 1 mL of 1% to 2% lidocaine is deposited along the lateral aspect of the digit aiming slightly medially and anteriorly toward the lateral aspect of the flexor tendon sheath where the proper palmar digital nerves and arteries are located. The

needle is partially withdrawn; then, an additional 1 mL of 1% to 2% lidocaine is deposited dorsally crossing the digit to the contralateral needle entry site to block the dorsal digital nerves. The needle is then completely withdrawn and an additional 1 mL of anesthetic solution is deposited at the contralateral entry site, again aiming slightly medially and anteriorly toward the lateral aspect of the flexor tendon sheath on the opposite side of the digit.

Comments

Note the following important guidelines with digital blocks:

1. Do not use epinephrine-containing solutions!

2. Always aspirate first to avoid an intravascular injection.

3. Limit the overall volume of anesthetic solution on a given digit to 5 mL or less (to avoid occluding or restricting blood flow to or from the digit, as can occur with high-volume injections); usually, 3 to 4 mL should suffice.

4. Do not inject through infected tissue (poor block efficacy).

5. Massage the digit after the injection to assist with the distribution of the local anesthetic agent.

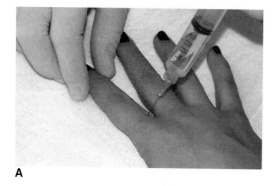

A

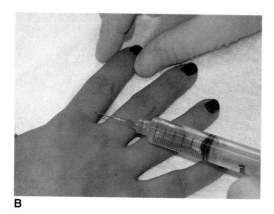

B

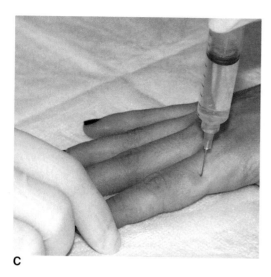

C

Figure 69.10
A, **B**, and **C**: Digital nerve block technique.

6. Remember that the loss of sensation progresses from proximal to distal (i.e., the tip numbs last).

Of note, the thumb is typically more difficult to block than the other digits because the radial palmar digital nerve of the thumb lies in a somewhat more ulnar location on the digit than is usually appreciated. The palmar portion of this block is usually most successfully accomplished by entering from the webspace between the thumb and index finger. Begin by palpating the flexor pollicis longus tendon of the thumb, and then deposit 2 mL of 1% to 2% lidocaine over the tendon sheath area at the level of the proximal digital crease. An inverted U-shaped field block of the dorsal and lateral portions of the thumb is necessary to complete the block and provide complete sensory anesthesia. This is accomplished with the injection of an additional 2 to 3 mL of 1% to 2% lidocaine.

Superficial Radial Nerve Block

Clinical Utility

Superficial radial nerve block is used in repair of dorsal hand injuries on the radial aspect of the hand.

Nerve to be Blocked

The superficial branch of the radial nerve is blocked.

Area of Anesthesia

The area of anesthesia includes the dorsal hand from the radial aspect of the thumb (with varying amounts of the thenar eminence) to the midline of the fourth digit, excluding the dorsal distal portions of the second, third, and fourth digits. (See Fig. 69.8.)

Block Technique

Superficial radial nerve block is demonstrated in Fig. 69.11. Flex the wrist to find the bulge of the flexor carpi radialis tendon on the volar radial surface of the wrist. Find the proximal wrist crease (the first horizontal skin crease noted when the wrist is held

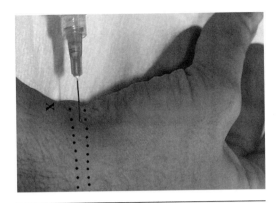

Figure 69.11
Superficial radial nerve block technique. X marks the location of the flexor carpi radialis tendon. The outlined area marks the region where the anesthetic agent is deposited.

in flexion). Beginning just radial to the flexor carpi radialis tendon, deposit a subcutaneous "garter" of 5 to 7 mL of 1% lidocaine around the wrist at the level of the anatomic snuffbox out to the mid dorsum of the wrist.

Comments

This block usually requires three needle-sticks for effective coverage. Use of a longer needle, such as a 25-gauge 1 1/2-inch needle, can decrease the number of needlesticks required. Given the proximity of the radial artery, it is important to aspirate before each injection. Remember that you are essentially depositing a garter of anesthetic agent in the superficial soft tissue perpendicular to the course of the branches of the superficial radial nerve to create this distal field block.

Ulnar Nerve Block

Clinical Utility

Ulnar nerve blocks are used in repair of injuries of the fifth digit or the ulnar portion of the palm and in reduction of fifth metacarpal fractures.

Nerves to be Blocked

Palmar and/or dorsal branches of the ulnar nerve are blocked.

Area of Anesthesia

The area of anesthesia includes the ulnar aspect of the palmar and dorsal aspects of the hand from the wrist to the axial midline of the fourth digit. (See Fig. 69.8.)

Block Technique

Palmar branch of the ulnar nerve lies superficial to the flexor retinaculum of the wrist and is located just radial to the flexor carpi ulnaris tendon and ulnar to the ulnar artery. Hold the wrist in flexion and ulnar deviation to palpate the flexor carpi ulnaris tendon. Two approaches are possible; both are performed at the level of the proximal wrist crease: (a) from the ulnar aspect of the wrist with the needle directed horizontally and radially under the flexor carpi ulnaris tendon or (b) from the volar wrist, perpendicular to the skin, entering just radial to the flexor carpi ulnaris tendon. Use a 25-gauge 5/8-inch needle, aspirate first because of the close proximity of the ulnar artery, and then deposit 2 to 3mL 1% to 2% lidocaine for either approach (Fig. 69.12).

Dorsal branch block (not shown) is achieved where the nerve passes subcutaneously just distal to the ulnar styloid process, a bony landmark readily palpable on the dorsal ulnar aspect of the wrist. Subcutaneous deposition of the anesthetic solution should begin on the volar aspect of the wrist at the level of the proximal wrist crease just ulnar to the flexor carpi ulnaris tendon. A subcutaneous garter of 5 to 7 mL of 1% to 2% lidocaine is then deposited around the wrist at this level, wrapping around dorsally out to the mid dorsum of the wrist.

Comments

If you inadvertently puncture the ulnar artery, remember to apply pressure for 5 minutes.

Median Nerve Block

Clinical Utility

Median nerve block is used in repair of radial palmar and digital injuries, multiple finger

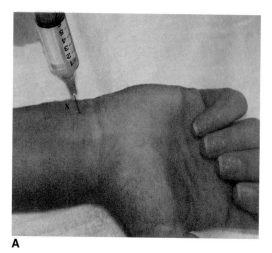

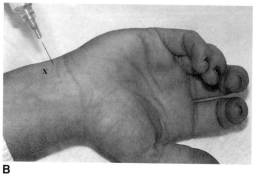

A   **B**

Figure 69.12
Ulnar nerve block technique, palmar branch, two approaches. **A**: Volar. **B**: Lateral. X marks the location of the flexor carpi ulnaris tendon.

injuries, and reduction of second and third metacarpal fractures.

Nerve to be Blocked

The nerve that is blocked in median nerve block is the palmar portion of the median nerve, a large sensory nerve with a small associated recurrent motor branch, which supplies motor function to the muscles of the thenar eminence.

Area of Anesthesia

The area of anesthesia includes the radial palmar surface of the hand to the midline fourth digit with varying coverage of the thenar eminence, which is often supplied by the superficial radial nerve. Dorsal distal sensation also is affected in digits two, three, and the radial distal half of digit four. (See Fig. 69.8 for details.)

Block Technique

Median nerve block technique is demonstrated in Fig. 69.13. Begin at the proximal wrist crease, and find the palmaris longus tendon in the midline wrist by opposing the thumb and fifth digit with the wrist flexed. The median nerve is located just radial to the palmaris longus tendon *below*

the flexor retinaculum. In the 20% of the population who are missing this tendon, you can aim just radial to the midpoint of the wrist at the level of the proximal wrist crease.

Enter perpendicular to the skin and deposit 1 mL of 2% lidocaine solution subcutaneously to anesthetize the small palmar branch of the median nerve, which provides sensation to the proximal mid palm. Advance the needle another 1 cm through the flexor retinaculum, where an additional 3 to 5 mL of 2% lidocaine is deposited with a 25-gauge 5/8-inch needle. If

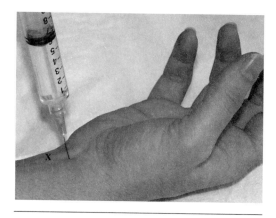

Figure 69.13
Median nerve block technique. X marks the location of the palmaris longus tendon.

paresthesias are obtained, reposition the needle slightly before injecting to avoid an intraneural injection. If significant resistance is met to injection, reposition the needle to avoid injecting into a tendon. Motor function of the thenar eminence (served by the recurrent branch of median nerve) is blocked with this technique as well.

Comments

This block, in conjunction with a block of the palmar branch of the ulnar nerve, provides anesthesia of most of the palmar surface of the hand. As noted previously, the radial portion of the thenar eminence is variably innervated by the superficial radial nerve and may need to be blocked separately for complete palmar surface anesthesia.

Regional Anesthesia of the Foot

Five nerves (the sural, superficial peroneal, saphenous, anterior tibial, and posterior tibial nerves) must be blocked for complete sensory anesthesia of the foot. Figure 69.14 illustrates the sensory territory supplied by each of these nerves. As with the hand, however, these nerves are usually blocked selectively depending on the location of the injury or pathology being addressed.

In clinical practice in the ED, the two most common foot blocks performed are either the superficial peroneal nerve block or the posterior tibial nerve block. These two nerves supply sensation to most of the dorsal and plantar surfaces of the foot, respectively. As with hand injuries, selective blockade of portions of the foot depend on the nature and location of the clinical problem addressed. Some injuries are adequately anesthetized with a single block, but others require deposition of the local anesthetic agent at multiple sites for effective anesthesia.

Anesthesia of the Dorsal Surface of the Foot

Clinical Utility

Anesthesia of the dorsal surface of the foot is used during repair of injuries to that area.

Nerves to be Blocked

Nerves blocked in the dorsal surface of the foot include primarily the superficial peroneal nerve (dorsal sensory supply); occasionally, the sural nerve (lateral sensory supply) and the saphenous nerve (medial sensory supply) are blocked.

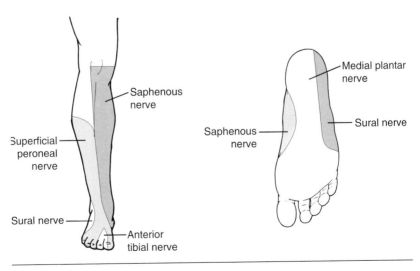

Figure 69.14
Sensory map of the foot.

Area of Anesthesia

The area of anesthesia includes most of the dorsal surface of the foot from the ankle mortise to the toes (excepting half of the first and second toes and the web space between them, which receives its innervation from the anterior tibial nerve).

Block Technique

A subcutaneous garter of 10 mL of 1% lidocaine deposited circumferentially at a level several centimeters above the lower border of the malleoli extending anteriorly from one side of the Achilles tendon around to the other provides sensory anesthesia of nearly the entire dorsal surface of the foot. However, selective blockade of just the superficial peroneal nerve is the more common clinical scenario.

For injuries that lie within the sensory territory of the *superficial peroneal* nerve, the subcutaneous deposition of the anesthetic solution is predominantly anterior, extending from the posterior border of the lateral malleolus to the anterior border of the medial malleolus, as demonstrated in Fig. 69.15.

If additional or selective sensory blockade is desired in the territory of the *sural* nerve, the block should begin at the same horizontal level above the malleoli but with the needle entry just *lateral* to the Achilles tendon and the subcutaneous garter of anesthesia extending around anteriorly to the lateral malleolus.

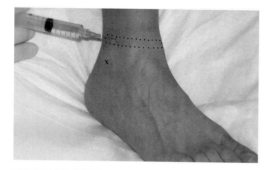

Figure 69.15
Superficial peroneal nerve block. X marks the location of the lower border of the lateral malleolus. The outlined area marks the region where the anesthetic agent is deposited.

If additional or selective sensory blockade of the *saphenous* nerve territory is desired, the block should begin at the same horizontal level above the malleoli but with the needle entry point now just *medial* to the Achilles tendon and the garter of anesthesia extending around anteriorly to the anterior border of the medial malleolus.

A small area supplied by the *anterior tibial* nerve—providing sensation to half of the first and second toes and the web space between them—are not anesthetized with the techniques described previously. Although much less frequently used, this nerve can be blocked at a level several centimeters above the lower border of the malleoli between the extensor hallucis longus and tibialis anterior tendons (have the patient extend the great toe and ankle, respectively, against resistance to locate these tendons). A 25-gauge 5/8-inch needle is advanced all the way to the tibia, where the anterior tibial nerve lies *under* the extensor retinaculum. Aspirate first, because the anterior tibial artery lies adjacent to the nerve, and then deposit 3 to 5 mL of 1% to 2% lidocaine.

Comments

With all foot blocks, aspirate first to avoid an inadvertent intravascular injection.

Anesthesia of the Plantar Surface of the Foot

Clinical Utility

Anesthesia of the plantar surface of the foot is used during repair of lacerations to that area and during foreign body removal.

Nerves to be Blocked

The medial, lateral, and calcaneal branches of the posterior tibial nerve are blocked in this technique.

Area of Anesthesia

The area of anesthesia includes most of the sole of the foot (usually, all except the lateral heel and sole).

Block Technique

Block technique is demonstrated in Fig. 69.16. In the classic posterior tibial nerve block, the needle entry is from behind the ankle. Ideally, the patient is supine with the knee flexed and the foot somewhat plantar flexed. A skin wheal of anesthetic solution is raised with a 25-gauge 5/8-inch needle just *medial* to the Achilles tendon or just behind where the posterior tibial artery pulse is palpated at a level approximately 2 cm above the lower border of the medial malleolus. A 22-gauge 1 1/2-inch needle is then directed in an anterior, slightly medial direction and perpendicular to the medial malleolus. Note that the posterior tibial nerve and artery lie beneath the flexor retinaculum. Proceed until bone is contacted or paresthesias are elicited, then withdraw several millimeters, aspirate to avoid an intravascular injection, and deposit 5 to 10 mL of 1% to 2% lidocaine.

Comments

Avoid this approach in someone with severe peripheral vascular disease or diabetes. Paresthesias are frequently obtained at this site but are not necessary for block efficacy and should not be actively sought. The time required for full block efficacy can range from 5 to 15 minutes and is determined primarily by how close to the nerve the anesthetic solution was deposited. Again, as with all foot blocks, aspirate first to avoid an inadvertent intravascular injection.

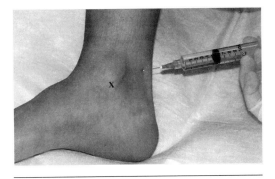

Figure 69.16
Posterior tibial nerve block. X marks the location of the lower border of the medial malleolus.

Anesthesia of Toes

Clinical Utility

Anesthesia of the toes is used in the following situations: paronychia drainage, ingrown toenail removal, nail bed repair, laceration repair, and reduction of toe dislocations.

Nerves to be Blocked

The dorsal and plantar digital nerves are blocked in anesthesia of the toes.

Area of Anesthesia

The area of anesthesia includes the base of the toe to the tip.

Block Technique

The cross-sectional location of the dorsal and plantar digital nerves in the toes is similar to that found in the fingers. The same ring block technique described for finger anesthesia can be used. Most of the pathology encountered is in the first toe, where one is frequently called on to remove an ingrown toenail. The size and thickness of the first toe often necessitates a slight modification of the finger block technique described previously. Using a 25-gauge 1 1/2-inch needle and beginning at the base of the toe in the dorsal midline, several milliliters of 1% to 2% lidocaine are directed both medially and laterally, aiming toward the plantar surface of the toe. Additional anesthesia is then deposited from the lower lateral and medial aspects of the toe, aiming toward the flexor hallucis longus tendon. Injection volume should be limited to approximately 5 mL; massage of the toe at its base can facilitate diffusion of the agent and hasten onset of the block.

Comments

Avoid toe blocks in patients with severe peripheral vascular disease or diabetes. In these situations, a more proximal block is warranted because abscesses and ulcerations can occur when needles are inserted into relatively ischemic distal parts of the extremities. In addition, epinephrine-containing solutions should not be used in the toes.

Suggested Readings

Adriani J. *Labat's regional anesthesia: techniques and clinical applications,* 4th ed. St. Louis: Warren H. Green, 1985.

Capan L, Patel K, Turndorf H. Regional anesthesia in the emergency department. In: Roberts JR, Hedges JR, eds., *Clinical procedures in emergency medicine.* Philadelphia: WB Saunders, 1998:430–462.

Christoph RA, Buchanan L, Begalla K, Schwartz S. Pain reduction in local anesthetic administration through pH buffering. *Ann Emerg Med* 1988;17(2):117–120.

Earle AS, Blanchard JM. Regional anesthesia in the upper extremity. *Clin Plastic Surg* 1985; 12:97–114.

Jenker FL. *Peripheral nerve block.* New York: Springer Verlag, 1977.

Snow JC. *Manual of anesthesia,* 2nd ed. Little, Brown and Company, 1982.

Stromberg BV. Regional anesthesia in head and neck surgery. *Clin Plastic Surg* 1985;12:123–136.

Wetchler BV, ed. *Anesthesia for ambulatory surgery.* Philadelphia:Lippincott, 1985.

CHAPTER 70

Wound Care

Sangeeta Kaushik, MD, Judith A. Linden, MD

The primary objective of wound care is to provide an optimal environment for the natural reparative process to occur. Proper cleaning, wound preparation, and aftercare instructions are equally important to a good cosmetic closure. This chapter reviews the normal wound healing process, wound evaluation, anesthesia, wound preparation, débridement, closure techniques, and aftercare.

Wound Healing

The normal response to injury can be divided into four phases: inflammation, epithelialization, collagen synthesis, and wound maturation. These phases proceed along a continuum unless interrupted by infection, devitalized tissue, inhibitory drugs (e.g., steroids), or underlying patient conditions (e.g., diabetes).

The inflammatory phase (0 to 3 days) is marked by activation of complement, prostaglandins, and cytokines. Polymorphonuclear leukocytes and macrophages migrate into the wound to clear debris and phagocytose dead tissue and bacteria. Macrophages also play a critical role in angiogenesis and fibroblast replication.

During epithelialization (1 to 2 days), epithelial cells begin migrating over the wound surface. Within 24 to 48 hours, a normal layer of epidermis is reestablished. During the collagen synthesis phase (3 to 24 days), fibroblasts are responsible for collagen synthesis, peaking 5 to 7 days after injury. Neovascularization is most active by day seven and is responsible for bringing oxygen and nutrients to the healing wound. During the final phase, wound maturation (24 days to 1 year), collagen fibers become cross-linked and aligned along tension lines. A wound will have only 5% of its original strength at 2 weeks, 70% by 6 to 8 weeks, and 100% by 5 months.

Wound Evaluation

Complete wound evaluation includes a thorough history and examination for associated injuries and foreign bodies. The history should include the time elapsed from injury, the mechanism, location, hand dominance (in hand injuries), and the patient's occupation. Information about the presence of systemic illnesses (e.g., diabetes, human immunodeficiency virus [HIV] infection, steroids), prior first aid applied to the wound, allergies, and tetanus status should also be obtained. The time since the wound occurred is critical because the risk of infection increases with time to wound closure. The "golden hour," or optimal time window for wound closure, is dependent on factors such as mechanism of injury, level of contamination, and body part wounded. In general, a wound should be closed within 6 to 8 hours. Clean facial lacerations, however, may be closed for up to 24 hours. A guiding principle is that if you can restore a wound to fresh, slightly bleeding, nondevitalized appearance, through aggressive cleaning and irrigation, it can be closed primarily.

The history should also include mechanism; for example, a laceration sustained from broken glass would increase the suspicion for a retained foreign body. Location is important in determining safe time to closure and associated injuries. Lacerations over the dorsal metacarpals are suspicious for injuries sustained during a fight, resulting from the teeth impacting on the knuckles. These wounds are handled with extreme care, with antibiotics and close monitoring for infection.

Physical examination should note location, depth, shape, size, and degree of contamination. Maintain a high degree of suspicion for associated injuries such as fractures, organ injuries (e.g., in abdominal and chest wall lacerations), tendon, nerve, or vascular injuries. Once prepped and draped, the extremity should be inspected over its full range of motion for tendon and bone violation. Nerve function (motor and sensory) should be fully tested before anesthesia.

Wounds may be closed immediately (primary closure), left open to heal secondarily (secondary closure), or closed later (tertiary closure). Primary closure (healing by primary intention) is achieved by staples, tissue adhesive, tape, or sutures and should only be done on relatively clean wounds with minimal

tissue loss. Secondary closure (healing by secondary intention) occurs when the wound is not closed and heals gradually by granulation, eventual reepithelialization, and wound contraction. Examples of wounds that should be allowed to heal by this method are ulcerations, abscess cavities, puncture wounds, and partial thickness tissue loss.

Delayed primary closure (tertiary closure) is appropriate for wounds that are heavily contaminated and have an increased risk of infection if closed. These wounds are cleaned, irrigated, débrided, packed with saline-moistened mesh, covered, and watched for 4 to 5 days. The wound is then sutured on the fourth to fifth day, if there is no evidence of infection and the patient does not report increased discomfort. Oral antibiotics (dicloxacillin or cephalexin) may be given during the wait for delayed closure.

Anesthesia

Anesthesia may be achieved by local injection, topical application, or regional nerve block (see Chapters 65 and 69). The most common method used is local injection. Topical anesthetics (e.g., tetracaine, adrenaline/epinephrine, and cocaine [TAC] or lidocaine, epinephrine, and tetracaine [LET]) may be used in children and in smaller wounds. Regional nerve blocks are useful for wounds in cosmetically important areas where less distortion resulting from local injection is desired (e.g., on the face), where larger areas can be anesthetized through regional block (e.g., hand or ear wounds), or where local injection is difficult (e.g., the plantar aspect of the foot).

In choosing a local anesthetic, it is important to consider onset of action, duration, and toxicity.

True allergic responses are rare and occur in less than 1% of patients receiving local anesthesia; however, other reactions include delayed rashes or generalized urticaria. If the patient describes a true allergy, there are several options available. Diphenhydramine (Benadryl) may be used as a local anesthetic; 50 mg (1 mL) of diphenhydramine is diluted

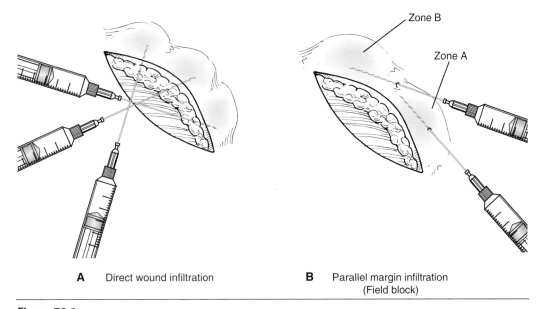

A   Direct wound infiltration   **B**   Parallel margin infiltration
                                                       (Field block)

Figure 70.1
A: Direct infiltration of wounds. **B**: Parallel margin infiltration of wounds.

with 4 mL of normal saline to produce 1% solution, to be used for local infiltration. Infiltrating with normal saline alone as an agent, although not ideal, may provide just enough anesthesia for small wounds.

Anesthesia may be infiltrated directly into the wound or parallel to the wound margins, as shown in Fig. 70.1. Direct infiltration is better for minimally contaminated wounds. When injecting directly into the wound, the needle is placed just under the dermis. Infiltration outside of the wound is the preferred method for grossly contaminated wounds. The plane of injection is the same with parallel margin infiltration, except that you infiltrate through intact skin. The pain of injection may be decreased by using a very small infiltration needle (30 gauge), by injecting slowly (over 10 seconds), by warming the anesthetic solution, and by buffering the lidocaine with sodium bicarbonate (1 mL of sodium bicarbonate to 9 mL of 1% lidocaine; the buffered solution should be discarded after 24 hours).

Options for topical anesthesia include LET and TAC. Neither agent should be used on mucous membranes, or in areas with end arteries (fingers, toes, penis, nose). LET is currently the most commonly used. It is cheaper than TAC and does not contain a controlled substance (cocaine). LET is dripped into the wound and then applied with cotton that is left in place for 20 minutes. TAC is less frequently used because of an increased risk of serious side effects such as seizures, respiratory arrest, and death (most commonly in children). Eutectic mixture of local anesthetics (EMLA) is an emulsion mixture of lidocaine and prilocaine in an ointment form. Although EMLA provides excellent analgesia (within 1 to 2 hours) for procedures such as lumbar puncture and intravenous cannulation, current indications exclude application to open wounds.

Wound Preparation

Wound irrigation is the most effective way to remove debris, decrease bacterial counts on the wound surface, and reduce the risk of infection. The wound is first cleansed with an aseptic solution. Povidone-iodine is the most commonly used solution for most body parts except the face, because it stains. When indicated, the wound periphery is cleaned in a circular motion. The circles gradually become larger without retouching each previous circle as you move away from the wound. A 1% povidone-iodine solution should be used. The standard solution, supplied at 10%, is toxic to the tissue inside a wound and must be diluted 1:10 with sterile saline for safe use. Povidone Scrub solution is a detergent that is toxic to wounds and should not be used inside wounds. After preparation of the periphery, the wound is then irrigated with high-pressure streams of normal saline. Pressure of 15 lb/in^2 cleans out approximately 85% of infectious debris in a wound. Using a 60-mL syringe with an 18-gauge catheter or splash shield device, irrigate with 250 mL of solution or more, depending on wound size and contamination (approximately 50 mL/cm for clean wounds and 100 mL/cm for contaminated wounds).

Hair does not have to be removed before wound closure, because it does not increase infection rates. If the wound is in a technically difficult area, you may cut the hair to better visualize or to prevent tangling with the suture material. Hair can be moved away from the wound edges by slicking it down with antibiotic ointment or lubricating jelly. Hair on the eyebrow should *not* be removed because this may prevent proper alignment of wound margins, and the hair may grow back thinner and irregularly.

Irrigation removes most foreign material and debris from the wound. If the suspicion for a foreign body remains high or if the patient feels something within the wound, then direct visualization and removal may be indicated. If the foreign body is inert (metal), the decision to remove it must be weighed against the potential damage created by searching for it. Foreign bodies are notoriously difficult to locate despite x-ray films that demonstrate the foreign body. Inert objects usually become encapsulated within soft tissue and cause few problems. Although you should attempt to remove glass foreign bodies, small insignificant pieces can be left behind. Organic objects (wood splinter or thorns) must be removed completely, because they increase the risk of infection and may form foreign body granulomas or draining fistulas. Radiographs can be helpful in locating the foreign body. Taping an open paper clip near the wound

before x-ray examination may help in orienting the foreign body. Metallic foreign bodies are the easiest to visualize on radiograph, but larger pieces of glass may also be visible. Wood foreign bodies remain difficult to detect on standard radiographs. Ultrasound shows promise for evaluation for foreign bodies and guided removal.

Wound Débridement

Wounds should be débrided of devitalized tissue before suturing while preserving as much tissue as possible to prevent a gaping wound. Devitalized tissue is blue or black but may not demarcate until 24 hours after the initial injury. Simple débridement consists of removing devitalized and soiled subcutaneous fat with a tissue forceps and scissors. In excising epidermis or dermis, tissue scissors or a number 15 blade should be used. Remove as little tissue as possible when débriding the epidermis or dermis, leaving as much tissue to work with as possible. The wound edges should be cut at a slight angle so that the skin edge protrudes slightly out, as shown in Fig. 70.2. This allows for natural eversion with proper suture placement. Hand wounds should not be

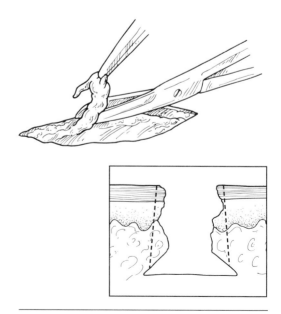

Figure 70.2
Excision of devitalized tissue.

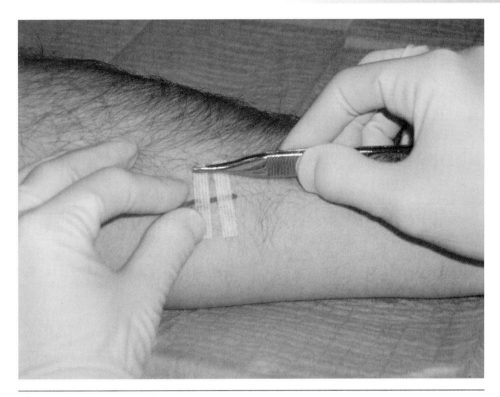

Figure 70.3
Application of Steri strips.

débrided by the emergency physician, because of the presence of many vital structures in close proximity.

Undermining is a technique used when wounds are under too much tension to allow good closure. The technique involves blunt separation of the dermis from the subcutaneous fat along the margins of the wound and the corner. Not all wide gaping wounds require undermining. If there is good opposition by using deep sutures and intradermal sutures, there is no need for undermining.

Methods of Closure

Options for wound closure include adhesive strips, staples, tissue adhesive (Dermabond), and sutures.

Adhesive Strips

Adhesive strips are useful for superficial wounds under little tension and in the elderly or steroid dependent patient with thin,

fragile skin. Once the wound has been properly prepped, benzoin is applied around the wound and allowed to dry. Be careful not to get benzoin into the wound. The tape is cut, allowing for 2 to 3 cm overlap of the sides of the wound. Individual pieces are removed by forceps and applied to one side. The opposite edge is apposed with a finger and the tape is secured, as shown in Fig. 70.3. Adhesive strips should not be used over joint surfaces, gaping wounds, the scalp, or areas that cannot be freed of blood or secretions. Tape does not work well on oily or hairy skin. Adhesive strips may also be used to reinforce the wound after suture removal.

Staples

Staples are best used to close linear lacerations over the scalp, neck, extremities, trunk, and buttocks. The cosmetic result is similar to sutures, and the amount of time to closure is about five times shorter than sutures. Staples should be avoided if you may need to

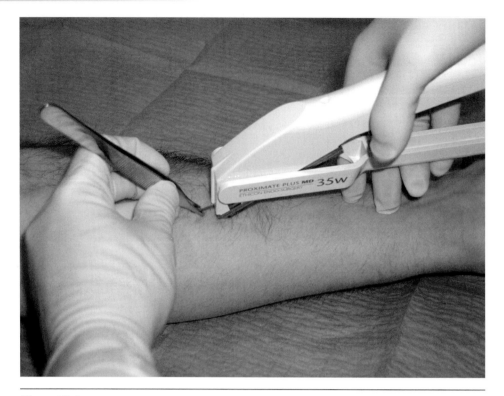

Figure 70.4
Application of staples.

image the area with computed tomography (CT) or magnetic resonance imaging (MRI). When using a stapling device, forceps help evert the wound edges, as shown in Fig. 70.4. Do not push down too hard with the stapler, because this may result in staples placed too deeply. Staples remain in place for the same length of time as sutures and require a staple remover for removal.

Tissue Adhesive

Tissue adhesives were first approved for use in the United States in August 1998. Tissue adhesives contain liquid monomers made from a combination of formaldehyde and cyanoacetate. One such adhesive is 2-octylcyanoacrylate (Dermabond), which polymerizes with hydroxyl ions found in blood and water, allowing it to bind to skin. Tissue adhesives are for topical use only and should not be placed within wounds. They are best used for short, linear lacerations in areas with little skin tension. The application

of tissue adhesives is fast and painless, and the adhesive sloughs off within 7 to 10 days. Cosmetically, Dermabond is equivalent to suturing. It comes in a single-use violet-colored ampule, which is crushed to begin the polymerization process. The adhesive is painted on while the edges of the wound are manually approximated (Fig. 70.5). If better control is needed for application, the adhesive may be drawn into a 5-mL syringe with an 18-gauge needle. Then a 22-gauge or 25-gauge Angiocath tip is attached, allowing for a smaller amount to be placed in the correct spot. Be sure to cover the patient's eyes with gauze when working on the face. Dermabond is excellent for children because it is relatively painless and does not require a revisit for suture removal.

Sutures

Suturing is the most commonly used method for wound closure. There are a wide variety

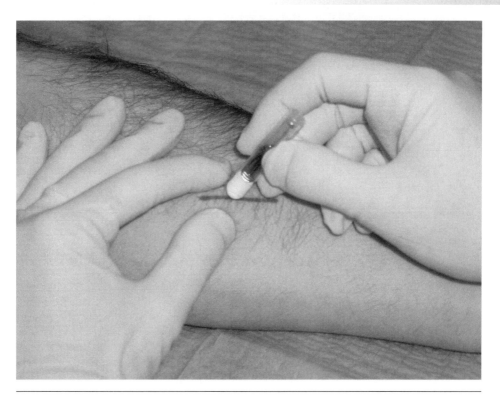

Figure 70.5
Application of Dermabond skin glue.

of suture materials available (Table 70.1). There are two main classes of sutures: absorbable and nonabsorbable. The proper suture material depends on location of the wound and the type of closure.

Absorbable sutures are made of materials that are rapidly degraded in tissues. Examples include polyglycolic acid (PGA), plain gut, and chromic gut. PGA (Dexon) is a synthetic absorbable suture that is less

Table 70.1.

Suture materials

Suture Type	Trade Name	Generic
Nonabsorbable	Ethilon	Nylon
	Dermalon	
	Prolene	Polypropylene
	Novofil	Polybutester
Absorbable (dermal closure)	Dexon	Polyglycolic acid
	Vicryl	Polyglactin 910
	PDS	Polydioxanone
	Maxon	Polyglyconate
Absorbable (mucosal closure)	Gut	
	Chromic gut	
	Vicryl	

reactive to tissue (than gut sutures) and has excellent knot security, but is difficult to work with because it has a high friction coefficient (the material drags through tissues and snags). Dexon Plus is a modified type of PGA, which is coated with a substance that reduces drag through tissues. Gut sutures incite more tissue reaction as they are digested by white blood cell lysozymes in 10 to 40 days. Chromic gut lasts 15 to 60 days and is used mainly to close oral lacerations, which heal rapidly and require little support. Newer synthetic monofilament absorbable sutures, such as polyglyconate (Maxon) and polydioxanone (PDS), have stronger tensile strength, knot security, and lower friction coefficients.

Nonabsorbable sutures maintain their tensile strength for more than 60 days. The most commonly used nonabsorbable sutures are made of synthetic monofilament nylon (Ethilon, Dermalon). This material is relatively nonreactive and has great tensile strength. The disadvantage is in knot security, because monofilaments have greater memory (tendency to return to the original packing shape). If not tied correctly, the knots will unravel. It takes at least four to five throws to achieve a secured final knot. Polypropylene (Prolene) is another monofilament that is stronger than nylon but more difficult to work with because it has greater memory. Polybutester (Novofil) is a new type of suture material that is stronger and has less memory than the others. It also has the unique property of stretching. In situations in which wound edema occurs, it stretches; when the edema subsides, this material resumes its original shape. Silk sutures maintain their tensile strength for almost 1 year. Although silk is easy to work with and has excellent knot security, it causes more skin reactions. In most situations, synthetic suture materials are preferred.

All suture materials evoke host defenses and produce inflammation. This reaction is related to the quantity of suture material and to the chemical composition of the suture. The strength of a suture material is proportional to the square of the diameter of the thread (thread size). Thus, thread size is a measure of the tensile strength of the suture material. A standard nomenclature set forth by the government differentiates between different sized sutures. Therefore, a 4-0 suture of any type is larger and stronger than a 6-0 suture. Generally, 5-0 and 6-0 sutures are used for closure in cosmetic areas such as the face. In most situations, 3-0 and 4-0 sutures are used in the repair of fascia and skin that is subjected to stress (i.e., over joints). Otherwise, 4-0 and 5-0 sutures are used for subcutaneous and skin closure. Many wounds in the emergency department require a layered closure. For that reason, one would have to pick an absorbable as well as nonabsorbable suture material to close the wound. Closing the dead space within a wound with deep sutures helps relieve skin tension and reduce hematoma formation. However, hand wounds should almost never be closed in layers.

Bite Wounds

All animal bites are considered contaminated with potentially pathogenic bacteria. Common pathogens include *Staphylococcus aureus, Staphylococcus epidermis, Enterobacter,* and other anaerobes. *Pasteurella multocida* is another pathogen found in up to 50% to 80% of cat bites and to a lesser extent, dog bites. *Pasteurella* is suspected in bites that show signs of local infection with intense inflammatory reactions within 24 hours and is often characterized by a gray, serosanguinous exudate. Puncture wounds resulting from fangs are at the greatest risk for becoming infected because they are difficult to adequately cleanse, irrigate, and débride. Snake and other reptile bite wounds should always be radiographed because the small teeth may break and be left inside the wound.

Cat bites and scratch wounds should be left open, because there is a higher incidence of infection. For that reason, prophylactic antibiotics should also be given. Antibiotic coverage must include *P. multocida* coverage. Amoxicillin-clavulanic acid is the antibiotic of choice. Erythromycin is recommended for penicillin-allergic patients (although many strains of *Pasteurella* are resistant).

Table 70.2.		
Rabies preexposure prophylaxis schedule, United States, 1999		
Type Vaccination	Route	Regimen
Primary	Intramuscular (IM)	HDCV, PCEC, or RVA; 1.0 mL (deltoid) one each day on days 0, 7, and 21, or 28
	Intradermal (ID)	HDCV; 0.1 mL, one each on days 0, 7, and 21, or 28
Booster	IM	Same as primary, day 0 only
	ID	Same as primary, day 0 only

HDCV, human diploid cell vaccine; PCEC, purified chick embryo cell vaccine; RVA, rabies vaccine adsorbed.
From ACIP guidelines: rabies prevention—US. *MMWR* 1999;48:1–20.

There is considerable controversy whether dog bites should be sutured. In general, wounds that would cause marked cosmetic deformity in a visible area are sutured (e.g., on the face). If the wound is sutured, deep sutures are avoided because they provide a nidus for infection. Sutured wounds should be covered with prophylactic antibiotics for 4 to 5 days. Amoxicillin-clavulanic acid is recommended. Clindamycin plus ciprofloxacin or trimethoprim-sulfamethoxazole is given to the penicillin-allergic patient.

Human bites are considered serious injuries. As a rule, these wounds are left open. *Eikenella corrodens*, a gram-negative, facultative anaerobe, is often found in human bite wounds. It is standard practice to treat human bites with antibiotics, such as amoxicillin-clavulanic acid, that cover *S. aureus* as well as *Eikenella*. Clindamycin plus ciprofloxacin or trimethoprim-sulfamethoxazole is given to penicillin-allergic patients.

Rabies prophylaxis should be given in all animal bites in which there is a suspicion of rabies. For a discussion of rabies, see Chapter 61. Rabies prophylaxis guidelines can be found in Table 70.2.

Puncture Wounds

Puncture wounds require special management. Puncture wounds are at high risk for retained foreign bodies and infection. After administering local anesthesia, these wounds must be explored. To get better exposure, the edges of the puncture wound can be ex-

cised as shown in Fig. 70.6. The subdermal area is then explored and irrigated under high pressure. Prophylactic antibiotics are not recommended for puncture wounds. Patients should be instructed to return for any sign of infection (i.e., redness, discharge, pain, or swelling). Puncture wounds to the plantar aspect of the foot (e.g., after stepping on a nail) have additional complications. In addition to the usual pathogens present on skin flora, *Pseudomonas aeruginosa* is an important cause of plantar puncture wound osteomyelitis. This pathogen is found in soil, water, and the damp environment of sneakers. Prophylactic antibiotics

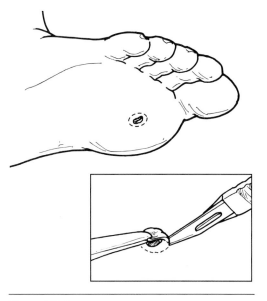

Figure 70.6
Débridement of puncture wound.

Table 70.3.

Routine diphtheria, tetanus, and pertussis vaccination schedule for persons ≥ 7 years of age, 1991

Dose	Age/Interval	Product
Primary 1	First dose	Td
Primary 2	4–8 wk after first	Td
Primary 3	6–12 mo after second	Td
Booster	Every 10 yr after last dose	Td
	Prolonging the interval does not require restarting the series	

Td, tetanus-diphtheria.
From Centers for Disease Control. Diphtheria, tetanus, and pertussis: recommendations for vaccine use and other preventive measures: recommendations of the Immunization Practices Advisory Committee (ACIP). *MMWR* 1991;40(No. RR-10):1–28.

are not routinely recommended for puncture wounds on plantar surfaces but may be considered. Good follow-up, proper wound care, and ensuring tetanus immunization are crucial. Puncture wounds of the hand may seem trivial but must be inspected with care so as not to miss a transected nerve or tendon or retained foreign body.

Wound Aftercare

Discharge instructions should include care of the wound (dressing and antibiotic ointment), signs of infection (fever, pus, redness, swelling, warmth, and increased pain), proper follow-up, and timing for suture removal. Tetanus prophylaxis should be addressed in every patient who visits the emergency department for wound care. Tetanus occurs among patients who have never been immunized or have been incompletely immunized. Most cases occur in people older than the age of 50, who often have lower levels of serum tetanus antibody. In general, a tetanus booster should be administered if the last tetanus immunization was more than 10 years in clean wounds and more than 5 years in a dirty contaminated wound. Tables 70.3 and 70.4 present guidelines regarding tetanus prophylaxis.

Table 70.4.

Summary guide to tetanus prophylaxis in routine wound management, 1991

Clean, minor history of absorbed tetanus toxoid (doses)	All Other Wounds		Wounds(*)	
	Td (+)	TIG	Td (+)	TIG
Unknown or Three (&)	No (@)	No	No (**)	No

*   Such as, but not limited to, wounds contaminated with dirt, feces, soil, and saliva; puncture wounds; avulsions; and wounds resulting from missiles, crushing, burns and frostbite.

+   For children older than 7 years; DTP (DT, if pertussis vaccine is contraindicated) is preferred to tetanus toxoid alone. For persons less than or 7 years of age, Td is preferred to tetanus toxoid alone.

&   If only three doses of fluid toxoid have been received, then a fourth dose of toxoid, preferably an absorbed toxoid, should be given.

@   Yes, if less than 10 years since last dose.

**   Yes, if less than 5 years since last dose. (More frequent boosters are not needed and can accentuate side effects).

Table 70.5.

Suture removal guidelines

Location	Suture Size	Suggested Time for Suture Removal
Face	6-0, 7-0	3–5 days
Scalp	3-0	5–8 days
Trunk	4-0, 5-0	7–10 days
Hand	5-0	7–10 days
Foot	3-0, 4-0	7–10 days
Over joints	3-0, 4-0	10–14 days
Upper and lower extremities	4-0	7–10 days

The use of prophylactic antibiotics in wound care management is controversial. Each case must be decided individually. Certain wound characteristics warrant antibiotic prophylaxis, such as mammalian bites (especially human and cat bites); significantly contaminated wounds; involvement of joint spaces, tendon, bone, or cartilage; and wounds in patients with impaired host defenses (e.g., patients with diabetes).

The antibiotic of choice should have activity against gram-positive and gram-negative organisms. For wounds not associated with bites, penicillinase-resistant penicillins such as dicloxacillin are a reasonable choice, as are first-generation cephalosporins such as cephalexin (Keflex). Erythromycin should be used in penicillin-allergic patients. Prophylaxis is usually administered for 3 to 5 days.

The timing of suture removal is dependent on the location of the wound and the presence of infection or complications. Timely removal of sutures prevents the formation of visible scars from the suture punctures. Facial sutures are removed fairly quickly despite the fact the wound has not regained any tensile strength. Table 70.5 shows the recommended times for suture removal. In areas of the body where cosmesis is not a prime issue, sutures can remain in longer. Suture removal is a simple technique, as shown in Fig. 70.7. It may be necessary to remove some of the coagulum from wound to prevent pulling. This is accomplished by cleaning the suture line with cotton swabs soaked in hydrogen peroxide.

There are a few things that a patient can do to minimize scarring. While the sutures are in place, the wound should be cleaned daily with cotton swabs soaked in hydrogen peroxide, which may discolor some of the suture materials. Studies have demonstrated that antibiotic ointments (e.g., bacitracin) applied to the wound edges aid in healing. However, antibiotic ointments must not be applied to wounds closed with tissue adhesive, because the petroleum base will dissolve the glue. After suture removal, the scar should be kept out of the sun. Some authorities recommend massaging the wound with vitamin E oil or lotion every day for up to 6 months after the sutures have been removed.

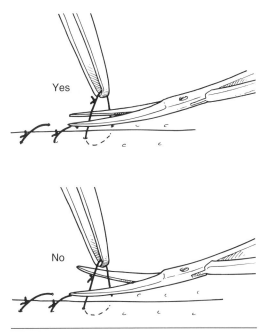

Figure 70.7
Suture removal technique.

Suture Techniques

This section covers some basic suturing principles and techniques. Although it is important to develop proper technique in the beginning, it takes time and practice to master these skills. You may want to practice on orange rinds or fresh pig's feet from a local butcher.

Suture techniques covered in this chapter include the following:

- Simple suture (percutaneous) and instrument tie

- Continuous (running) suture

- Vertical and horizontal mattress suture

- Corner stitch

- V-Y flap closure

- Correction of a "dog ear" deformity

Before beginning the simple suture, the correct technique of handling the needle holder should be used, as shown in Fig. 70.8. The needle should be placed in the needle holder close to the suture end. Fingers should be placed on the midshaft of the needle holder, instead of through the rings, allowing for greater ease and speed of suturing. When suturing, the needle should enter the skin at a 90-degree angle to the epidermis. This produces a stitch that is deeper than it is wide, allowing for more subcutaneous tissue to be incorporated. The needle is driven through tissue by flexing the wrist and supinating the forearm. The angle of exit should be the same as the angle of entrance so that identical amounts of tissue are contained on both sides, as shown in Fig. 70.9.

The Simple Suture and Instrument Tie

The most frequently used suture to close wounds is the simple interrupted suture. Each suture is tied individually so that, if one fails, the remaining sutures continue to hold the wound together. Figure 70.10 shows the technique of the simple suture. As the needle is driven downward, the needle

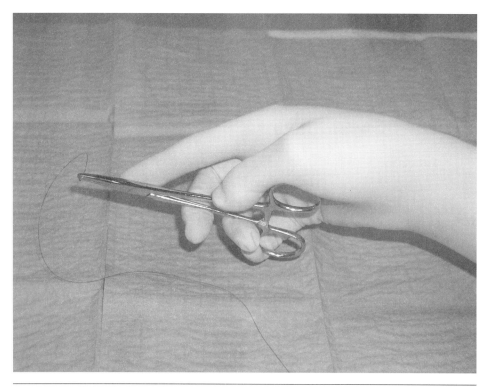

Figure 70.8
Correct technique for using the needle holder.

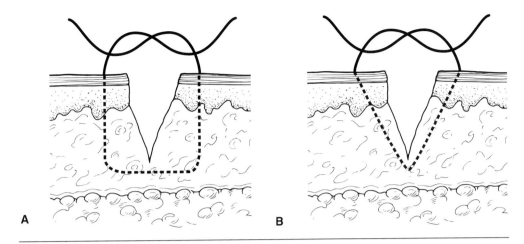

Figure 70.9
Configuration of suture in tissue. **A**: Correct configuration of suture in tissue. **B**: Incorrect configuration leads to inversion of edges and "pitting" of the scar.

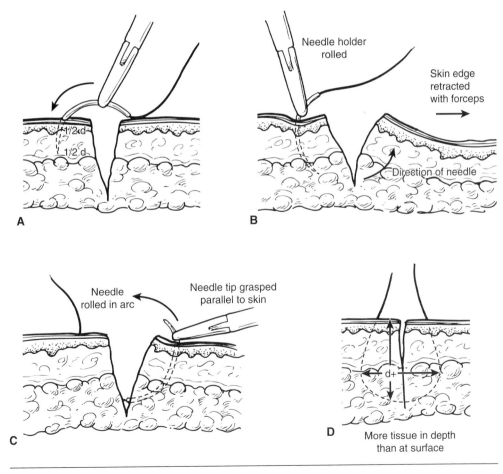

Figure 70.10
Simple suture technique. The correct sequence is shown in panels **A–D**.

may be advanced straight to the opposite side if the distance across the wound is not too great. Retracting the skin edge on the opposite side helps with controlling the path or arc of the needle. If necessary, the needle may be removed from the first side, reloaded on the needle holder in the center of the wound, and taken through the opposite side. The needle is driven upward starting from the same depth as the depth of the other side of the wound and exiting the surface the same distance from the wound edge as the opposite side.

An instrument tie secures the suture ends. In this method, as shown in Fig. 70.11, the needle driver is placed between the needle end and the free end of the suture. The needle end of the suture material is looped around the needle driver toward the free end. Then the free end is grabbed and pulled through the loop, in the opposite direction. When done correctly, the knot will lie flat across the wound. Two loops around the needle driver during the first tie help secure the knot. After that, the needle drivers are again placed between the two ends, and the suture is looped again toward the free end (this time, in the opposite direction). In this manner, alternating between clockwise and counterclockwise loops, the suture ends are tied. Your hands may need to cross to

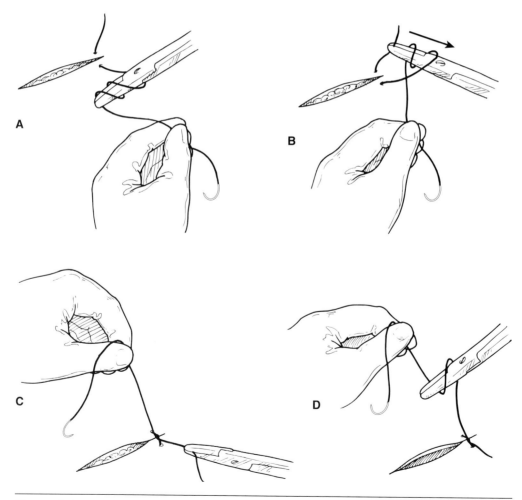

Figure 70.11
Correct technique for instrument tie. The correct sequence is shown in panels **A–D**.

lay the knot down flat. The number of knots tied is dependent on your suture material. Too many knots will weaken the suture at the knot site. Too few or improperly tied knots will cause the suture to unravel. Three square knots are used to secure a stitch with silk or other braided, nonabsorbable materials. Four knots are used for synthetic, monofilament absorbable, and nonabsorbable sutures.

Subcutaneous Closure

The subcutaneous closure is used to close the deep space of a laceration. The epidermis is brought closer together, resulting in a narrower scar. In this stitch, the suture is inverted, allowing the knot to be buried, or placed at the bottom of the wound. This prevents a painful, palpable nodule underneath the epidermis and keeps the foreign suture material away from the skin's surface. As shown in Fig. 70.12, the suture enters the subcutaneous layer at the bottom of the wound. The entry point on the opposite side should be at the same depth it exited. The ends are then instrument tied. One may elect to place the suture at an oblique angle to facilitate instrument tying. This layer is easiest closed in segments by starting in the middle. Each segment is then bisected in this manner until the layer is closed. Place only the minimum number of sutures, because each stitch acts as a foreign

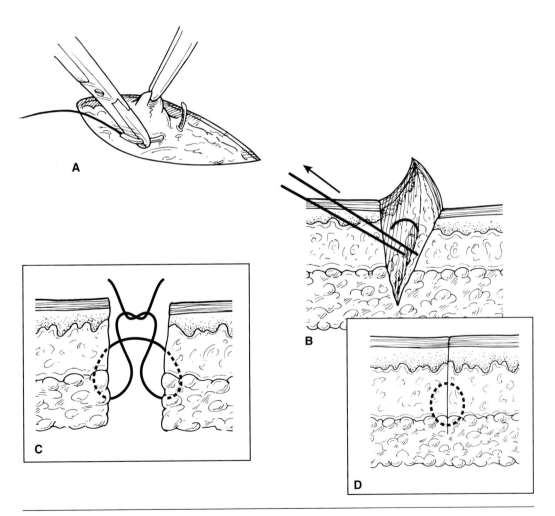

Figure 70.12
Technique for placing a subcutaneous (deep) suture. The correct sequence is shown in panels **A–D**.

body and can predispose to infection. Subcutaneous sutures must not be used in closing hand lacerations. A granuloma will form, which is problematic given the number of important structures within a small space.

Continuous Stitch

Also known as the running stitch, the continuous stitch can be done faster than a series of single interrupted sutures. The tension is evenly distributed along the entire length. More effective hemostasis is provided, and fewer knots are used (which are weak points). The major disadvantage of this stitch is that if one suture breaks, the entire closure unravels. In addition, if infection develops, the entire suture line must be removed, rather than a limited number of individual sutures. This stitch is best used for clean wounds that are under little tension on immobile skin surface in people without conditions that would impair wound healing.

As shown in Fig. 70.13, the continuous stitch starts with a single interrupted stitch in which only the free end is cut. Suturing continues with the needle passing at a 45-degree angle to the wound direction. The cross stays of the suture will be at a 90-degree angle to the wound direction. The suture material is held out of the way with the

nondominant hand and is slightly taut. The last stitch is placed just beyond the wound and is left as a loop. The last loop serves as the tail end in the instrument tying of the knot, as shown in Fig 70.14.

One variation of this stitch is the interlocking technique. As the suturing continues, the needle is taken through the loop being held in the nondominant hand. This method is useful for an irregular laceration.

Vertical Mattress Stitch

The vertical mattress stitch is usually reserved for single-layer closure of wounds under great tension, in areas that have lax skin (e.g., the elbow). It produces effective eversion of skin edges but also causes more ischemia and necrosis within its loop. This stitch is started a generous distance away from the wound edge and exited in the same manner. Then, the stitch is entered only 1 to 2 mm from the wound edges, as shown in Fig. 70.15 on page 630. An easy way to remember the stitch sequence in the vertical mattress is far-far-near-near. Mattress sutures should never be used on the face.

Horizontal Mattress Stitch

The horizontal mattress stitch also helps achieve wound eversion. The horizontal mattress suture is theoretically preferred to

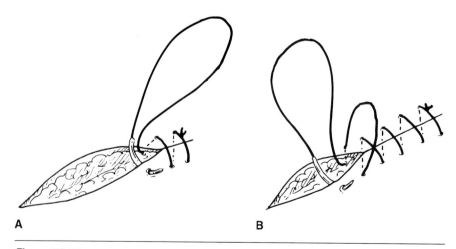

A   **B**

Figure 70.13
A running suture. The correct sequence is shown in panels **A** and **B**.

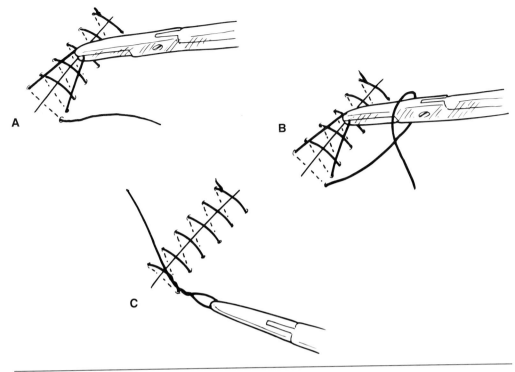

Figure 70.14
End a running suture with an instrument tie using the last stitch and the remaining suture. The correct sequence is shown in panels **A–C**.

the vertical mattress, because there is less interruption of circulation and necrosis at wound edges. In this technique, the needle in introduced into the skin as in the simple suture. After the needle is brought out the other side, a second bite is taken adjacent to the exit, as shown in Fig. 70.16 on page 631. The needle is then brought back through to the original starting side.

Corner Stitch

Also known as the half-buried horizontal mattress suture, corner stitch is used to close complex flaps. It does not interrupt the small capillaries at the tip, thus reducing the chance of tip necrosis. The suture is introduced in a non-corner portion of the wound. The needle is then brought out through the dermis and passed horizontally through the flap, as shown in Fig. 70.17 on page 631. When passing the suture horizontally, it should be at the junction of the epidermis and dermis. The stitch is then passed out through the dermis on the other non-corner side of the wound. In this manner, half of the suture will be above the skin and the other half buried below. If the entry and exit wounds are not at the same level of the epidermal-dermal junction, then the wound edges will be uneven. Once the tip is in place by the corner stitch, then the remainder of the flap can be closed, making sure the remaining sutures are placed far enough from the tip to allow unrestricted dermal circulation.

V-Y Flap Closure

Some flaps or corners have nonviable edges. The edges need to trimmed; however, with the smaller amount of tissue, it will be difficult to close the defect. In these instances, the V flap is converted to a Y flap, as shown in Fig. 70.18 on page 632. The corner stitch is then used to close the Y flap. The remain-

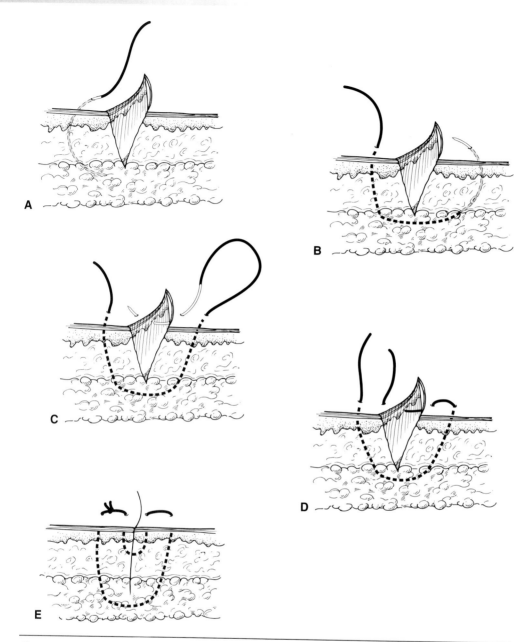

Figure 70.15
Vertical mattress stitch. The correct sequence is shown in panels **A–E**.

der of the wound is closed with small-bite percutaneous sutures.

Dog-Ear Closure

Closure of a laceration can lead to bunching at one end, referred to as a dog ear. This tends to occur with wounds that have a curve. The technique for correction of this problem is shown in Fig. 70.19 on page 633. An incision is made at a 45-degree angle on the same side as the excess tissue. The redundant tissue is excised along the 45-degree angle to the wound. The wound is closed, with the resulting laceration assuming a curved appearance.

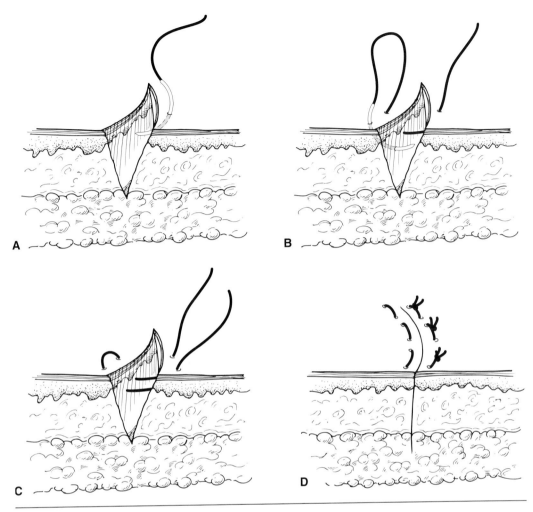

Figure 70.16
Horizontal mattress stitch. The correct sequence is shown in panels **A–D**.

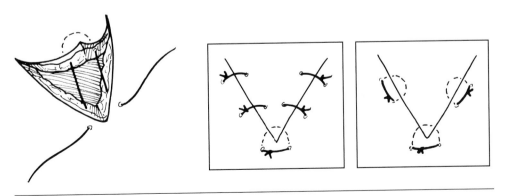

Figure 70.17
A corner stitch. The box on the left shows simple sutures at the straight edges with a corner stitch closing the flap. The box on the right shows three half-buried corner stitches closing the entire flap.

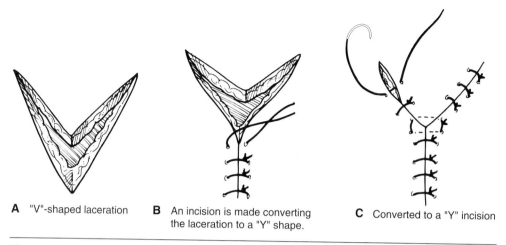

A "V"-shaped laceration   **B** An incision is made converting the laceration to a "Y" shape.   **C** Converted to a "Y" incision

Figure 70.18
Creating a V-Y flap and its closure, is shown in figures **A–C**.

Special Areas

Scalp

All scalp lacerations should be explored for foreign bodies and galea interruption and palpated for skull fractures. Figure 70.20 on page 634. shows the cross section of the scalp. Lacerations of the galea must be repaired. The galea inserts into the frontalis muscle and failure to repair it can lead to asymmetric contraction. The scalp is extremely vascular, and uncontrolled bleeding may lead to hypovolemic shock. If pressure and elevation of the head of the bed do not help, local injection of lidocaine with epinephrine is effective. The galea is repaired with 3-0 or 4-0 absorbable sutures. Staples or nonabsorbable sutures are then used to close the skin. After repair, a pressure dressing is helpful to reduce hematoma formation.

Oral Cavity

Lacerations of the buccal or gingival mucosa generally heal without repair. Large or gaping wounds can be closed with absorbable chromic gut or Vicryl. Oral cavity tissues heal quickly. Tongue lacerations are treated in the same manner. If they need to be closed, obtaining the trust of the patient makes the situation easier. The tongue can be controlled by holding it with dry gauze, or using two 2-0 silk sutures through the side borders. The area must be anesthetized before the placement of these retention sutures. An assistant may be needed. Absorbable sutures such as 5-0 chromic gut or Vicryl are used to close lacerations of the tongue and oral mucosa. The patient should be instructed to take soft foods or liquids for the first several days and to rinse the mouth after eating.

Cheek and Zygomatic Area

Uncomplicated lacerations may be closed with 6-0 nonabsorbable sutures. There are two structures just anterior to the ear that can be injured by penetrating lacerations: the parotid duct and the facial nerve. If there is any doubt about damage to these structures, consult an oral or plastic surgeon. If the parotid duct is injured, salivary fluid may be seen leaking from the wound or bloody salivary fluid can be seen coming from the opening of the duct in the buccal mucosa at the level of the second molar tooth. All five branches of the facial nerve should be tested. Wrinkling the forehead and elevating the brow tests the temporal branch. Having the patient open and close the eyes tests the zygomatic branch. Having the patient smile and frown tests the buccal and mandibular branches. The cervical branch is tested by contraction of the platysma with neck shrugging.

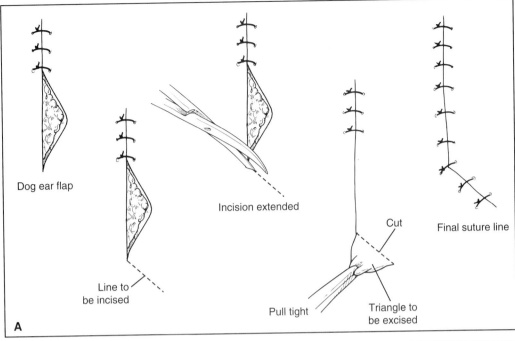

Dog ear flap

Line to be incised

Incision extended

Pull tight

Cut

Triangle to be excised

Final suture line

A

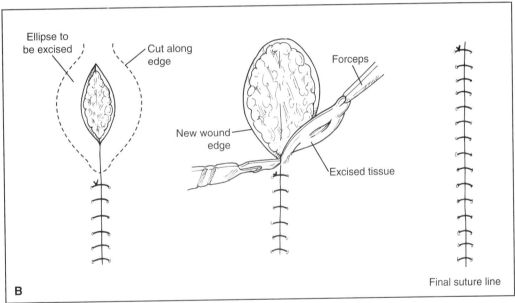

Ellipse to be excised

Cut along edge

Forceps

New wound edge

Excised tissue

Final suture line

B

Figure 70.19
Correction of the dog ear deformity can be accomplished by two methods, as illustrated in **A** and **B**.

Lips

Lip lacerations are cosmetically important. A misalignment by even 1 mm of the vermilion border is easily noticed. The vermilion border is the white line around the lips. This de-fect is not amenable to revision once primary healing has happened. Repair begins with the first suture aligning the vermilion border on each side (Fig. 70.21, page 634). Once the vermilion border is aligned, the

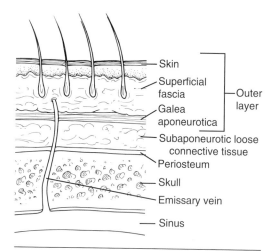

Figure 70.20
Cross section of the scalp.

remainder of the wound is closed. If the mucosal border is damaged, it must also be aligned with meticulous care. Lacerations

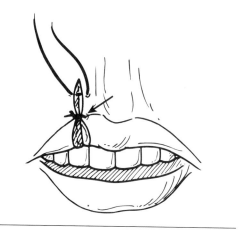

Figure 70.21
Correct closure of the vermilion border of the lip.

that extend into the mucosa are repaired with absorbable suture. Antibiotics are recommended for full-thickness lacerations that penetrate the cheek into the oral mucosa.

Suggested Readings

ACIP guidelines: diphtheria, tetanus and pertussis. Guidelines for vaccine prophylaxis and other preventative measures—US. *MMWR* 1991;40:1–28.

ACIP guidelines: rabies prevention—US. *MMWR* 1999;48:1–20.

Edlich R, Thacker J, Rodeheaver G. Wound management and skin closure. In: Hardwood-Nuss A, Linden C, Luten R, et al, eds. *The clinical practice of emergency medicine*, 2nd ed. Philadelphia: Lippincott-Raven, 1996:392–403.

Griego R, Rosen T, Orengo I, et al. Dog, cat, and human bites: a review. *J Am Acad Dermatol* 1995;33:1019–1029.

Hollander JE, Singer AJ. Laceration management. *Ann Emerg Med* 1999;34:356–367.

Markovchick V. Suture materials and mechanical after care. *Emerg Med Clin North Am* 1992; 10:673–688.

Mortiere M. *Principles of primary wound management*, 3rd ed. Fairfax, VA: Clifton, 1996:6–92.

Roberts J, Hedges J, eds. *Clinical procedures in emergency medicine*, 2nd ed. Philadelphia: WB Saunders, 1991.

Singer AJ, Hollander JE, Quinn JV. Evaluation and management of traumatic lacerations. *N Engl J Med* 1997;337:1142–1148.

Trott A. *Wounds and lacerations*, 2nd ed. St. Louis: Mosby, 1991:2–31.

Soft Tissue Infections

Jeffrey I. Schneider, MD

Patients presenting with cutaneous abscesses are frequently encountered in the emergency department (ED). They seek medical assistance because of pain, swelling, constitutional symptoms, or cosmetic disfigurement that result from such soft tissue infections. This chapter discusses the etiology, pathogenesis, bacteriology, and management of the cutaneous abscess. Incision and drainage (I&D) procedures are discussed in general, and specific techniques involving commonly presenting disease entities are presented in some detail.

Definitions

An *abscess* is essentially a walled-off collection of pus. Clinical presentation usually includes a painful, fluctuant mass surrounded by erythema and induration.

Fluctuance is noted when one is able to feel a fluid component at the center of an inflammatory mass.

Induration refers to the firm, tender, erythematous area of skin and is a sign of active inflammation that has not yet progressed to necrosis and liquefaction.

Beneath the skin, one generally finds a pocket of fluid and cellular debris that is interrupted by projections of granulation tissue and pus, which extend along the tissue planes that offer the least resistance.

Conversely, *cellulitis* is typically defined as a superficial infection of the skin, resulting in edema and erythema, with little exudate, and no necrosis of underlying structures.

Abscess Formation

Localized skin infections can be found in any region of the body and are usually a direct result of failure of normal epidermal defense mechanisms. This breakdown in the body's protective covering allows indigenous flora to invade, and, as a result, bacteria that are native to the particular location on the body colonize most abscesses. Thus, unlike other bacterial disease processes, abscesses are generally identified by their site, rather than the specific etiological agent.

Several factors must occur to allow bacteria on the skin's surface to penetrate into the deeper soft tissues. It has been demonstrated that a high concentration of pathogens alone is generally insufficient, because of the skin's natural defenses. There also must be interruption or obstruction of the skin's ability to drain, and disruption of the corneal layer of epithelium. These circumstances allow for the generation of a moist environment in which bacteria can multiply in the presence of nutrients and pass through the skin barrier. Those bacteria that initially may cause a cellulitis continue to multiply and begin an enzyme cascade that results in necrosis, liquefaction, and buildup of cellular debris and leukocytes. When this collection becomes sealed off, an abscess has formed.

These conditions can be created in many ways: via the person who works with his or her hands, by the intravenous (IV) drug user who injects into his or her veins, or by people who shave their axillae or wear clothes that prevent normal aeration of skin folds, leading to maceration and skin breakdown. Additional host factors, such as poor blood supply to certain areas, immunocompromise (e.g., diabetes, human immunodeficiency virus [HIV] infection), or septic emboli from endocarditis may provide additional risk factors for the development of abscesses.

Bacteriology

There have been several studies attempting to describe the microbiology of cutaneous abscesses. In one of the larger published series, investigators cultured abscesses from 135 patients who underwent routine I&D. Material from the abscesses was immediately aspirated and injected into culture containers. Although the study is dated (published in 1978) and not all data points were collected (admitted and immunocompromised individuals excluded), several important characteristics of the flora of abscesses were identified.

To start, Meslin and colleagues demonstrated that most abscesses of the trunk, axilla, extremities, and hand, contained mixed aerobic bacteria. In those cultures that did grow only one species, *Staphylococcus aureus* was identified in 72% of cases. Significantly, *S. aureus* was the most commonly isolated aerobic strain; it was seen in 24% of all abscesses. Perianal cultures, however, were

more likely to grow anaerobic species; one third contained anaerobes exclusively, and the remainder had mixed flora. The most commonly isolated anaerobes included several *Bacteroides* subspecies, *Peptococcus* species, *Peptostreptococcus* species, *Clostridium* subspecies, *Lactobacillus* subspecies, and *Fusobacterium* subspecies.

Subsequent studies, including those that examined cutaneous abscesses in children, revealed similar data. Brook and coworkers studied 209 abscesses in children age 7 days to 15 years and found that aerobic bacteria only were isolated in 46% of abscesses, anaerobic species only in 26%, and mixed bacteria were present in 28%. In addition, they reported that each abscess contained an average of 2.3 isolates (1.3 anaerobes and 1.0 aerobes). They suggested that anaerobic flora tended to be found in areas adjacent to mucosal membranes (i.e., perirectal) or in areas in children that often come in contact with these areas (i.e., nailbed infections that occur when children place their fingers in their mouths).

Intravenous Drug Users

Those who use IV drugs represent a slightly different population by their risk of developing subcutaneous abscesses and by the bacteriology of their pus collections. Of the numerous medical complications of parenteral drug abuse, the development of infection represents 28% of all hospital admissions for addicts, and most of these admissions are due to the development of an abscess at the site of injection. In one series of 77 patients admitted for abscesses secondary to parenteral drug use, 18 abscesses were identified in the hand; 9 in the wrist or forearm; 18 in the elbow; 26 in the arm and deltoid region; 6 in the flank, thigh, or knee; 7 in the leg; and 1 in the foot (several patients had more than one abscess).

These patients had their infections drained (the majority were performed in the operating room), and the fluid collections were sent for aerobic and anaerobic culture. The investigators reported that they were able to identify 128 separate organisms from the 86 abscesses. Of the abscesses that were cultured before the initiation of antimicrobial therapy, 44% grew a single pathogen (44% *S. aureus*, 33% β-hemolytic streptococci, 22% microaerophilic streptococci), and 49% had polymicrobial isolates. Interestingly, 32% of the isolates obtained from patients older than 40 years contained an aerobic gram-negative rod, whereas only 6% of those obtained from patients younger than 40 years had similar organisms.

Diagnostic Evaluation

Laboratory investigation has little role in the treatment or evaluation of abscesses. Currently, no evidence-based conclusions can be drawn from the results of any laboratory tests. (Some might argue that a blood glucose value might indicate the presence of diabetes in an individual who had previously gone undiagnosed.) Most patients with a simple cutaneous abscess have a normal complete blood cell count and do not have systemic symptoms.

Similarly, a Gram stain is only appropriate in those individuals who are immunocompromised, appear toxic, or who will be receiving prophylactic antibiotics (i.e., those with prosthetic heart valves). If one does wish to culture a wound, the most accurate results are achieved when aspiration with a needle and syringe is attempted before I&D.

Incision and Drainage

Surgical I&D is the definitive treatment of cutaneous abscesses; antibiotics alone are ineffective. Patients who have their infections drained experience a rapid improvement in symptoms and generally have the natural history of the disease process altered and shortened. Care must be taken, however, not to attempt I&D of an abscess prior to the localization of pus. Premature surgical intervention may not only fail to be therapeutic, but might allow proliferation of the infection and subsequent bacteremia. Occasionally, application of moist heat to an "early" abscess

may lessen symptoms, and contribute to the localization and accumulation of pus.

Many cutaneous abscesses are amenable to ED I&D, whereas others may mandate operating room intervention. Factors that may influence the ED physician's choice of treatment include location of the abscess (in close proximity to major neurovascular structures), size of the abscess, or the inability to obtain adequate anesthesia to allow complete I&D.

Preparation and Anesthesia

Although many EDs use prepackaged suture trays, one can easily gather the equipment necessary for the I&D of an abscess. Useful instruments include needle and syringe for local anesthesia, scalpel, hemostat, gauze, and packing material. It is impossible to complete this procedure with complete sterility. Nevertheless, you should attempt to prevent contamination of the surrounding tissue. Although many ED physicians prepare the skin with an antiseptic solution (e.g., an iodine-based solution), there are no data to support such an intervention.

Anesthesia is discussed elsewhere (see Chapters 65 and 69); adequate anesthesia is often difficult to obtain in the setting of an abscess. Reasons include the weak activity of local anesthetics in the acidic environment of infected tissues and the pain associated with injection of medication into a closed space that is already distended by pus. As a result, anesthesia of the overlying skin is generally sufficient, whereas that of the abscess cavity is often suboptimal.

Some suggest that anesthesia is best obtained by attempting to inject subcutaneously over the dome of the abscess. This can be accomplished by delicately directing a small (i.e., 25 gauge) needle just below the skin (the syringe should be held parallel to the skin surface). This technique is demonstrated in Fig. 71.1. As the anesthetic solution dissects through the subcutaneous plane, one often sees a blanching of the skin. Tissues can be highly vascular in the regions of many abscesses. The anesthetic agents you are using may be absorbed into the

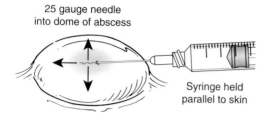

Figure 71.1
Local anesthesia is obtained by injecting lidocaine across the dome of the abscess. The needle should be parallel to the skin.

bloodstream. You must be diligent and strictly adhere to maximum doses of local anesthetics. For those patients in whom pain or anxiety limits the ability to deliver adequate analgesia, conscious sedation with IV narcotics and/or opiates (see Chapter 65) or general anesthesia and operative intervention may be warranted.

Incision and Blunt Dissection

Generally, a number 11 or 15 scalpel blade is used to cut the skin at the area of greatest fluctuance. With the expression of pus, the incision should be extended over the entire length of the abscess (Fig. 71.2). The incision should traverse the *entire* length of the abscess, *not* the area of induration, which is substantially bigger. When you are beginning these procedures and are less experienced, you may be tempted to make only a

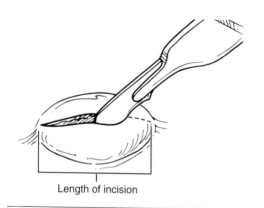

Length of incision

Figure 71.2
The incision is made across the length of the abscess.

small stab wound over the abscess. Although pus may be seen initially, the small incision does *not* provide an adequate mechanism for continued drainage of the pus and cellular debris. There is the chance that the stab incision you made will heal before the inside of the abscess closes to the surface of the skin. The result is that the abscess may form again in the same location.

Extreme care must be taken in areas such as the groin, popliteal, antecubital fossae, and neck so that nearby neurovascular structures are not violated. If possible, you should attempt to direct those incisions in the same direction as the skin creases or tension lines to minimize scarring.

In regions such as the face, in which cosmesis is of crucial importance, or on extensor surfaces, in which skin tension is high, you can be less aggressive in making an incision. Instead, an initial aspiration or small incision may be made with the understanding that repeated interventions may be necessary. Carefully explain to the patient the possibility that further treatment may be needed.

Some clinicians advocate cruciate (cross-shaped) incisions or elliptical excisions, in which an elliptical piece of skin is cut away from the surface of the abscess. These techniques do not confer any great advantage to a simple straight incision. The tips of cruciate incisions are at higher risk for necrosis, and elliptical excisions often result in larger scars.

After using the scalpel to penetrate the skin over the abscess, it is best to use blunt dissection to probe the extent of the cavity and disrupt any loculations (walled-off areas of pus within the abscess cavity) that may be present and might inhibit continued drainage. Classically, it had been taught that a gloved finger was the appropriate tool for this process. However, this practice is strongly discouraged, if not forbidden, given the risks of injuring yourself on retained foreign bodies such as needle fragments.

Instead, use a hemostat or a hemostat wrapped with gauze. It should be advanced through the skin incision opening and gently swept around through a complete circle. As discussed previously, anesthesia within the abscess cavity is often difficult to obtain; consequently, this aspect of the procedure is often the most painful for patients. This crucial step, however, should not be limited; additional systemic analgesia may be necessary.

Irrigation

Although the washing out of debris and "cleansing" of the infected space may make intuitive sense, there are no improved outcomes by irrigating within the abscess cavity.

Wound Packing, Dressing, and Follow-up

Packing a wound serves several purposes. Most importantly, it maintains a tract by which material can continue to drain. There is plain packing strip gauze (available in a variety of widths) or gauze impregnated with an iodine-based solution. There are no data to suggest that either material is superior. The goal is to place enough packing material within the cavity so that it is in contact with the inner walls of the abscess but not so much that extreme pressure with the cavity may result in further tissue necrosis.

A perfectly packed abscess cavity will have an elliptical or "fish-mouth" appearance from the pressure of the gauze within it forcing the edges of the incision to separate. This will allow the abscess cavity to heal from the inside up to the surface before the incision site closes and heals. A small piece of packing strip should be left exiting from the wound (the "wick") to further promote drainage and preservation of a pathway exiting the cavity. Over this, place a generous amount of absorbent gauze dressing to soak up any drainage or blood. If needed, the body part may be splinted.

Pain control, elevation, and follow up in 24 to 48 hours are the hallmarks of outpatient abscess therapy. Decisions regarding specific follow-up intervals should be based on immune status (e.g., diabetes, HIV), patient compliance with instructions, abscess size and volume of drainage, and abscess location. Patients should be instructed to leave the wick in place until the wound is reexamined.

In some institutions or clinical settings, patients return to the ED for continued wound management; at others they may be instructed to follow up with a specialized clinic such as those staffed by nurse practitioners or nurses. For those who do return to the ED, the packing is generally replaced within the first 1 or 2 days and then approximately every 48 hours. The primary goal for the packing is to keep the surgical wound open. Once the edges of the incision have sufficiently contracted and granulated, the wound will remain open on its own and does not require further packing.

If the packing strip has dried, moistening it with saline may allow for an easier and less painful removal process. If the packing was placed so that it was in contact with the walls of the abscess, removal should provide for some débridement of additional dead tissue.

Are Antibiotics Needed?

Simply stated, there exist no conclusive data demonstrating that antibiotics are necessary in healthy, immunocompetent patients, without valvular heart disease, who undergo routine I&D of cutaneous abscesses. However, those who are at risk for endocarditis (i.e., prosthetic heart valves, cyanotic congenital heart disease, previous infective endocarditis) should be treated before abscess incision.

Studies have confirmed detectable bacteremia following I&D procedures. Some have suggested providing patients who are immunocompromised (i.e., those with diabetes, acquired immunodeficiency syndrome, those on immunosuppressive drugs, alcoholics) and those with significant cellulitis or systemic symptoms such as fever and chills with antibiotics. Generally, a first-generation cephalosporin provides sufficient antimicrobial coverage.

Special Considerations

Although the general principles of cutaneous abscess therapy in the ED remain true irrespective of the location of the pus collection on the body, several specific areas warrant special mention and consideration.

Perirectal Abscesses

Perirectal abscesses are complex; entire book chapters are dedicated to discussing them. For the purposes of this text, you should understand that perirectal infections are a diverse group of disease entities, ranging from those that are within the realm of ED physician intervention to those that are potentially life threatening and require timely surgical consultation.

An understanding of the anatomy of the anus and rectum is crucial in comprehending the etiology and spread of perirectal abscesses. Briefly, it is believed that the mucus-producing glands at the base of the rectal *columns of Morgagni* located at the dentate line are responsible for the pathogenesis of perirectal abscesses. These glands become blocked, which, in turn, leads to destruction of normal host defense mechanisms and overgrowth and invasion of indigenous bacteria. Depending on the direction of spread of infection, the development of an ischiorectal, intramuscular, intersphincteric, pelvirectal, or perianal abscess occurs.

Adequate drainage is the hallmark of effective treatment. These abscesses are extremely painful and difficult to anesthetize in an awake patient. Even performing a rectal examination of the patient with a perirectal abscess is often impossible without sedation or spinal or general anesthesia. Consequently, unless the abscess is clearly superficial and/or you have the time and sufficient nursing staff in the ED to do conscious sedation, most patients will need to go to the operating room for appropriate treatment.

An incision should be made across the length of the fluctuant area, as described previously. Blunt dissection is used to break up loculations, and the wound is packed with gauze. Follow up should occur within 24 to 48 hours for wound check and repacking. Antibiotic therapy is generally not indicated.

Breast Abscesses

Abscesses located peripherally in the female breast should be treated in the standard fashion with a linear incision that radiates from the nipple. Local anesthesia may be complemented by using topical agents, such as eutectic mixture of local anesthetics (EMLA) cream; however, adequate analgesia is often difficult to obtain.

Those abscesses located centrally or near the areola require care that is more specialized. Specifically, these collections of pus include multiple organisms (including anaerobes) and tend to form deeper, less palpable abscesses. There is a high rate of chronic infections and subsequent ductal ectasia. Consequently, drainage often mandates complex incisions and general anesthesia. Similarly, abscess formation as a result of postpartum mastitis usually requires operating room management.

Infected Sebaceous Cysts

Sebaceous cysts, which are often present for years, usually go unnoticed until they become infected. At that time, patients may present to the ED complaining of a painful, red lesion where a small "bump" had been present earlier. These cysts, which result from obstruction of sebaceous gland ducts, become filled with a thick, cheesy material that can be seen seeping out from within. When the contents become infected, pain and erythema are the result.

Initial treatment of an infected sebaceous cyst is similar to that of all other soft tissue infections: I&D. However, two important caveats must be remembered. The first is that you must try to express as much of the thick contents of the cyst as possible. The viscosity of the substance may make spontaneous drainage unlikely. The second is that an infected sebaceous cyst has a capsule that lines the interior of the pocket. The definitive management of the cyst is extraction of this capsule. This is most often performed by a surgeon at a later date, once the infection has cleared.

Pilonidal Abscess

Abscesses in the sacrococcygeal region are referred to as pilonidal abscesses and are believed to be secondary to blockage of a pilonidal sinus. These sinuses are common malformations that occur during embryogenesis.

Obstruction of the sinuses, often by hair, may lead to infection, resulting in a painful and extremely tender area at the lower back. The mainstay of therapy is I&D.

After initial incision, be sure to explore the cyst, because subcutaneous extension of the pocket is often not evident from superficial examination. After determining the full extent of the cyst, the incision should be extended to allow adequate drainage. The wound, which is often large, should be packed, and the patient instructed to follow up in 24 to 48 hours. Recurrence is the rule with pilonidal abscesses, and surgical consultation should be arranged after the initial inflammatory process has resolved to excise the entire sinus tract.

Paronychia

Localized infections of the nailbed are termed paronychia. Patients present to the ED complaining of a red, extremely tender swollen area at the base of the nailbed. Paronychia are relatively common and thought to be a result of trauma to the fragile skin that is present between the fingernail and the cuticle. *Staphylococcus* is the predominant organism, but anaerobes and group A β-hemolytic streptococci have also been cultured from these infections (likely as a result of contact between oral flora and hands during activities such as nail biting).

As with other abscesses, a focal collection of pus and palpable fluctuance is often preceded by soft tissue swelling and erythema. If patients present during this early portion of the disease process, instruct them to soak their finger frequently in hot water and administer oral antibiotics such as cephalexin or dicloxacillin. This may result in a cure without needing to incise and drain the pus.

Once an abscess has formed, drainage is the only effective treatment. Generally, this can be accomplished without skin incision or removal of the nail. As with other soft tissue infections, creation of a tract for pus drainage is the key. With paronychia, this is accomplished by lifting the skin edge off the nail. Often, if done with care, you may gently lift the skin at the area of maximal fluctuance

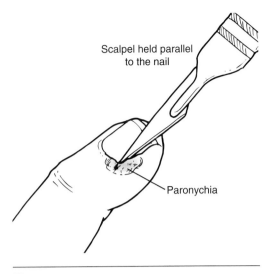

Figure 71.3
To drain a paronychia, direct a number 11 scalpel parallel to the nail surface and lift the eponychium at the area of maximum fluctuance.

using a large-gauge needle (e.g., 18 gauge) without anesthetizing the finger. If this proves painful for the patient, then do a digital block (see Chapter 69); once the area is blocked, you may use a number 11 scalpel and advance it under the skin parallel to the nail and under the eponychium at the area of most prominent swelling (Fig. 71.3). Pus should be expressed easily, and the patient should have relatively swift pain relief. If there is concern that there may be a larger pocket of pus, the area can be gently explored by sliding the instrument under the eponychium (maintaining a plane parallel to the nail). If drainage is continued, a small piece of packing gauze may be placed in the drainage tract to maintain its patency. Although systemic antibiotics are often prescribed, there are no data to support their use. Patients may be told to begin warm soaks after 24 hours, remove the gauze themselves if present, and cover the digit with a clean dressing. Topical antibiotics have no proven benefit (other than they may prevent the bandage from sticking to the wound).

If purulence is observed beneath the nail, further intervention is required to ensure adequate drainage. Specifically, one must either remove a portion of the nail, or alternatively, place several holes in the nail to allow the pus to drain. The holes may be created with either a prefabricated electrocautery device (sold commercially) or a paperclip that has been heated sufficiently. If a piece of the nail is to be removed, you should aim to remove only the proximal portion. This is done by elevating the eponychium, as described for the initial I&D, until the proximal edge of the nail is visualized. The nail may then be gently separated from the nailbed, and the proximal portion resected with scissors. Care should be taken to avoid damaging the nail matrix, and a small piece of gauze may be placed beneath the eponychium to allow for continued drainage.

It is generally recommended that simple paronychia be treated in a nail-sparing manner initially. Recurrent infections, or those having spread beneath the nailbed, may require partial nail removal. In addition, most paronychia resolve within several days of treatment; those that persist should be evaluated for osteomyelitis of the distal phalanx (a known complication of even correctly drained paronychia).

Felon

Another soft tissue infection deserving special mention is the felon. Typically, these are the result of invasion by *Staphylococcus* or *Streptococcus* species that invade the pulp of fingers after local trauma. Infection may spread to involve the distal phalanx of the finger, where increasing pressure in the enclosed space may lead to ischemic injury, compounding the damage of the infection.

This topic is not covered in detail, but important aspects of the management of the felon include those typical of other abscesses: digital nerve block to allow for adequate I&D, search for foreign bodies, packing, and

close follow up. Although there are several approaches to the therapeutic incision, all stress the importance of avoiding injury to digital nerves, blood vessels, and flexor tendon mechanisms.

Suggested Readings

Blumstein, H. Incision and drainage. In: Roberts JR, Hedges JR, eds. *Clinical procedures in emergency medicine*, 3rd ed. Philadelphia: WB Saunders, 1998:651–653.

Brenner BE, Simon R. Anorectal emergencies. *Ann Emerg Med* 1983;12:367–376.

Brook I. Microbiology of non-puerperal breast abscesses. *J Infect Dis* 1988;157:377–379.

Brook I, Finegold SM. Aerobic and anaerobic bacteriology of cutaneous abscesses in children. *Pediatrics* 1981;67:891–895.

Burney RE. Incision and drainage procedures: soft tissue abscesses in the emergency service. *Emerg Med Clin North Am* 1986;3:527–542.

Carson SC, Prose NS, Berg D. Infectious disorders of the skin. *Clin Plastic Surg* 1993;20:67–76.

Dixon JM. Outpatient treatment of non-lactational breast abscesses. *Br J Surg* 1992;79:56–57.

Lewis RC. Infections of the hand. *Emerg Med Clin North Am* 1985;3:263–274.

Llera JL, Levy RC. Treatment of cutaneous abscesses: a double-blind clinical study. *Ann Emerg Med* 1985;14:57–61.

Meislin HW. Pathogen identification of abscesses and cellulitis. *Ann Emerg Med* 1986;15:329–332.

Meislin HW, McGehee MD, Rosen P. Management and microbiology of cutaneous abscesses. *J Am Coll Emerg Physicians* 1978;7:186–191.

Meislin HW, Lerner SA, Groves MH, et al. Cutaneous abscesses: anaerobic and aerobic bacteriology and outpatient management. *Ann Intern Med* 1977;87:145–149.

Musculoskeletal Emergencies

Lumbar Puncture

Joel M. Wassermann, MD

The lumbar puncture (LP), or spinal tap as it is commonly known, is a common procedure in the emergency department (ED) and a useful diagnostic tool. Prompt cerebrospinal fluid (CSF) analysis is necessary in the ED to assess for several potentially life-threatening diseases. Although it has the stigma of being an uncomfortable and dangerous procedure, when performed correctly the LP is neither.

Indications for Lumbar Puncture

LP as a tool of neurologists has many varied indications. In the ED, however, there are only a few clinical indications for LP. A principal indication is the patient presenting to the ED with suspected meningitis, (Chapter 30) especially bacterial. These patients classically have symptoms of fever, neck stiffness, signs of meningeal irritation, and may have altered mental status. However, patients may present atypically with or without any of these symptoms. In the immunosuppressed or elderly patient, the physician must have a higher index of suspicion for meningitis. Furthermore, LP is a crucial part

of the workup in infants younger than 3 months presenting with fever. Early antibiotic coverage should be initiated and can be started up to 2 hours before performing an LP without affecting its sensitivity, although the antibiotic may alter culture results.

Another indication for LP in the ED is to rule out a subarachnoid hemorrhage (SAH) in the patient who presents with the sudden onset of a severe headache (see Chapter 28). These patients should all have a computed tomography (CT) scan of the head before LP. The CT scan is approximately 91% sensitive for SAH. The sensitivity of CT is diminished for very small hemorrhages or those presenting later than 24 hours. The most important reason for performing an LP in the patient with a sudden severe headache is to attempt to detect a small leak of blood from an aneurysm (a "sentinel bleed"), which may precede rupture of a cerebral aneurysm.

Contraindications for Lumbar Puncture

The only absolute contraindication to LP is infection of the LP site. Relative contraindications to an LP are mainly related to any pathology increasing intracranial pressure (ICP). Increased ICP with subsequent LP may release pressure lower in the spinal cord, theoretically causing cerebellar herniation leading to seizures, cardiopulmonary collapse, and death. In any patient with suspected increased ICP, head CT scan should be performed before the LP to rule out a space-occupying lesion. There is debate about the necessity of a head CT scan before performing an LP in the young healthy patient with suspected meningitis. However, a head CT scan must be done before LP in patients with focal neurological deficits; elderly patients; immunocompromised patients; patients with recent head trauma; or any patient with suspected cerebral infarct, hemorrhage, abscess, or tumor. A relative contraindication is the patient on anticoagulation secondary to the risk of creating an epidural hematoma. If absolutely necessary, reversal of coagulation defects has been shown to be effective if done before LP.

Procedure

After the patient is told the essential elements and potential complications of the procedure and informed consent is obtained, the LP can be performed. The standard LP kit contains all the necessary equipment except povidone iodine solution. Proper sterile precautions should be taken, including gown, cap, mask, and sterile gloves, none of which are included in the kit.

Positioning

Proper position is most important for ensuring a successful tap. The patient should be arranged in the lateral decubitus position, with the patient's back to the physician and the patient's lumbar spine bowed out toward the examiner (Fig. 72.1). The spine should be flexed to the maximum tolerable by the patient to open the intervertebral spaces, facilitating easier access to the spinal

canal. Alternatively, the patient can be arranged in a sitting position with the head leaning over a table that is covered with a pillow. This position allows the physician to better judge the patient's midline, and may be particularly helpful in the obese patient. However, in this position, opening pressure measurements may differ by a few millimeters. If pressure result is critical, patient may be carefully placed in the decubitus position with the needle in place, and pressure recorded in this position.

Preparation

After the physician is properly gowned with sterile precautions, the patient is prepped with Betadine solution. To sterilize the area properly, concentric circles of povidone iodine solution wash should be made outward from the prospective insertion site. At least three swaths of antiseptic should be made. The patient can then be draped with the sterile cloths provided in the kit. Excess povidine iodine solution can be wiped from the site of insertion with a piece of sterile gauze.

Localization of Interspace

Once the patient is prepared sterilely, the site of insertion should be found. The spinal canal should be accessed below the level of the termination of the spinal cord. In most adults, the spinal cord ends at the level of L1, although in up to 31% of patients the cord will extend to the level of L2. Therefore, the needle should be inserted at the level of the

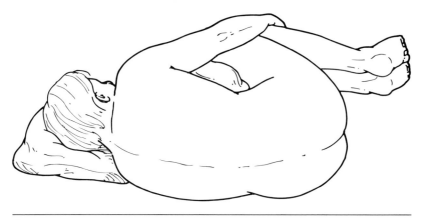

Figure 72.1
Proper positioning in the lateral decubitus position.

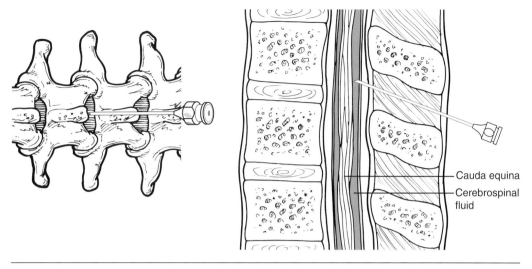

Cauda equina
Cerebrospinal
fluid

Figure 72.2
Insertion site between vertebrae.

L3-4 intervertebral space, although the column can be accessed one level above or below. The cauda equina is the only element of the spinal cord at this point; theoretically, the needle should push apart the fibers and therefore cause no harm. In infants or children, the cord extends further distally and the spinal needle should be inserted at the L4-5 or L5-S1 interspace. The level of L4 is found by palpating the level of the iliac crests bilaterally; midline at this anatomic mark is L4. The spinous processes can then be palpated, with the insertion site being midline between adjacent spinous processes (Fig. 72.2).

Anesthesia

Proper anesthesia is important for patient satisfaction and facilitates a successful LP because a comfortable patient is better able to lie still during the procedure. After the planned insertion site is located, anesthesia with 1% lidocaine without epinephrine is administered. Most kits include a 2-mL vial of lidocaine; however, more may be needed if the examiner is inexperienced or the patient is obese. Additional lidocaine can be withdrawn sterilely with the help of an assistant. At the insertion site, place a wheal of lidocaine subdermally

with the small-bore needle provided in the kit and then proceed deeper into the subcutaneous tissue in the direction the spinal needle will presumably travel. This facilitates a track of anesthesia, which the spinal needle can then follow. In larger patients, use a 22-gauge needle to facilitate anesthetizing deeper tissues. When advancing the needle, withdraw on the syringe to create negative pressure before injection to avoid injecting lidocaine into blood vessels. A eutectic mixture of local anesthetics (EMLA) cream can be applied 60 to 90 minutes before LP in infants to alleviate the pain of the procedure.

Lumbar Puncture Technique

After anesthetizing the patient, have a three-way stopcock ready, vials set up in proper order, and equipment for measuring opening pressure. The spinal needle is inserted midline between the spinous processes and advanced slowly, aiming toward the umbilicus. Usually the standard 20- to 22-gauge, 1.5-inch needle is adequate; however, a longer (2.5-inch) spinal needle may be needed in obese patients. When the dura is entered, a "pop" may be felt and the stylet should be removed. However, the pop is often not felt, and the stylet must be removed periodically to allow the examiner to assess for fluid retreating from the catheter. Always replace the stylet before further manipulation of the spinal needle. If there is no CSF return, the needle can be advanced until the spinal column is accessed or bone is hit, in which case the spinal needle should be removed to just below the skin surface and then redirected. If multiple attempts are unsuccessful, another physician can attempt the LP one interspace higher after anesthetizing to avoid a traumatic false-positive spinal tap.

Pressure and Fluid Collection

After accessing the CSF, place the three-way stopcock on the catheter's end and attach the opening pressure column. Measure the opening pressure by waiting until the column no longer advances upward. Normal pressures range from 80-180mm H_2O. Then, fill each vial with 1 to 2 mL of CSF to be sent for laboratory analysis (Table 72.1). Most standard LP kits have four tubes with numbers from one through four already etched into the tubes. It is crucial to fill the tubes with CSF in the order in which they are numbered. If the tap is traumatic, when the laboratory evaluates red blood cell count you will see a significant drop in the number of red cells counted from tube one to tube four, as the local bleeding has stopped. This is known as the CSF "clearing" from tube one to four. After all four tubes are filled, replace the stylet within the needle, withdraw the needle, and apply pressure to the site. An adhesive bandage, usually included in the kit, is applied.

The patient should lie supine for approximately 1 hour to minimize the postprocedure complication of spinal headache. A spinal headache results from puncture of the dura and CSF leakage. The headache is classically much worse when sitting up and resolves with lying flat; it can be managed with caffeine, nonsteroidal antiinflammatory drugs, or a blood patch. A blood patch is usually performed by an anesthesiologist, in which a few milliliters of the patient's peripheral blood are injected through an epidural needle at the exact same site as the LP. The blood clots around the dura where the CSF is leaking, thus stopping the leak and curing the headache.

LP is an important clinical procedure used often in the ED for diagnosing potentially life-threatening diseases. If performed well, it can be only slightly uncomfortable for the patient and should be approached as such. The procedure may be more difficult to perform in patients who are uncooperative, obtunded, or obese; however, a successful LP can be facilitated with a good patient interaction, proper positioning, accurate identification of landmarks, and the use of adequate anesthesia. In the patient who is nonobtunded but uncooperative, sitting the patient up can facilitate identifying the midline. In the morbidly obese patient, ultrasound can be a useful adjunct to map the vertebrae before antiseptic preparation of the patient.

Table 72.1.

Lumbar puncture studies by tube number

Tube Number	Laboratory Test
1	Cell count and differential
2	Glucose and protein
3	Gram stain and culture or other studies: India ink, viral studies, fungal/cryptococcal antigen studies, acid fast stain for TB, *Borrelia* antibody, counterimmune electrophoresis
4	Cell count and differential; may also send for Gram stain and culture if tube 3 is needed for special studies

TB, tuberculosis.

Suggested Readings

Kanegaye JT, Soliemanzadeh P, Bradley JS. Lumbar puncture in pediatric bacterial meningitis: defining the time interval for recovery of cerebrospinal fluid pathogens after parenteral antibiotic pretreatment. *Pediatrics* 2001;108: 1169–1174.

Kooiker JC. Spinal puncture and cerebrospinal fluid examination. In: Roberts JR, Hedges JR eds. *Clinical procedures in emergency medicine,* 3rd ed. Philadelphia: WB Saunders, 1998.

Levine DN, Rapalino O. The pathophysiology of lumbar puncture headache. *J Neurol Sci* 2001; 192(1-2):1–8.

Sames TA, Storrow AB, Finkelstein JA, Magoon MR. Sensitivity of new-generation computed tomography in subarachnoid hemorrhage. *Acad Emerg Med* 1996;3:16–20.

Silverman R, Kwiatkowski T, Bernstein S, et al. Safety of lumbar puncture in patients with hemophilia. *Ann Emerg Med* 1993;22:1739–1742.

CHAPTER **73**

Arthrocentesis

Lynn C. Dezelon, MD, Katherine Manzon, MD, Sandra Najarian, MD

Chapter Outline

General Principles

Pain is the most common complaint of patients who come to the emergency department with joint problems. These can be either exacerbations of chronic conditions or acute problems. It is important to confirm previous diagnosis in the patient presenting with joint symptoms.

First, it is necessary to differentiate between an articular and periarticular process. Arthrocentesis (aspiration of synovial fluid from a joint) only aids in diagnosis of the former. True articular processes (gout, infection, arthritis, hemarthrosis) manifest as diffuse pain, perhaps with warmth, erythema, and swelling. This is in contrast to the more focal findings of tendonitis, bursitis, or local cellulitis of a periarticular process.

Next, the pattern of joints involved (migratory, monoarticular, or polyarticular) should be considered. For instance, involvement of multiple proximal interphalangeal joints is common with rheumatoid arthritis, whereas isolated first metatarsophalangeal joint (MTP) involvement should provoke suspicion of gout.

Finally, fever, systemic illness, and patterns of injury must also be considered. For instance, fever in a child who is limping or unable to bear weight on a lower extremity should prompt the clinician to rule out a septic joint. A history of nephrolithiasis in a patient with monoarticular arthritis should raise suspicion for gout. Arthralgias, tenosynovitis, or hemorrhagic pustules in a sexually active patient with urethral discharge should alert the clinician to disseminated gonococcal disease. Articular pain and effusion following trauma may represent fracture or ligamentous injury.

Informed Consent

As with any invasive procedure, informed consent must be obtained before performing arthrocentesis. The clinician must explain the risks and benefits of the procedure in a manner that the patient can understand. Benefits include examination of the synovial fluid to rule out fracture, inflammatory process, hemarthrosis, or presence of limb- or life-threatening joint infection. Risks include iatrogenic infection, bleeding, cartilage damage, bruising, or anesthetic reactions. These are small risks, and complications can be minimized if a thorough history is obtained and proper technique is used.

Indications

Diagnostic Tool

Arthrocentesis is a useful tool for diagnosis and treatment of various types of arthritis. Arthrocentesis may confirm the diagnosis of a traumatic bony or ligamentous injury. Aspiration of blood and fat globules in synovial fluid indicates the presence of an intraarticular fracture. Analysis of the synovial fluid also helps differentiate between various nontraumatic joint diseases. For example, a crystal-induced arthritis and a septic arthritis are often indistinguishable clinically. Both diseases may present with a warm, erythematous, painful, swollen joint. Septic arthritis is a medical emergency, and prompt arthrocentesis provides the definitive diagnosis.

Therapeutic Tool

Arthrocentesis may also be therapeutic. It can help relieve pain and pressure from a traumatic hemarthrosis or large effusion. Arthrocentesis can also provide a means for instillation of medications into a joint for relief of pain and inflammation from acute and chronic arthritis. For example, intraarticular injection of corticosteroids may provide pain relief for those with severe rheumatoid arthritis. This should only be considered if joint infection has been ruled out. Intraarticular injection of lidocaine may provide symptomatic relief in patients with a painful, traumatic joint injury. This may also facilitate obtaining a better examination of the affected joint.

Contraindications

Arthrocentesis is contraindicated in the presence of overlying skin or soft tissue infection, such as cellulitis or abscess. Bleeding diatheses, anticoagulation, and the presence of a prosthetic joint are no longer considered absolute contraindications but should be taken into consideration as relative risks. A tense hemarthrosis in patients with hemophilia may be aspirated if appropriate blood products and clotting factors are administered before the procedure. Prosthetic joints may be tapped if the clinician is ruling out an infection. In a prospective study of anticoagulated patients on warfarin, Thumboo and O'Duffy showed that joint aspirations are associated with a low risk of hemorrhage, are diagnostic and are often therapeutic.

Sterile Technique

Adherence to strict sterile procedure when performing arthrocentesis is essential. It is important to palpate bony landmarks and position the patient appropriately before sterile preparation. Most joints are tapped on the extensor surface to avoid major vessels, nerves, and tendons that often lie on the flexor surface.

Once the patient is positioned appropriately and the puncture site has been selected, the skin should be prepped with a povidone-iodine solution, and a large sterile drape should surround the prepped area. The subcutaneous tissue at the selected puncture site should be infiltrated with a local anesthetic agent such as 1% or 2% lidocaine. Next, an appropriately sized needle attached to a syringe should be introduced through the anesthetized skin and subcutaneous tissue and into the joint space. Avoidance of bony surfaces is imperative. Bone contact by the needle causes pain and can damage the articular cartilage.

Complete aspiration of the fluid is the goal. Occasionally, the needle tip orientation must be slightly adjusted if the fluid stops flowing. After the synovial fluid is aspirated, the needle and syringe are removed. After hemostasis is achieved, a sterile dressing may be applied to the puncture site.

Synovial Fluid Collection

Once the synovial fluid is obtained, the fluid should be sent in a sterile container for the appropriate laboratory tests. Common studies include cell count with differential, crystal analysis, Gram stain and culture, and glucose. Other specialized tests may be obtained and should be tailored to the clinical situation. Therapeutic aspiration does not require laboratory evaluation.

Table 73.1.

Synovial fluid interpretation

	Normal	*Aseptic Inflammation*	*Crystal-Induced Inflammation*	*Septic Inflammation*
Gross appearance	Clear, straw-colored	Turbid	Turbid	Turbid, purulent
Cell count (WBC/mm³)	<200 (<25% PMN)	2,000–100,000	2,000–100,000	10,000–>100,000 (>80% PMN)
Glucose	Equal blood glucose	<Blood glucose	<Blood glucose	<<<Blood glucose
Crystals	Negative	Negative	Positive	Negative
Gram stain	Negative	Negative	Negative	Positive

PMN, polymorphonuclear neutrophil leukocytes; WBC, white blood cells.

Interpretation of the synovial fluid is summarized in Table 73.1.

Considerations for Specific Joints

First Metatarsophalangeal Joint

A frequent site of gouty arthritis, the first MTP joint is easily aspirated for synovial fluid. Locate the landmarks of the metatarsal head, the base of the proximal phalanx, and the extensor hallucis longus

tendon. Applying linear traction to the toe, insert a 22-gauge needle between the metatarsal head and base of the proximal phalanx. The needle is inserted perpendicular to the dorsal surface of the toe and medial to the extensor hallucis longus tendon (Fig. 73.1A and B).

Ankle

Although the ankle joint can be entered medially or laterally, the anteromedial approach

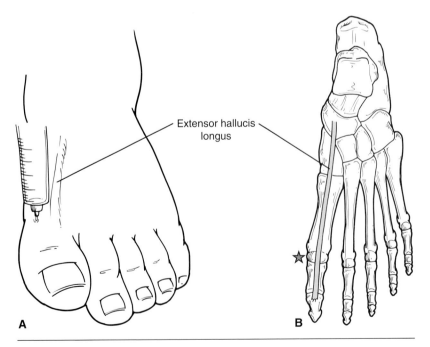

Extensor hallucis longus

A   B

Figure 73.1
A: Arthrocentesis of metatarsophalangeal joint. **B:** Site of injection, metatarsophalangeal joint.

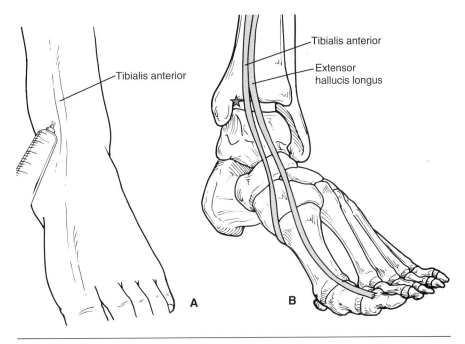

Figure 73.2
A: Arthrocentesis of ankle, medial approach. **B:** Site of injection, ankle.

is preferred. Locate the landmarks of the distal medial malleolus, tibialis anterior tendon, and the extensor hallucis longus tendon. With the ankle plantar flexed, insert a 20-gauge needle medial to the tibialis anterior tendon and extensor hallucis longus tendon to enter the tibiotalar space. Direct the needle slightly cephalad in line with the medial malleolus (Fig. 73.2A and B).

Knee

Several different approaches may be used to aspirate the knee. The parapatellar approach is most commonly used. With this approach, lay the patient supine with the knee fully extended. Introduce the needle medially or laterally at the midpoint or superior one third of the patella, approximately 1 to 2 cm inferior to the patellar edge. Direct the needle at approximately 30 degrees from horizontal, toward the intracondylar femoral notch just posterior to the undersurface of the patella (Fig. 73.3A and B). The infrapatellar approach involves hanging the leg over a table with the knee flexed at 90 degrees. Direct the needle perpendicularly toward

the intercondylar fossa at the midpoint of the patellar tendon. An 18-gauge needle is preferred.

Wrist

Using a 22-gauge needle attached to a syringe, the wrist is entered dorsally. Two sites of entry may be used. The first is the pollicis longus tendon. Lister's tubercle is palpable in the middle of the distal radius. Wrist flexion and longitudinal manual traction or finger traps help to open the joint space. The second entry site is located between the fourth and fifth extensor compartments, using the distal ulna as the bony landmark. Again, manual traction facilitates aspiration (Fig. 73.4A and B).

Elbow

The landmarks for aspirating the elbow include the head of the radius, the lateral epicondyle of the humerus, and the tip of the olecranon. With the elbow flexed 90 degrees and the forearm pronated, these landmarks form a triangle at the lateral surface of

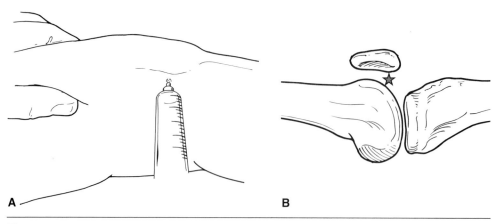

Figure 73.3
A: Arthrocentesis of knee. **B:** Arthrocentesis of knee. Site of injection.

the elbow. Insert a 22-gauge needle in the center of this triangle, perpendicular to the radial head and distal to the lateral epicondyle, directing medially (Fig. 73.5A and B).

Shoulder

The patient should be seated with the shoulder externally rotated. A mark should be made just medial to the humeral head and inferior and lateral to the coracoid process. A 1.5-inch 20- or 22-gauge needle attached to a syringe is then inserted at the mark and directed posteriorly, superiorly, and laterally. If contact with the bone is made, then the needle should be redirected slightly into the joint space. Arthrocentesis of the shoulder is difficult and may require ultrasound or fluoroscopic guidance (Fig. 73.6A and B).

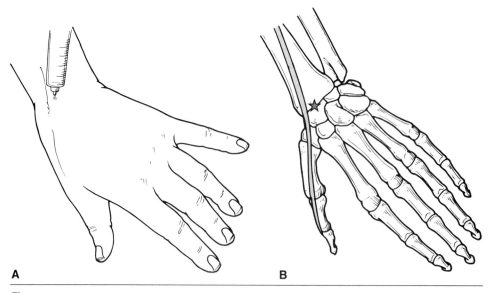

Figure 73.4
A: Arthrocentesis of wrist. **B:** Arthrocentesis of wrist. Site of injection.

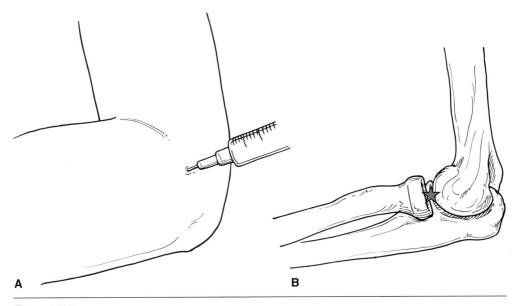

Figure 73.5
A: Arthrocentesis of elbow. **B:** Site of injection, elbow.

Hip

Ultrasound or fluoroscopic guidance is recommended for aspiration of the hip. Two approaches are commonly used, each using a 20-gauge 3.5-inch spinal needle. For the anterior approach, place the patient in the supine position with the lower extremity extended and externally rotated. A mark is made 1 inch lateral to the femoral arterial pulse and 1 inch below the inguinal ligament. At this site, the needle is inserted at a 60-degree angle to the skin and directed posteriorly and medially until contact with bone is made. Then withdraw the needle slightly to aspirate the joint fluid.

The alternative, lateral approach allows the needle to "follow" the femoral neck. Again, position the patient supine with the

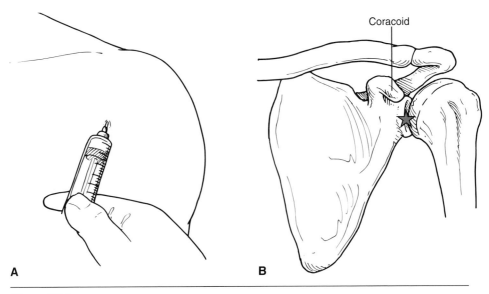

Figure 73.6
A: Arthrocentesis of shoulder. **B:** Site of injection, shoulder.

lower extremities fully extended. The hip is internally rotated with toes touching, facing together. The greater trochanter is palpated, and the needle is inserted anterior and superior to this point. With the needle parallel to the table, it is directed medially and 45 degrees cephalad. This technique is difficult if the patient has large thighs.

Ultrasound is extremely helpful in the detection of fluid and in determining other pathophysiology in the hip such as abscess, osteomyelitis, and tenosynovitis, thereby preventing unnecessary joint aspirations.

Suggested Readings

Benjamin GC. Arthrocentesis. In: Roberts JR, Hedges JR, eds. *Clinical procedures in emergency medicine*, 3rd ed. Philadelphia: WB Saunders, 1998:919–932.

Berman L, Fink AM, Wilson D, et al. Technical note: identifying and aspirating hip effusions. *Br J Radiol* 1995;68: 306–310.

Harcke HT, Grissom LE. Pediatric hip sonography: diagnosis and differential diagnosis. *Radiol Clin North Am* 1999;37:787–796.

Owen DS. Aspiration and injection of joints and soft tissues. In: Ruddy S, Harris ED, Sledge CB, eds. *Kelly's Textbook of Rheumatology*, 6th ed. Philadelphia: WB Saunders, 2001:583–585.

Thumboo J, O'Duffy JD. A prospective study of the safety of joint and soft tissue aspirations and injections in patients taking warfarin sodium. *Arthritis Rheumatol* 1998;41:736–739.

Till SH, Snaith ML. Assessment, investigation, and management of acute monoarthritis. *J Accident Emerg Med* 1999;16:355–361.

Wang SC, Chhem RK, Cardinal EA, et al. Joint sonography. *Radiol Clin North Am* 1999; 37:653.

CHAPTER 74

Dislocations

Mark Bracken, MD, Tri C. Tong, MD

Chaper Outline

Joint dislocations are commonly encountered in the emergency department (ED). The spectrum of injury runs the gamut from a simple jammed finger resulting in an interphalangeal (IP) dislocation to a serious motor vehicle collision (MVC) causing a hip dislocation. It is important to search for associated life- and limb-threatening injuries, particularly in dislocations that result from high-energy transfer such as hip, knee, and sternoclavicular. No matter what the mechanism, however, certain principles apply to all dislocations.

General Principles

The terminology of dislocations is based on the anatomic position of the displaced bone. The distal segment is described in relation to the proximal, normally located structure. Therefore, in an anterior shoulder dislocation, the humeral head lies anterior to the glenoid fossa. The definitive treatment of a dislocated joint is reduction. Most dislocations can be achieved by closed reduction. Open reduction (operative repair) is indicated only if closed reduction attempts fail or if the closed reduction is unstable. A detailed neurovascular examination must be performed before and after attempted reduction.

Radiographs are indicated before and after joint reduction. The series of x-ray films required depends on the particular joint but generally includes an anteroposterior (AP) and a lateral view. There are certain situations in which prereduction x-ray films are not necessary. These include field settings where x-ray examination is unavailable and clinical conditions in which there is vascular compromise or threatened skin penetration.

Reduction should not be attempted until the patient is adequately prepared. The key to a successful joint reduction is good muscle relaxation. This can be achieved by anything from hypnosis to general endotracheal anesthesia in the operating room. Anesthesia in the ED usually consists of a combination of intravenous benzodiazepine and narcotic analgesic, although the anesthetic agents etomidate and propofol are gaining popularity. Numerous reduction techniques are found in the literature and in common practice, and every physician has his or her favorite. In general, the sooner the reduction is attempted, the less the degree of muscle spasm, and the greater the likelihood of success. The ideal technique should be efficacious, easy to perform, require as little analgesia as possible, and have a low complication rate.

After reduction has been attempted, the physician should recheck the patient's neurovascular status. The reduced joint should be splinted, and x-ray films obtained to check for proper positioning and to assess for fractures.

It is beyond the scope of this book to review all types of dislocations. However, we have attempted to include those dislocations seen most commonly and those presenting as true emergencies.

Shoulder Dislocation

The shoulder joint is notable for both its range of motion and its relative instability. The head of the humerus sits in a shallow glenoid fossa, encompassed by a loose joint capsule. Although this arrangement allows for a mobile shoulder, it leaves the glenohumeral ligament as primary barrier to anterior dislocation. Anterior dislocations of the shoulder are far more common than posterior dislocations because of the support of the scapula and the muscular structures that surround it.

Anterior Shoulder Dislocation

Of all the major joint dislocations encountered in the ED, anterior shoulder dislocations are by far the most common. These injuries often result from a combination of abduction, extension, and external rotation of the shoulder. Less often, they are the result of a direct blow to the posterior elements. In individuals with a history of recurrent dislocations, the inciting force may be minor. In this population, simple external rotation while in bed, or raising the arm,

may elicit separation and then dislocation of the joint. The younger the patient is at the time of the first dislocation, the higher the incidence of a recurrent similar injury.

Clinical Features

Visually, an anterior shoulder dislocation presents as an obvious deformity. The shoulder appears less rounded as the humeral head tucks beneath the deltoid muscle and the acromion juts out into a prominent position. Typically, the patient also leans forward to support the injured side and is unable to reach across his or her chest to grasp the opposite shoulder with the affected hand.

Initial evaluation of the shoulder must include a careful neurological and vascular assessment. Injuries to the axillary artery are rare but can be assessed easily by palpating a radial pulse. An axillary nerve injury is the most common neurological complication in anterior dislocations. Testing sensation over the lateral deltoid assesses the axillary nerve. The motor component can be assessed through measurement of deltoid muscle strength. Neurological deficits do not necessarily preclude reduction. However, it is important to document and inform the patient of all such deficits before performing a closed reduction.

Radiology

A typical x-ray series of the shoulder includes AP, scapular Y, and axillary views. The grossly obvious anterior dislocation can be seen on a simple AP view. Posterior dislocations can be much more difficult to diagnose and require additional radiographic angles (Fig. 74.1).

Nearly one fourth of all anterior shoulder dislocations have associated fractures. Fortunately, most of these are fractures of the greater tuberosity, which usually heal well after closed reduction. If the fracture is displaced more than 1 cm, an orthopedic consultation is indicated. Unlike tuberosity fractures, those of the humeral neck may lead to avascular necrosis of the humeral head. Postreduction radiographs serve the dual purposes of clearly establishing a suc-

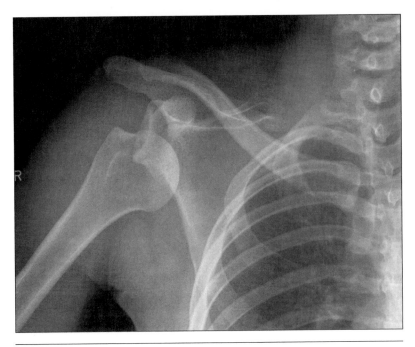

Figure 74.1
The humeral head is sitting below the glenoid fossa, where it usually articulates.

cessful reduction and of detecting fractures not initially evident.

Reduction

Many different reduction techniques have been reported with variable success. Adequate analgesia and sedation are usually required to overcome pain and spasm. Alternatively, or in addition to systemic analgesia, intraarticular injection of 10 to 20 mL of 1% lidocaine may be helpful. (See Chapter 73.)

STIMSON MANEUVER

In the classic technique known as the Stimson maneuver, the patient is placed prone on a stretcher and weights are attached to the wrist on the affected arm. Slow, steady traction exerted by the pull of the weights can often lead to successful reduction in 15 to 20 minutes. The reduction may be facilitated by gentle external rotation of the arm. The advantage of this technique lies in the ability of an operator to perform it without the aid of additional personnel. Disadvantages include the time required for success-

ful reduction, the hazards of placing a patient on the edge of a bed, and the resources required of a busy ED to monitor progress.

SCAPULAR MANIPULATION TECHNIQUE

Often described as simple to perform and with few complications, the scapular manipulation technique focuses on repositioning the glenoid fossa rather than the humeral head. The easiest variation of this technique positions the patient in a prone position on a stretcher with the arm dangling, as in the Stimson maneuver. One operator places traction on the overhanging arm as a second operator rotates the exposed scapula externally, that is, pushing the inferior tip medially toward the spine while stabilizing the superior aspect with the other hand. This technique may be performed with the patient in a sitting position, although this is technically more difficult. Often, the resultant reduction may be so subtle as to go undetected by the operator; therefore, careful palpation of the subclavicular aspect should be used to confirm reduction.

EXTERNAL ROTATION

Another technique that can be performed with one person involves the slow and gentle external rotation of a fully adducted arm (proximal arm to side of chest). In a variation of the maneuver, the patient lies supine, and the elbow is flexed to 90 degrees as the operator holds the elbow in an adducted position against the chest. With his or her other hand, the operator grasps the patient's wrist and slowly rotates the arm externally with the end point of shoulder reduction or when the wrist passes through the coronal plane. No traction is applied to the arm, and at all times, rotation is temporarily halted if the patient indicates pain. Again, reduction with this technique is subtle and may occasionally be noted with internal rotation of the arm.

MILCH TECHNIQUE

The Milch technique is characterized as abduction, external rotation, and longitudinal traction Performed correctly, the maneuver simulates a reach motion for an abject above one's head. The first step is to secure the head of the humerus with the thumb by gripping the affected shoulder. The next step is to fully abduct the arm above the head while keeping the head of the humerus in the same position. The patient may be asked to reach behind and grasp the back of his or her head. Once this is accomplished, the thumb can be used to push the head of the humerus back into its anatomic position. A slightly different version of the Milch technique used first at Hennepin County has been nicknamed the Hennepin technique (Fig. 74.2). Instead of using your hand to move the head of the humerus back into position, traction is placed in a longitudinal direction, while the forearm is gently rotated externally. If reduction does not occur, the humeral head can be gently pushed back manually into the glenoid fossa.

TRACTION-COUNTERTRACTION

Classic and familiar to many practitioners, the traction-countertraction method necessi-

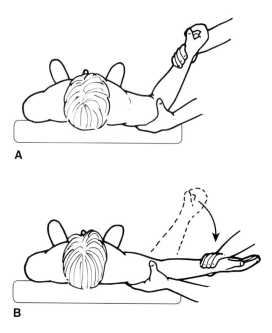

A

B

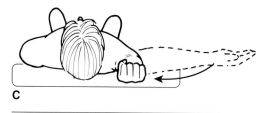

C

Figure 74.2
The Hennipen technique of shoulder reduction.

tates at least two individuals who exert counter force to reduce the dislocation (Fig. 74.3). Many patients will complain of discomfort, because considerable force is often required. With the patient first placed in a supine position, one sheet is wrapped around the upper chest and axilla of the patient and is used to apply countertraction by an assistant. The operator then applies traction to the arm. Although technically the traction can be done manually, this is usually better accomplished by placing a sheet around the patient's forearm and then looping it around the operator's waist. A steady backward force is applied to fatigue the muscles of the shoulder and allow the humerus to reduce. The operator must wait patiently for the reduction. When successful reduction occurs,

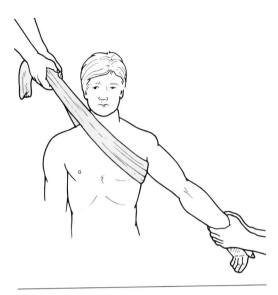

Figure 74.3
Traction-countertraction method of shoulder reduction.

there may be a slight lengthening of the arm or a "plunk" sound as the shoulder relocates. The greatest barrier to success is patient discomfort and muscle spasm, and appropriate sedation is mandatory.

Postreduction

Confirmation of a successful reduction includes relief of pain, resolution of a gross deformity of the shoulder (return of normal rounded appearance), and improved passive motion in the shoulder. Placing the shoulder through a limited range of motion should not be harmful. A fast and reliable method of determining reduction success is to have the patient place the hand on the affected side onto the opposite shoulder.

Shoulder immobilization with a sling and swath minimizes external rotation and abduction. Follow-up in 1 week is prudent, with earlier reevaluation for patients older than 60 years who require more rapid mobilization of the arm. Rotator cuff injuries are seen in more than one third of cases and may complicate healing.

Analgesia is always appropriate following dislocation. In the event that a patient with a successful reduction returns to the ED, the shoulder must be examined for evidence of a hemarthrosis (blood in joint). In this event, aspiration of the blood may be helpful, as are intraarticular injections of lidocaine.

Posterior Shoulder Dislocation

Accounting for less than 5% of all shoulder dislocations, posterior dislocations can often be missed in the clinical setting. Mechanism of injury is almost always indirect and may occur following an event such as a fall or a seizure, in which the shoulder is adducted, internally rotated, and flexed.

Clinical Features

Posterior dislocations may often be misdiagnosed as a contusion or a shoulder strain. The arm is typically positioned in an internally rotated and adducted position. Movement may elicit pain, and inspection of the shoulder may reveal flattening anteriorly with a rounded prominence posteriorly. As in any situation, comparison should be made to the opposite unaffected limb, and a careful neurovascular examination should be performed.

Radiology

Diagnosing a posterior dislocation from a simple AP radiograph can be misleading. Clues to the presence of such an event should be a widened articulation between the humeral head and the glenoid rim, and a symmetric appearance to the humeral head that has been internally rotated ("rifle-barrel" or "light-bulb" appearance). An axillary view is generally diagnostic and can obtained with minimal abduction of the shoulder.

Reduction

Closed reduction generally consists of traction on the internally rotated and adducted arm with simultaneous pressure placed on the humeral head posteriorly. Late reductions should be attempted in a closed manner but often may require an open procedure.

Postreduction

Given the rarity of this dislocation, an early orthopedic consultation might be considered. As with all reductions, careful neurovascular examinations must be performed.

Inferior Shoulder Dislocation

Inferior dislocations are rare but are generally obvious on presentation. The patient will present with an injured arm in abduction and his or her flexed forearm placed behind the head or just lateral to the head. Reduction consists of overhead traction on the forearm in the longitudinal direction with cephalad pressure on the head of the humerus.

Elbow Dislocation and Subluxation

The most common joint dislocation in children, the elbow is second only to the shoulder as the most commonly dislocated joint in the adult. Anatomically, it is a relatively stable joint, with the distal intercondylar groove of the humerus articulating onto the olecranon fossa of the ulna to form a hinge. Significant soft tissue injuries often accompany elbow dislocations because of the force required to dislocate this joint. There are several different types of elbow dislocations, but the most common are categorized as anterior and posterior types.

The vascular structure of greatest concern is the brachial artery. An injury to this artery may not be immediately apparent, but clues such as expanding soft tissue may be present. Admission for observation should always be considered. Injury to the median and ulnar nerves must also be considered. Any deficits before and after reduction must be documented carefully.

Posterior Elbow Dislocation

Posterior dislocations are the most common types of elbow dislocations. Typically, the mechanism is a fall on an outstretched, extended arm. Clinical examination is generally sufficient for diagnosis, because the normal angular relationship between the olecranon and the distal epicondyles of the humerus

is contorted, resulting in a foreshortened arm held in flexion.

Radiology

A single AP and lateral view is generally sufficient to assist in the diagnosis of posterior dislocations. Because studies have indicated that up to 30% of elbow dislocations are associated with fractures, there must always be a careful, systematic review for fractures. In children younger than 14 years, a medial epicondyle dislocation is often present, because the epiphyseal plate of the medial epicondyle often separates before the medial collateral ligament fractures. Figure 74.4 demonstrates a posterior elbow dislocation with associated radial head fracture.

Reduction

Reduction of the elbow tends to be quite uncomfortable, and intravenous sedation is often necessary. Many clinicians also inject 3 to 5 mL of 2% lidocaine to maximize the analgesic effect, and wait 10 to 15 minutes.

TRACTION METHOD

Reduction of the posteriorly dislocated elbow may be achieved through a simple traction method with the patient in a supine position. An assistant should stabilize the humerus, while the operator grasps the affected wrist and applies slow and steady in-line traction. The elbow may be slightly flexed, and if reduction does not occur within a short time, increased flexion may be helpful. Occasionally, downward pressure on the proximal forearm may be helpful as well. Successful reduction is often accompanied by a "clunk" sound.

PRONE TECHNIQUE

There are several alternatives to the classic traction technique. In the prone technique for elbow reduction, the patient can be allowed to sit or lie in the prone position with the affected arm hanging by the bedside (Fig. 74.5 on page 664). The humerus is then stabilized distally by an assistant positioning himself or herself behind the arm. The assis-

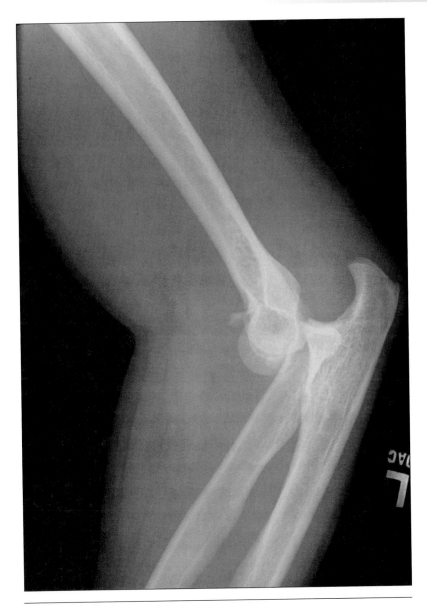

Figure 74.4
Posterior elbow dislocation with associated radial head fracture.

tant should exert pressure on the olecranon with his or her thumbs. The operator then applies longitudinal traction on the forearm with the arm in a slightly flexed position.

Postreduction

Following reduction, the elbow should be placed through gentle range of motion to ensure stability of the joint. Inability to move the elbow through a limited range of motion may indicate a medial epicondyle fracture that would require surgical intervention. Otherwise, if range of motion is possible, the elbow should then be immobilized in 90 degrees flexion.

A complete neurovascular reassessment must be performed. If evidence of delayed vascular compromise is present, typically loosening the splint or lessening the flexion should be attempted first. In-ED or in-hospital observation should be considered if the concern for vascular compromise exists.

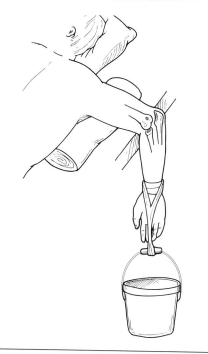

Figure 74.5
The prone technique for elbow reduction.

Anterior Elbow Dislocation

An anterior dislocation of the elbow invariably involves significant force, thus predisposing the elbow to other injuries. The typical dislocating event is a posterior blow to the olecranon with the elbow in flexion. Neurovascular injuries are more likely in anterior dislocations, as are disruptions of muscular insertions.

While an assistant grabs hold of the humerus, the operator provides in-line traction and backward pressure on the proximal forearm. Early consultation with an orthopedic specialist should be considered, given the rarity of this injury and the force required to induce it.

Radial Head Subluxation

A common problem in pediatric presentations, radial head subluxation (also known as "nursemaid's elbow") classically occurs because of longitudinal traction on a pronated wrist. The pathological event is a tear in the annular ligament, which is attached to the radial periosteum. This torn segment then becomes lodged between the head of the radius and the capitellum.

Clinical Features

The child, generally 1 to 3 years of age, may present with a described mechanism typical for this injury. Alternatively, there may be simply a history of a fall or no identifiable trauma in children younger than 6 months. Typically, the injury will not elicit any signs of distress or overt trauma. The patient often will have the injured arm slightly flexed, pronated, and hanging at the side. The patient may refuse to use the affected arm.

Care should be taken to examine the child's clavicle and distal radius for fractures. In the absence of findings concerning for other injuries, reduction may be performed safely without radiographs.

Radiology

The diagnosis of subluxation is typically made based on clinical impression. Because the radial head epiphysis is not calcified, the subluxation will not be radiographically visible. External signs of trauma (bruising, swelling, deformity) or the child's refusal to use the arm normally after the reduction attempt are indications for radiographs.

Reduction

Before any reduction attempt, the operator should explain to the guardian that reduction might cause some transient discomfort to the child. To begin the procedure, the child is placed on the lap of an assistant who stabilizes the humerus. With the arm adducted to the body and the thumb of one hand placed over the radial head, the arm is gently supinated. Generally, the arm is then flexed, with the thumb monitoring for the reduction click. Nearly one third of all children require a repeat maneuver after 10 to 15 minutes if a reduction click is not heard and the child does not use the arm. Painful passive supination may be an indication of failed reduction. Reduction of radial head subluxation is demonstrated in Fig. 74.6.

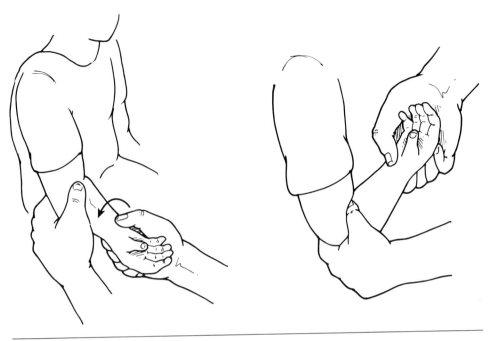

Figure 74.6
Reduction of radial head subluxation (nursemaid's elbow).

Postreduction

If painless function returns, follow-up is generally not necessary. Documentation of the child's normal unrestricted use of the arm must be made, because a few other conditions (e.g., occult fracture, osteomyelitis, joint infection, and tumors) can mimic this condition.

If after a few attempts the child has not regained use of the arm, radiographs can be performed. More than half have spontaneous recovery of function, whereas the remainder have recovery after additional manipulation. A 24-hour follow-up should be arranged. Immobilization with a posterior splint in the patient with residual discomfort or with a history of repeated subluxations is advisable; its benefit is equivocal in the painless but not fully functional elbow.

Hand Dislocation

Because of the vital role the hand plays in daily living, it is frequently injured. It is imperative that major disability be avoided through proper diagnosis and care. There are numerous types of hand dislocations involving the carpals, metacarpals, and phalangeals. Some of the more common types are presented here.

The digital joints are supported by fibrous volar plates, to which two lateral ligaments are affixed. The joints themselves are hinged with tongue-and-groove articulations. Traumatic disruption of the volar plate occurs in posterior dislocations, whereas lateral joint dislocations result in damage to the collateral ligament. Generally, x-ray films of suspected injuries must include at least two views of the injured site, with particular attention given to lateral views to assess for presence of fractures or intraarticular fragments. Anesthesia can be achieved with regional blocks.

Thumb Dislocation

Because of its exposed position, the thumb is vulnerable to numerous injuries.

Interphalangeal Joint Dislocation

In general, dislocations of the IP joint of the thumb are open. This occurs because tremendous force is required to disrupt the strong ligamentous support unique to the thumb (generally dorsal dislocations). Reduction involves recreating the mechanism of dislocation by distracting the finger in a longitudinal fashion and hyperextending the joint, followed by pressure at the base of the distal joint. Postreduction care involves splinting the joint for 3 weeks and orthopedic follow-up. All open dislocations require orthopedic consultation.

Metacarpophalangeal Joint Injuries

DORSAL DISLOCATION

There are two types of dorsal dislocation injuries, both of which are caused by hyperextension. The first, in which the proximal phalanx lies dorsal to the first metacarpal, may be amenable to closed reduction accomplished by hyperextension of the thumb with flexion at the wrist and direct pressure on the base of the proximal phalanx. In the second, more complex type, the volar plate may become entrapped within the metacarpophalangeal (MCP) joint, preventing reduction. In this case, surgical intervention will be required. One clue about the presence of a complex fracture is the reduced angulation of the proximal phalanx. Simple MCP injuries require immobilization for 3 weeks and orthopedic follow-up.

ULNAR COLLATERAL LIGAMENT RUPTURE

Rupture of the ulnar collateral ligament often presents with the MCP joint reduced but with local pain in the area. This "game-keeper's thumb" often results from direct force laterally on the MCP joint, such as occurs in MVCs in which the thumb is solely draped over the steering wheel. Stress testing is best performed with the MCP joint in full flexion (to minimize the stabilizing effects of the volar plate) and assessing instability with lateral movement. X-ray films may show avulsion fractures. Although complete ruptures require surgical repair, partial injuries require casting for up to 3 weeks and orthopedic follow-up.

Finger Dislocation

The anatomic structures of the fingers are similar to those of the thumb, and the basic principles of evaluation and treatment are similar. However, MCP dislocations are less common because there is typically more lateral support in the finger MCP joint than in the thumb.

Proximal Interphalangeal Dislocation

When examining a proximal interphalangeal (PIP) injury, one must assess for degree of hyperextension (an indication of a volar plate injury), inability to actively extend (extensor tendon central slip rupture), and laxity of lateral movement with passive stress (potential collateral ligament injury). These features must also be examined in the postreduction joint to assess for stability.

DORSAL PROXIMAL INTERPHALANGEAL DISLOCATION

One of the most common joint dislocations seen in the ED, dorsal PIP dislocation usually presents after an axial load blow to the finger end. The middle phalanx repositions dorsally to the proximal phalanx and the volar plate is always disrupted. If there is an associated fracture that is more than 33% of the joint surface, operative repair may be necessary for stability. Reduction in the absence of a major fracture involves analgesia with a finger block followed by an exaggeration of the injury through hyperextension and distraction. Reduction occurs with downward pressure at the base of the middle phalanx. The affected digit should be splinted in 20 to 30 degrees of flexion and the patient should follow up with orthopedics in 3 weeks. Figure 74.7 demonstrates PIP joint dislocation of the fifth finger. Figure 74.8 demonstrates reduction of a dorsal PIP dislocation.

LATERAL PROXIMAL INTERPHALANGEAL DISLOCATION

Typically obvious on presentation or already reduced, lateral PIP dislocations are fairly common and involve collateral ligament injury. Reduction of the still dislocated joint involves recreating the injury with longitudinal traction. Buddy-tape with an unaffected

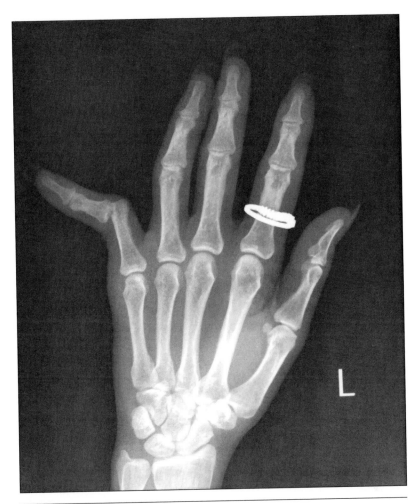

Figure 74.7
Proximal interphalangeal (PIP) joint dislocation of the fifth finger.

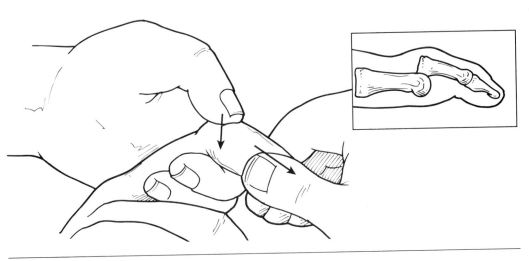

Figure 74.8
Dorsal proximal interphalangeal (PIP) joint reduction.

finger and follow-up examination in 3 weeks is generally recommended.

Distal Interphalangeal Dislocation

Dislocations of the distal phalanx are typically open because of their close attachment to skin. As with other dislocation injuries of the finger, the typical mechanism is a blow to the fingertip causing a dorsal dislocation. Lateral radiographs often are needed for diagnosis of dislocations of the distal interphalangeal (DIP) joint because some movement may still be preserved even in the unreduced position. Reduction is similar to other finger joints and involves recreation of the dislocating event and longitudinal distraction.

Metacarpophalangeal Dislocation

MCP dislocations of the finger are treated and managed like those of the thumb. It is important to recognize that reduction may convert a simple MCP dislocation into a complex one. As such, the initial motion of reduction should be hyperextension, rather than traction. Buddy taping following reduction should be sufficient to stabilize the joint.

Hip Dislocation

Hip dislocations, once an uncommon injury resulting from significant force, have become much more commonplace with the advent of the prosthetic joint. The anatomy of the hip lends itself to stability. The femur sits deep in the acetabulum where it is anchored by strong ligamentous support. However, when that support is disrupted, as with hip replacement surgery, dislocations can result from a relatively minor mechanism of injury. The annual incidence of prosthetic hip dislocations is approximately 11.5%. Figure 74.9 demonstrates dislocation of a prosthetic hip.

The mechanism of injury for native hip dislocations usually involves MVCs, motorcycle accidents, falls, and rarely, sports injuries. Because these dislocations are associated with a high-impact mechanism, it is important to examine the patient for other limb- and life-threatening injuries. In fact, there are associated fractures in up to 88% of hip dislocations.

There are two types of hip dislocation: anterior and posterior. Different classifica-

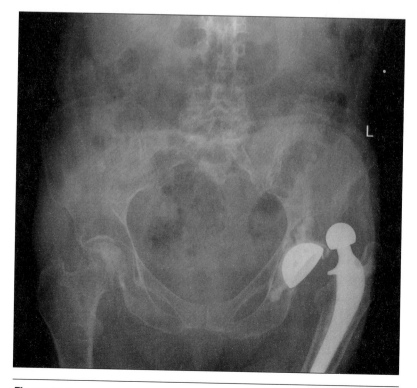

Figure 74.9
Dislocation of prosthetic hip.

tion systems exist. Thompson and Epstein developed the following criteria for both anterior and posterior injuries:

I: Dislocation with no associated fracture

II: Irreducible dislocation

III: Unstable hip after reduction, or incarcerated fragments of cartilage, labrum, or bone

IV: Dislocation associated with acetabular fracture requiring reconstruction

Posterior Hip Dislocation

The vast majority (90% to 95%) of hip dislocations are posterior. The mechanism of injury involves a force on the flexed knee with the hip in some degree of flexion at the time of impact. This has been called the "dashboard dislocation" because it occurs most commonly when the patient's knee strikes a car dashboard during an MVC. The greater the degree of hip flexion at the time of impact, the more likely a simple dislocation (without associated acetabular fracture) will result.

Clinical Features

The affected leg will be shortened, internally rotated, and adducted. On examination, particular attention should be paid to the sciatic nerve, because compression and traction injuries occur in 10% to 14% of cases. Both motor and sensory components of the sciatic nerve can be assessed grossly by knee flexion and light touch over the posterolateral leg and foot. The knee should also be examined carefully, because the incidence of knee injury in hip dislocation is about 25%.

Radiology

AP and lateral views are necessary. However, the diagnosis is often obvious on an AP view of the pelvis alone. On the AP view, the posteriorly dislocated femoral head looks smaller, and the anteriorly located one looks larger than the unaffected side. This disparity is due to the relative distance between the x-ray cassette and the femoral head. Figure 74.10 illustrates a posterior dislocation of the left hip.

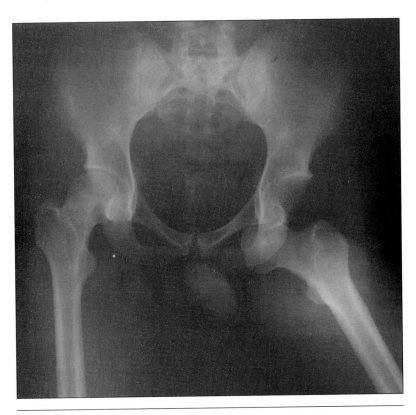

Figure 74.10
Posterior dislocation of left hip.

Reduction

The key to a successful reduction is adequate analgesia. Proper anesthesia is especially important in hip reduction because of the force that is often required to relocate this large joint. Hip dislocations usually require either conscious sedation or general anesthesia to achieve a successful reduction. There are numerous reduction techniques. Many older techniques have been modified over the years.

BIGELOW AND ALLIS TECHNIQUES

Bigelow described the first hip reduction strategy in 1870. The patient lies supine while a distraction force is applied to the hip and a counterforce to the pelvis. The hip is then flexed to 90 degrees or more on the patient's abdomen, externally rotated, abducted, and then extended. Allis, in 1893, described a similar technique that has endured until today. In the Allis technique, the patient is supine (Fig. 74.11). An assistant provides downward stabilization of the pelvis while the operator exerts upward traction in-line with the deformity. The hip is then internally and externally rotated until successfully reduced.

STIMSON TECHNIQUE

Unlike Allis and Bigelow, in 1889, Stimson described a reduction technique in which the patient is placed in the prone position. The patient's distal pelvis hangs over the edge of the stretcher and the hip, knee, and ankle are all flexed to 90 degrees. Downward pressure is applied to the proximal posterior tibia, followed by internal and external rotation of the hip. The femoral head can be pushed into place directly by an assistant. Figure 74.12 illustrates the Stimson reduction technique.

Over the years, several modifications to these three original techniques have been described in the literature. In 1992, Howard added lateral traction to the Allis technique and reported success in five traumatic and three prosthetic hip dislocations. In a paper in 1992, Bassi et al. described the addition of direct pressure on the femoral head to the Allis technique. They reported 26 successful reductions with this technique. Also in 1992,

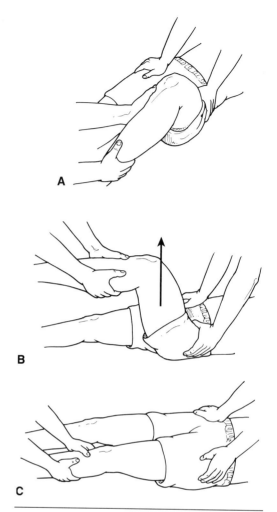

Figure 74.11
Allis hip reduction technique.

Herwig-Kempers et al. described a modified Stimson technique in which the operator grasps the patient's ankle and places his or her knee in the patient's calf, using his or her own body weight to exert downward pressure. Regardless of the strategy chosen, traumatic dislocations of a native hip requires a greater amount of prereduction analgesia and a more forceful approach than the prosthetic dislocations.

Anterior Hip Dislocation

The anterior hip dislocation is a far less common injury, occurring in only 5% to 10% of hip dislocations. Although the Thompson-Epstein classification system applies here, these are also described anatomically.

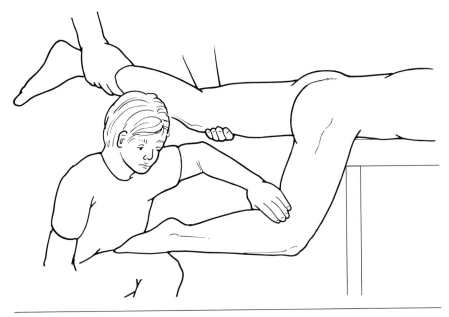

Figure 74.12
Stimson hip reduction technique.

I: Obturator

II: Iliac

III: Pubic

The obturator type is the most common of these injuries. The type name identifies the position of the head of the femur in the anteriorly dislocated hip. In the obturator type, for instance, the femoral head sits anterior to the obturator foramen, and so forth.

Clinical Features

The mechanism of anterior dislocation involves a forced abduction of the hip caused by a fall or MVC. The presentation depends on the type of dislocation. In the obturator type, the patient's affected leg is abducted and externally rotated. In the iliac and pubic types, the affected leg is extended and externally rotated. Anterior dislocations tend to have a much higher incidence of vascular injuries than posterior injuries because of the anterior location of the femoral neurovascular bundle.

Reduction

The techniques used are modifications of the Allis and Stimson methods. In the modified Allis, the patient is supine. An as-

sistant applies lateral countertraction to the thigh while the operator provides traction in the long axis of the femur. The leg is then adducted and internally rotated to effect reduction.

Indications for open reduction include (a) unsuccessful closed reduction, (b) unstable reduction, and (c) fracture fragments entrapped in the joint postreduction.

Postreduction

The affected leg must be immobilized with a pillow or Charnley wedge between the patient's knees. Light skin traction, otherwise known as Buck's traction, can also be used (Fig. 74.13). Buck's traction is an apparatus used to apply longitudinal traction on the leg with weights on a pulley system, secured to the leg with tape or other adhesive.

Patients with hip dislocations require hospital admission and commonly have protracted recovery times. Patients should be non-weightbearing from 3 to 6 months.

Complications

The most significant and debilitating complication of hip dislocation is avascular necrosis (AVN). The incidence of AVN after

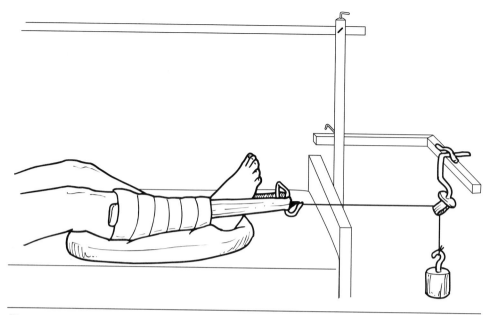

Figure 74.13
Buck's skin traction.

hip dislocation typically ranges from 6% to 40%. AVN ensued in the aftermath of the hip dislocation of Bo Jackson, one of the more notable athletes of our time. Most authors advocate early hip reduction to decrease the incidence of this devastating complication. It has been found that delayed reduction, greater than 12 hours after the injury, has been associated with a threefold increase in the incidence of AVN. Osteoarthritis is another common complication. The incidence of osteoarthritis of the hip is thought to be at least 20% for patients with a history of hip dislocation.

Knee Dislocation

Femoral-Tibial Dislocation

Knee dislocations are true orthopedic emergencies. Although the knee is a hinge joint, it is well protected by strong ligamentous support. The major ligaments that bolster the knee are the anterior cruciate ligament (ACL), the posterior cruciate ligament (PCL), the lateral collateral ligament (LCL), and medial collateral ligament (MCL).

Because most knee dislocations have spontaneously reduced by the time the pa-

tient presents to the ED, one must have a high index of suspicion based on history and physical examination. Neurovascular injuries are common, with the incidence of popliteal artery injury ranging from 20% to 40%.

Classification
Femoral-tibial knee dislocations can be classified as anterior, posterior, medial, lateral, and rotary. Anterior and posterior types constitute almost all knee dislocations. Anterior dislocations are slightly more common than posterior ones.

Knee dislocations are quite rare. When they do occur, however, they usually result from a significant force. The common etiologies are MVCs, vehicle-pedestrian accidents, motorcycle accidents, and sporting injuries. Knee dislocation has also been described as resulting from a relatively minor force, such as stepping off a curb or into a hole.

ANTERIOR-HYPEREXTENSION INJURY

Anterior-hyperextension injury may occur when a patient is tackled or steps into a hole while briskly walking. The result is a tear of the posterior capsule and the PCL, with rupture of the ACL. There is a high incidence of associated vascular injuries. The popliteal artery is commonly contused or intimal injury occurs to the artery as it is stretched anteriorly.

POSTERIOR INJURY

Posterior injury occurs when there is a posteriorly directed force on the tibia of a flexed knee. This is commonly seen when the patient's flexed knee strikes the dashboard in a car crash. The resulting injury involves a rupture of the posterior capsule and complete ACL and PCL tears. The popliteal artery is frequently fractured or transected by the posterior displacement of the tibia.

LATERAL, MEDIAL, AND ROTARY INJURY

Lateral, medial, and rotary injuries are rare. They involve a combination of ACL, PCL, and collateral ligament tears. These dislocations are commonly associated with peroneal nerve injuries.

Clinical Features

If the knee is already reduced on presentation to the ED, it is incumbent on the physician to rule out a dislocation. Often, this is challenging. There may be no obvious deformity. Swelling may be absent because a tear in the joint capsule allows the synovial fluid and blood to dissipate into the adjacent soft tissue. Studies have shown that a severely unstable knee is associated with a similar incidence of popliteal artery injuries. A severely unstable knee is defined as recurvatum (hyperextension) greater than 30 degrees and medial joint opening with stress on a knee in full extension.

A good physical examination includes inspection, palpation, and neurological and vascular assessments. The vascular examination is extremely important in a patient with a knee dislocation. The distal pulses (dorsalis pedis and posterior tibialis) must be assessed and compared with the unaffected side. Doppler ultrasound is often required to make an accurate analysis. Ankle-brachial indices (ABI) should also be done on these patients. The ABI compares ankle systolic blood pressure with that of brachial in a ratio of ankle over brachial. The systolic blood pressure is higher in the lower extremities than the upper. Therefore, a normal ABI is greater than 1.0. Any value below 0.95 is considered abnormal and suggests damage to the popliteal artery and/or its branches. The popliteal artery is commonly injured because it sits posterior to the knee joint fixed proximally and distally in a fibrous tunnel. Popliteal artery injury is associated with a high amputation rate because of poor collateral circulation around the knee.

Neurological examination is also important. The peroneal nerve crosses the lateral aspect of the knee and is particularly vulnerable in rotatory, lateral, and medial type dislocations. This injury has an incidence of 14% to 35%. On examination, these patients have hypoesthesia of the first web space and/or a loss of dorsiflexion.

Radiology

Prereduction and postreduction standard AP and lateral films looking for associated fractures are indicated in knee dislocation.

Many advocate arteriography for all knee dislocations with abnormal ABIs or suspected arterial injury. The difference between early and late treatment of popliteal artery injuries is often the difference between functionality and amputation. Operative exploration should not be delayed for arteriography if ischemia is present. One study compared injured patients who had surgery within 8 hours with those who either had no surgery or had surgery after 8 hours. The results demonstrated a 15% amputation rate in the early surgery group compared with an 80% amputation rate in the delayed group. The results of this study and others like it suggest that all patients with knee dislocation should undergo arteriography unless ischemia is clinically present, in which case the patient should go promptly to the operating room.

Reduction

Expeditious reduction is particularly important in the knee where joint relocation may reestablish distal blood flow. The techniques

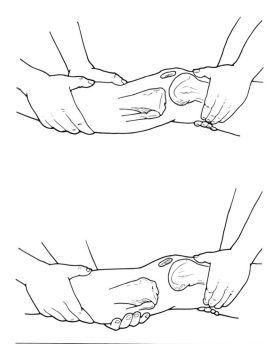

Figure 74.14
Reduction of a posterior knee dislocation.

for anterior and posterior dislocations are similar. In the anterior type, the assistant provides longitudinal traction while the operator lifts the femur anteriorly. Attention should focus on avoiding pressure on the popliteal space. In the posterior type, an assistant again provides longitudinal traction while the operator lifts the tibia anteriorly (Fig. 74.14).

Postreduction

The vascular examination should be rechecked, and postreduction radiographs should be done. The knee should be immobilized in 15 degrees of flexion in a Bledsoe brace or plaster. These patients need to be admitted for serial neurovascular assessments. In the long term, the ligamentous damage incurred will require surgical repair.

Patellar Dislocation

Dislocation of the patella is a far more common and less debilitating injury than dislocation of the knee. Patellar dislocation is pri-

marily an injury of young adolescents. There are certain body types that are predisposed to dislocation. Patients with genu valgum or femoral anteversion have a much higher incidence of dislocation. These conditions lead to excessive lateral stress on the knee.

The anatomy of the patella is important to review in describing the mechanism of injury. The patella is anchored into place by the vastus medialis muscle, medial retinaculum, and medial and lateral patellofemoral and patellotibial ligaments. The vastus lateralis is usually a bulkier and stronger muscle than its medial counterpart. The mechanism of injury often involves a powerful quadriceps contraction combined with some valgus stress and external rotation. As the quadriceps contracts as a single unit, a disproportionate amount of force is applied laterally. This commonly occurs while "cutting" while playing a sport or dancing. Rarely, it can result from a direct blow to a flexed knee.

Clinical Features

The diagnosis is usually obvious. The patient's knee is held in flexion and the patella is seen or palpated laterally. Often, as with the knee dislocation, the patella has already been reduced on presentation to the ED. Some clues can aid in the diagnosis. There is a history that the knee "went out." There is usually a joint effusion and tenderness along the medial border of the patella. A useful diagnostic test is the Fairbanks test or patellar apprehension sign. When the patient's patella is pushed laterally, the patient will grab his or her knee as he or she feels the sensation of a repeat injury.

Radiology

Adequate x-ray films are often difficult to obtain because the patient's knee is in flexion. Consequently, if the diagnosis is clinically apparent, prereduction radiographs are unnecessary. One caveat is that this injury is primarily one of the young, and any diagnosis made in an older patient should be done with caution. Postreduction films are useful to document proper reduction and to check for associated fractures, which may be pre-

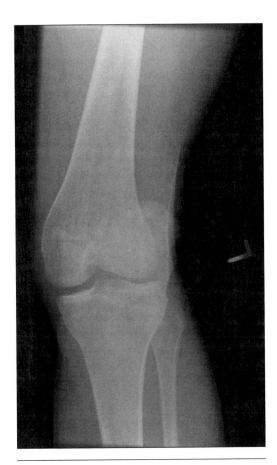

Figure 74.15
Lateral patellar dislocation.

sent in 5% of cases. Figure 74.15 demonstrates a patellar dislocation.

Reduction

The technique for reduction is quite simple. Premedication is often not even required. The steps are as follows: (a) extension of the knee and (b) gentle medial pressure to the patella (lifting the lateral edge over the femoral condyle).

Postreduction

The knee should be immobilized in full extension. Because these injuries are associated with a high rate of persistent instability and recurrent dislocation, prompt orthopedic follow-up is recommended. Routine patellar dislocations do not require hospital admission.

Ankle Dislocation

The ankle is a modified hinge joint with strong ligamentous support. Pure dislocations are very rare. When they do occur, they involve the disruption of some combination of the following ligaments: deltoid, anterior tibiotalar, anterior and posterior talofibular ligaments. Associated fractures are common. Arterial injury can occur, particularly in anterior dislocations.

The relation of the talus to the tibia describes ankle dislocations. Lateral dislocations are the most common, followed by posterior, anterior, and superior types. Figure 74.16 shows a posterior ankle dislocation.

In the reduction of posterior dislocations the patient is supine and knee flexed to relax the Achilles tendon. The operator grasps the affected foot with both hands, one on the heel and the other on the forefoot. The foot is flexed slightly plantar

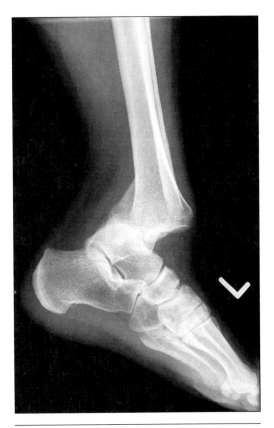

Figure 74.16
Posterior ankle dislocation.

while longitudinal traction is applied to the foot. The assistant applies downward pressure to the tibia as the operator moves the heel anteriorly to effect reduction. Reduction of a lateral dislocation uses the same positioning with the foot distracted and directed medially. Figure 74.17 demonstrates the reduction technique for a lateral ankle dislocation: traction is applied with the foot in a plantar flexed position.

The same positioning is used for reduction of anterior dislocations as with the posterior technique. Dorsiflexion rather than plantarflexion is used in this case to free the talus. The assistant applies upward pressure to the tibia while the operator moves the foot posteriorly.

Foot Dislocations

These are divided into hindfoot and forefoot injuries. Hindfoot injuries include subtalar and talar dislocations, whereas forefoot injuries include metatarsophalangeal (MTP) and IP dislocations.

Subtalar Dislocation

Subtalar dislocation is a very uncommon injury associated most frequently with high-energy mechanisms including MVC, significant falls, and sports. The injury results from severe foot inversion or ever-sion, causing medial or lateral dislocation, respectively. Medial dislocation occurs 85% of the time. Clinically, the calcaneus, navicular, and forefoot are all displaced from the talus. The talus is usually prominent, often tenting the skin.

After initial radiographs and analgesia, reduction is attempted by placing the patient supine with the knee flexed to relax the Achilles tendon. The operator places one hand on the forefoot and the other on the patient's heel. The deformity is increased as the operator applies longitudinal traction. For a medial dislocation, the foot is inverted initially and then everted to affect reduction. The opposite is done for a lateral dislocation.

Metatarsophalangeal and Interphalangeal Dislocation

MTP dislocations are usually caused by hyperextension, resulting in dorsal displacement of the proximal phalanx in relation to the metatarsal bone at the MTP joint. IP dislocations occur by axial load, such as kicking a hard object. Reduction is achieved by increasing the deformity through hyperextension, applying traction on the phalanx, and pushing down on the base of the dislocated proximal phalanx. Postreduction treatment includes buddy taping the affected toe to its neighbor for 2 to 3 weeks and placing the patient in a hard-soled shoe for comfort.

Suggested Readings

Bassi JL, Ahuja SC, Singh H, et al. A flexion adduction method for the reduction of posterior dislocation of the hip. *J Bone Joint Surg* 1992;74B:157–158.

Bucholz RW, Heckman JD. *Rockwood & Green's fractures in adults*, 4th ed. Philadelphia: Lippincott-Raven, 1996:1756–1803, 2110–2114, 2299–2302, 2318–2320, 2337–2338.

Harris H, Harris W. *The radiology of emergency medicine*, 4th ed. Philadelphia: Lippincott, Williams & Wilkins, 2000.

Herwig-Kempers AH, Veraart BE. Reduction of posterior dislocation of the hip in the prone position. *J Bone Joint Surg* 1992;75B:328.

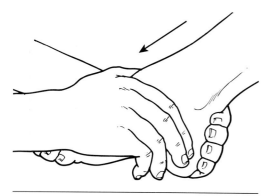

Figure 74.17
Reduction technique of a lateral ankle dislocation: traction is applied with the foot in a plantar flexed position.

Howard CB. A gentle method of reducing traumatic dislocation of the hip. *Injury* 1992;23: 481–482.

Kendall RW, Taylor DC, Salvian AJ, et al. The role of arteriography in assessing vascular injuries associated with dislocations of the knee. *J Trauma* 1993;35:875– 878.

Nordt WE. Maneuvers for reducing dislocated hips. *Clin Orthoped Related Res* 1999;360: 260–264.

Roberts JR. *Clinical procedures in emergency medicine*, 3rd ed. Philadelphia: WB Saunders, 1998: 818–852.

Rosen P. *Emergency medicine: concepts and clinical practice*, 4th ed. St. Louis: Mosby-Year Book, 1998:55–761, 786–810, 821–835, 800–801, 842–843, 851–852.

Simon R, Koenigsknecht S. *Emergency orthopedics*, 3rd ed. Norwalk: Appleton & Lange, 1996:326–329, 336–340, 486–489, 430–436, 463–469.

Extremity Splinting

William E. Baker, MD

Indications

Splints are often used in emergency medicine to immobilize an injured extremity. Symptoms of extremity injury following trauma include pain with or without deformity. Signs of injury may include deformity, swelling, bruising, crepitation, instability, or limitation of range of motion. Splinting reduces pain and may limit or prevent further bleeding and vascular or neurological damage associated with movement at the site of injury. Splinting may also prevent a closed injury from converting into an open injury. This chapter focuses on extremity splinting within the emergency department.

General Principles

All fractures that are appropriately treated by casting may be adequately immobilized by splinting in the emergency department. This is the standard of care provided by most emergency medicine clinicians and is usually the more desirable initial approach compared with casting. A cast applied on an acutely swollen extremity may fit poorly several days later when swelling subsides. Further swelling often occurs in the subsequent hours after an acute injury, and a circumferential cast applied under these circumstances may contribute to the development of a compartment syndrome.

Materials

Plaster of Paris

Plaster of Paris (gypsum) has been used by generations of clinicians for splinting and casting. It has the advantage of being inexpensive and molds well. Orthopedic plaster is supplied in the form of flexible, thin, plaster-impregnated gauze-like material in rolls or slabs of various widths. Water is added to the plaster, causing it to crystallize and become rigid (set). You have several minutes in which to apply the flexible wet plaster before it sets. Cool water, clean water, table salt, and a clean container retard plaster setting and lengthen working time. Warm water, water previously used for plastering, and a dirty mixing container accelerate plaster setting. Consider these factors when splinting. A slower setting plaster may be more desirable for a splint in which further fracture manipulation may take place. A faster setting mix

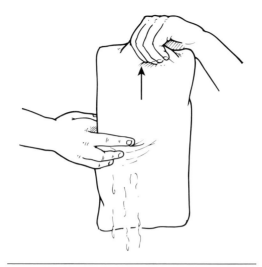

Figure 75.1
Wet plaster thoroughly and laminate between two fingers to eliminate all excess water.

may be more desirable for a splint requiring no manipulation. Always thoroughly soak the plaster and laminate by rubbing the layers together between your fingers (Fig. 75.1) for good strength, being careful not to rub too much of the plaster off into the bucket.

Fiberglass

Fiberglass is another splinting material that is supplied in thin flexible rolls impregnated with polyurethane resin that hardens when exposed to moisture. Although it is more expensive and harder to mold than plaster, it sets more quickly (in 3 to 4 minutes) and is lighter and stronger than plaster. Fiberglass is not weakened by water and is more radiolucent. Newer, non-fiberglass polyurethane resin-impregnated materials that mold more like plaster have been marketed recently.

The skin must be protected from direct contact with plaster or fiberglass with wadding, either alone or in combination with stockinette. Wadding is composed of either synthetic (polyester) or natural (cotton) materials in the form of rolls and is available in various widths. Stockinette is constructed of a thin layer of knit polyester or cotton tubes and comes on a large roll in various widths. Wadding is especially useful in protecting

bony prominences and may be rolled back over the ends of the splint to provide a soft durable edge. Although some clinicians apply stockinette against the skin and cover it with wadding before applying fiberglass or plaster, many simply use padding.

Elastic wrap is most commonly used as a final external layer to complete the splint. Commonly available elastic wrap contains latex and must be avoided in patients allergic to latex. Latex-free elastic wraps (e.g., Cohesive) are available. Some clinicians prefer to use nonelastic wrap, such as roll gauze, to minimize the risk of creating a compartment syndrome. Each layer of elastic wrap adds to this risk, and it is easy to apply elastic wrap too tightly.

Splint Construction and Application

Splints may be constructed from 8 to 10 layers of suitably wide plaster or fiberglass (forming a slab) placed over wadding and covered with gauze (or wadding) and finally elastic wrap. The wadding over the wet plaster prevents the elastic wrap from sticking to the plaster, thus enabling one to remove and reapply the elastic wrap if needed to adjust the splint. Do not wrap the elastic wrap too tightly. Fiberglass and plaster are also supplied as prefabricated splinting material in various widths with padding on both sides. Examples of specific brands of fiberglass splints include Ortho-Glass and 3M Scotch-cast splints.

Upper Extremity Splints

Volar Splint and Volar-Dorsal Splint

The volar short arm splint (Fig. 75.2) is used to immobilize wrist sprains, hand injuries, and some carpal fractures (i.e. triquetrum fractures). The splint controls wrist flexion-extension but does not effectively control pronation-supination. Construct the splint from 3- to 4-inch plaster and measure from just proximal to the volar aspect of the metacarpophalangeal (MCP) joints

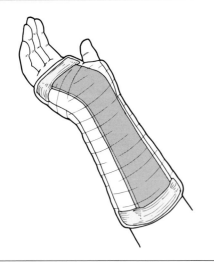

Figure 75.2
Volar splints should immobilize the wrist in
15 degrees of extension and neutral with respect
to ulnar or radial deviation.

and extending to the proximal volar surface
of the forearm. The splint should not impede motion of the thumb, MCP, or elbow
joints. The MCP joints lie along a line drawn
from the radial edge of the distal palmar
crease to the ulnar edge of the proximal palmar crease (Fig. 75.3).

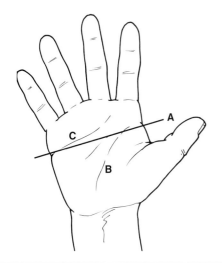

Figure 75.3
The surface landmarks for the metacarpophalangeal joints are approximated by a line (**A**)
drawn from the radial border of the proximal palmar crease (**B**) to the ulnar border of the distal
palmar crease (**C**).

Occasionally (for soft tissue injuries),
the fingers may be immobilized by extending the splint distally and placing padding
between the fingers to avoid maceration.
The wrist should be held in 15 degrees of
extension and the forearm positioned with
the thumb pointing upward.

A second slab may be placed dorsally in
conjunction with the volar slab starting at the
level of the MCP joints and extending to the
proximal forearm. This splint functionally re-
sembles a cast, which is bivalved (or cut with
a saw on two sides). The volar-dorsal short
arm splint controls pronation-supination to a
certain extent, which is important in some injuries such as distal radius fractures.

Sugar-Tong Forearm Splint

The sugar-tong splint (Fig. 75.4) is used to
immobilize fractures of the distal radius and

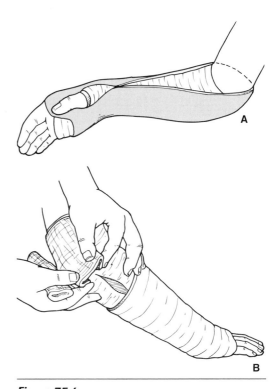

Figure 75.4
A: The sugar-tong forearm splint should hold the
wrist in neutral position or slight extension (for
nondisplaced fractures) with the thumb pointing
upward. **B**: Excess splint material is folded and
tucked as the splint circles the elbow.

ulna (e.g., Colles' fractures) and provides excellent control of wrist flexion-extension and pronation-supination. Construct the splint from a 3- to 5-inch slab, measuring from the MCP joints dorsally, over the flexed elbow, and extending to MCP joints on the volar surface (see volar splint section for landmarks). The wrist may be placed in neutral position or in slight extension with the thumb pointing upward. Common mistakes in constructing this splint are to measure the plaster too short, thus not effectively immobilizing the wrist or extending the volar slab too far, impeding MCP joint motion. A sling must be used with this splint, because the splint partially immobilizes the elbow.

Short Arm Gutter Splints

Gutter splints (Fig. 75.5) are often used to treat metacarpal and some phalangeal fractures. Construct the splint from a slab either over the radial or ulnar aspect of the forearm, measuring from the fingertips to two thirds of the way up the forearm. The slab should be wide enough (4 to 5 inches) to cover the volar and dorsal aspects of the metacarpals to be immobilized (second and third for radial slabs and fourth and fifth for

ulnar slabs). The wrist should be held in 15 degrees of extension and the MCP joints in flexion. Place cotton wadding between the fingers, and a thumbhole must be carefully cut and padded for radial gutter splints.

Spica Splint

Spica splints (Fig. 75.6) are used to immobilize the wrist and thumb and are often used to treat scaphoid, first metacarpal or thumb fractures or thumb ulnar collateral ligament injuries. Construct the splint from a 3- to 4-inch slab. Place the slab over the dorsal thumb, extending over the radial side of the wrist and forearm, holding the wrist and thumb in the "wine-glass position." The splint should control motion at the wrist and first metacarpal-carpal and MCP joints. For scaphoid fractures, we suggest adding a well-molded dorsal or volar slab to assist in controlling forearm pronation-supination. The interphalangeal joint of the thumb need not be immobilized unless one is treating a thumb phalanx fracture.

Long Arm Splint

Long arm splints (Fig. 75.7) are used to immobilize the wrist (also limiting supination

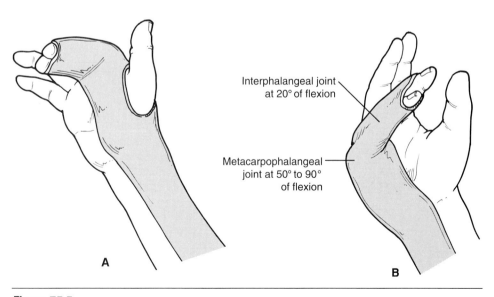

Interphalangeal joint at 20° of flexion

Metacarpophalangeal joint at 50° to 90° of flexion

A

B

Figure 75.5
The radial gutter (**A**) and ulnar gutter (**B**) splints should immobilize the wrist in slight extension, the metacarpophalangeal joints in flexion, and the interphalangeal joints in extension.

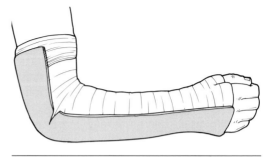

Figure 75.7
The long arm splint immobilizes the wrist in slight extension and the elbow at 90 degrees with the thumb pointing upward.

Upper Arm Sugar-Tong Splint

Upper arm sugar-tong splints (Fig. 75.8A) are used to immobilize humeral shaft fractures. Construct the splint from a 4- to 5-inch slab. The slab should wrap around the elbow, starting from the deltoid area, extending distally, wrapping around the elbow, and extending proximally toward the axilla. Make certain that the elastic wrap is not applied too tightly as this will exacerbate the tendency for these injuries to swell significantly. The weight of the splint will assist in distracting the fracture fragments. The forearm is supported by a collar-and-cuff sling, which may be constructed from stockinette. This sling supports the forearm through a narrow cuff, and differs from a traditional sling in that the cuff solely supports the forearm and allows the weight of the upper arm and splint to "hang" and maintain fracture alignment. The location of the cuff on the forearm will assist in maintaining an adequate reduction (see Fig. 75.8B).

Lower Extremity Splints

Short-Leg Posterior Splint

Short-leg posterior splints (Fig. 75.9) are used to immobilize a variety of ankle and foot injuries. Construct the splint from a 5-inch wide slab. Measure from the metatarsal heads over the posterior foot and ankle to the proximal calf. The slab is most easily applied with the patient resting prone on a stretcher with the affected extremity's

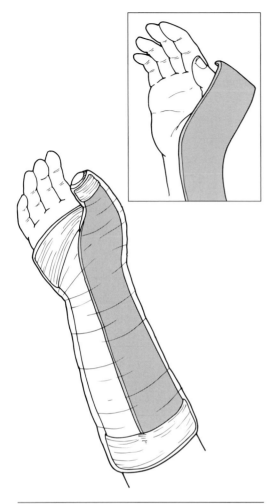

Figure 75.6
The spica splint immobilizes the wrist and thumb in the "wine-glass position," immobilizing the wrist and first metacarpophalangeal joint.

and pronation) and elbow. They may be used to initially stabilize forearm fractures or injuries about the elbow. Construct the splint from a 4- to 5-inch slab. Place the slab over the ulnar aspect of the hand and forearm, wrapping over the elbow and over the posterior aspect of the upper arm. The splint should extend from the MCP joints to the proximal aspect of the upper arm. The wrist should be held in 10 to 20 degrees of extension and the elbow should be held at 90 degrees with the thumb pointing upward. Movement at the MCP joints should not be impeded.

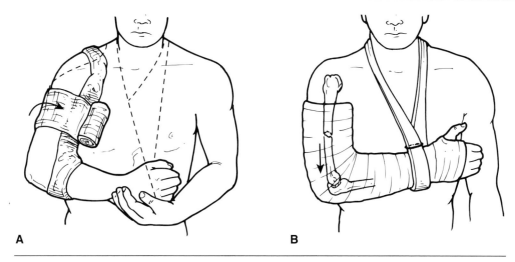

A   **B**

Figure 75.8
The upper arm sugar-tong splint should immobilize the upper arm, wrapping around the elbow (**A**).
The forearm is supported by a collar and cuff sling (**B**).

knee held in 90 degrees flexion. The ankle should be immobilized at 90 degrees. Place the slab over the plantar aspect of the foot beginning at the metatarsal heads, and wrap the slab over the posterior foot and lower leg, terminating over the proximal calf.

Short-Leg Stirrup Splint

Short-leg stirrup splints (Fig. 75.10) are used to immobilize ankle injuries and are more effective at controlling pronation and supination than a posterior splint. Position the patient as if applying a posterior splint. Construct the splint from a 4- to 5-inch wide slab. Apply the slab starting from just below the fibular head (just below the lateral aspect of the knee), wrapping over the plantar surface of the foot and extending proximally to just below the knee on the medial side of the leg. Avoid including the fibular head under the splint, as this will

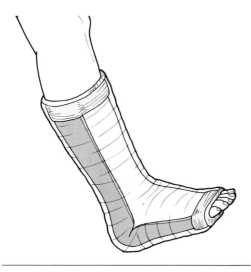

Figure 75.9
The short-leg posterior splint immobilizes the ankle at 90 degrees.

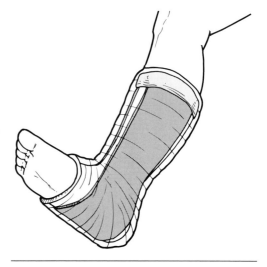

Figure 75.10
The short-leg stirrup splint immobilizes the ankle, effectively preventing pronation or supination.

increase the risk of injuring the peroneal nerve.

Long Leg Splints

Long leg splints are used to immobilize fractures around the knee and lower leg. The splint may be constructed using either a posterior or a stirrup technique as described in the previous sections, but extending the splint to the proximal thigh. The ankle should be maintained at 90 degrees and the knee in extension. The patient should be positioned supine. The splint ideally requires two assistants; one assistant lifts the leg and the other holds the slab while the clinician molds the slab and secures the splint with elastic wrap.

Complications

Compartment Syndrome

Compartment syndromes are rare, but serious complications associated with splints but are less likely than with circumferential casts. The initial symptom of increasing pain under a splint, especially pain distal to the injury, should be taken seriously. Elastic wrap and padding should be removed and the limb inspected.

Thermal Burns

Thermal burns may be caused by heat released during the curing process of plaster (less likely with fiberglass). Increasing the thickness of the splint (greater than 10 layers) and using warm water, or water previously used for splint construction (with respect to plaster splints), increases the risk of thermal injury. Inform the patient that the splint will "get warm," but remove the splint immediately if the patient complains of a burning sensation.

Compression-Related Injuries

Compression-related injuries may be caused by the hard surface of the splint pressing against a small area and resulting in skin breakdown. Such injuries are more likely to occur over poorly padded bony prominences, over wrinkles or "bumps" in the padding, or under dimples or ridges in the plaster or fiberglass. In addition, direct pressure over a nerve (such as the peroneal nerve) could result in a neuropathy without damaging the skin.

Splinting plays a vital role in the initial management of many orthopedic and soft tissue injuries. The emergency clinician must be aware of the indications for specific splints and potential complications. One must master the techniques of construction and application of extremity splints, one of the most frequently performed therapeutic procedures in emergency medicine.

Suggested Readings

Chudnofsky CR. Splinting techniques. In: Roberts JR, Hedges JR, eds. *Clinical procedures in emergency medicine*, 3rd ed. Philadelphia: WB Saunders, 1998:852–873.

McRae R. *Practical fracture treatment*, 3rd ed. New York: Churchill Livingstone, 1994.

Simon RR, Koenigsknecht SJ. *Emergency orthopedics*, 4th ed. New York: McGraw-Hill, 2001.

Index